FINANCIAL MANAGEMENT FOR NURSE MANAGERS

MERGING THE HEART WITH THE DOLLAR

SECOND EDITION

EDITED BY

JANNE DUNHAM-TAYLOR, PhD, RN

JOSEPH Z. PINCZUK, MHA

JONES AND BARTLETT PUBLISHERS

Sudbury, Massachusetts

BOSTON   TORONTO   LONDON   SINGAPORE

World Headquarters

Jones and Bartlett Publishers	Jones and Bartlett Publishers International	Jones and Bartlett Publishers Canada
40 Tall Pine Drive	Barb House, Barb Mews	6339 Ormindale Way
Sudbury, MA 01776	London W6 7PA	Mississauga, Ontario L5V 1J2
978-443-5000	United Kingdom	Canada
info@jbpub.com		
www.jbpub.com		

Jones and Bartlett's books and products are available through most bookstores and online booksellers. To contact Jones and Bartlett Publishers directly, call 800-832-0034, fax 978-443-8000, or visit our website, www.jbpub.com.

Substantial discounts on bulk quantities of Jones and Bartlett's publications are available to corporations, professional associations, and other qualified organizations. For details and specific discount information, contact the special sales department at Jones and Bartlett via the above contact information or send an email to specialsales@jbpub.com.

The authors, editor, and publisher have made every effort to provide accurate information. However, they are not responsible for errors, omissions, or for any outcomes related to the use of the contents of this book and take no responsibility for the use of the products and procedures described. Treatments and side effects described in this book may not be applicable to all people; likewise, some people may require a dose or experience a side effect that is not described herein. Drugs and medical devices are discussed that may have limited availability controlled by the Food and Drug Administration (FDA) for use only in a research study or clinical trial. Research, clinical practice, and government regulations often change the accepted standard in this field. When consideration is being given to use of any drug in the clinical setting, the health care provider or reader is responsible for determining FDA status of the drug, reading the package insert, and reviewing prescribing information for the most up-to-date recommendations on dose, precautions, and contraindications, and determining the appropriate usage for the product. This is especially important in the case of drugs that are new or seldom used.

Production Credits
Publisher: Kevin Sullivan
Aquisitions Editor: Emily Ekle
Aquisitions Editor: Amy Sibley
Associate Editor: Patricia Donnelly
Editorial Assistant: Rachel Shuster
Associate Production Editor: Amanda Clerkin
Marketing Manager: Rebecca Wasley
V.P., Manufacturing and Inventory Control: Therese Connell
Composition: diacriTech, Chennai, India
Cover Design: Scott Moden
Cover Image: © Eugene Kuklev-Dreamstime.com
Printing and Binding: Malloy, Inc.
Cover Printing: Malloy, Inc.

Library of Congress Cataloging-in-Publication Data
Dunham-Taylor, Janne.
    Financial management for nurse managers: merging the heart with the dollar/Janne Dunham-Taylor, Joseph Z. Pinczuk.
        p.   cm.
    Includes bibliographical references and index.
    ISBN-13: 978-0-7637-5713-7 (alk. paper)
    ISBN-10: 0-7637-5713-6 (alk. paper)
    1. Nursing services—Business management. 2. Nursing—Economic aspects. 3. Nurse administrators. I. Pinczuk, Joseph Z. II. Title.
    [DNLM: 1. Economics, Nursing. 2. Nursing Services—economics. 3. Nursing Services—organization & administration. WY 77 D917h 2009]
    RT86.7.D855 2009
    362.1068'1—dc22
                                        2008040211
6048

Printed in the United States of America
13 12 11 10 09   10 9 8 7 6 5 4 3 2 1

Contents

Chapter 5   *Pinpointing Evidence-Based Information: How to Find the*
Needle in the Information Haystack *153*

Rick Wallace, MA, MDiv, MAOM, MSLS, EdD, AHIP
Martha Whaley, MSLS
Nakia Joye Carter, MSIS, AHIP
Janne Dunham-Taylor, PhD, RN

Part III   **Workload Management** **181**

Chapter 6   *Workload Management* *183*

Kathy Malloch, PhD, MBA, RN, FAAN
Janne Dunham-Taylor, PhD, RN
Janelle Krueger, MBA, BS, RN

Chapter 7   ***Ethics in Nursing Administration*** *243*

LOIS W. LOWRY, DNSc, RN, ANEF
JO-ANN SUMMITT MARRS, EdD, RN

Chapter 8   ***Contemporary Legal Issues for the Nurse Administrator*** *263*

FRANCES W. "BILLIE" SILLS, MSN, RN, ARNP, LNC

Part IV   Healthcare and the Economy **291**

Part V   Budget Principles 367

Chapter 12   Budgeting 369

R. PENNY MARQUETTE, DBA
JANNE DUNHAM-TAYLOR, PhD, RN
JOSEPH Z. PINCZUK, MHA

Chapter 13   Budget Development and Evaluation 397

JANNE DUNHAM-TAYLOR, PhD, RN
JOSEPH Z. PINCZUK, MHA

Chapter 20   *Financial Analysis: Improving Your Decision Making* *583*

PAUL BAYES, DBA ACCOUNTING, MS ECONOMICS, BS ACCOUNTING

Contributors

Paul Bayes, DBA Accounting, MS Economics, BS Accounting, is formerly Chair and Professor of Accountancy at East Tennessee State University. Dr. Bayes earned his Bachelor and Doctorate degrees in Accounting from the University of Kentucky. He also holds a Master's in Economics from Indiana State University. Dr. Bayes has published and presented over 50 articles for both practitioner and academic organizations and has published an Accounting Information Systems Case textbook with co-author Dr. John Nash.

Sandy K. Calhoun, PhD(c), MSN, RN, CPHQ, is a doctoral candidate at East Tennessee State University (ETSU). Sandy's research focus is transition to professional nursing practice for accelerated second-degree baccalaureate graduate nurses. In 2007 she was one of four scholars selected nationally to receive a National League for Nursing Foundation dissertation scholarship. She has 33 years of nursing experience with concentrations in nursing administration, leadership, quality management, risk management, and education. Sandy serves as an assistant professor at ETSU College of Nursing and in nursing administration at Mountain State Health Alliance, both located in Northeast Tennessee.

Nakia Joye Carter, MSIS, AHIP, is a Clinical Reference Librarian at East Tennessee State University Quillen College of Medicine Library. She attends clinical rounds with Family Medicine, Pediatrics, and Surgery. She coordinates the Medical Library's Database Instruction/Evidence-Based Medicine Classes, along with working in Consumer Health, Reference, and Outreach. Nakia is currently working on her Master's in Public Health.

Janne Dunham-Taylor, PhD, RN, teaches nursing administration graduate courses at both master's and doctoral levels at East Tennessee State University. She has been a head nurse, nursing supervisor, and director of nursing in a state hospital, a university hospital, and a teaching hospital. She has been an assistant dean and has held two acting dean positions, as well as being a chair, in university settings. She has taught nursing administration courses for 25 years. Her research has been concerned with transformational leadership at the CNO level nationally. She has numerous publications on various nursing administration topics. Dr. Dunham-Taylor is a co-author of this book and has previously co-authored two books: *Health Care Financial Management for Nurse Managers: Merging the Heart with the Dollar*; and *Health Care Financial Management for Nurse Managers: Applications in Hospitals, Long-Term Care, Home Care, and Ambulatory Care*, published by Jones and Bartlett in 2006.

Joellen Edwards, PhD, RN, is Professor, Family/Community Nursing and Director, Center for Nursing Research at East Tennessee State University. She teaches health policy and research methods courses in ETSU's PhD in Nursing program and provides support to nursing and interdisciplinary faculty members in the development and implementation of their research. During her nearly 20 years at ETSU, Dr. Edwards has served as Chair, Department of Family/Community Nursing; Associate Dean, College of Nursing; Dean, College of Nursing; and Interim Vice President, Health Affairs. Before her appointment at ETSU, she served as a faculty member in nursing at both Ohio University and Clemson University. She was instrumental in establishing a large nursing faculty practice network at ETSU, which now serves rural, migrant, homeless, and uninsured populations in northeast Tennessee. Her personal research interests include rural women's health and related policy issues and measurement of clinical outcomes in primary care. Dr. Edwards' most recent publications are in the areas of rural women's health, primary care outcomes in nurse-managed clinics, faculty practice, and interdisciplinary collaboration in health professions education. She was a founding member of the Rural Health Association of Tennessee, member of the National Advisory Committee on Rural Health and Human Services, and has served as a consultant for foundations, schools of nursing, and state and national agencies.

Patricia A. Hayes, PhD, RN, is an Associate Professor of Nursing at East Tennessee State University. Her current research centers on the development and implementation of a case management model for the frail elderly in public housing, which won the Virginia Stone Scholar Award of the American Nurses Foundation. She teaches case management and philosophy of nursing science, as well as theory and research.

Janelle Krueger, MBA, BS, RN, has been a registered nurse for over 20 years, specializing in critical care and long-term acute care. She held corporate level and regional level clinical and quality positions for 10 years in a multihospital organization before starting her independent consulting work. Her experiences include program management for ENEPCS®, training and education of clinical information systems and hospital administrative roles. She has her CCRN certification and collaborated with Kathy Malloch in the writing of a chapter on patient classification systems. Janelle received her MBA from the University of Phoenix.

Catherine B. Leary, MSN, RN, CNAA, works as an independent nursing consultant. She is the co-author of *A Charge Nurse's Guide: Navigating the Path of Leadership*, published by the Center for Leader Development Press in Cleveland, Ohio. While with the Regional Cleveland Clinic hospitals, she held many leadership positions, including Charge Nurse, Nurse Manager, Chief Nurse Executive, Vice President of Patient Care Services, and Chief Operating Officer. Ms. Leary holds a Master of Science in Nursing degree, a nursing diploma, and a Bachelor of Arts degree in Psychology. In addition, she has completed numerous graduate semester hours in the areas of education and business. She holds nursing licenses in Ohio and Wisconsin and is a member of Sigma Theta Tau International honorary nursing society. She is board certified as a Nursing Executive, Advanced. Ms. Leary is a nurse who is very proud of her profession. Experience has taught her that effective nursing leaders are the key to high-quality health care.

Linda Nash Legg, MSN, RN, is a registered nurse with a total of 27 years in the nursing profession. During her career she has been employed in the positions of Perinatal Staff Nurse, Maternal-Child Clinical Educator, Nurse Manager of Obstetric and Pediatric Nursing Units, Nurse Educator, and Director of Planetree and Volunteer Services.

Lois W. Lowry, DNSc, RN, ANEF, is Professor Emerita at East Tennessee State University. She was rewarded for 30 exemplary years of teaching students from associate, baccalaureate, master, and doctoral degree programs by induction into the inaugural class of the Academy of Nursing Education in 2007. Dr. Lowry was director of the DNS program at East Tennessee State University for its first 6 years. Her greatest expertise is in the area of theory development in which she publishes extensively. Further, Dr. Lowry has been instrumental in designing interdisciplinary courses for students within the health care profession in the areas of law and ethics. Currently, she is engaged with nurses in Magnet hospitals as they seek to apply ethical principles in nursing practice.

Dru Malcolm, MSN, RN, CNAA-BC, CPHRM, is currently Chief Nursing Officer and Assistant Administrator at Indian Path Medical Center, a facility of Mountain States Health Alliance. She celebrates 25 years of nursing experience with a focus in emergency nursing, emergency preparedness, quality, risk management, and administration. She holds a Master of Science in Nursing Administration, certification as a Certified Nurse Administrator Advanced (CNAA-BC) and Certified Health Care Professional in Risk Management (CPHRM), has been selected as an examiner for TNCPE, and serves as adjunct faculty at East Tennessee State University.

Kathy Malloch, PhD, MBA, RN, FAAN, is president of Kathy Malloch & Associates, a national health care consulting firm providing innovative leadership and insight into effective systems, decision making, futures strategy, and new model creation. Before her focus on consulting and education, she held positions of staff nurse, nurse manager, director of nursing, and vice president for patient care services. She is a recognized expert in leadership and the development of effective evidence-based processes and systems for patient care. Her uncanny focus on accountability and results is the hallmark of her practice. Her expertise in the identification of organizational, clinical, productivity, and financial indicators/variables for the analysis and evaluation of futuristic health care systems engaged in evidence-based facility design has been useful to many organizations across the country. Most recently, Dr. Malloch has served as program director for the Arizona State University, College of Nursing, Master's in Healthcare Innovation program. This innovative, multi-disciplinary program is the first of its kind in the country.

A nationally known writer and speaker, Dr. Malloch has been a registered nurse for 35 years. Kathy has published extensively in proctored health journals. She is a frequent presenter and author on leadership topics, healing environments, professional nursing practice, and patient classification systems. Her textbook, *Quantum Leadership*, co-authored with Tim Porter-O'Grady, is a best seller and is currently used in over 60 graduate programs. *Quantum Leadership* received the American Journal of Nursing Book of the Year award in 2005. Most recently, *Introduction to Evidence-Based Practice in Nursing and Healthcare*, published with co-author Dr. Porter-O'Grady, received the 5-Star Doody Award for best publication. She is sought after as a consultant and has worked with many large health systems on issues of shared leadership, workload, and organizational effectiveness.

Dr. Malloch is a graduate of Wayne State University, College of Nursing, received an MBA from Oakland University, and a PhD in nursing from the University of Colorado. She is a member of the American Academy of Nursing. Currently, Dr. Malloch serves as Member and Past President of the Arizona State Board of Nursing; Senior Consultant for Tim Porter-O'Grady Associates; Director, Master's in Healthcare Innovation, Arizona State University, College of Nursing and Healthcare Innovation; and Area I Director, National Council of State Boards of Nursing Board of Directors.

R. Penny Marquette, DBA, presently retired, was a KPMG Peat Marwick Faculty Fellow in Accounting and a Professor in Accounting at the University of Akron, Akron, Ohio. She has also taught at Cleveland State University in Cleveland, Ohio and at Kent State University in Kent, Ohio. She has a DBA in Accounting with a Finance Minor at Kent State University, an MBA at the University of Akron in Accounting, and a BS in Journalism and English from the University of Florida in Gainesville. She has authored numerous publications.

Jo-Ann Summitt Marrs, EdD, RN, is presently a professor in the Professional Roles and Mental Health Nursing Department at East Tennessee State University College of Nursing. Jo-Ann holds a Doctor of Education in Public Health and a Master of Science in Nursing from the University of Tennessee. She acquired her Family Nurse Practitioner certificate from Pittsburg State University and is presently practicing in one of the College of Nursing's nurse managed clinics for Hispanic women and children. She has served in an administrative capacity since 1987. Her main interest is in the area of moral turpitude and licensure for nurses. She has led a national campaign for background checks and fingerprinting to be a requirement for admission to nursing schools.

Joseph Z. Pinczuk, MHA, presently retired, held executive positions overseeing finance, administration, and operations for 29 years. He has a Master's of Professional Management in Hospital Administration from Indiana Northern University and a Bachelors of Business Administration in Accounting from Cleveland State University. He has been a Chief Financial Officer (CFO) in hospitals ranging in size from 55 beds to serving as the CFO of the Tri-County Hospital Group in Ohio consisting of three hospitals with a total of 254 beds. He also served as CFO of a Continuing Care Retirement Community consisting of 285 resident units, 75 skilled nursing, and 24 assisted living beds. He has served as Director on the Board of the Healthcare Financial Management Association Northeast Ohio Chapter and received the Follmer Bronze, Reeves Silver, and Muncie Gold Awards for his contributions to the organization. A former Adjunct Professor of Nursing, College of Nursing, University of Akron and a co-author of an article "Surviving Capitation," *American Journal of Nursing* (March 1996), Mr. Pinczuk is a co-author of this book and has previously co-authored two books: *Health Care Financial Management for Nurse Managers: Merging the Heart with the Dollar;* and *Health Care Financial Management for Nurse Managers: Applications in Hospitals, Long-Term Care, Home Care and Ambulatory Care*, published by Jones and Bartlett in 2006.

Tammy Samples, MSN, RN, is currently Assistant Professor of Nursing at Milligan College, teaching Maternal Child Health and Pediatrics. She holds a Master's of Science degree in Nursing with a concentration in Nursing Administration, and graduate certificate in Health Care Management. Her past 23 years of experience were focused in neonatal intensive care and pediatrics. Her experience includes nursing supervision, Children's Hospital educator, and Neonatal Outreach education.

Mary Anne Schultz, PhD, MBA, MSN, RN, is nurse-scientist and a tenure-track faculty member of the Nursing Department at California State University, Los Angeles. Her specialties are Nursing Administration, Nursing Economics, and Nursing Informatics. She holds a Master's in Nursing degree from Case Western Reserve University in Cleveland, Ohio and an MBA degree from the Peter Drucker Management Institute of the Claremont Graduate University in Claremont, California. In her doctoral work at the UCLA School of Nursing, she examined economic factors of California hospitals impacting adverse patient outcomes such as unexpected death and complications. She also works as a Staff RN for a nursing registry in direct care and served as a Volunteer Nurse for Hurricanes Katrina and Rita. She has held many elected and appointed positions in Sigma Theta Tau chapters, the American Nurses Association, and the American Nurses Association of California. Her current professional activities include her work as a Steering Committee member for Sigma Theta Tau's first Virtual Honor Society and as a member of the Association of California Nurse Leaders' Health Policy group.

Frances W. "Billie" Sills, MSN, RN, ARNP, LNC, received a diploma from St. Mary's School of Nursing in Rochester, Minnesota; a Bachelor of Science degree in Nursing at the University of Miami, Coral Gables, Florida; and a Master of Science degree in Nursing as a Clinical Nurse Specialist/Advanced Registered Nurse Practitioner with a double major in administration and education at the University of Alabama. She is a retired Air Force Flight Nurse and has held nursing administrative positions at various settings including a 1,200-bed teaching hospital, a 180-bed comprehensive freestanding rehabilitation hospital, and a 120-bed long-term care facility. She has met the challenges, the rewards, and the multiple changes that have occurred in health care over the last few decades first hand. She is very active in professional organizations, having held several positions in state nursing associations, Sigma Theta Tau, Association of Rehabilitation Nurses, Case Management Association, and was past president of the American Association of Neuroscience Nurses. She served on the American Hospital Association Council for Rehabilitation and Long-Term Care. As an Assistant Professor at the University of Texas, Houston, she was responsible for undergraduate and graduate courses and served as the Director of Student Affairs. She has presented both nationally and internationally on advanced practice, leadership, case management, and gerontology. She presently teaches in the College of Nursing at East Tennessee State University and serves as an expert witness for nursing practice in the areas of neuroscience, orthopedics, rehabilitation, and long-term care.

Karen W. Snyder, MSN, RN, is currently working in the role of Facility Education Coordinator for an acute care hospital system. Her 26 years of nursing experience include critical care, active duty time in the U.S. Army Reserve, staff development, and more recently as the Education Coordinator for roll out of the electronic health record across an 11 hospital system. She holds a Master of Science in Nursing Administration.

Norma Tomlinson, MSN, RN, CNA, is a registered nurse with over 30 years of professional nursing experience. As a staff nurse, her practice included medical-surgical and orthopedic nursing, children's psychiatric nursing, and geriatric skilled nursing. She has been a staff development instructor in a general hospital and developed and administered a Medicare-certified, hospital-based home health agency. She has experience as the Director of Medical-Surgical Nursing in both a large urban hospital as well as in a hospital system. She has served as the Vice-President of Clinical Services in hospitals in Ohio, Michigan, and Tennessee. She is currently the Associate Vice-President, Associate Executive Director, and Chief Nursing Officer at University of Toledo Medical Center in Toledo, Ohio. She holds an Associate degree in Nursing from Purdue University, a Bachelor of Science degree in Nursing from Youngstown State University, and a Master of Science degree in Nursing from the University of Akron. She is a member of Phi Kappa Phi, American College of Health Care Executives, Sigma Theta Tau, and is currently president-elect for Zeta Theta Chapter, AONE, and OONE. She served for several years as the president of the Akron-Canton Regional Organization of Nurse Executives and on the Board of OONE.

Patricia M. VanHook, PhD, MSN, RN, FNP-BC, has 25 years of nursing management experience in acute care, specifically critical care. She has managed in rural and urban community hospitals. She served as the Magnet coordinator for the first hospital in Tennessee to be designated as Magnet. She is active in state and national efforts to reduce stroke through evaluation of systems and design of systems to improve access and the delivery of care across the continuum. She currently is Assistant Professor at East Tennessee State University's College of Nursing.

Rick Wallace, MA, MDiv, MAOM, MSLS, EdD, AHIP, is the Assistant Director for the Quillen College of Medicine Library. The library provides services to hospitals, clinics, and public health departments in 48 Tennessee counties.

Martha Whaley, MSLS, has worked in the Quillen College of Medicine Library since 1976. As Technical Services Coordinator, she manages the selection, acquisition, cataloging, and processing of print and electronic library materials. She is director of The Museum at Mountain Home, which is housed in an early 20th century clock tower building at the James H. Quillen VA Medical Center. The Museum chronicles the development of health care in South Central Appalachia. She also manages the library's historical book and journal collection, which is housed in an early 20th century Carnegie Library.

Preface

Janne and Joe have been working together for years. It all started when the CNO at Joe's hospital invited Janne (an experienced nurse administrator teaching at the local university) to work with the hospital's nurse managers to enhance their knowledge about budgeting. When Janne met Joe (the CFO), she realized that he was an unusual CFO because he both understood and supported the "care" side of health care. She found out that he was a former respiratory therapist and married to a registered nurse. Joe thought that Janne's information for the nurse managers was important, and it was evident that the CNO and CFO worked well together.

Then Joe began to regularly come to talk to graduate nursing administration students in Janne's fiscal course. He could clearly explain financial terms, the way the finance department worked, and the future implications of reimbursement and how it would affect the healthcare organization, nurses, patients, and community.

Gradually, the ideas for this book began to take root and blossom. Janne and Joe knew they did not want to create the typical financial book that kept finances in a silo. Instead, they wanted to present finances in the larger dimension—as a part of a greater whole. They also both felt strongly that regular dialogue and respect between finance and nursing were critical to the success of a health care organization. Their goal was to provide nurse administrators with information so they can be more effective in their roles.

This book has been a labor of love but has been fraught with delays. Janne moved to another state. The original contract was with Aspen Publishers, and when halfway finished there was an 18-month delay until Jones and Bartlett purchased Aspen's book division. Then when finished, the book was too long, so what started as one book became two—both titles starting with *Health Care Financial Management for Nurse Managers*. This became the first book, *Health Care Financial Management for Nurse Managers: Merging the Heart with the Dollar*, with a broader focus on all that affects finances in an organization. The second book is *Health Care Financial Management for Nurse Managers: Applications in Hospitals, Long-Term Care, Home Care, and Ambulatory Care*, providing specific financial applications in those settings.

Because of the acceptance of the first book, we are now updating and including new information in this second edition.

This book is made richer by the many contributors who have shared their expertise on certain subjects. Joe and Janne thank them for all their time, knowledge, and dedication to this book.

Joe and Janne hope that this book is both practical and helpful for you. They have tried to provide other wonderful references—but, of course, cannot possibly do justice to the many additional resources available.

Acknowledgments

We would like to thank the other people who made this second edition possible. First, a big thanks to all the author contributors in this book. Thanks to Ms. Phyllis Danner, Ms. Sarah Hill, Ms. Phyllis Livesay, and Ms. Sandra Tucker for their secretarial support with this endeavor.

Dedications

This book is dedicated to the many nursing administration students and nurse administrators who have touched our lives. We learned a lot from you and we salute you.

—JDT & JZP

Thanks to Mom, Dad, and the family for all your support and encouragement in completing this venture.

—JDT

I want to thank Rosemary, my wife and best friend, for encouraging me in this labor of love. It is through her patience and understanding that I was able to complete this project.

—JZP

Every Management Decision Has Financial Implications—Every Financial Decision Has Management Implications!

Janne Dunham-Taylor, PhD, RN

Joseph Z. Pinczuk, MHA

This book addresses healthcare financial management issues for nurse managers although, in many cases, this information is also helpful for the chief nursing officer or other nurse administrator roles. Nurse managers/administrators can be found in a variety of settings—hospitals, ambulatory/outpatient clinics and centers, long-term care, and home care. This is written to provide helpful information that pertains to each of these settings.

To be successful in financial management, nurse administrators must understand, regardless of setting, what impacts the healthcare environment and the financial implications that result from these forces. The nurse administrator needs to express what must happen not only for good nursing practice but also for the financial aspects involved. To be most effective in this new century the nurse administrator needs to operate from a new knowledge base using different skills. This is further complicated by the financial implications.

Leaving Our Silos Behind!

We all need to break down our silos. The problem with the financial aspect of healthcare is that it is often viewed as a separate silo—a silo where nurses do not enter and one where financial personnel reside. Meanwhile, nurses are in their own silo, and financial personnel are not found there. As co-authors of this book we, a nurse administrator and a chief financial officer, believe that it is time to break down, and to end, this silo mentality. Our effectiveness in healthcare demands that we interface regularly with each other and truly have dialogue about the issues that we both face. We are most effective if we can face these issues together using the strengths of both our professions.

Nurses need to express themselves more effectively using financial principles and data; financial personnel need to more effectively understand the "care" side of healthcare. Because this book is written for the nurse administrator, we give our emphasis to the first. We hope this book will be helpful for financial personnel as well.

A problem that occurs when nurses and financial people try to have dialogue together is that financial officers often think in a linear way. When they talk to each other, they talk about numbers, ratios, and stats. On the other hand, nurses think in an abstract, interpersonal way. When nurses talk to each other, they talk about how someone feels, how someone will be affected by a certain treatment, or whether tasks have been accomplished.

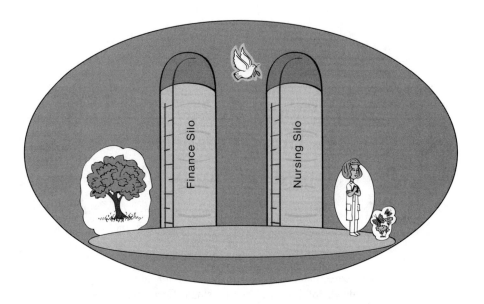

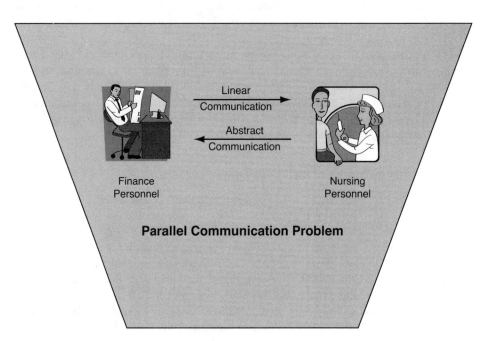

The breakdown in communication occurs when nurses talk to financial people using abstract language and financial people talk to nurses using linear language. The conversations run parallel to each other, with both sides not understanding what the other side is talking about. Nurses complain that financial people never think about anything but the bottom line; financial people complain that all nurses do is whine about quality. True dialogue and communication do not occur.

This book gives examples that nurses can use to better communicate with financial personnel, as well as with other linear-thinking administrators. In addition, we recommend that if a nurse administrator really wants to talk effectively with financial administrators, he or she should think of ways to communicate the abstract information using linear language (i.e., numbers that will be affected by something that has occurred or that is being planned, specific amounts of money needed to implement a project, and so forth).

Abstract thinking is an effective way for communication with nurses and physicians. However, it is often ineffective when communicating with the finance department. And concepts like "care" will not have meaning to a finance officer. Caring is an abstract term. Exceptions occur when a financial person experiences a serious illness or when, in the past, the financial officer has been a healthcare professional.

At times this communication problem can be compounded by simple differences in male and female communication (remember *Men Are From Mars, Women Are From Venus* [Gray, 1992]), especially if the chief financial officer is male and the chief nursing officer is female. This is changing with less gender-specific roles in the workplace. In the past, a male chief nursing officer often had an edge because he could be "one of the boys." This is also slowly changing.

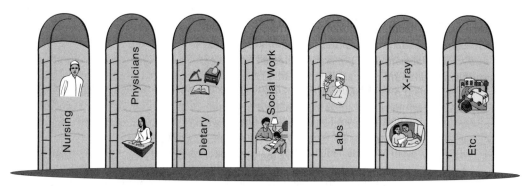

Organizational Silos

Other silos can impact a healthcare team's effectiveness. Chances are other departments have structures that need to be broken down as well. This book discusses various organizational processes that can actually cause errors to happen, putting a patient's life at stake—not to mention resulting lawsuits occurring from the errors. Although one person may have made the mistake, when the team analyzes what occurred, most often personnel from several departments and/or physicians contributed to the error. We advocate that if each member can bring his or her expertise to the table and work as members of a team, everyone benefits—patients, staff, and physicians as well as the bottom line. Additionally, all the team members get a larger, more accurate assessment of the organization as a whole.

Solutions are always better when the people directly involved are part of the team that is coming up with the solutions. Therefore we advocate that staff, as well as administrators, come to the table on issues and decide on the best way to accomplish the work. This gets rid of another silo—that administrators are to handle all this, not delegate to others. And under the old system, staff implement whatever the administrator decides is best and blindly follow the administrative edicts. This old patriarchal (or matriarchal in nursing) authoritarian model is not effective. This is another silo that is disintegrating and needs to disappear. It is a leftover from the previous century.

Another silo is the concept that finances are a separate issue. By this, we mean that financial decisions belong in the finance department, management decisions belong to the administrative

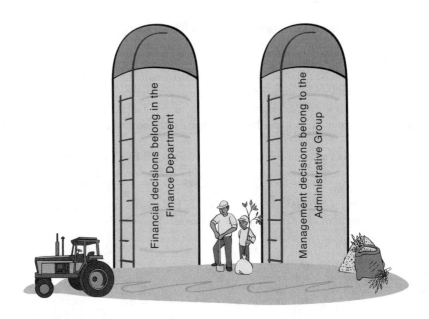

group, and so forth. The reality is that *every financial decision has management implications, and every management decision has financial implications*. If we properly prepare the nurse manager/administrator, this person must be able to make the interface between finance and nursing management and make decisions based on both perspectives. This person needs to understand both the financial situation and the nursing situation. In addition, both groups need to have a better overall organizational perspective because there are other stakeholders in the mix.

To break down this silo we turn to clinical decision making. In Part Six we discuss the importance of staff having a heightened awareness of the financial implications involved in clinical practice. This is another area that the nurse manager will need to work on with staff.

Financial Know-How

Knowledge of the current healthcare financial overview and healthcare economics allows nurse managers to effectively manage and anticipate appropriate actions in response to a changing financial environment. But understanding is not sufficient. To respond effectively and to work successfully with the financial arm of the healthcare entity, nurse managers must understand financial concepts such as staffing, budgeting, identifying and analyzing variances, measuring productivity, costing, accounting, and forecasting.

A critical element for success is the ability to effectively interface with finance department personnel. An unusual feature of this book is that it contains both typical nursing administration terminology and financial accounting terminology. Suggestions are given to the nurse manager to more effectively communicate and to maximize understanding of concepts and issues, with financial personnel who may come from different backgrounds and attach different meanings to the same terms. This book provides nurse managers with a view from both the nursing and the financial sides—and gives suggestions for successfully integrating these viewpoints. This realistic integration of nursing and finance enhances nurse manager effectiveness.

This book covers a wide range of financial information. All chapters cover information that is important regardless of healthcare setting. Concepts are presented followed by examples. Although many of the examples have an inpatient focus, there are also examples from other healthcare settings such as ambulatory care, home care, and long-term care. For example, individual chapters on health-care finance, economics, budgeting, workload management systems, and providing what the patient values present useful information applicable to all settings.

As information is presented in each chapter, it is important to note that much of this information is interrelated. For example, when discussing budgeting one must be concerned with staffing, patient acuity, and productivity of staff as well as with quality standards. Although finance and accounting terminology are interspersed throughout all the chapters, specific chapters on account-ing and assessing financial performance are included.

In the complementary text, *Health Care Financial Management for Nurse Managers: Financial Applications in Hospitals, Long-Term Care, Home Care, and Ambulatory Care* (Dunham-Taylor & Pinczuk, 2006), specific examples are given that illustrate the nurse manager role in specific settings. This information expands and tailors the principles in this book to the unique rules and regulations, or the way of measuring services, for hospitals, long-term care, home care, and ambulatory care.

An enormous challenge in the current healthcare climate is achieving quality service while keep-ing expenses down. An infinite number of strategies can be used toward achieving this end. The healthcare industry has a long way to go, and every nurse manager and every healthcare adminis-trator needs creative solutions to better meet the goal of quality service at an acceptable cost. This book discusses strategies used within the healthcare industry as a whole, as well as specific strate-gies for the nurse manager.

A Systems Approach

This book takes a systems approach to analyzing the financial impact of healthcare decisions. Although there are specific chapters on certain financial aspects, a nurse manager cannot make the mistake of ignoring the whole while dealing with the individual parts. After all, *every management decision has financial and budgetary implications, and every financial decision has management implications*. Too often decisions are made in isolation, ignoring the secondary or feedback effects of those decisions. Often, such isolated decisions yield short-term improvement followed by a long-term worsening of the underlying situation.

For example, prospective payment has mobilized administrators in healthcare organizations to identify effective and efficient processes that cost less yet deliver quality care. Nursing comes under scrutiny because a large part of the operating budget is devoted to nursing staff costs. When health-care administrators do not really understand the patient care side of business, it is easy for them to come to the conclusion that considerable cost savings can be realized by cutting the nursing serv-ice budget. And if nursing is not paying attention to efficiency and cannot articulate effectively how massive cuts will impact the organization, chances are that big cuts will occur—and not necessar-ily in ways that best serve the patient.

It has become essential that the nurse administrator understand, and can articulate, how the dol-lars and cents of the healthcare business impact the entire business. And, in the process, it may be necessary to more directly show other administrators what patient care is really about and how cost cutting needs to account for patient outcomes.

By viewing the healthcare organization as an integrated system and involving staff who directly work with patients, we can help nurse managers avoid these pitfalls. In an integrated system no one department, profession, or organization can stand alone. To be most effective, there needs to be constant dialogue between all segments of the organization, along with an open dialogue with the community being served.

There is a ripple effect. If one department is not functioning adequately, the whole organization is affected. Worse yet, patients receiving services are affected. The impact may extend beyond the healthcare entity to affect suppliers such as physicians. Ultimately, the long-term effects could include decreased patient safety, more patient complications, less patient satisfaction with services, fewer patients coming to the healthcare organization, physicians choosing to refer patients elsewhere, more lawsuits, increased staff turnover, and other problems. Obviously, this cycle can dramatically affect revenues. If competing sources are available and the problems are significant enough, the healthcare organization could even go out of business.

It is easy for nurse managers to get so caught up in the day-to-day details of running their department or division(s) that they become isolated from the larger picture. This is dangerous and can have deleterious effects on the organization. Let's take an example.

Nurse managers frequently believe they are "between a rock and a hard place." On the one hand, they are involved in patient care, constantly working with staff members who provide direct service to patients. On the other hand, they must effectively interface with other disciplines and with administrators at higher levels in the organization, individuals who are somewhat distanced from patient care. Often, the nurse manager is caught between two groups wanting diametrically opposed solutions to existing problems. The best way to resolve such dilemmas is to get back to basic values—what is best for the patient? The purpose of this book is to help the nurse manager increase her or his knowledge base, learn techniques, and develop additional skills to be more effective in acting as the link between direct patient care and the financial administration of the entity.

For effective financial management, it is necessary for the nurse manager to

- Be an effective leader
- Have an organizational/systems perspective
- Achieve quality standards understanding the importance of what the patient values
- Be conversant in financial practices and techniques
- Understand how all this fits within the community and society

It is a tall order for a person who may have had no management training.

Discussion Questions

1. What silos exist in your workplace?
2. What actions further the silo concept?
3. Identify some strategies that can help to break down the silos.
4. Give an example where a nurse administrator effectively expresses a need to the finance department using numbers and dollars.
5. State an administrative decision and explain the financial implications of the decision.
6. Describe a financial decision, giving the administrative implications of this decision.
7. Describe a management decision, giving the financial implications of this decision.
8. Describe an administrative/financial decision and map out the ripple effect of this decision.

References

Dunham-Taylor, J., & Pinczuk, J. (2006). *Health care financial management for nurse managers: Applications from hospitals, long-term care, home care, and ambulatory care.* Sudbury, MA: Jones and Bartlett.

Gray, J. (1992). *Men are from Mars, women are from Venus.* New York: HarperCollins.

PART I

Necessary Essentials for Financial Viability—or If Not Fixed It Will Cost More Money

Some may wonder why we have included the chapters in Part I in a financial management book. After all, why aren't we getting right into finances and budgeting? Actually, we start with these chapters for a very specific financial reason. As will become clear in later chapters, *any time we make the finances, or bottom line, come first, we will create more financial problems*—things will become more expensive. So for the most effective bottom line, the bottom line ***cannot*** be first priority! It has to become second behind some VERY important issues.

Part I was given first placement in this book because the issues discussed here are most important. If we do not pay attention to every aspect in Part I, we will lose money! However, if these aspects are in place, we will realize financial success.

Part I starts with a letter to nurses about doing what is right for the patients, written by a hospital chief operating officer who is also a nurse. The message behind the letter is, *If we do what is right for the patient, the money will follow*. We found this letter to be energizing and personally moving. We hope you do too.

The second chapter is concerned with leadership. If the administrative leadership is broken at any level—especially at the top—everything else is broken within an organization, and the organization will lose A LOT of money. *Fish rots from the head*. But money is only a minor problem compared with patient outcomes. Patients will be in more jeopardy if the leadership is inadequate. This chapter is next deliberately because we need to fix our administrative leadership before we can expect others to improve! If the administrative leadership is broken at any level in the organization, other financial problems will occur that could have been prevented if we had fixed the leadership problem(s).

Leadership starts from within, so the first part of the chapter is concerned with personal mastery. The second part of leadership involves the effectiveness of our relationships with others. It is leadership that must emphasize, in actions as well as in words, that the top priority is doing what is right for our patients. The second priority is the money available and how to best use it to achieve the patient goal. Our leadership role has changed and will continue to change. Can we keep up with it?

Authoritarian leadership, along with "control" and language like "subordinates" and "superiors," is a thing of the past. Can we let all that go and truly empower and trust others to give their best?

The third chapter is concerned with organizational strategies. First, it is important that all live by the core values of what is best for the patient. Second, an administrator (at any level) needs to accurately assess the organization and can accomplish this only if each administrator does regular, frequent rounds. Next, it is important to examine organizational processes or relationships that can impede progress. Shared governance, interdisciplinary teamwork, and promoting healthy collaborative cultures are all part of our administrative work as we design the organization. As we deal with needed changes, we must avoid "quick fixes" that worsen problems rather than fix them, and we may need to effectively turn dysfunctional groups around.

These first three chapters set the stage for the basics of effective financial management. Financial viability follows all this. It never should be top priority, or all the rest of this will not be in place and finances will suffer.

CHAPTER 1

An Open Letter to Nurse Leaders:
If We Do What Is Right for the Patients,
Financial Well-Being Will Follow

Catherine B. Leary, MSN, RN, CNAA

DRG, RBRVS, BBA, APC, ABN, HMO, MCO, OSHA, LMRP, HIPAA . . . in the final years of the 20th century our daily bread was served up with a bitter alphabet soup. The same trend continues at the start of this new millennium. Program after program is launched to control the runaway costs of health care and to increase fiscal accountability for the use of the health care dollar.

These years have been hard for nurses. Our health care organizations reacted to diminishing fiscal resources by downsizing and reengineering. Doing more with less became a route to survival. In this time of crisis, we nurses have come close to the edge—the edge of losing control of our values and of our ability to make a difference.

Nurses are good people—compliant to the rules. We want to do the right thing and be team players. In these years of declining reimbursement, however, we have sometimes been led to believe that we should make our decisions on behalf of dollars instead of patients. We have become followers instead of leaders.

This letter is a call to leadership and a call to believe in yourself and the nurses you lead. As the gospel hymn says, "We are the people we've been waiting for."

Our calling in life is to do what is right for our patients. And it has been my experience (and that of many others) that doing what is right for the patient leads to a positive bottom line. *Make decisions on behalf of the patients and the dollars will follow*; "a good outcome leads to a good income" as one of my friends declares.

All nurses know this is true—we have seen it with our own eyes. The relative value of nursing care is huge. There is no substitute, and there are no shortcuts. It is up to you and other nursing leaders in your organization to carry this message to all corners of your realm of influence—to the community in which you work, to the board that directs your organization, to the physicians, to the patients, and to the nurses whom you lead.

Now is the time. We are fortunate to be experiencing a return to a values-based workplace in this country. Scan the shelves of the business section in your local bookstore. People are seeking a reconnection between their personal and work lives. We are awakening to a need for principles and values to breathe spirit and meaning into what we do with our lives. This belief is a natural fit for nurses because it is what we have always believed.

It is easy to catch the wave but difficult to stay on top of it. It takes courage, persistence, and a lot of hard work. It requires that you align your daily work with the dictates of your heart. Having blind faith without looking back helps a lot when you champion a cause. Always remember that you and your nurses embody the standard of care. Couple that thought with the message that a high standard of care leads the organization to a profitable position. *Reflect on what is right for the patient in everything you say and do.* It is a winning formula. I guarantee it. Say it out loud a lot. People want to hear it. And best of all, it is catching. Soon you will hear people around you saying it and acting it out.

Another current trend that supports the cause is patient safety—the prevention of errors. The research literature, as well as the popular media, concludes that patients must come first. Errors not only harm patients, but they also cost more. Doing what is right for the patient saves money. Staffing with an adequate number and mix of registered nurses (RNs) prevents errors. Arm yourself with all the objective data and information you can get your hands on to prove your point. We nurses have always known this information in our guts; now there are studies to prove it. There are a few other ways to prepare yourself for this crusade on behalf of the patients. Know your business. Be credible. Be smart. And most of all develop relationships. Health care (as with most things in life) is about relationships. Let me explain what I mean.

Mission

To be successful, know (and feel) the relationship between the organization's mission and your own mission. **Exhibit 1–1** illustrates this idea.

Exhibit 1–1 Translating a Mission into Desired Outcomes

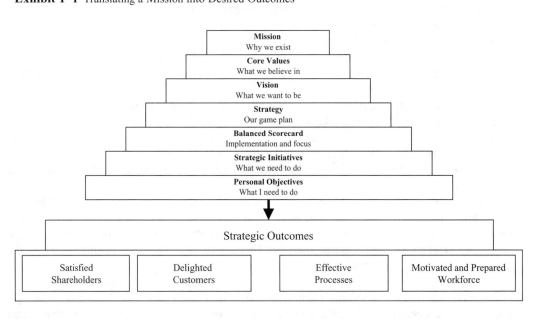

Source: Reprinted by permission of *Harvard Business School Press.*
From: Kaplan, R. & Norton, D. (2001), *The Strategy-Focused Organization: How Balanced Scorecard Companies Thrive in the New Business Environment.* Boston: Harvard Business School Press, p. 73.
Copyright © 2004 by the Harvard Business School Publishing Corporation; all rights reserved.

Spend some time thinking about this, reflecting on it, and discussing it with others in your workplace. It is important to personally embrace the alignment and to understand how what you do supports the mission. To feel a resonance between your spirit and the cause of the organization is very powerful. If you believe in what you are doing, work becomes a joyful thing. Your role as a nurse leader is to develop a unit-based mission that supports the organization's mission and strategy. The most effective approach is to engage your team in this effort. Personal involvement for each nurse inevitably leads to buy-in and success. It takes a lot of time up front, but there is a huge return on this investment, because each heart connects personally to the mission. **Exhibit 1–2** is an example of a hospital's mission and scorecard.

You can see how this can be carried to the unit level. Regular and timely reporting on progress toward goals helps to keep nurses engaged in the process. Pride in their unit grows with the realization that everyone has value to the organization as a whole.

Staffing Model

Another key to success is to thoroughly know and understand how your area delivers patient care. What exactly are the needs of each patient population that your unit serves? What are the needs of the unit as a whole? Ask all the questions you need to develop a comprehensive construct of staffing requirements. Next, sort this out in terms of skill mix. What delivery-of-care method should you use? Try several ideas. How many RNs do you need? Be reasonable. There really is a shortage of labor and revenue. Be able to justify your request for high-priced personnel to senior management. Know the hours per patient day or relative value units that are required to deliver excellent patient care. Know this by day, by shift, and by hour. Know exactly what skill mix you need. Be able to visualize who will do what on each shift. What exactly is the role of the RN, and what exactly is the role of everyone else? And finally, how do these roles mesh to deliver safe, seamless care that satisfies the customer? This exercise, of course, is the first part of the budgeting process. To do it as a group project with your staff is the most effective method. Everyone can then understand where the budget (the staffing) comes from and how important it is to work as a team to care for patients. When they are involved in the process, nurses start to feel more like participants and owners of the process and less like victims of it.

The Budgeting Process

Often, the annual budget is developed without input from managers. Historical performance is used in the forecast, and some adjustments are made based on economic predictions. If this is the case for you, you still have two opportunities for influence.

To be effective you need to have inside knowledge of the budgeting process. Find out who develops the wage and salary budget. It may be a management engineer or someone in the human resource department. The best way to find out is to ask the chief financial officer (CFO). CFOs are usually delighted that someone is interested in learning more about the budgeting process. It is likely that he or she will candidly and eagerly answer all of your questions.

Developing a partnering relationship with the CFO is key. You need each other to be successful. The CFO is often the pivotal contact between the board and the organization. Even if most board members have little health care experience, they usually have a lot of expertise with financial reports. Therefore they scrutinize expenditures and want explanations. The budget for nursing is often one of the biggest, and the CFO must be prepared to defend it. With input from the chief nursing officer (CNO) as a primary "business partner," the CFO is well equipped to defend the nursing budget—pointing out the direct link between nursing care and excellent patient outcomes.

Exhibit 1–2 Duke Children's Hospital—Balanced Scorecard

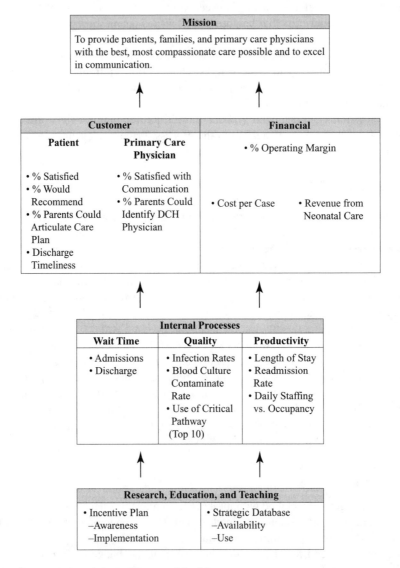

Get involved in forecasting the budget at the very beginning. If your organization's fiscal year coincides with the calendar year, this may be as early as the middle of the third quarter. Make recommendations to the appropriate person for the staffing your unit needs. Be detailed—include full-time equivalents, skill mix per shift, allocation to each shift, and so on. Be sure to include a line item for education and development. It is a good idea, too, to compare your staffing tables with benchmarks recognized as respectable in the industry. This helps you verify your work to yourself, your nurses, the CFO, and the board. You may not find exact comparisons, but you will be able to find scenarios close enough to your own to be helpful. If you can get both staffing numbers and information about patient outcomes from the benchmark, you are well on the way to building the case for putting patients first.

Most organizations expect managers to review the first draft of the budget before it is finalized. This is another opportunity for you to give valuable input. However, you may need to negotiate with your peers at this late point in the allocation process. In other words, the size of the pie has been determined. All that remains to decide is the size of the slice for each department.

The Nursing Team

There is significant power in having a strong nursing leadership team. Rally around each other. Know your strengths. Know your plan. Stand as one. In unity there is strength. Be the world's best champion for front-line nurses and for patients. Be quite clear on who your customers are and how to delight them. Meet frequently as a team and share your progress toward goals. Celebrate. Have fun. Incredible synergy and creativity will emerge. Get worked up. Be excited. Your work is very meaningful. It is a cause worthy of your best effort. Nursing is the noblest calling—serving human kind. What could be more important? Be positive and optimistic! Fall in love with nursing again. A strong visionary team can master any challenge.

Group Think

A potentially powerful attribute of having a strong leadership team is the ability to make good decisions. When resources are scarce, every decision about their use must be a careful one. A team that recognizes the strengths of each member and is open and trusting is a vehicle to success. Problems can be explored from different perspectives. Divergent opinions and disagreements can stimulate spirited dialogue and new ideas will emerge. Concurrence and convergence on a plan of action will result in an even stronger team. Every decision should be tested for its possible short-term and long-term consequences. For example, a short-term plan of conservative staffing to save money may result in a long-term result of poor staff retention and cost more money in the long run. The more good minds you bring to bear on a problem, the better your decisions will be, as long as you are nimble and quick in getting to the plan of action.

Other Relationships

Depending on your perspective, just about everyone is your partner and/or your customer. The personal relationships you develop with each and all are an important part of your base of power. Nursing leaders usually have excellent interpersonal skills; building relationships is probably second nature. Capitalize on this skill. Use every opportunity to communicate and educate. You are the nursing expert. You, better than anyone, can explain why nursing is the backbone of the organization—the key to impeccable patient care and financial health.

Following are some suggestions on leaders in your organization who can be pivotal to your (nursing's) success. Cultivate these relationships:

- **Chief Administrator (CEO, COO, CAO):** This person wants to be credible in the eyes of the board and the physicians. His or her goal is to ensure that high-quality health care is provided in a fiscally responsible manner. If you succeed in this goal, it is a done deal.
- **Chief Nursing Officer (CNO):** The same thoughts apply here. If you report to the CNO, always know what goals the CNO is working toward and mesh into those.
- **Human Resources Director:** There are several key roles here—recruiting the best people, establishing competitive wages, offering benefits that retain and satisfy employees, developing feedback methods that reinforce goal-oriented performance, gathering information about employee satisfaction, and helping in the process of severing from the organization employees who do not share the values and the goals of the organization.
- **Staff Educators:** These people need to be your best friends. The nurses of the organization are their most important asset. Invest in their education heavily. Start with a stellar orientation—a little extra time and effort up front will pay off handsomely. Offer education abundantly. Nurses like to keep learning. They also like to teach. Pay them a stipend when they mentor new employees. Excellent experienced nurses are the standard of care. Reward them for passing on their knowledge.
- **Chief Information Officer:** An important key to the future lies here. We need to push the "e-envelope" for nurses. Time-saving and error-preventing information systems, monitoring systems, and documentation systems are an absolute necessity. Ideally, you will find a nurse on your staff, or on your leadership team, who is a nursing informatics fanatic. Get this person involved in decisions about the organization's investment in information systems that ease the paper burden on our nurses.
- **Physicians:** As our colleagues at the bedside, if you consistently provide excellent patient care, they can be your greatest ally. It is more effective if they are beholden to you and not the opposite. Nursing alone cannot be successful. Everyone needs to embrace the thought that patients come first. Your job is to get all departments to support the work of the nurses. This is not easy to do if you appear superior or demanding. Express your appreciation. Celebrate successes. Share progress toward goals as a mutual endeavor and accomplishment.
- **Governing Board:** The governing board is our ultimate partner and customer. Remember, The Joint Commission on Accreditation of Healthcare Organizations requires that the voice of nurses be heard at the board level. Ideally, the CNO attends all board meetings. At the least, the CNO should report regularly to the board. Use this forum wisely. Report progress on established goals. Emphasize improved performance. Using objective data, make your needs known—better staffing, better wages. No whining allowed. Never undercut the CEO. Rehearse your presentations. Remember that you are equal. Do not be intimidated. Study after study has shown us that nurses are the most respected of all professionals. Let your presence reinforce that well-deserved stature.

Keep Your Promises

Strive tirelessly to meet and exceed the goals you establish. This is sometimes the hardest part—especially if you have set "stretch" goals (and you should). In linking mission to strategy to goals, you develop a dashboard of indicators that help you steer your course. These should include patient outcomes that reflect excellent nursing care, such as skin integrity, patient education, and so on.

Keep track of indications of the well-being of your nurses—things like retention rate, employee satisfaction, and hours of nurse education. And, of course, keep track of data that tell you about adherence to your staffing plan—hours per patient day, skill mix, agency hours, and overtime hours. Review your progress frequently. It is essential that you share timely information with your staff. Celebrate successes. Develop action plans with staff input when you get off track. A good rule of thumb is that three data points are a trend. If you have three data points off track, it is time to act. Remember also that flexibility is important. That is not to say that you should ever lower the standard of care. Impeccable patient care is sacred. However, health care is changing so fast these days that a goal established 6 months ago may no longer be applicable. Change your plan if the plan no longer fits.

Though objective measurable goals are essential in securing the resources you need and in measuring your success, subjective feedback is also very valuable. Listen carefully to what your customers are saying—the patients, their families, your nurses, and the physicians. You will hear compliments and complaints. Pass the compliments on to those who have earned them. Consider the complaints as gifts. This is often free advice on how to make things better. There is a grain of truth in every complaint. Do not let complaints get you down. Remember this: When people bring their concerns to you, they believe in you. They know that you have the power to make a difference. I believe that, too. Godspeed.

There is one question, one answer, one passion: **What is right for the patient?**

Discussion Questions

1. The author refers to "make decisions on behalf of the patients and the dollars will follow." What does this statement mean to you as you approach your management responsibilities to provide patient care?
2. Based on your experience or understanding, what would you say is the winning formula for achieving good patient care outcomes?
3. Some would say that you can catch more flies with honey. As a nurse administrator how would you implement this approach?
4. What are the critical statistics that you should have on the tip of your tongue when you are justifying your needs to provide safe quality care for your patients?
5. As the nurse manager of your unit, give examples of what elements are important for you to provide to achieve an appropriate budget. How will you use your influence as a manager to present your budget to Administration to achieve the best possible outcome for your unit?
6. Communication with your nursing team is critical. Remembering that your front-line nurses are most important for your success and good care for your patients, who are other critical partnerships that you should establish to ensure successful patient care outcomes?

CHAPTER 2

Quantum Leadership: Love One Another

Janne Dunham-Taylor, PhD, RN

Why have a chapter on leadership in a financial book? Because poor leadership at any level of the organization loses money—and it can be *considerable* budget dollars, not to mention valuable resources. Financial effects of poor leadership include decreased satisfaction levels from patients and their families, staff, physicians, and other interdisciplinary team members that result in fewer patients wanting to come back; higher staff turnover; disgruntled physicians; more unsafe situations; more patient complications; and more legal issues. All this dramatically affects the bottom line. Thus it is very important to pay attention to the quality of the leadership at all levels in an organization.

The leadership problem may have to be fixed by improving or changing unit leadership, or it may be a much larger systems problem. "Rotten to the core" does not just refer to fruit! In this case, fixing the leadership problem may extend to those above the nurse administrator—including the chief executive officer (CEO) and the board. When poor leadership is not recognized or is allowed to continue, the message to staff, physicians, patients, and families is that poor job performance is acceptable behavior. Employee retention becomes a problem as qualified, high performing staff find another workplace that better matches their needs.

> Leadership is a journey. It is not a trip, with an identifiable destination and triptiks to keep you on the right road. A journey unfolds gradually. It meanders. You stop and start, take side roads, get bogged down. You meet travel companions and sometimes stay with friends for a while. A journey is not predictable, even though there may be an end goal. On a journey, the process of getting there is part of the overall goal....
>
> Our leadership journeys are only at *midpoint* when we have achieved a position of power.
>
> The second half of the leadership journey comes once we admit our first feelings of dissatisfaction with our leadership, for it is then that we have the opportunity to lead from our souls.... Soul leadership begins to emerge when we find our existing leadership style less rewarding, less satisfying than it was; when we must either shift to the inner leadership journey or recycle to an earlier leadership style which is more comfortable and predictable.
>
> The leadership journey is a matter of the soul and that is where the energy and the focus have to be.... This is more about inner courage and peace than it is about strategic planning. It is not about skill development, it is about facing fear, letting go of control, gaining self-worth and inner strength, finding inner freedom and moral passion—the things you learn only after you think you know it all. This journey takes you to your core, including your dark core (shame, fear of abandonment, rage), wherein lies the raw power of transformation. It is not an easy journey, and the goal is not to be successful in the traditional sense; it is to be faithful to the journey itself. The only requirement is courage (Hagberg, 2003, pp. 273–274).

So What Is Good Leadership Anyway?

Love One Another

This is such a simple concept, yet it is something that we may work at for a lifetime and still be able to do better! This is what soul leadership is all about, for love needs to permeate everything we do. Love dissolves conflicts. We feel better when we are loved and when we are loving. Victor Frankl discusses this in his book, *Man's Search for Meaning*, written as he experienced a concentration camp during World War II: "Then I grasped the meaning of the greatest secret that human poetry and human thought and belief have to impart: The salvation of man is through love and in love" (1984, p. 57). It is such a simple statement yet so complex to implement every moment of our lives.

The word "love" has different meanings for different people and is easily misunderstood. Some people would define love as a physical union of two bodies and the pleasure derived from that physical union. That is not the meaning we refer to here. Nor is love merely a sentimental feeling. The definition here is about a more mature love, which grows stronger as we progress through life. It is a love that abides regardless of circumstances or popularity. It is whatever feels right at the "gut level" and is in harmony with the universe. Love gives respect to each person. When love is present, it is possible to achieve very difficult goals.

Love starts internally because one must love and respect oneself before one is able to truly love another. Love is not always pleasant and wonderful. It can demand sacrifices. Love can be selfless, meaning that one makes personal sacrifices for another, but one still loves and respects oneself in the process. Think of a mother protecting her child or insisting that the child behave a certain way. To achieve this, the mother has to personally give up certain things.

Love is honest and straightforward. Honesty can be difficult at times, especially when it involves sharing unpleasant realities. This requires a maturity on the part of the leader to know what is best to share and how to share it. The truth can be painful yet may be necessary to achieve a higher goal.

In nursing love is expressed as *caring*. Many of those we serve are vulnerable, so it is important to serve them to the best of our ability and protect them from harm, helping them to remain true to themselves. When one has empathy and a genuine concern for others, this (love) gains support and loyalty from others. This is why some leaders are so effective.

When one is in an administrative role, it is important that the intention behind every thought, word, and action is love. A leader's actions always mirror the intention. People sense the intention rather than the words. Teamwork is strengthened by this mature love. People are willing to make sacrifices for causes when love is present.

When one is in harmony with the universe, this unswerving love actually protects an individual. Correspond this with someone out of harmony with the universe who draws negativity back from the universe. What we put out there is what comes back. So it is important to remain positive and loving, regardless of the negativity that others may choose to express. Love and compassion protect one from harm and, in addition, are contagious. We all function best when we can be in a loving environment.

Our present research gives us some other clues about love. Based on a quantum perspective, we are all interconnected. Each small effort we make is linked with the whole global system. As a nurse administrator provides effective leadership, the quantum view is that this energy combines with the energy of other leaders around the globe—all contributing to an improvement of the human condition and the earth as a whole.

Although this may sound rather far-fetched, it is actually based on 20th century research that Margaret Wheatley describes in her book, *Leadership and The New Science*. Wheatley (2006) presents current scientific thought in an understandable way and applies this to leadership and organizations:

> Changes in small places… affect the global system… because every small system participates in an unbroken wholeness. Activities in one part of the whole create effects that appear in distant places. Because of these unseen connections, there is potential value in working anywhere in the system. We never know how our small activities will affect others through the invisible fabric of our connectedness (p. 45).

The Berlin wall exemplifies one example of this quantum view. It came down even though the powers that be did not want this to occur. Local efforts—and other similar energies around the world—combined until they were finally strong enough to tumble the wall, even though the government officials wanted the wall to remain. Think of the possibilities that confront us; think of what we could do to improve our world as we know and experience it.

Our interconnectedness affects each of us. It is reflected in energy fields flowing both through us and all around us. Each of us bumps into and merges with others' energy fields. For instance, how is it that a parent who is not present is able to know that his or her child is in danger? How does a nurse know when a patient is nearing a crisis or death? The energy fields transmit this knowledge. This is why it is important to stay positive. Our thoughts create our reality. Negative thoughts—anger, hate, jealousy, revenge—come back to us. Positive energy—love and compassion—come back to us. What reality do we want to have next? The biblical story about Job exemplifies this. Because he worried about various calamities (the calamities were strongly in his thoughts), they became his reality. It is better to replace a worry (negative) with a picture of something positive. This puts strength into the positive so that it will manifest.

This concept is introduced in a wonderful, entertaining book, *Zapp! Empowerment in Health Care* (Byham, Cox, & Nelson, 1996). In this book—written as a novel—as certain events occur, a nurse manager begins to realize that specific negative interactions sap the energy of the people involved, whereas people become energized by other positive interactions (zapp). It provides an actual example of true empowerment, described later in this chapter.

The quantum view of leadership is a dynamic process that varies with different groups of people. No leader is the same. No group is the same. What works well with one group will fail abysmally in another. However, there are certain landmarks, such as *love one another*, that every leader needs to observe to be effective, regardless of how each person implements leadership or love.

Dynamic leadership involves seeing the whole and understanding how we fit in it. For instance, in quantum leadership the organization is a flexible whole, ever changing, both internally and externally. The people we serve—and their needs—change; we change, our work group changes; the community changes; and societal expectations change. Our work is fluid and ever-changing. *Everyone we come in contact with is a valuable resource, necessitating our need to change to accomplish the best outcomes.* There is always more to do to make things better. Staff, physicians, and patients are equitable and accountable partners with administrators. They can think of better ways to do things or have new ideas that never occurred to the administrator. All are leaders. Each has definite things to do that benefit everyone else—and that will not be done by anyone else. All need to be empowered to go ahead with the work.

In fact, *dynamic leadership is needed from every person on earth.* Leadership occurs at all levels in an organization—from the patient or housekeeper to the board chairperson. Patients and their families are leaders as they make decisions about what they need and want. Housekeepers are leaders as they perform various cleaning activities. Staff nurses are leaders as they determine priorities and provide care to patients.

We have many practices in health care that do not encourage patient leadership, such as having to wear hospital gowns, setting visiting hour limitations, or automatically putting heavy patients on 800-calorie diets at a time when they are experiencing a health crisis and have not chosen to lose weight. It is important to think about how our decisions and policies either limit or enhance patient autonomy and, thus, patient leadership.

Leadership Fallacies

All the results of good nursing may be spoiled or utterly negated by one defect—petty management—or, in other words, by not knowing how to manage so that what you do when you are there is done when you are not (Nightingale, 1869).

Now let's turn to leadership fallacies that can negatively affect leadership effectiveness. Fallacies, as shown in **Exhibit 2–1**, are traps that cause us to get derailed or become less effective. Once understood, fallacies can be overcome and our leadership will improve.

Perhaps it is best to start with our language, which can enhance or detract from our leadership effectiveness. There are a few words—popular in current business journals—that do not support quantum leadership. The terms *subordinate* and *superior* indicate that one person is better than another. The authors recommend that an effective leader *never* use such terms. Each person in an organization has gifts and abilities that benefit everyone else. The housekeeper is just as important as the CEO. After all, if the wastebaskets are not emptied and the bathrooms not cleaned properly, we all suffer. Everyone uses leadership to more effectively accomplish their work. In this book, even when quoting other authors from the business journals that use these terms, we have substituted the terms *staff* and *supervisor, administrator* or *boss* for *subordinate* and *superior*.

Another example of problematic language is to call everyone *my* staff or *girls/boys/kids*. In the first case, although we all might be in the same work group, no one belongs to anyone else, including the leader. In the second case, it is demeaning to call someone by a child title. This indicates that we do not believe they are capable adults. We enhance this concept in the nursing profession when we use such expressions as *girls*, implying that staff are little children, have not yet grown up, and need parenting. However, in an effective organization staff at all levels are leaders.

Another word commonly used in business literature is *control*, such as the span of control of a manager. In fact, according to some of the management literature, a managerial function is *control*. Control is a myth. We suggest not using this term. After all, controlling ourselves is hard enough! Think of our inability to turn down a wonderful dessert full of sugar and lots of calories. How well do we *really* control *ourselves*? It is a fallacy to believe that we control others. Dictators have tried—and continue to try—but no one has achieved it. After all, a controlling manager is an ineffective one. We suggest the word *responsibilities* as a better word for *control*. We could list a manager's responsibilities rather than saying span of control.

Another problematic term used in health care is *noncompliance*. Most often we say that patients are noncompliant, meaning that the patient did not follow our treatment regimen. This can be a serious problem, especially when a patient starts an antibiotic, feels better, and stops taking it before the prescribed time is completed. But the use of this term also smacks of saying, "Do this *my* way." What about the patient's point of view? Was this considered before deciding what treatment regimen to use?

Another misconception people can get from the business literature is the implication that the administrators (especially CEOs) are the leaders, all others being followers. In reality all staff and patients need to be leaders as well.

Exhibit 2–1 Leadership Fallacies

Leadership Fallacies	Replace by
Subordinate and *superior* are appropriate labels for people within organizations, as are *my* staff and *girls, boys, kids.*	Language can enhance effectiveness. Use the words *staff; supervisor or administrator*; and *women* or *men.*
Control is a component of effective leadership.	Control of others is impossible. Staff are equitable and accountable partners in the work.
Patients are described as being *noncompliant.*	What about the patient's point of view?
The administrators are the leaders while other staff are followers.	Everyone is a leader.
Leaders have inborn qualities. Leadership cannot be learned.	Leadership can be learned by anyone. It has more to do with our gifts and life purpose.
Leadership is better than management.	Actually we need a combination to effectively accomplish work. The problem occurs when someone is predominantly transactional, not taking into account others' perceptions, ideas, knowledge, and relationships.
The leader, or CEO, has all the answers.	We have some of the answers, but other answers will come from other people around us—including those reporting to the leader.
When everyone is empowered and there is effective leadership, the result is peace and harmony.	Actually the result is that not everyone agrees. Conflicts occur necessitating dialogue to work through issues. Better solutions result.
There is one right way to do the work.	There are many ways that are effective.
What works well in one group will work well in another.	People are different and thus groups of people differ as well. What could work effectively with one group might not work with another.
Administrators strive to have everyone like them.	This is not possible. A better goal is that everyone *respects* the administrator because the administrator consistently supports the core value.
Effective leaders always use a participative leadership style, involving staff in every decision.	There are times, such as in an emergency, when being participative is not an effective method. In this case someone must make a decision quickly.
A leader must always win.	This is not humanly possible.
Claim another person's idea or work as one's own.	Integrity is important. Give credit where credit is due.
Do not want staff to outshine oneself or are threatened by more competent people.	Competent staff increase a leader's effectiveness, and make the work group look more effective.
Leaders do not fear anything.	It is important to recognize our fears and deal with them.
Charisma is an essential aspect of leadership.	The core values are the essential part of leadership.

continued

Exhibit 2–1 Leadership Fallacies (continued)

Our leadership is perfect; the problems are caused by everyone else's behaviors.	Our actions may be causing the problem. Thus we always need to examine whether we are contributing to the problem.
We have always done it this way.	The only constant is change.
We think we are better than others because of our administrative title or our degree.	Everyone is equally important.
Pursue one's own selfish agendas.	Think about how each action affects others.
Gender or race bias issues can contribute to erroneous decisions.	It is better to base our assessment of others based on their gifts and contributions.
Successful managers/people are promoted before effective managers/people.	Effective managers/people do a better job.
A manager who politicks regularly with the supervisor is effective.	The supervisor needs to always do regular rounds to determine manager effectiveness.

There is a question by some as to whether leadership can be learned. Some say that leaders have inborn qualities that cannot be taught to others. However, *leadership can be learned*, and we can always improve our leadership, regardless of inborn leadership qualities. This learning can happen serendipitously and can happen in infinite ways as we experience life. Mentoring has become so popular because we can learn from effective leaders who feel a special affinity to help us learn more about the role. The more important point here is that each of us has certain gifts. If we pay attention to the gifts, we can be leaders in those areas. This is not to say that everyone should be an administrator. There are some people who are very unhappy in the administrative role because it is not a match with their gifts.

Another issue is that leadership is more important than managing day-to-day activities. Both are important, and an effective leader knows when to do each. In fact, the work needs to be done. We need a combination of both to achieve this work being done most effectively. The problem occurs when someone is predominantly managing, because this person is not tuning into others' perceptions, ideas, and knowledge. *The ideal is to more predominantly lead while still managing.*

Along the same lines, another fallacy is that the leader has all the answers. Because we are human, we will never achieve this. In administration there is always a new or different twist to situations that must be taken into account. Many times the best answer will come from another person or some event that triggers us to think about the problem differently. It is okay for a leader not to know what to do. It is okay to say, "I do not know what I will do yet. I need to think about this and get back to you." Or, "Do you have any suggestions or solutions to this problem?" This is all part of the *dialogue* that *produces more effective solutions* to problems.

Another fallacy is to assume that when all in the work group are empowered, the result is peace and harmony! Instead, many times, there is conflict. Establish a dialogue with each other on the conflicts. *Disagreement and healthy argument on issues provide different perspectives and help a group move to better outcomes* that would not have occurred without the disagreement. Thus continuous improvement is achieved.

Another erroneous leadership expectation is that there is one right way to do the work. Expecting others to "do it *my* way" does not necessarily achieve the best possible result. People differ. Work groups are never the same.

It is a mistake for a leader to think that what works well with one group will work equally well with another. What might work effectively with one group could bomb with another. It is important for an effective leader to know each person in the work group as well as to know how group members work together. Then the leader can better anticipate what might work effectively with that group.

Some administrators want everyone to like them. This can be very dangerous because, realistically, everyone will not. It may be as simple as we resemble Aunt Alice or Grandpa Mike, who treated the person badly in the past. If an administrator wants everyone to like him or her, then the administrator may change decisions depending on what the current individual or group wants. This will cause a lack of consistency in the administrator's actions. People will see this. The administrator will be ineffective. This is a trap. A better option is to have staff respect making decisions that support the core value: *what is best for the patient*. Sometimes staff disagree with the administrator's decisions. Such is life. This is okay. Even though they may disagree, staff will respect the administrator because they know the administrator consistently supports the core value.

Another fallacy is that effective leaders *always* use a participative leadership style, involving staff in every decision. If an administrator never makes a decision without having staff discussion and getting a staff vote, this is not effective leadership. There are times, such as an emergency situation, when the administrator needs to make decisions and proceed without participation or to make decisions based on current data. The key here is that the administrator knows when it is best to just make the decision, when it is best to have dialogue about a situation, and when it is best to have staff decide what to do (see Decision Making, later in this chapter).

Another trap is the belief that one must always win. First, this does not represent life very accurately. How important is the incident? Is it something that we will even remember 10 years from now? Invariably, there are conflicts at the workplace. It is not humanly possible to resolve every conflict. If some issue is really important, such as a life or death situation, it is important that a decision be made. However, if it is a trivial issue, it may be best to just overlook the situation. Second, how do we know that we have the best solution? Maybe someone else has a better one. Third, as people share ideas with us it may be better to encourage them to try their own ideas—and not add how we might do it. If people interpret the leader's comments as saying that their idea really isn't very good, people will not be as committed to the idea as they were at the beginning of the conversation. Fourth, as we lose, it can teach us a lot—things like humility or not doing something a certain way again.

Sometimes, a manager takes another person's idea or work and claims the success as her or his own. This selfish action does not demonstrate integrity. Generally, word will get out, the manager will be "found out," and others will lose respect for the manager. When we do not give another person credit for work, we are not effective as leaders. Integrity, discussed later in this chapter, is important. We must always give credit where credit is due.

Some administrators do not want staff to shine or to look better than they do. Usually, this happens when someone who seems very competent threatens the administrator. The administrator is ruled by fear because the competent person looks better than the administrator or might even upstage the administrator. In this case, the administrator will be drawn to, and hire, incompetent people. Is it any wonder that such a work group usually has problems, being mediocre at best? This administrator may need to be replaced or will need to do a lot of work to change such behavior.

Another fallacy is that the leader does not fear anything. Fear is a human trait. Fear of any kind interferes with our leadership effectiveness. When we fear anything, we must stop and catch ourselves. Fear causes a downward spiral in our choices of actions and only worsens with time. The best way to deal with the fear is to realize that feeling and then find a way to deal with the fear. For instance, in the Judeo-Christian tradition, one comforting place to turn is Psalm 91.

Charisma has been identified by some people as being an important component of effective leadership. There has been a lot of research measuring charisma. Some confuse charisma with convincing others to do what we want them to do. Instead, we need to ask, "How do we know that what we want to do is best? What harmful side effects might be caused by this? What will people do when we are not around?" This is like control—we cannot control others. In actuality, many researchers have concluded that being charismatic is not an essential part of effective leadership and can, in fact, be detrimental to a company (Collins & Porras, 1994; Khurana, 2002). Instead, the important factor is really the commitment of the leader to the mission and values and that the leader is living the values consistently and humbly. This then inspires and motivates others.

We must never consider our leadership to be perfect or assume problems are caused by everyone else's behaviors. Sometimes, administrators do not realize that they operate using this fallacy, which can be very dangerous. As discussed previously in this chapter, we always must first examine how we might have contributed to the problem. We all have "Achilles' heels." Our own actions may actually be causing the problem. Others may do those things better or think of better ways to handle situations. A wonderful book presented by the Arbinger Institute, *Leadership and Self-Deception* (2002), discusses how in the midst of tensions, conflicts, and problems the first thing we need to look at is *ourselves*. We need to determine if we are the cause of, or contributing to, the problem. The people around us every day—staff, colleagues, family members—can give us the best feedback on our issues for improvement. For example, say one realizes that one does not listen to customers enough. One could go to seminars on customer improvement. However, isn't the best way just to make it a point to talk directly to customers? Aren't they the best source of information on customer needs? Or perhaps one decides to change some behavior. After accomplishing the changes, it can help to get feedback from colleagues as to their perception about the change. Have they noticed that we made the change? This is the real test as to how effective we have actually been in the change.

We should avoid the fallacy that because we have always done something a certain way, that way is best. Although it is best to get to know the history behind certain actions, this perspective means that the person or group saying it is probably ineffective, as the only constant is change.

Falling into the importance of the title, such as vice president or manager, or degree, such as getting a master's degree, and believing we are better than others is another fallacy. Actually, everyone is equally important.

Along this line, it can be tempting to pursue our own selfish agendas, not thinking of how this may affect others. People do not thrive under dictators unless they support the dictator's views. And even then, they must be careful not to say or do something unacceptable to the dictator, so even the supporters do not really thrive.

Another fallacy can revolve around gender or race bias issues. Some people do not believe women or people of a certain race can lead effectively. Or people feel more comfortable dealing with others who are like them. For example, within nursing we have some among us who discriminate against male nurses. On the other hand, female applicants for an administrative position may not be considered, with preference given to the male applicant. In nonleadership research, it has been shown that when resumes are reviewed, if one can tell whether the person is male or female, the female is rated lower than the male, by both men and women. Unfortunately, this is equally true in racial situations. All this creates unnecessary conflicts but, unfortunately, is a fact of life. We have not yet achieved perfection societally. Biases still exist. The place to start is to change within ourselves. It is a better policy to treat everyone with respect and to give *all* equal treatment based on each person's gifts, abilities, and experiences.

At times, research on administrator effectiveness shows differences in leadership styles based on gender. For instance, in business research, studies consistently show that women are more transformational (transformational leadership is explained in the next section) than men (Sharpe, 2000). However, in studies examining nurse executive leadership, the results consistently show that it does not matter whether one is male or female, nor is effective leadership determined by one's race. When one looks at who is most effective in these studies, it can be any of the above. Somehow, there is a factor in nursing that makes both men and women equally transformational in their leadership style.

Another issue with leadership is identified by Luthans (1988). In an observational study, Luthans discovered a distinct difference between what he labeled *successful* versus *effective* managers. Some managers were able to achieve both, but more often managers exhibited one trait more predominantly:

> *Successful managers* give relatively more attention to networking (socializing, politicking, and interacting with outsiders)… and give relatively little attention to human resource management activities (motivating/reinforcing, managing conflict, staffing, and training/development) (p. 127).

Yet *effective* managers have a very different work style:

> *Effective managers* give by far the most relative attention and effort to communicating (exchanging information and processing paperwork) and human resource management activities and the least to networking (p. 127).

According to this study a *successful* manager is promoted relatively quickly, whereas the *effective* manager may not be promoted quickly but has "satisfied and committed" staff who achieve higher quantity and quality in their work performance. So if there is a leadership problem, the manager may be more like the *successful* manager Luthans identified. If so, it might be helpful to coach this person to pay more attention to *effective* management activities.

There is another pitfall for supervisors. A successful manager, by politicking with the supervisor, may be perceived to be a better nurse manager than is actually the case. This is where it is so important for administrators at all levels to regularly do rounds. In doing rounds effectively, it can become readily apparent that there is a leadership problem, whereas one might not recognize this problem if only hearing what the manager has to say.

Another way to determine an administrator's effectiveness is evaluative feedback on a yearly basis from the individuals who report to that administrator (a 360 evaluation). To be most effective this needs to be handled confidentially. This feedback can provide helpful information for an administrator to improve certain areas and to provide confirmation that his or her leadership is effective. If the feedback identifies real problems, the administrator's supervisor must take action.

By understanding leadership fallacies, we can avoid possible traps that will make us less effective. Now we turn to leadership excellence.

Quantum Leadership Excellence

> Excellent nursing leadership is orchestrating your professional practice climate in such a way that the system moves effectively in the caring of patients, and is cost effective, yet your hand is hardly noticed.
>
> *—Anonymous*[1]

---

[1] This quote is from a nurse executive interview as part of a research project. Confidentiality was promised so the person cannot be named here.

Now let's turn back to the positive—effective leadership, *Love one another* Quantum leadership is dynamic. It changes as we grow both individually and societally. Because leadership is a dynamic process, it is hard to capture it on a two-dimensional page. What is here represents where we are currently. We learn from what is. We are in various stages of learning because a whole range of leadership styles exist. (Actually, some of the styles, such as dictatorships, are not effective, and one hesitates to call them leadership.) Our leadership knowledge base is expanding and ever-changing as we all learn and contribute to it. We are in a time of discovery and we need more research to provide us with better answers.

The *dynamic* role of leadership also means that various components of leadership need to be *integrated* into a dynamic whole. For a while leadership research focused on leadership traits. The problem with this research was that initially no one realized the connections between all these traits, which can then be linked with outcomes. Effective leadership is when all leadership components are present and integrated appropriately in one's day-to-day activities.

Now, in quantum leadership, we realize that if any one leadership component is weak or missing, the entire process is affected. The same is true when certain leadership components are used too much or at the wrong time. In interviews with "excellent" nurse executives,

> [T]hey described their leadership style as a dynamic process. Their leadership style was rather amorphous having no regular structure, yet having a number of leadership characteristics that must all be present and intermesh with one another. For example, while making a difficult decision that supported their vision, their integrity was always intact. They were "deadly serious" about the various aspects of leadership. If a characteristic was missing or overused, a leader would not be effective.... All characteristics were required together and all needed to be used at appropriate times (Dunham-Taylor, 1995, p. 25).

Research began to reflect this dynamic quality of leadership, first calling it transformational leadership and later quantum leadership. Transformational leadership was more concerned with the process an effective leader used to achieve a positive outcome. A transformational leader

- Had integrity
- Was committed to end values that the people following that leader also were committed to
- Established trust
- Identified a vision of where the group wanted, or needed, to go next
- Intellectually stimulated followers
- Gave individualized consideration to followers
- Was a role model for followers
- Provided meaning and challenge for followers' work
- Empowered followers
- Approached situations using appropriate first- or second-order change (Bass, 1998; Bennis & Nanus, 1985; Burns, 1978; Watzlawick, Weakland, & Fisch, 1974).

Along with transformational leadership, an administrator needs to manage. As transformational leadership (leading) gained in popularity, it was corresponded with transactional leadership (managing). Transactional leaders were more like the traditional manager. They might use contingent reward, only give feedback to others when things go wrong, or even be laissez-faire (doing nothing) rather than having transformational qualities. In reality, a leader tends to exhibit both types of leadership, transformational and transactional, but has an overall leadership style that is more like one or the other. Transformational qualities are preferable, but both qualities are needed to get the work accomplished.

Research shows that predominantly transformational leadership leads to a better bottom line (Bass, 1998). Simons' (2002) research, which examined managers' behavioral integrity (part of quantum leadership discussed later in this chapter), found the following (p. 18):

> The ripple effect we saw was stunning. Hotels where employees strongly believed their managers **followed through on promises** and **demonstrated the values they preached**, [the hotels] were substantially more profitable than those whose managers scored average or lower. So strong was the link, in fact, that… a profit increase of more than $250,000 per year [was noted]. No other single aspect of manager behavior that we measured had as large an impact on profits. [Bold type added by author.]

Quantum leadership research shows that organizationally there are other positive outcomes. *Fortune* provided survey results from their "Most Admired Companies" survey. These companies

- Are far more satisfied with the quality and breadth of leadership at both their executive and senior management levels
- Are less tolerant of inappropriate leadership behavior to meet their numbers
- Place more value on leadership development and put more emphasis on ongoing development efforts that are linked closely to strategic business goals and supported by formal rewards programs
- More frequently use competency models and various developmental programs in selecting and advancing their leaders
- Have leaders who are perceived as demonstrating more emotional intelligence (Stein, 2000)

In another study McClelland (1973) found that, *"when senior managers had a critical mass of emotional intelligence capabilities their divisions outperformed yearly earnings goals by 20%"*. So what is emotional intelligence? "Emotional intelligence is the capacity for recognizing our own feelings and those of others, for motivating ourselves, for managing emotions well in ourselves and in our relationships" (Snow, 2001, p. 441).

Goleman's (1998) book, *Working with Emotional Intelligence*, outlines four capabilities that are present when one has emotional intelligence: Self-Awareness, Self-Management, Social Awareness, and Social Skills. Here it is important to have an awareness of self within as well as socially with others. Self-Awareness has three components:

- *Self-Confidence*: Certain of one's own expertise
- *Accurate Self-Assessment*: Conscious of one's limitations
- *Emotional Self-Awareness*: Cognizant of one's positive and negative biases (Snow, 2001, p. 442).

Self-Management has three components:

- *Self-Control*: Remaining poised even when under pressure
- *Adaptability*: Welcoming new ideas
- *Trust worthiness*: Displaying honesty/integrity (Snow, 2001, p. 442).

Then using this awareness one's actions need to translate it into action. Social Awareness is displayed in two ways:

- *Empathy*: Learning from other people's experiences, expertise
- *Organizational Awareness*: Remaining cognizant of organizational life, politics (Snow, 2001, p. 442).

And when with others one needs the Social Skills:

- *Visionary Leadership*: Inspiring and executing effective tactics
- *Communication*: Establishing positive relationships and managing expectations
- *Conflict Management*: Developing consensus and mitigating conflicts (Snow, 2001, p. 442).

Vitello-Cicciu (2002, pp. 441–442) also defined emotional intelligence:

> Emotional intelligence is the ability to manage ourselves and our relationships effectively. Each capability is composed of a set of competencies. Emotional intelligence skills and cognitive skills are synergistic; top performers have both. The more complex the job, the more emotional intelligence matters…. Emotional competencies cluster into groups…; each is based on a common underlying emotional intelligence capacity. The underlying emotional intelligence capacities are vital if people are to successfully learn the competencies necessary to succeed in the workplace. [For example,] if they are deficient in social skills,… they will be inept at persuading or inspiring others, at leading teams, or catalyzing change. If they have little self-awareness, they will be oblivious to their own weaknesses and lack the self confidence that comes from certainty about their strengths. None of us is perfect in using all of the emotional competencies; we inevitably have a profile of strengths and limits. *However, the ingredients for outstanding performance require only that we have strengths in a given number of these competencies (at least six or so), and that the strengths are spread across all four areas of emotional intelligence.*

Goleman's (1998) and McClelland's (1973) research show a "strong link between an organization's success and the emotional intelligence of its leaders. The research also demonstrates that if people take the right approach, they can develop their emotional intelligence. The research supports the idea that leaders are not born but that people can learn how to manage their emotions and how to motivate people they lead" (Snow, 2001, p. 441). This research has helped to explain how leaders who are very different can be very effective.

Emotionally intelligent nursing leaders help their organizations create competitive advantage through the following:

1. Improved performance of nursing personnel, leading to more satisfied patients, physicians, and families
2. Improved retention of top talent
3. Improved teamwork among nurses
4. Increased motivation by team members
5. Enhanced innovation in the nursing group
6. Enhanced use of time and resources
7. Restored trust between nurses and their leaders (Snow, 2001, p. 443).

Recent neurobehavioral research on the limbic system indicates that emotional intelligence can be learned through motivation, extended practice, and feedback. Goleman (1998) contends that to enhance emotional intelligence, one must break old behavioral habits and establish new ones through an individualized approach. He also states that "building one's emotional intelligence will not happen without a sincere desire or concerted effort on the part of an individual. A brief seminar won't help or a how-to manual. Learning to internally empathize as a natural response to people is much harder to learn than regression analysis" (Vitello-Cicciu, 2002, p. 207).

New aspects about effective leadership are continually identified. Meanwhile, all of us must stay in touch with our intuitive, inner core to achieve more effective leadership. This can be difficult in the frantic pace of the workplace. Each of us needs to find our way to stay in touch with this core. Tall order, isn't it?

> With a quantum sensibility, there are new possibilities for how to create order. Organizational behavior is influenced by the invisible. If we attend to the fields we create, if we help them shine clear with coherence, then we can clean up some of the waste of organizational life.... In a field view of organizations, we attend first to clarity. We must say what we mean and seek for a much deeper level of integrity in our words and acts than ever before. And then we must make certain that everyone has access to this field, that the information is available everywhere. Vision statements move off the walls and into the corridors, seeking out every employee, every recess in the organization .... We need to imagine ourselves as beacon towers of information, standing tall in the integrity of what we say, pulsing out congruent messages everywhere. We need all of us out there, stating, clarifying, reflecting, modeling, filling all of space with the messages we care about. If we do that, a powerful field develops—and with it, the wondrous capacity to organize into coherent, capable form. Let us remember that space is never empty. If it is filled with harmonious voices, a song arises that is strong and potent. If it is filled with conflict, the dissonance drives us away and we don't want to be there. When we pretend that it doesn't matter whether there is harmony, when we believe we don't have to "walk our talk," we lose far more than personal integrity. We lose the partnership of a field-rich space that can help bring order to our lives (Wheatley, 2006, pp. 56–57).

Effective leadership is like quality. No matter how effective we become, we can always improve. Good leadership can be taught and learned. So do not become discouraged when we stray from the path once in a while; it's human. When we realize this has happened, start back on the path and be open to new ideas and new ways of doing things.

Our present model of dynamic leadership is all of the above plus listening to our intuitive center. The emotional intelligence research suggests that effective leadership starts with work we accomplish within ourselves. As Snow (2001) pointed out, none of us achieves perfection, but we can improve our own personal mastery. We further learn when we work with others, the social awareness occurs, along with relationship management skills defined in the emotional intelligence research.

Developmental Levels of Leadership

Kuhnert and Lewis (1987) identified several developmental levels of leadership. At the *first* level, leaders are only concerned with their "personal goals and agendas" (p. 652). This approach is a selfish one. The *second* developmental level occurs when the leader is able to see that joining a group and having mutual goals and partnerships are more advantageous than the selfish goals present at the first stage. The problem with the second stage is that sooner or later one is torn between two groups. For example, a nurse manager might realize that staff wants something that is the antithesis of what the higher level administrative group wants. The *third* stage of leadership resolves this dilemma. At the third stage the leader has developed end values—doing what is best for the patient—that "transcend" the leader's own goals and agendas. Even though the staff and the higher level administrative groups do not agree on a goal, the leader makes a decision based on the end value of what is best for the patient.

Dunham-Taylor (1995) identified four stages of leadership among nurse executives. The *first* group "influences others on a situational basis, is action oriented, is still learning, experiences emotional discomfort, and is working on personal change" (p. 31). At the *next* stage the nurse executives "used common sense; were not afraid to fail and admit mistakes; lacked a leadership definition; thought leaders were born, not made; had difficulty with balance; were aware of strengths and weaknesses; and were inconsistent" (p. 30). The *third* stage, which is highly transformational, leaders "enjoy 'cleaning up' difficulties; underestimate their own abilities; are not maintenance people [meaning that they will not stay in the same position for years]; hire the best staff possible; work to develop staff; have people skills; are visionary; have perseverance; enjoy analyzing problems with staff, discussing alternatives, and then have staff decide what to do; want staff to let them know when something goes wrong; are not as balanced; personalize issues; and can become easily frustrated if standards are not met" (pp. 26–27). In the *fourth*, or highest, stage leaders "achieved more balance, were always striving for higher quality—both organizationally and personally, possessed humility, had a dynamic leadership definition and style, were deadly serious about their work, felt that their work mattered, were comfortable with change, had integrity, identified values, experienced intuitive decision making, were a coach and mentor to others, were humanistic, had humor, had charisma, were visionary, and were aware of their own humanity" (p. 29). They often were in executive positions for years and always believed that there was more that needed to be accomplished.

The Only Constant Is Change

> As we discuss leadership excellence, there is a theme that we consider a given in life. Change is not a thing or an event; it is instead a dynamic, the major element of a universe that is still unfolding.... Change is the major motivator of life and movement in the universe. People have no control over the condition of change but do influence its circumstances and actions. In short, people don't make change, they simply give it form. Change is not something we define; it is more something we discern... The direction change takes, its application in human experience, and its impact are what humans can influence and affect (Porter-O'Grady, 2003b, p. 59).

All through this book, it is evident that *the only constant in life is change*. As we work to take on the administrative role, we realize that everything, including ourselves, changes, with the possible exception of end values and the need for integrity and love. Hopefully, one's integrity and love grow over time. We all change—whether we want to or not—and the environment around us changes. When we specifically do not want to change, we change by becoming more rigid.

When we flow with change that seems right for the moment, we are more balanced and in tune with the world. This dynamic permeates everything. In fact, in a leadership role we even become catalysts, either initiating or managing change. Because we have said that everyone in an organization needs to be a leader, this is a tall order. The goals we are working to achieve change, both success and failure result from change, our relationships with people change, the people around us change, our leadership changes, our work environment changes, and we can always improve ourselves or our environment—another change.

> Schrodinger, a famous middle 20th century physicist, proved with his famous "Schrodinger's Box" analogy that there are two prevailing realities that operate at any given time: actual reality and potential reality.... The former is the reality that currently occupies our immediate experience and moments; the reality in which our senses and awareness are presently engaged. Potential reality is inevitable, on the other hand, is current and present to us at any given moment but, while present, is not yet experienced. Potential reality is inevitable and just as current and applicable as actual reality; it is just not yet experienced. Until applied, it is still potential; present but waiting for the right

moment of its expression when it will then become actual much like a stop sign in the street can be seen long before it is responded to by a driver....

It is in this arena of potential reality that leadership takes its form. The leader is differentiated from the follower in that the leader derives the preponderance of his or her role within the scope of *potential reality*. It is the leader's role to engage unfolding reality in advance of others experiencing it; to see it, note its demands and implications, translate it for others, and then guide others into processes that will act in concert with the demands of a reality that is not yet present but inexorably and continuously becoming (Porter-O'Grady, 2003b, p. 59).

Our leadership role means that we need to keep abreast with this unfolding reality, bringing it out for others to see, hear, and experience, lifting all of us to new levels not yet achieved. When we are in the middle of experiencing unfolding reality, it can be very difficult to discern where we are headed.

For instance, there are less invasive treatment modalities, a wealth of outcome research data becoming readily available, and information/information technology barraging us at every turn. All these changes are forcing us to change the way we work and communicate with one another. This translates into an adaptation of both how we care for patients (e.g., telehealth) and how we communicate with others.

This high level of change can be overwhelming. I am reminded of my grandmother who first experienced electricity (for lighting, appliances, and so forth) and a motorized car rather than a horse and buggy. Our ancestors came through rapid changes just fine, and we can too. The main point is to remain open to what is in that potential reality. One change within nursing is that our patients are generally not with us for long amounts of time. So we do not know them as well as we did. Someone can come in for an operation and go home the same day. Nurses, and other interdisciplinary workers, come and visit us in our homes to follow up on the surgery or treatment needed. This is an enormous change in the way we care for patients. As leaders, we need to help staff understand these changes and develop new work expectations and new ways of working with patients who will not be with us as long. An excellent reference on this subject is the book, *Quantum Leadership: A Resource for Health Care Innovation*, by Tim Porter-O'Grady and Kathy Malloch (2007).

In this chapter we discuss several aspects of leadership that are part of the fluid experience of change. One way of thinking about change is to examine first- and second-order change (Watzlawick et al., 1974). In *first-order change*, a method or person changes. Here, when one asks the question "why?" The solution is based on common sense. Many changes are actually first-order changes. For example, if there is not enough light in a room so I can read, I can ask, "Why isn't there enough light?" I then decide to add a lamp to supply the needed light and the problem is solved.

At times though, first-order change does not accomplish anything. Asking "why?" does not solve the problem. For instance, during layoffs some employees in an outpatient department were asked to describe an outpatient role they would like to do, to decide on what they would charge to do the role, and to give all these details to the administrator by a certain date. Otherwise, they would be laid off. Being told this, several employees asked, "*Why* are you doing this to us?" They became stuck in first-order change and could not get beyond the question "why". Eventually, they were laid off.

However, a few employees realized that asking "why" did not result in their keeping their jobs. They turned to the question of "what": "What do we need to do?" When using the question "what," they turned to *second-order change* and reframed the situation. Reframing (Watzlawick et al., 1974) demands creativity and getting out of the box. Reframing involves looking at a situation differently. An example is if we look into a house through one window and get one perspective; then we look in another window to get a different perspective. The employees who turned to second-order change began to imagine their work roles in a different way, a way that they had not imagined before. They began to devise the role, develop costs for their services, and give it in writing to the administrator by a certain date. The employees choosing to use second-order change still had jobs and were not laid off.

Second-order change often means we need to get out of the box for the solution. For example, during Nazi occupation of Denmark in World War II, King Christian was told to issue a decree that all his countrymen should wear the Star of David armband if they were Jewish. King Christian did not want to do this, yet the Nazis in occupation would enforce it even if he refused—a dilemma. Instead, King Christian used second-order change by very effectively getting out of the box. He issued a decree that all countrymen would wear the Star of David armband. The Nazis soon rescinded the order.

Using a health care example, a nurse administrator was working with a medical chief of a service. He was wonderful with patients and really cared about their receiving good treatment. However, he had a flaw that could sometimes cause a problem. When a nurse had not made appropriate decisions, thus causing a problem with a patient, or the nurse's decisions had made a bad situation worse, this medical chief would lose his temper in the nurse's station, saying in a loud, angry voice that the nurse should be fired. Thus the nursing staff had decided that they did not like this medical chief and wanted the nurse administrator to do something about it. This situation presented dilemmas for the nurse administrator. First, the physician's behavior was a problem. Staff observed consistency in the behavior when difficult situations occurred. Second, staff wanted the administrator to be the parent and take care of the problem—with staff not assuming any responsibility to work out a solution to the problem.

The nurse administrator realized that the staff picture of this physician was negative because of his angry behavior. It would be necessary to help staff reframe the situation. The physician was not a bad person; in fact, the physician really cared about giving good care to patients. The problem was the physician's behavior in these difficult situations. The administrator decided to try a potential solution, asking staff to call the administrator the next time such an incident occurred. At this point the administrator located the medical chief in his office and broke the news to him there. The medical chief was able to rant and rave in the administrator's presence, but no one else heard what was said. When the physician had calmed down a bit, the administrator began to discuss what could be done to deal with the incident. After some dialogue, the two could go together to the unit and discuss what to do with the staff and with the patient and/or family. This worked.

After that success, the administrator encouraged the nurse manager to use this approach with the medical chief if and when the next incident occurred. Then, the nurse administrator and nurse manager discussed this physician with staff who had labeled him to be a "bad" physician. The process of reframing was discussed with staff. They agreed that he did give really good care to patients and really cared about the patients. They also noticed the difference in the physician's behavior. After several incidents, even staff members were able to take the physician aside when an incident occurred, so the incident would be discussed in a private area. Eventually, the nurse administrator could bring up this approach with the physician, asking the physician if he realized how his behavior had affected everyone. The physician was able to change.

Personal Mastery

Know thyself.

Effective leadership starts from within. We change as we begin to know ourselves better. This internal process is called *personal mastery*. Personal mastery does not occur immediately in life but follows a great deal of personal work. Even then we are continually working to better our personal mastery if we choose to increase our effectiveness. This continual work can occur as we work internally to improve ourselves or can occur as we experience various difficulties we encounter in our environment.

Sometimes hard environmental lessons, or personal crises, bring about a change within us even when we did not plan to change.

Personal mastery may not mean what is perceived as success in our society. It is not having a title, getting rich, being popular or liked, achieving physical beauty, or getting an advanced educational degree. Instead, personal mastery is what is present inside us, what is there despite events going on around us.

Because each of us is different with different gifts, personal mastery is an individual process. We are most effective if we can be brutally honest with ourselves about our life purpose, our gifts, and our personal strengths and weaknesses. When we are aware of our gifts, we see ways we can make the world better and understand what we need to do next. The amazing thing is that if each of us explores our special gifts, everything fits together beautifully. One person's gifts make a contribution because no one else is meeting that particular need. Thus if we all can stay in tune with our gifts and creativity, it all fits together so that we have all we need to live full, productive lives.

As we realize that we are not perfect and that there is always more to learn, our personal mastery and leadership improve. Personal mastery is something that we can get closer to but never totally achieve in our lifetime. It is elusive, just like continuous improvement. As we become more and more effective and closer to personal mastery, there are new nuances and directions that we realize we need to master. Our cues come from all over. It is amazing how *what one needs at any point in time will suddenly emerge when one needs it.*

SELF-AWARENESS

Although we never know ourselves completely, we must be able to accurately assess our strengths and weaknesses, know how we respond to certain situations, and be aware of our internal states and resources, our emotional awareness, our spiritual beliefs, our preferences, our biases, and our intuitive capabilities. If we do not realize what our weaknesses are, our judgment could be faulty, our interpersonal relationships may suffer, and we will not achieve our life purpose as well, or at all.

> Goleman (1998) found that people who are competent at self-assessment are: (a) aware of their strengths and weaknesses; (b) reflective, learning from experience; and (c) open to candid feedback, new perspectives, continuous learning, and self-development. Honest self-awareness may be a challenge for some leaders to achieve. Howlin and Hickok (1992) identified several factors that may discourage executives' self-awareness:
>
> - The power of their position may isolate them from criticism.
> - Expectations of high performance may cause executives to continue to do what they've done well in the past.
> - The nature of many executive jobs leaves little time and provides few rewards for introspection.
> - Successful executives learn to focus and build on strengths and may be unaware of their own weaknesses.
>
> … In a study of top executives who failed,… the two most common traits… were:
>
> 1. *Rigidity*—an inability to adapt to changes in organizational culture or to respond to feedback about traits that need to be changed or improved.
> 2. *Poor relationships*—being too harshly critical, insensitive, or demanding; ultimately alienating those they work with.
>
> Other characteristics identified… include poor self-control, reacting defensively to criticism, being ready to get ahead at the expense of others, and poor social skills (especially lacking empathy and sensitivity) (Snow, 2001, p. 442).

Kerfoot (1997) describes three situations that can cause good leaders to stumble:

1. Interpreting present-day events in terms of past successes.
2. Not being open to new ways of filtering information; processing information through old paradigms.
3. "Egotistical invincibility," which is resting comfortably on one's past success p. 275.

The Johari Window provides a nice depiction that can be used in self-assessment and is displayed in **Exhibit 2–2**. Quadrant 1 consists of the information that we know about ourselves that others also know about us. Quadrant 2 contains aspects about ourselves that are unknown to us (we are blind to them) but that others know about us. Quadrant 3 encompasses hidden information that we know about ourselves that others are not aware of. Many of our beliefs and assumptions are in this quadrant. Opening these up to others can help one examine and possibly be challenged by others. But it keeps us from being blindsided by others when we are able to more clearly define these beliefs even under fire. Sometimes we can be blinded by our own perceptions that cause us to respond to situations in a certain way. Quadrant 4, the unknown area, is the part that no one knows about.

Three principles may help one understand how the self functions in this representation:

1. A change in any one quadrant will affect all other quadrants.

2. The smaller the first quadrant, the poorer the communication.

3. Interpersonal learning means that a change has taken place so that quadrant 1 is larger, and one or more of the other quadrants are smaller (Sundeen, Stuart, Rankin, & Cohen, 1985, pp. 62–63).

Exhibit 2–2 Johari Window

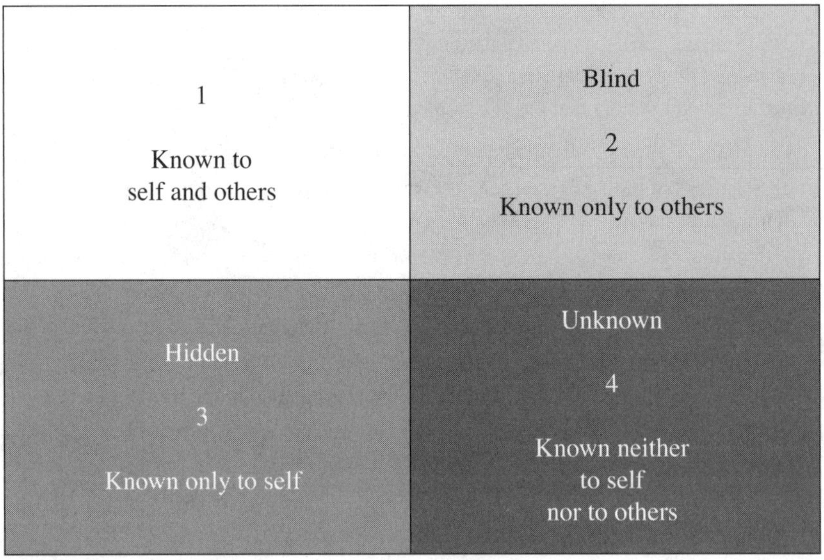

1 Known to self and others	Blind 2 Known only to others
Hidden 3 Known only to self	Unknown 4 Known neither to self nor to others

Source: Sundeen, S. Stuart, G. Rankin, E. & Cohen, S. (1985). *Nurse-Client Interaction, Implementing the Nursing Process* (3rd Edition). The C.V. Mosby Company.

As you can see in **Exhibit 2–3**, quadrant 1 is smaller when we lack self-awareness; in **Exhibit 2–4**, quadrant 1 gets larger when we are more self-aware and have achieved better personal mastery. When we remain blind to information in either quadrant 2 or 4, we cannot grow.

Additional personal feedback can be gained by taking work style inventories, such as the Myers-Briggs[2] or the Life-Styles Inventory[3] from Human Synergistics. These inventories can be used to identify what styles one uses when approaching life or work. Then one can determine how we work, how this differs from other styles, and how people with this style interact with people who have different styles. This gives us a better understanding of ourselves. These data can be used to change how we respond to situations. The Life-Styles Inventory can also be used by staff directly reporting to a manager. Here staff members rate their perception of their manager's leadership. This provides a "360 evaluation." This view can help supervisors who may not perceive leadership problems and provide the manager with ways to improve effectiveness.

Once we possess self-awareness and expand our positive capabilities, our self-confidence and self-worth increase. We begin to be able to regulate our internal states, our impulses, our internal resources. We have more self-control, keeping disruptive emotions and impulses in check.

Exhibit 2–3 Johari Window

When a person has little self-awareness

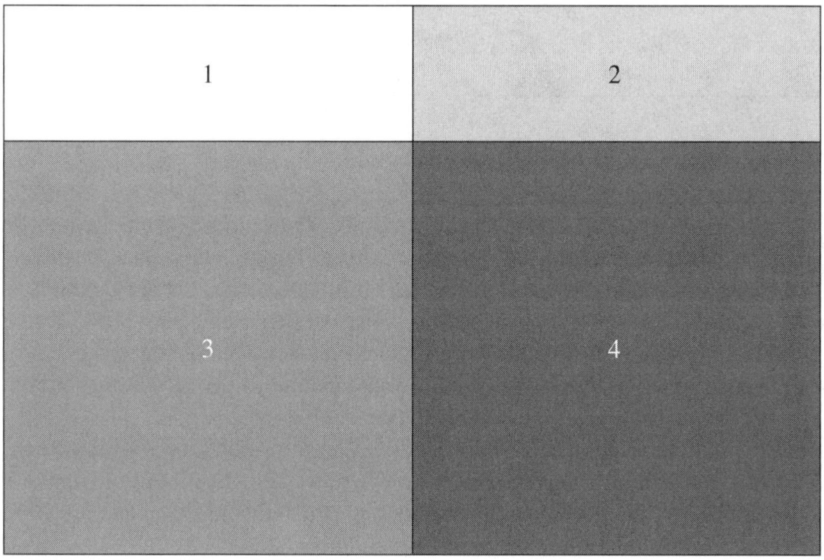

Source: Sundeen, S. Stuart, G. Rankin, E. & Cohen, S. (1985). *Nurse-Client Interaction, Implementing the Nursing Process* (3rd Edition). The C.V. Mosby Company.

[2] This is widely available. One source is Keirsey and Bates (1984) or go to http://www.humanmetrics.com/cgi-win/JTypes1.htm

[3] Available from Human Synergistics International., 39819 Plymouth Rd., C-8020, Plymouth, MI 48170, Tel: 800-622-7584 or 734-459-1030, Fax: 734-459-5557, e-mail: info@humansynergistics.com, website: http://www.humansynergistics.com

Exhibit 2–4 Johari Window

When a person has a great deal of self-awareness

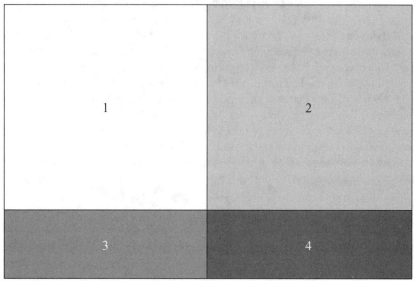

Source: Sundeen, S. Stuart, G. Rankin, E. & Cohen, S. (1985). *Nurse-Client Interaction, Implementing the Nursing Process* (3rd Edition). The C.V. Mosby Company.

We strive to improve. We handle change better because we are more adaptable and flexible. We can become more comfortable with new information, different approaches, or novel ideas that help us to be more innovative. We can experience optimism—that "can do" attitude. A growing awareness of our gifts and our life purpose develops. We then can start to manifest these gifts. We can become more persistent in pursuing our goals even when obstacles cross our path or when we experience setbacks. This knowledge increases our ability to better relate to the world at large.

All of this is an individual choice; it is like a spiral. The spiral can move upward toward personal mastery or downward in a more negative direction where we become more rigid and entrenched in our beliefs, lose integrity, and become a dictator. Pessimism and depression can result. However, at any point we have a choice and can change the direction of the spiral.

As we identify bad or destructive habits in ourselves, it is important to stop these behaviors as well as to be vigilant in identifying bad habits as we move through life:

> Just say no to them. It is the strength to shift behavior and refuse to participate in actions that do not serve us well. This shortcoming could be anything that doesn't work, such as an uncontrolled temper, failure to meet deadlines, an unwillingness to work with others, or being "too busy" to make patient care rounds or spend time with faculty and students. Any of these habits may violate professional standards, and curtailing or stopping these habits creates an opportunity to strengthen character (Kowalski & Yoder-Wise, 2003, p. 27).

As we work on problems, forgiveness of both ourselves and others is important. If we do not do this, we may become so bogged down in our thoughts that we do not deal with the problem areas effectively. Forgiveness in a larger sense is also important in personal mastery:

> There are times when each of us are hurt by others or hurt others. If we respond with resentment and the desire for revenge in the first instance or smugness and glee in the second instance, weakened character results, and we are less human than we could be. Forgiving those who hurt us is paramount. At the same time, asking for forgiveness when we hurt someone is equally important. Another aspect of forgiveness, forgiving ourselves, after committing a hurtful act toward another or making a grievous error of omission or commission is critical to personal growth in the leadership role. It is difficult to let go of self-condemnation, yet it is essential to continuing development as a leader (Kowalski & Yoder-Wise, 2003, p. 27).

A positive belief in self is essential when pursuing personal mastery. In the emotional intelligence research, self-confidence, being certain of one's own expertise (Snow, 2001), is part of personal mastery. We achieve success in meeting our life's goals when we believe we have the capability to succeed, are able to seize the opportunities, act on them, and work with or around the obstacles. When we can picture the outcome, we are more likely to achieve it. One effective nurse executive said, "There's nothing I can't do if I don't want to, except sleep."

Our self-confidence can also be enhanced by our environment and by our own presentation. If we find comfort being around water, perhaps living where there is a view of water will be helpful. How we dress or fix our hair can enhance or detract from our self-confidence as well as give out a message to others. Presentation is also important in our work. As we write a report, if it is clear, succinct, and well presented, chances are it will be more favorably received, as opposed to one having a sloppy appearance or having a less coherent approach.

FINDING OUR LIFE PURPOSE

Part of self-awareness is identifying our life purpose. The problem is that we often do not have a clear idea about our life purpose until we are well into our thirties—and sometimes it can occur much later. In our younger years our picture is still clouded, and as we experience life a clearer picture begins to emerge. At times we may believe that we have a clear picture, but we learn that we did not fully understand the picture or even that we need to go in an entirely different direction.

The best answer always lies within. What feels right? When things are clouded, then it is not yet time to understand. Once we understand, we have a choice. Do we follow what our inner core tells us? Or do we ignore it? If and when we do follow that inner guidance, the world becomes clearer, and more opportunities, including the challenges, occur to enhance our achievement of our life's purpose. Brooks (1966) suggests that through stillness we can find the answers:

> The cultivation of inner quiet, so that in a true sense one can become all eyes, as one sometimes calls a heightened receptivity. ... As long as the head is still busy, full sensory receptivity is impossible, while with increasing stillness in the head, all perception, traveling unimpeded through the organism, automatically becomes sharper and more in context. In this new stage of more awareness and permissiveness the self-directive powers of the organism reveal themselves ever clearer, and we experience on a deeper level the unexpected transformations we can undergo.... [When] one reaches a state of relative balance, simultaneous changes happen throughout the whole person. The closer we come to such a state of greater balance in the head, the quieter we become, the more our head 'clears', the lighter and more potent we feel. Energy formerly bound is now more and more

at our disposal.… We find ourselves being more one with the world where we formerly had to cross barriers. Thoughts and ideas "come" in lucidity instead of being produced. We don't have to try to express ourselves… but utterances become just part of natural functioning. Experiences can be allowed to be more fully received and to mature in us. As Heinrich Jacoby once remarked: "Through becoming conscious we have been driven out of paradise, through consciousness we can come back to paradise" (pp. 502–503).

In the West we do not value contemplation. Yet it is a major way to decrease stress.

In addition to listening to our inner core, we can turn to many helpful people—significant relatives, mentors, teachers, as well as other references concerned with personal mastery. For example, one wonderful reference, among so many possibilities on personal mastery, is a book written by Morris (1994), *True Success: A New Philosophy of Excellence*. Morris organized the mastery process into seven elements: a conception of what we want, a confidence to see us through, a concentration on what it takes, a consistency in what we do, a commitment of emotion, a character of high quality, and a capacity to enjoy.

BALANCE

Inner quiet is intertwined with balance, another aspect of personal mastery. When balance is achieved, we are calm yet have energy for whatever we believe is important at that moment. When we are not balanced, we experience stress and anxiety and our performance suffers. In fact, a popular phrase, "living in the moment," is useful for achieving balance and personal mastery. Living in the moment means just what it says: giving our attention to what is happening at that moment, leaving other cares or worries elsewhere. It is not remembering the past—that has already happened and we cannot change it. It is not thinking of the future—that has not happened and is yet to be.

Achieving balance at all times is the ultimate goal. Some helpful hints are as follows:

- Accept that administration is generally a multitasked job—we handle multiple inputs and tasks simultaneously. We start one thing, get interrupted by another, and so forth.
- We achieve our goals, but it may neither happen the way we picture it nor happen when we believe it *should* occur. *Shoulds* do not "go with the flow." It may not be the divine plan to achieve something in the way or at the moment when we have decided it should be achieved.
- Part of the leadership role is learning to respond to what seems to be the most important issue in that moment. There are days when personal goals may not be achieved at all because one is so busy responding to others' issues or crises. Balance is when we are not bothered by such unexpected events but go with the flow.
- Balance is when we choose to take care of something because our intuition tells us to do it, and vice versa.
- Balance *keeps things in perspective*. When something goes wrong, it can be helpful to think ahead 5 years. How important will this issue be then? Perhaps we will not even remember the incident. Or perhaps this incident will lead to something unexpected but better.

As we discuss balance, we cannot avoid the issue of what causes stress. This varies for different people. Actually, there is "eustress," which is wonderful, and "distress", which is not desirable. Stress is useful when it mobilizes us to take action. It is harmful when it buries us in negativity. Negative stress can affect our immune system and create disease. What causes stress in one person may not in another. Why is that? It depends on our perspective about issues confronting us. I am reminded of a woman who suddenly lost her son in a tragic accident. She said, "It's amazing to think about what used to cause me stress. It was little things that I won't even remember tomorrow. Those things are not important in the scheme of life. Now I realize that *only the far more important matters are stressful issues*."

So we have a choice whether to become stressed; it is a personal experience. How empowering. I can choose whether to be stressed; I can choose detachment and calmness—it is up to me. If what we picture is what materializes, I would choose to be *calm*.

Stress can also be caused by fear and worry. Fear is very negative and hurts us. People's fears vary greatly, but one commonality is that many of their fears are of things that may never happen. We put energy into them anyway, which is more likely to make them occur. *So the question is whether we want to put energy into such negative things.*

Various coping mechanisms can help one keep in balance. First, it is important to always remain positive: "everything will work out perfectly" or "I am in perfect health." Coping mechanisms differ for each person, ranging from swimming, walking, or running to meditation and prayer to sitting on a mountain looking at the view to regulating breathing. It is best if this can occur on a regular basis. In fact, to decrease stress and encourage health in employees, some companies encourage staff to exercise in facilities provided by the employer, to not take work home in the evening, to engage in counseling made available for employees, to provide massage therapy for employees, and to have better health habits such as eating more nutritious foods, not smoking, and so forth.

Balance harmonizes left brain/masculine/yang and right brain/feminine/yin. **Exhibit 2–5** illustrates these attributes. This is a subtle process where we need to choose the appropriate characteristic for each moment. Each trait is wonderful when used at the right time and is inappropriate when used at the wrong time. This supposes that we have the capability to access both sides at all times. Have you noticed how certain people seem to be dominant on one side or the other? This is not balanced, because these people are not using a good part of the energy within themselves. These traits are not determined by our biological sex. The attributes are all present in each of us. It is up to each of us whether we use them or not. The knowledge of which attribute to use at what time is deep within ourselves if we choose to tune in to it.

Balance also involves recognition that because everything is constantly changing, a bad situation will change. It will not last forever; happiness will not last forever either. In this world there is duality. Sometimes we experience sadness and sometimes happiness. Neither will last forever. Actually, balance often is the area in between the extreme high and the extreme low. Balance is when we experience calmness.

Exhibit 2–5 Left-Brain and Right-Brain Attributes

Left Brain (Masculine)	Right Brain (Feminine)
Conscious mind	Subconscious mind
Aggressive/Assertive	Passive/Receptive
Logical/Analytical	Emotional/Sensitive
Intellectual	Intuitive
Mental	Psychic
Objective	Subjective
Giving	Receiving
Will	Creation
Force	Power
Knowledge	Wisdom
Voluntary systems	Involuntary Systems
Separate/Individualized	Inclusive/Unifying
Sun	Moon
Yang	Yin

Balance not only occurs internally—with feminine and masculine traits or with the analytic/ cognitive and emotional/feeling parts—but includes balancing life issues. Balance includes such things as balancing the personal life with the professional life; balancing different groups that we are a part of; and balancing personal, organizational, professional, societal, and spiritual commitments (Dunham-Taylor, 1995, p. 25). Specific ways to achieve balance, as well as encouraging others to achieve balance, are infinite.[4]

Achieving balance is most often a process of becoming. At times we are better with achieving it; at other times we relapse. The goal is to become balanced as we experience each moment and not think about the past or future.

FULFILLMENT: ACHIEVING ONE'S POTENTIAL

Contemplation and balance can be helpful in bringing about life purpose awareness. Once we understand our life purpose, it becomes a powerful motivator as we proceed through life. We can then more fully use our talents, capacities, or potentialities. Life purpose provides a powerful work ethic. This is what Maslow called *self-actualization*. "There is increasing agreement among psychologists that the greatest satisfaction and experience of fulfillment in life is reached by bringing one's best potentials to materialization" (Buhler, 1966, p. 19). At first in life we may be unaware of our full potential, and it may remain latent throughout life. However, when activated, our imagination lights up, releases creative energy, and new ideas result. We become enthusiastic about it. Thus we achieve fulfillment by maximizing our potential and realizing and using our gifts. Fulfillment can be that wonderful feeling when we achieve something we have worked hard to bring to fruition; it also can involve very difficult, life-threatening goals, such as sacrificing one's life to save another's. Our actualized gifts contribute to our society.

As we begin to understand our full potential, we become more creative. We experience a passion for our life's work. We appreciate new ideas, concepts, feelings, and spiritual beliefs that can change our perception of life and the way we interact with the world. This awakening helps us to understand what we need to create. In the popular phrase, this helps us "to get out of the box." We troubleshoot more effectively. We pay more attention to our intuition and know what is right or what to do next. We become more aware of other areas to explore. We learn how others might fit into this dynamic process.

Sometimes difficulties we face lead us in creative directions we never would have considered otherwise. When we experience failures, we can develop humility. Maybe we are going to need to try again to see if we can do it better. Occasionally, obstacles are significant crucible events:

> Our recent research has led us to conclude that one of the most reliable indicators and predictors of true leadership is an individual's ability to find meaning in negative events and to learn from even the most trying circumstances. Put another way, the skills required to conquer adversity and emerge stronger and more committed than ever are the same ones that make for extraordinary leaders....
>
> For the leaders we interviewed, the crucible experience was a trial and a test, a point of deep self-reflection that forced them to question who they were and what mattered to them. It required them to examine their values, question their assumptions, hone their judgment. And, invariably, they emerged from the crucible stronger and more sure of themselves and

---

[4] For a perspective on balance in nursing leadership, see Distefani and Bledsoe's article, "A balanced approach to leadership" (2003).

their purpose—changed in some fundamental way. Leadership crucibles can take many forms. Some are violent, life-threatening events. Others are more prosaic episodes of self-doubt.... A crucible is, by definition, a transformative experience through which an individual comes to a new or an altered sense of identity. It is perhaps not surprising then that one of the most common types of crucibles we documented involves the experience of prejudice.... Some crucible experiences illuminate a hidden and suppressed area of the soul. These are often among the harshest of crucibles, involving, for instance, episodes of illness or violence.... Fortunately, not all crucible experiences are traumatic. In fact, they can involve a positive, if deeply challenging, experience such as having a demanding boss or mentor....

So, what allowed these people to not only cope with these difficult situations but also learn from them? We believe that great leaders possess four essential skills, and, we were surprised to learn, these happen to be the same skills that allow a person to find meaning in what could be a debilitating experience. First is the ability to engage others in shared meaning.... Second is a distinctive and compelling voice.... But by far the most critical skill of the four is what we call "adaptive capacity." This is, in essence, applied creativity—an almost magical ability to transcend adversity, with all its attendant stresses, and to emerge stronger than before. It's composed of two primary qualities: the ability to grasp context, and hardiness. The ability to grasp context implied an ability to weigh a welter of factors, ranging from how very different groups of people will interpret a gesture to being able to put a situation in perspective. Without this, leaders are utterly lost, because they cannot connect with their constituents.... Hardiness is just what it sounds like—the perseverance and toughness that enable people to emerge from devastating circumstances without losing hope.... It is the combination of hardiness and ability to grasp context that, above all, allows a person to not only survive an ordeal, but to learn from it, and to emerge stronger, more engaged, and more committed than ever. These attributes allow leaders to grow from their crucibles, instead of being destroyed by them—to find opportunity where others might find only despair. This is the stuff of true leadership (Bennis & Thomas, 2002, pp. 39–45).

COMPETENCE

Personal Competence. Personal competence is necessary to achieve *effective* leadership. This includes such capabilities as a good memory and being able to have good concentration as one accomplishes work. It is being goal-oriented and losing our sense of self in the accomplishment of something. It is being completely serious, or motivated, about our work and keeping a sense of humor. Research has shown over and over again that humor, and laughing, relieves stress. When we are fulfilling our life purpose—at home or at work—we are more likely to be happy, motivated, enthusiastic, optimistic, and enjoy life. Life flows more freely.

It is seeing opportunities and challenges as stimulating or, at least, as *something that we can successfully deal with*. (A world view of *abundance* is preferable to one of *scarcity*.) Personal competence also involves knowing when it is time to leave a position, such as when issues cease to be challenges, when we are tired of dealing with issues, and when we have grown stagnant on the job, or when we physically can no longer do the work.

Clinical/Administrative Competence. In the nursing profession, fulfillment comes from serving our clients. This means that we have clinical knowledge that is ever-changing and that needs to be updated. This is coupled with the need to talk with our customers so that we can understand what they need. The more we understand about our customer—patient, resident, client—the more effective we are in delivering appropriate care to that customer. Then we can deliver the care needed or make sure that they receive the care they need. In Benner's (1984) work, she identifies how we start as a novice and gradually, as we get more experience, become an expert.

Having clinical skills enhances our ability to anticipate patient needs and to understand why there is no one best practice for a patient with a certain diagnosis. After all, we treat the whole patient with all the baggage they bring to us. The baggage differs, as does the patient response to certain treatments. Clinical competence is necessary to understand processes, procedures, standards, methods of treatment, and technologies related to the care and then to choose the best options for each patient's individual needs.

When we are in administrative roles, clinical competency enables us to be more effective managers. When we can pitch in and help with patients when the going gets rough, we earn staff respect and trust because staff can see that the nurse manager can provide safe, competent patient/resident care. As one moves up the ladder in administrative positions, clinical competence in all the areas we may supervise becomes impossible. At this point, we must continue to learn and enhance our clinical competence but also trust other's expertise to best manage patient care.

When we are in an administrative role, having an understanding of the patient experience enables us to be more effective. It is important that we talk regularly with our customers as well. They are very helpful to identify issues that are important for us to resolve in the work setting. In addition, we need to stress the importance of staff dialogue with customers as well. One problem that occurs regularly with health care administrators is that those who do not have a health care background cannot understand the service side—what patients experience—of the health care business. Unfortunately, that is why at the executive level it is often only the chief nurse officer who can identify what is best for the patient. When administrators are clinical professionals, they have the added patient care dimension that makes them more effective in health care administration. They understand the "care" side of our business. Healthcare administrators who lack this dimension can have an eye-opening experience when they experience a life-threatening illness and suddenly see the service side from the patient perspective. They often become more effective administrators after having had this experience. (Actually, this is sometimes the case for nurses and physicians as well!)

This clinical competence expertise, along with regular dialogue with patients and families, gives us many clues for ways we can improve our clinical effectiveness as well as the health care - environment. Too often our goals for the customer do not fully match theirs. In fact, we remain in our box and do not even perceive some of the problems that need to be resolved. For instance, *we make people wait to see us*. (Do you remember how frustrating it is to have a 2 p.m. appointment at a clinic, having taken off time at work, and to still be waiting to see a health care professional at 3 p.m.?) Or we *do not treat people with dignity*. (Have you ever worn a hospital gown that might flap open in back as you are walking down the hall?) And *we do painful invasive procedures*. (It is not fun being poked and prodded.) We may make choices the patient does not want, such as not recording his or her wishes regarding life-saving measures in life-threatening situations.

From a marketing perspective, most of our customers are not saving their dollars because they are looking forward to buying hip replacement surgery. They may be saving for a new car or in case they experience catastrophic illness, but it is more of a worry that illness will deplete their funds rather than something they look forward to with anticipation. Yet when experiencing a health crisis, suddenly people want our help.

Organizational Awareness. Organizational awareness is one of the emotional intelligence competencies, defined as being cognizant of organizational life and politics (Snow, 2001). Actually, organizational awareness extends beyond the organization. It includes a picture of how the organization fits into the community and how larger societal issues impact the organization.

Continual Learning. No matter how competent we are, there is always more to learn. Every moment in our lives provides the teaching most needed. It gives us the opportunity to constantly grow and learn. Our choice is to trust the process and allow the lesson to seep in or to fight it or ignore it. Learning is dynamic. Our learning changes too. What may interest us at one point in our lives may not later. Then we can learn about something new or different, or we can appreciate certain nuances that we were unaware of before. As we learn, we acquire more wisdom, accomplish our work more effectively, and become more proficient in life. There can be joy in learning new things—exploring new vistas—especially when our explorations match our gifts and interests.

This is also true on an organizational level. In a study with nurse executives identified as "excellent," interviews revealed that, "No matter how much things improved, there always was more that could be achieved. This did not produce frustration, but provided an ongoing commitment. These executives were highly satisfied personally and professionally—yet they balanced this with more to be accomplished" (Dunham-Taylor, 1995, p. 25). Research has found that people like to have something different to do in their work or they get bored. Therefore, remember that no matter how much things improve, there is always more that can be achieved. Status quo is the kiss of death. Change keeps us alive. There is no single best way to do anything. Each of us responds differently to situations. Creativity is part of the process because constant improvement has to be improvisational. (This is not to say that some consistency is helpful, because too much change all at once can be overwhelming.)

Learning can challenge and stretch us. It can offer new opportunities. We can strengthen areas that have been weaknesses. However, the joy of learning can be extinguished by life circumstances, illnesses, or even past educational experiences. Sometimes the most profound learning happens when we experience difficulties or make mistakes; it is the conflicts we face and the people that we have conflicts with that teach us the most. These challenges can be reframed and are wonderful opportunities for further learning. No matter what we have or have not done, there is always hope, for anyone can learn and improve.

We learn in many ways. Learning is more than just passively being a sponge. It involves listening, asking questions, processing information, identifying patterns of similarity, and reflecting on events, processes, issues, or other things that have presented themselves to us. It is actually trying things, changing our behavior when warranted, and learning from the experience.

As we talk about continual learning, we need to consider our mind and its potential. According to various research studies, we use only 5% to 10% of our brains. Think of this untapped resource within each of us. We have so much more potential that could be used as we live our lives! Our minds are capable of things like superlearning where one listens to certain music (i.e., the Mozart effect), and in this relaxed state, one has the potential to learn more effectively.

There are many opportunities for learning in our work life. This starts with self-evaluation. For example, we could ask ourselves why we do things the way we do them. Becuase we all wear our blinders that keep us "in the box," we need to question our basic assumptions. For instance, a nurse administrator could ask such questions as

- Why do I procrastinate and wait until the last minute to complete something?
- Why do we need shifts? Why does everyone have to work an 8- or 12-hour day?
- Why do we need a policy and procedure for everything—do nurses really use them? Aren't nurses professionals? If so, why do we need more policies and procedures for the registered nurses than we do for the aides?
- Why do we teach using only a lecture format? What is the best method for us to learn about something new?

As we help others in the work group to achieve better leadership in their work roles, they need opportunities for learning, just as we do. I continue to be amazed to hear wonderful staff nurses say they are not leaders and that leadership content does not apply to them. This seems to be a common misconception. Staff nurses, in actuality, are leaders as they go about their work each day. For that matter, there are wonderful aides that provide the backbone of the day-to-day care that would not describe themselves as leaders either. Yet they (or the housekeepers) are often the person who is the most significant to an inpatient or resident.

WISDOM

Wisdom is the result of much learning, often enhanced by such things as encountering a crucible experience or achieving a quietness within, that helps us to lose our sense of self (as contained in selfish), gaining our sense of selflessness, and realizing our interdependence with the world.

One bonus of the quest for personal mastery is that it leads to wisdom. Interestingly, as we become wise and possess wisdom in some areas, chances are we are beginning learners in other areas. After all, there are so many things to explore in this world. Wisdom is enhanced when we develop a broad knowledge base and possess practical knowledge based on life experience, yet have insights about situations or people or can perceive the motivations of others. It is a road that spirals ever upward if we are paying attention to what is within.

> Ultimately we have just one moral duty: to reclaim large areas of peace in ourselves, more and more peace, and to reflect it towards others. And the more peace there is in us, the more peace there will also be in our troubled world.
>
> —Etty Hillesum, Holocaust Victim (from *Real power: Stages of personal power in organizations*, Hagberg, 2003, p. 273)

HUMILITY

> In past research interviews with "excellent" nurse executives, they were comfortable with themselves, but ego was not a part of this process. In fact a quality of humility... was evident. Perhaps this is why their own transformational scores were lower than staff ratings of them. They did not see themselves at the top of a pyramid in power positions but saw staff members as pivotal to organizational success. Their role was to support and facilitate staff members within the organization. They also freely admitted and owned their mistakes (Dunham-Taylor, 1995, p. 25).

We remain aware of our vulnerabilities and weaknesses during personal mastery. We are aware there is still so much more to learn and improve about ourselves. This self-awareness in the emotional intelligence research includes accurate self-assessment, being aware of one's limitations (Snow, 2001), and emotional self-awareness, where one accurately knows one's positive and negative biases (Snow, 2001). As this awareness grows, we become more humble.

As one approaches personal mastery, one becomes more influential within the world and yet still understands that one is only a very small part of it. Part of humility is assuming responsibility for our personal performance, having high standards, and being conscientious. We are harder on ourselves than others will be. We are brutally honest about our motivations. We are committed to our life purpose. At the same time we begin to see in the scheme of things how insignificant we are. "It means to act according to one's conscious conviction, but still always having the humility to keep the door open and be proved wrong" (von Franz, 1980, p. 145).

Eisenhower never fell into the trap,… believing the rules no longer applied to him or that he was better than anyone else.… He was never arrogant or condescending, and he was thoroughly honest.… Humility like Ike's, which conveys absolute assurance but at the same time acknowledges a leader's equality with followers, can be truly inspiring (Gergen, 2003, p. 21).

INTEGRITY

The bedrock of both personal mastery, and of effective leadership, is *integrity*—remaining true to oneself while doing what is best for everyone concerned. Integrity is morality, or what is good or right for people as they interact together. Integrity respects everyone. It occurs when one can be empathetic with other people and understand why they are doing what they are doing. One can separate the behavior from the person. (It does not mean that we judge others because we have not walked in their shoes.) We understand their position or their choices—even when we may not agree. We are compassionate. It represents justice and fairness. It does not violate anyone's rights or personal welfare. When we live it, we are strong and balanced. We are *tuned in to that inner core* that lets us know what is right in a situation. There is a oneness within ourselves. As we work toward this wholeness, every situation we encounter helps us to better understand and reach toward this wholeness.

Integrity becomes our choice each moment in our lives. It's a series of choices, each adding to the other. It is incremental. It spirals. In a previous leadership study with "excellent" nurse executives, they stressed the importance of having very high professional, moral, and ethical standards—and stressed the importance of *not compromising* these standards. In other words, they stressed integrity. A wonderful book, written as a story, further explores leadership and integrity: *Leading with Soul: An Uncommon Journey of Spirit* (2001) by Bolman and Deal.

INTUITION: PAYING ATTENTION TO OUR INNER CORE

Intuition (listening to our inner core) is another capability that we can enhance. We can start by just paying attention to our gut level and the direction it leads us. Have you ever had the experience where you wake up in the morning and suddenly you know what to do about a certain problem or situation? Or had a dream where you know that your child is in danger while on his bike? Or suddenly you start thinking about someone and then they call you, or you know that you need to call them? Or you know that you will be safe in some scheduled surgery? Or you know that a patient is "going bad?" All this information comes from our intuition.

In nursing, we have been more aware of our intuitive capabilities because we are involved with so many people experiencing life-threatening events. Intuition is what helps us deal more effectively with ambiguity, with situations where we do not have all the facts, when there is uncertainty, or when there is complexity. Intuition can also lead us to have better timing in our actions. Our "gut level" tells us what is right and when the right time is to do something.

Our intuition, or inner core (if we tune in to it), is a wonderful gift. Our gut level signals us, if we listen to it, and tells us what is right in each life situation. Some situations are rather mundane, so following our inner core is quite easy; at other times we are really tested. For example, in interviews with nurse executives, many of them said that in our present volatile work situations, they knew they might lose their job at any moment. When something happens that is ethically wrong, they face a choice. What should they do? Confront it or overlook it? If one decides to confront it, one may need to go against a powerful physician, or one may not have the support of the CEO, chief operating officer, or board. Several executives discussed confronting such situations and leaving their positions because they could not get support to do what was ethically correct. In other situations, both the executive team and physician group rallied around, doing what was right, with the nurse executive continuing to work there. Health care is fraught with such ethical dilemmas.

The bottom line is always, "Can I live with my decision?" Ironically, even when something awful happens to us (like suddenly losing our job or resigning unexpectedly), if we have followed our inner core, it will always lead us to something better—something we may never have found if this situation had not happened. So in the midst of difficulties and crises, there is hope. Our choice at each step is whether to pay attention and support our inner core or to ignore it. A helpful resource on developing, or tuning into, our intuition can be found in Schultz (1965), *Awakening Intuition: Using Your Mind–Body Network for Insight and Healing*. This book discusses research on intuition and gives personal stories as well.

Persistence

When something is important yet we are not able to achieve it easily, it becomes important to have persistence. We are like a river that flows along and when there is an obstruction, the water tries to find a way around the obstruction—or flow under or over the obstruction, causing its meandering course. Life is like a river. As we are obstructed in pursuing our life purpose, persistence is needed as we meander around the obstruction or overcome the obstacle. Sometimes we find that we have created the obstruction within ourselves. In this case, persistence means working through our own obstruction. Occasionally, there is a large enough obstruction that we cannot find a way around it. At this point, we must accept what is and move on from there. It does not make sense to continue to knock our heads against the obstruction. However, if something is really important, persistence may well be necessary before one can achieve one's objective.

A wonderful, easy-to-read book about such issues is Johnson's (1998) *Who Moved My Cheese*, written about how we respond to change. This book shows how persistence under the wrong circumstances does not change the present circumstances. The theme of the book is illustrated by this excerpt: "change happens (they keep moving the cheese); anticipate change (get ready for the cheese to move); monitor change (smell the cheese often so you know when it is getting old); adapt to change quickly (the quicker you let go of old cheese, the sooner you can enjoy new cheese); change (move with the cheese); enjoy change (savor the adventure and the taste of the cheese); and be ready to quickly change again and again (they keep moving the cheese)" (p. 74).

Relationship Effectiveness

Now that we have discussed internal personal mastery issues, we can turn to the way we interact with the world around us. Leadership involves working closely with people in the external environment. We recognize the connectedness between all of us. This external capability allows us to be able to effectively work with, and build relationships with, people and groups with various personalities or characteristics. Building relationships is an important administrative competence. Collaboration increases as relationships deepen. This is relationship effectiveness. Emotional intelligence research has labeled this external function as involving social awareness and social skills. Certainly, this interpersonal effectiveness component is an important part of dynamic leadership. As with personal mastery, this external leadership capability can be learned and improved.

Social awareness and social skills develop as we mature. We exist in interdependent relationships where each person influences others. Close relationships are important for human survival; thus we build bonds, nurturing instrumental, authentic relationships. These relationships are strengthened when we have empathy for each other and understand each other and the predicaments that we all face. As we experience relationships, it is helpful if we have some social competence and political awareness and have a certain adeptness at knowing when to accept the course others are taking, or know when to inspire or persuade others to take a different approach or respond differently to something.

As one experiences relationships, it is inevitable that conflicts occur. This occurrence does not mean that we have been ineffective leaders but does require us to respond to the conflicting issues that result from differences. When negotiating conflict, effective leaders create an environment where people respect each other and can openly discuss their differences, ideas, and perceptions. This can lead to finding ways to resolve conflicts or to at least better understand where others are coming from in their relationships with us:

> This role competence requires the leader to communicate effectively with others in a way that anticipates and, as necessary, disarms the potential for conflict. This leader focuses on establishing relational and emotional bonds in the team that develop the emotional maturity of team members and facilitate the stability of positive and effective relationships. The enthusiastic, caring, and supportive leader generates those same feelings throughout the team. This individual supports the power of humor, kindness, communication, and availability to others in a way that creates a context of inclusion and caring (Porter-O'Grady, 2003a, p. 109).

It is important to note here that both the external and internal components of leadership have to be integrated together. Thus we continue to respect each person, be honest, possess integrity, and be trustworthy. In our relationships, we encourage everyone to find meaning in his or her life and work—even when this may cause us some difficulties as leaders. For instance, it may be best to encourage a valuable staff member to take another job more suitable to his or her gifts and life purpose, even when this means we will have to replace that person.

DIALOGUE

Relationships are established and strengthened by dialogue. The word *dialogue* is used consistently in this book to mean the process of honest communication where everyone discusses their ideas with one another as well as respects and listens to one another. It is a *two-way process* that is a very important component of effective leadership. This form of dialogue, or the Socratic method, so-called because it came from Socrates in ancient Greece, is very important, not only to leadership effectiveness but to an organization or work group. Effective leadership involves constant dialogue both written and verbal, coupled with good interpersonal skills.

An effective leader exhibits good interpersonal skills with others, both individually and in groups, recognizing that we have different personalities and come from different backgrounds. This means that we are effective communicators—in expressing ourselves, in listening openly and intently, in actively seeking feedback from others, and in wanting to better understand others. Communication is one of the competencies identified in emotional intelligence research. This is defined as establishing positive relationships and managing expectations (Snow, 2001). "If your words don't stick, you haven't spoken" (Useem, 2001, p. 56).

When a problem occurs, there are usually many different perceptions about the problem. It can be very dangerous making a decision about an issue when only one perspective has been heard. Instead, one should find out different points of view about the matter before making a decision.

Part of the dialogue process includes listening to what others communicate both verbally and nonverbally. Then one can ask the right questions to further clarify the situation. For instance, sometimes a presenting problem is not the real issue. A leader may intuitively sense this or may find out by asking some questions—such as *Why has this become such an important issue?*—to get to the bottom of the issue. Questions, both from the leader and from others in the environment, can help to identify additional factors that need to be considered before making a final decision. The best way to achieve this is through dialogue.

Once the decision is made, the person or people making the decision must effectively communicate this decision to others so that they can best understand it. This is also an important part of the dialogue process or the decision cannot be implemented, or implemented properly.

Sometimes communication is most effective when stories are shared. Some people learn by experience, some by hearing, and some by seeing. Stories can achieve learning for each of these learning styles and thus may be the most effective way to communicate what is important. People may remember the story, and the meaning of the story, for a long time, long after a discussion of just the principles involved within the story would have been forgotten. Stories can also enhance our relationships with others.

When all from the top down use this method, there is better communication and fewer roads to Abilene. Harvey (1988) explains this concept. This article discusses how no one really wants to go to Abilene for dinner, but all are afraid to speak out and say so when one person suggests they go. Thus all go to Abilene and come to find out, if they had honestly discussed the question, none would have chosen to go.

As we discuss issues together honestly, we come up with better ideas and better methods of doing things. As we know each other better, we work together better, so teamwork improves. We tend to know each other's gifts and preferences and divide the work accordingly. No matter how much or how well we communicate, we have never communicated enough. Communication should be direct and stay in the present. No one, including the leader, should play games. Good communication is knowing when to say something, when to be silent, and when to listen. It is authenticity.

We take a risk when we expose our thoughts and feelings, but this sharing leads to achieving better decisions and more effective teamwork. Thus when conflicts occur, the leader needs to encourage appropriate expression of conflict as a way to achieve better decision making. No one is wrong or right; there just needs to be dialogue with each person sharing his or her perceptions and ideas about how to resolve issues. It is not a shouting match but rather a dialogue carried out using the adult. Let me explain.

Staying in the Adult. Looking at **Exhibit 2–6**, the *P* stands for the *parent* part of us. This side has many aspects. It can be nurturing and helpful. It can be judgmental and be full of "should" statements. The *C* stands for the *child* part of us. Children can be playful or angry. They can be loving and responsive. Children often need direction and attention from parents to grow. Finally, there is the *A*, or *adult*, part of us. This is the reasoning part. It is more like a computer in that emotion is not attached to it, whereas emotion is attached to the parent and child part.

Now let's use this exhibit and look at interactions between two people. If person A comes from the parent when communicating with person B, person B will probably respond from the child. If the parental communication is nurturing, the child response is loving and uses the information to learn more about the world. When the parental approach is judgmental, the child may feel ashamed or angry and respond based on that response. Emotion is involved in the conversation. The same thing happens if the supervisor comes from the parent when interacting with staff.

Now let's move to **Exhibit 2–7**. Here person A is coming from the child when communicating with person B. The communication coming from person A's child will hook into person B's parent. So person B will respond from their parent. If the child is angry, the parent may be angry. When anyone is angry, the person is not as effective in responding to situations. Anger causes more anger. Issues escalate. This is not desirable. Or the parent may be calm and try to stop, or ignore, the angry outburst. Again, emotion is part of the interaction.

Exhibit 2–6 Parental Approach

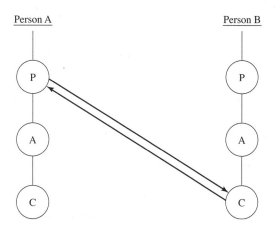

A parental approach will elicit a child response.

Key:

P = Parent
A = Adult
C = Child

Exhibit 2–7 Child Approach

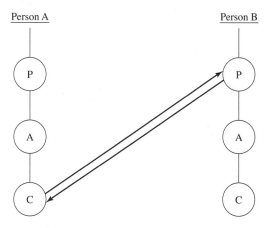

A child approach will elicit a parental response.

Key:

P = Parent
A = Adult
C = Child

In **Exhibit 2–8**, person A is in the adult when communicating with person B. This is most likely to hook into person B's adult. This is the reasoning, calm part of both individuals. Emotion is not involved. Person B still has a choice as to how to respond. If person B chooses to stay in the parent or child mode, his or her response may switch to that approach. However, the greatest likelihood is that each person will communicate from the adult. Ideally, the effective administrator uses the adult approach in communicating with others. In fact, when we feel ourselves responding to someone using emotion, this is a clue that we are either in the parent or child part of ourselves. This is a time to rethink, "Do I really want to be in the parent or the child?" It may be time to exit to a place where one can become more calm and balanced before continuing with the communication!

There is greater chance for success when one is able to stop and think before acting—or reacting—to a situation. If one is immediately emotional in a situation, it is generally better to wait, or step out of a situation, until one can get back into the adult before acting. Police know this—the best way to live to retirement is to remain calm in the midst of crises.

Even nurturing behaviors can get us in trouble. For instance, I often hear nurses say, "I will do this myself because I can do it better." This is their reason not to delegate tasks to others. This is dangerous because one person cannot possibly take care of everything alone! What the person often does not realize is the child message this gives to others, "You cannot do this as well as I can." In fact, this attitude is dangerous because then others do not learn. For example, a new nurse is not appropriately mentored about the role, or a patient does not learn how to give his own insulin or appropriately care for himself. Or the parental nurse manager expects that all staff will check to see what the manager wants to do before taking action. This is also a trap—what are staff members to do when the manager is absent? Thus staying in the adult is very important in quantum leadership.

Exhibit 2–8 Adult Approach

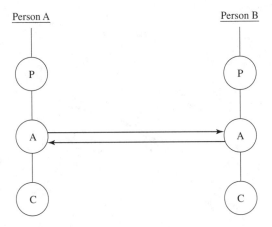

An adult approach will be more likely to elicit an adult response.

Key:

P = Parent
A = Adult
C = Child

Objectivity, or staying in the adult, is very helpful when in conflict. It is easy for people to see each other as without a redeeming quality, even though the conflict is only caused by a person's behavior or by differences in opinion. It is helpful to identify the real source of the conflict. In this case, discussing the problem and encouraging others to not attach the problem to the entire person can be helpful. It can be helpful to come back to the values when examining a conflict and dialogue, asking, "What is best for the patient?"

Objectivity leads to better conflict management and decision making. To a certain extent, our own life experiences always somewhat cloud our objectivity. But this is something that can be improved. Dialogue helps us to have a dynamic picture of the people involved, take into account all the different viewpoints, and stay in touch with what feels right intuitively.

Now that we are in the information age, our communication ability has been both greatly enhanced and yet it has become very impersonal, causing misunderstandings if clarification or dialogue does not occur. First, we need to have skill at various types of information technology—everything from the cell phone, to the personal data assistant, to the computer, to the Internet:

> The ability to communicate well… actually grows difficult as technology makes communication instantaneous, impersonal, and overwhelming. No longer needed to merely pass on information, this century's leader needs to help followers understand, frame, and manage the flood of information bombarding them, and listen to their concerns and issues. In today's email society, communication of meaning, previously done by gesture, tone, inflection, body language, and eye contact, is attempted by :), J, L, :-o, :-Q, :&, etc., and often is misunderstood. (Remember that capital letters mean you are shouting at the recipient.) Future leaders need opportunities to develop skill in all forms of electronic communication and encouragement to embrace new communication technologies (Nauright, 2003, p. 26).

AUTHENTICITY

Relationship effectiveness is actually a humanistic approach where we are *authentic* and appreciate authenticity in others. We put people first and often get recharged by people. This way we are able to accept, and even delight in, others' differences and successes; we also have empathy for problems that others face. This calls for honesty and sensitivity—accuracy in interpreting social cues, recognition of all the interconnections between us, treating everyone with dignity, and knowing that we need to build links between individuals, groups, the community, and society. "Interpersonal ineptitude in leaders lowers everyone's performance. It wastes time, creates acrimony, corrodes motivation and commitment, and builds hostility and apathy" (Snow, 2001, pp. 442–443).

One very important component of administrative competence is generating *trust*. We achieve this by being honest and by exhibiting consistent behaviors. What we say is what we do. Our actions match our words. For instance, if the administrator says there will be no layoffs during a budget cut, then no layoffs occur. Or if the administrator doesn't know what will happen, it is best to say so to staff. In the emotional intelligence research trustworthiness includes displaying honesty and integrity (Snow, 2001). *Every action the administrator takes, every word out of the administrator's mouth, needs to display honesty and integrity.*

Actions speak louder than words. Administrators may believe that all they have to do is give lip service to the values. Instead, staff will look at the leader's actions and quickly see whether or not the administrator actually means and lives by the values. And if the organizational leadership does not have integrity, this has a negative, downward spiral effect organizationally. *"A fish starts to rot from the head."* Trust is lost and probably will not be regained.

HUMOR

Relationship effectiveness is not humorless. Encouraging everyone's *humor* can enhance relationships. Humor can make the world a better place because it relieves tension. When we enjoy our work and those we work with, life is so much more fun. All can enjoy life, work, and the workplace when everyone can express their lighter side.

THE PYGMALION EFFECT

Within the interpersonal leadership environment, the Pygmalion effect is something very important for administrators to consider. This concept is discussed in detail in a classic *Harvard Business Review* article, "Pygmalion in Management" (Livingston, 2003). Research has shown that a supervisor's beliefs about the person being supervised become a self-fulfilling prophecy—even when the person may believe the opposite. In other words, if the nurse executive believes that a nurse manager is doing a poor job, even a high achiever will eventually be doing poor work. The same is true for a nurse manager. If the nurse manager believes that a staff member is a wonderful employee, this becomes a self-fulfilling prophecy. And, conversely, as in the movie *My Fair Lady*, even when the staff member believes he or she cannot do the job, as long as the supervisor believes the staff member can do the job, the staff member will successfully accomplish the work. This is why it is important to have good chemistry with your supervisor as well as with those who report to you. When this occurs, anyone can succeed given the values, support, and opportunity.

If an employee is having problems, the first thing we supervisors need to do is to examine our own beliefs about the person who is not performing adequately—a powerful message for any supervisory person! "Do I believe this person is doing well, or is capable of doing well, on the job? Do I believe this person can improve?" Self-examination about one's own likes and dislikes, as well as personal biases about each staff member, is the first step one must take when in the supervisory role. An administrator must be fair to each employee. Then anyone can succeed given the support and opportunity. The Pygmalion article finds that effective leaders provide "high performance expectations that [staff members] fulfill," whereas ineffective leaders "fail to develop similar expectations, and as a consequence, the productivity of their [staff] suffers" (Livingston, 2003, p. 122). Do we administrators set high performance expectations for staff—and expect that staff will accomplish these? When we care for the caregiver, the caregiver will then care for the patients.

POWER

Now let's examine our definition of power. Let's change "love of power" to **power of love**. Do you believe power is finite? If so, there is only so much of it. This means that for me to get more power, I must take it away from someone. The quantum view would say that power is infinite, that there is always more power available. So if I give it away by empowering others, there is still plenty left for me. In fact, if I encourage others' leadership, I will be enhancing my own leadership. The idea here is that the more I give away, the more power I create for myself. After all, continuing with the quantum view, we are all in this together. (Just as an effective leader possesses all aspects of leadership integrated within oneself, so are we all interrelated in this world of ours.)

This is why such wonderful energy can result when a group works together to accomplish a certain objective. All come with different perspectives that, when empowered, can lead the group as a whole to develop shared visions of the past, the present, and the future. The future vision is better than what any one person involved could have come up with alone, and all will have a more accurate picture of what this vision is because they participated in creating it.

Stages of Power. A wonderful resource on power representing the quantum perspective is Janet Hagberg's book (2003), *Real Power: Stages of Personal Power in Organizations*. It states that,

"Personal power is the extent to which one is able to link the outer capacity for action (external power) with the inner capacity for reflection (internal power)" (p. xxi).

Using that power definition Hagberg identifies six developmental stages of personal power (see **Exhibit 2–9**). The first three stages reflect the external power perspective, believing power is finite, whereas the last three stages become internally oriented, seeing power as infinite. The definition of power changes at each stage and has resultant positive and negative aspects that cause developmental dilemmas a person needs to resolve before moving on successfully to the next stage. One can manifest different stages of power when we experience different situations and people, yet we have a "home" stage where we tend to be most often.

When in *Stage One, Powerlessness*, people do not believe they possess much power. Because of this world view, they deal with the world using manipulation:

> Powerless people feel they are constantly being *manipulated by others*, pushed around, helped, controlled, duped, or taken care of, but they also find they depend upon manipulating others to get things done or to acquire things for themselves (Hagberg, 2003, p. 3).

Exhibit 2–9 Hagberg's Model of Personal Power

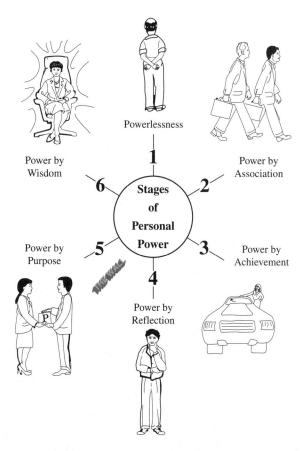

The struggle at this stage is to overcome dependence. Resolution begins when people start to feel good about themselves, develop self-esteem, and begin to use other more effective skills to deal with the world. In Stage One a person's most consistent deterrent is fear. When fear rules, a person will divert back to manipulation again.

When his or her skills increase, a person moves on to *Stage Two, Power by Association*. People at Stage Two "believe that certain people in the organization have the power, usually defined as control and influence, and they hope these people will notice them, lead them, nurture them, and reward them" (Hagberg, 2003, p. 26). Within an organization, people at this stage identify the people with the power and hope that maybe some of the power will rub off on them. Magic—their description of power—is expected. This is the stage where bosses take on the most significance. These people love to be mentored. To move on to Stage Three, one needs to further develop self-esteem and learn to have self-confidence—not have a need for the confidence or security gleaned from others.

Stage Three is *Power by Achievement*. "Stage Three is the dynamo stage.... [They] are in the thick of things. They know how the organization works and they help make it work better. The threes are in charge. They have the feeling that "this is it!" (Hagberg, 2003, p. 53). At this stage a person strives for something—a degree, a position, a special car, a fancy home, being rich—and, when attained, believes that he or she has "made it." These things become symbols of success. Threes enjoy showing off these symbols. Their description of power is control. They can become stuck at this stage because they like it. It often takes a crisis to move a person on to Stage Four. The crisis—whether internal or external—prompts the person to question how important these things really are. Then confusion begins. Up to this point their power definition has been provided externally by others. This confusion begins an internal search where one eventually arrives at Stage Four. Note that in the first three stages empowerment has *not* occurred.

In *Stage Four, Power by Reflection*, a person is competent and has developed his or her own leadership style. This style may or may not fit with organizational norms. These persons have integrity. Fours have a "reputation for sound judgment, fairness, and a listening ear" (Hagberg, 2003, p. 93). Yet they have inner unresolved dilemmas that may not be apparent to others. Thus it is a time for reflection. What is really important? Here true leadership begins—leadership that is based on *internal* values, not on *external* symbols or positions. At this stage "they can admit their mistakes without having to be found out first" (Hagberg, 2003, p. 106). They also are better risk-takers and are more courageous. True empowerment does not happen until one is at this stage.

When we empower others, it means that we trust them to accomplish the goal(s)/tasks. A Stage Four realizes that leaders succeed through the successes of others. Empowering others can involve several processes: mentoring and coaching others in their learning and development, fostering staff creativity, encouraging growth, determining and trying out new solutions, enhancing and recognizing staff successes, protecting staff from unnecessary work, and respecting and valuing staff contributions. Because each staff member has different gifts, this process varies with each person. Empowerment also occurs in times of trouble. Giving staff support and help when overwhelmed or experiencing a problem, discussing possible alternatives in a difficult situation, or even recognizing mistakes but making sure that someone is not devastated by what they have done, are all examples of empowerment.

A difficulty for Fours is their mismatch with the Stage Three environment and the lack of trust that that engenders between people as a result. The people at Stage Three wonder what Fours' agenda is because they are not used to Stage Four behavior. This is not a fault of the Fours but a by-product of being different from the norm. People who manage Fours soon realize that Fours are not motivated by the same things that Threes are. They cannot be persuaded to do things by the suggestion of rewards like money or promotions. Because their motives are not traditional, they are sometimes viewed suspiciously (Hagberg, 2003, pp. 114–115).

In Stage Four there are two traps—both coming from the ego. The first is just struggling with the ego. The second is they have not "experienced a need for a meaningful, other-oriented life purpose" (Hagberg, 2003, p. 123). Before one can move into Stage Five, one reaches **The Wall**. Here one comes face to face with his or her ego. At this stage the only way to overcome the ego is to go within. One needs to discover a meaningful life purpose. This process is different for everyone. There is no cookie cutter approach or one size fits all. The answer is found within.

Stage Five is *Power by Purpose*:

> Stage Five is unlike all of the preceding stages. Its uniqueness lies in the strength of the inner person relative to the strength of the organizational hold on that person. The guide for behavior in Fives is the inner intuitive voice. They trust it more than they trust the rules. Stage Fives are different internally *and* externally now. They are more congruent because they no longer have to live two separate lives as Stage Fours do. And it is even harder to spot Fives because they don't care if they're ever spotted. In fact, they may even hide a bit. Fives have a life "calling" that extends beyond them (Hagberg, 2003, p. 145).

Here is where the infinite power definition comes in. "Power is like love: You can't have it truly until you give it away or let it go, and the more of it you give unselfishly, the more it multiplies" (Hagberg, 2003, p. 146) and comes back to you in different ways. Fives let others lead. They believe that power is based on values—not on organizational norms or positions—and make decisions accordingly. "They do not attempt to gain or accumulate power because they find the other forms in which it reappears, like caring, appreciation, and friendship, more rewarding" (Hagberg, 2003, p. 146). They are humble and possess inner vision. They concentrate on the things that give meaning—both to them and to others. Their ultimate objective is to empower others. They do not need to be in charge, preferring to work behind the scenes. It is their faith, and their willingness to give up everything that is important to them, that moves them on to Stage Six.

People at *Stage Six, Power by Wisdom* possess inner vision. "Stage Six people are very involved with life yet detached from their involvement. They see from a different eye, hear with an unusual ear, and feel with a new heart. They are a paradox, even yet, at the same time, they are deeply moved by the pain and stress in themselves and in the rest of the world" (Hagberg, 2003, p. 177) and are willing to sacrifice themselves for a cause. They often spend a lot of time alone and gain strength from higher sources. They possess an inner calm and have quiet strength. These individuals often go unrecognized because they choose not to take prominent positions. Instead, they prefer to be alone, tuning into higher sources.

Using Hagberg's definitions of power, it becomes more obvious how to define effective leadership. "People can be leaders at any stage of personal power, but they cannot be TRUE leaders until they reach Stage Four—Power by Reflection" (Hagberg, 2003, p. 201). She portrays how a person at each stage leads in **Exhibit 2–10**. Looking at this, one can see that the authoritarian leader is actually at Stage One. However, leaders at Stage Two are not much of an improvement because they are playing by the rules. At Stage Three, though they still see power as external, they use personal persuasion to influence others. This is why empowerment does not occur until Stage Four, when a person begins to realize that power comes from internal sources. Thus leaders at Stage Four lead by modeling integrity, at Stage Five by empowering others, and at Stage Six by being wise. Wouldn't you rather lead from one of these last three stages? This is possible. No matter where we currently are, we can learn, grow, and change. As we do, this will be reflected in our leadership, which will become more mature.

Exhibit 2–10 Hagberg's Summary of Leadership and Power at Each Stage of Power

Stage	They lead by	They inspire	They require
Stage 1	Domination, force	Fear of being hurt	Blind obedience
Stage 2	Sticking to the rules	Dependence	Followers to need them
Stage 3	Charisma, personal persuasion	A winning attitude	Loyalty
Stage 4	Modeling integrity, generating trust	Hope for self and organization	Consistency, honesty
Stage 5	Empowering others, service to others	Love and service	Self-acceptance, calling
Stage 6	Wisdom, a way of being	Inner peace	Anything/everything/nothing

Source: Copyright © 2003 by Janet O. Hagberg.

Empowering Based on Gifts.

> By allowing others to shine that light will end up somehow reflecting back to you.
>
> —*Anonymous*[5]

From Hagberg's stages, then, we can see that effective leadership involves empowering staff to do work that is a match with their gifts and that a leader must at least be at Stage Four to begin empowering others. That is why "Maxwell hypothesized that being immensely secure in yourself is at the heart of serving people" (Kowalski & Yoder-Wise, 2003, p. 30). How wonderful it would be if all nurses, not to mention every other person working in health care organizations, were at least in Stage Four.

Bass (1998) has called this kind of empowerment *individualized consideration*. Individualized consideration is needed because people are in different places with different abilities and gifts. A leader delegates differently to different individuals. Leaders empower others by giving as much responsibility to staff and patients at all levels to make the most of whatever talents and experience staff have. It is best if people's abilities are stretched in an empowering environment. When we empower, or delegate, we trust. Our message is that we know they can accomplish the work successfully. (Remember the Pygmalion effect?)

The Pygmalion effect influences how effectively we are able to empower others. It is important that everyone be empowered to go ahead with their work in ways that support the core value, such as *what is best for the patient*. After all, all have something unique to offer based on their gifts.

The word "empowerment" has been a popular fad, yet many different definitions of empowerment abound. Two people using this term may mean very different things. Some administrators will say, "I empower staff. I let them do the work," meaning "I delegate the work but make sure you do it my way." In actuality, empowerment has a very different definition in quantum leadership.

---

[5] This quote is from a nurse executive interview. Confidentiality was promised so the person cannot be named here.

Empowering is effective because people want to make a difference. We want our lives to have meaning. Each of us comes to this world to accomplish something special that no one else will do. This serves a larger purpose, making this a better world. We reach our highest potential when we pursue and use our gifts. Identification of our personal gifts starts us on the road to achieving our life purpose.

> Man's search for meaning is the primary motivation in his life and not a "secondary rationalization" of instinctual drives. This meaning is unique and specific in that it must and can be fulfilled by him alone; only then does it achieve a significance which will satisfy his own will to meaning (Frankl, 1984, p. 121).

At times people are in jobs that are not a match with their gifts. They may not be performing well because they are not engaged in the work; the work does not tie in with their life purpose and their gifts. They are probably unhappy and are in the wrong place. As a leader, you may need to talk to a person when you perceive a mismatch with his or her work and gifts and then encourage a change in jobs to better achieve his or her life purpose.

Empowerment, at times, can achieve magical results. In past research conducted by the author, one hospital nurse executive described how the wheelchairs kept disappearing and were not in the locations where they were needed. An orderly approached the nurse executive and said that he would like to be put in charge of the wheelchairs. The nurse executive said, "Go to it," and put him in charge—announcing that the orderly was in charge of wheelchairs at the next set of meetings she had with staff on all shifts. Her comment to the researcher was, "I didn't know how to fix this problem and I didn't have the time to deal with it!" The orderly was proud of his responsibility, felt empowered, fixed the problem, and there were always wheelchairs where they were needed.

Just think of what could be accomplished if more empowerment occurred! When someone wants to try to improve something, why not encourage them as well as give them the time and the authority to do it? It is easy with circumstances that seem limiting—such as the nursing shortage—to say that there is no way this person can be given extra time. Somehow, if we really believe there is a solution to finding the time, there will be one. Job satisfaction studies show that people are more satisfied with their jobs when they do not consistently do the same things every day. All of us need challenges. In fact, challenges result in retention—a reason the person stays rather than moving on.

EMPATHY

Along with empowerment, empathy for each other and for the people we serve is very important. We are most effective when we can go beyond selfishness and connect with something that is larger than ourselves. This empathy, or sensitivity, or connection with others and their predicaments reflects an altruism that will better other's welfare. "Without feelings of deep sympathy and sorrow for others struck by misfortune and a genuine desire to alleviate suffering on the part of caregivers, patient care service would be no more than a robotic endeavor" (Porter-O'Grady & Malloch, 2003).

In emotional intelligence research, empathy means that we are able to learn from others' experiences and expertise (Snow, 2001) and that empathy is reflected in our actions. Empathy also reflects the connection between ourselves and a higher power, found in our integrity. It is the "caring" component so important in health care. It is what we give to others with no motivation other than what is best for them. Perhaps the best way to say this is we want what is best for everyone concerned.

Empathy occurs when we understand another person's perspective. To achieve this understanding we need to communicate with others. In fact, as we get to know each other, we become able to anticipate a person's response to a situation, decision, or action. It is important to understand why someone chose to take a certain action or to understand how a decision affects others. This understanding helps us to lead more effectively.

CONFLICT: A RICH RESOURCE!

Effective leadership means that we are comfortable with or at least realize the value of conflict. One mistake we often make is to believe that conflict is something to avoid. We caution that trying to force everyone to "get along" and brushing the conflict "under the carpet" is dangerous. Actually, differences in opinion are a natural occurrence, and they afford us many rich opportunities for different ideas, perspectives, and change. Conflict, like change, will always happen. (Wouldn't it be wonderful if everyone agreed with us? However, life doesn't work like that.) We are *not* a failure as a leader when conflicts occur in our work group. In fact, what measures our leadership effectiveness is that we encourage people to express their differences in appropriate ways in the workplace. All of us are flawed people, working together to provide care for others. These differences provide a rich resource of possibilities, improve decisions, processes, and relationships.

Thank goodness there is diversity in this world! Wouldn't this world be a dull place if everyone were exactly alike? Diversity means differences in our views of the world. For instance, cultural differences can become a strong source of conflict just because we do not understand someone's viewpoint. Such differences exist within work groups. Here is where empathy is put to the test. How well do we understand another person's perspective of the world? Are we comfortable to let them tell us about it, or are we so uncomfortable that we do not give them a chance to air their beliefs?

Healthy disagreements and honesty provide different perspectives. By paying attention to, and valuing, different points of view we can make better decisions. Thus conflict can be very helpful and, when handled appropriately, can help us determine better alternatives. Dialogue and disagreements allow us to consider other ramifications that could occur before choosing the action we will take. Thus, instead of reacting, we can more thoughtfully consider the situation.

The problem with conflict is that when it is inappropriately expressed, it can result in anger, jealousy, fear, pain, and violence. More often than not when this happens one of the parties in the conflict has more power, is stronger, or is in some way unequal. This inequality results in that person not being able to express viewpoints in a safe environment. If something can be done to create more equality, it is important to provide it. For instance, if there is a difficult situation with a physician, having medical staff and administrative support in dealing with the situation is helpful. (And smart!) It helps if all are working toward a value, such as *what is best for the patient*. It is best when physicians value and respect team members. Research shows that patient outcomes are better on units where this is true.

There are more unresolved conflicts happening in an unhealthy workplace. These cause higher staff turnover, and staff play more games, like being passive-aggressive, talking behind other's backs, and/or complaining, and nothing is done about poor performance. Most often, problems start with the leader, assuming the present leader is not trying to clean up issues a past leader has caused. In this situation one first needs to deal with the ineffective administrative leader and then start cleaning up other staff issues.

Conflicts can occur not only between people but can also be caused by *systems problems*. These can create barriers to getting the work accomplished. They can create unnecessary hassles that, when they occur day after day, prompt one to finally leave. Staff will grumble about these issues. If administrators are doing regular rounds, they will hear. Usually, these problems will need to be dealt with by an intra-organizational group, discussed in Chapter 3, representing different departments or professions, followed by change. And as the change is implemented, additional problems will probably occur that will result in further change before the systems problem can be fixed.

Another source of conflict can occur when our day does not go as planned. We come to work expecting to accomplish certain things. Then an emergency happens, or someone is distressed about something, or someone takes an action that adversely affects the patient. Sometimes the whole day passes with the planned activities not being accomplished. This can be upsetting. However, think back—we really did what was best at each moment in the day. Perhaps it was not *the right time* to do the planned activities. After all, there is a right time for everything—it just may not be today! We can either experience a great deal of conflict internally—everything kept interfering with the goals we had set—or we can actually have a rewarding day because we know that we responded effectively to more important issues.

As a nurse administrator, we want to create a safe environment for appropriate expression of differences of opinions or viewpoints. The environment is strongest when there is support at higher levels of the organization as well as from other departments for this kind of climate to occur. (If someone is more linear and does not appreciate this climate, it can make the situation more difficult to exist.) Dialogue is encouraged, team members feel *valued and respected* and value and respect each other, and better decisions result because all are listening to each other and then decide what is best.

This is much easier for leaders who are at Hagberg's Stage Four or higher. At Stage Four empowering others happens. One also realizes the value in differences of opinion and that differences in opinion are okay. (At a lower stage a person does not understand this.)

In Chapter 3, where we discuss Likert's systems, a participative system is best for this climate. Here people are not in power struggles but instead are part of a team, help each other as needed, and are proud of their team (and they may even express something like "We are the best unit," or "We do excellent work caring for *any* patient."). They can more comfortably discuss differences together. This does not mean that tension never exists. But discussion happens and is healthy. The result is better patient care and a happier work environment because people are heard.

In empowering environments, the work group can resolve many issues, *without* any intervention needed from the administrator. Effective leaders know when to get involved and when it is more appropriate to have others deal with the issue.

In reality, though, there will probably be other units, or other disciplines, or people at higher levels who do not value this climate. All this creates a source of conflict. It is still possible for a unit to achieve this climate, even without having support of all the other players. It is just more difficult when team members have a conflict with the person who does not value this, because they may not fairly and honestly deal with conflicts.

The actual conflict can lead us to determine who is the most appropriate person(s) to deal with and to resolve the conflict. Sometimes it is best for one person to make a decision, resolving the conflict, while at other times it is best for a group to come to agreement as to how to best handle a situation.

In a safe environment people feel free to *express disagreement*. This includes the leader having "a willingness to risk exposing thoughts and feelings and to acknowledge how these impact perception and behavior" (Perra, 2000). The more people are able to be honest about a situation in a calm manner, the better. The goal is to *stay in the adult*. To be "in the storm of conflict and at the same time out of it… watching it in serenity" (von Franz, 1980, p. 149).

Sometimes when we disagree with someone, we don't like the person. Often, it really is not the *person* we dislike, it is their words or their actions or their beliefs that we do not agree with. It is not the whole person. In fact, sometimes the conflict is just a difference in style—for instance, one person is very detail oriented, never seeing the big picture, whereas another sees the big picture and never pays attention to detail. Thus it is important to get to the *root cause* of the conflict.

Have you noticed that certain people or behaviors really hit your hot button? Learning is possible here too because these issues or people probably are a little too close to some problems that exist within ourselves that we have not yet resolved. Therefore an important competency includes encouraging people to discuss issues when they do not agree—and it starts with us. Who is pushing our hot button, and why? What do we need to face within ourselves? How is our problem affecting others? Are we willing to work on this issue, talk about it with others, and ask their help to deal with it?

While discussing disagreement, an effective leader knows that it is all right *for staff to disagree with the leader*. This is hard to understand until one achieves Hagberg's Stage Four. After all, why would we want people to disagree with us? If we listen, we can learn about our misperceptions or about issues we need to resolve. A result is that staff will have more respect for the leader. If someone does not allow others to disagree with them, chances are they are at one of the first three stages.

Porter-O'Grady and Malloch (2007) spend a whole chapter on conflict, an excellent resource. Sources of conflict are found in **Exhibit 2–11**. "The secret of good conflict management is simple, but the process is not. *The secret is to get the parties in conflict to discern the root issues and mutually agree on actions to be taken*. Actually building an effective process to accomplish this goal, however, is a complex task" (Porter-O'Grady & Malloch, 2007, p. 82).

Within nursing a lot of us are women. Women have had to learn to be assertive in society. Similarly, nurses have had to learn how to be more assertive while giving care because sometimes physicians, and administration, have been given more importance than nurses in health care organizations. Yet it is the nurses who spend more time with patients.

Assertiveness, or being able to objectively, yet respectfully, describe a problem situation directly with the person with whom one disagrees, is a very important skill. Assertion uses "I" statements, such as "I felt __ when __ happened," or "I thought ___ was the way we were doing ___." (Aggressive statements often use "You" statements while expressing disagreement, like "You did ___," often being accusing or angry. Or one might just be passive-aggressive in dealing with the situation.)

Assertiveness is a positive use of dialogue. In a disagreement it is very possible that once we understand the other person's perspective, we at least have a better understanding where he or she is coming from and why the other person doing something a certain way. It is also possible that by listening to each other, the conflict may be easily resolved. Also, after all the dialogue, we may just decide to continue to disagree! Honest dialogue brings people closer together. There is more trust between people. There is also a possibility that we may both arrive at a better way of doing things than either of us had thought of in the first place.

Conflict management (see **Exhibit 2–12**) is an important leadership competency. In the emotional intelligence research, this is further defined as *developing consensus* and *mitigating*

Exhibit 2–11 Sources of Conflict

Environmental Sources

- Ego
- Personality
- Identity
- Intimate relationships
- Beliefs
- Perceptions
- Perspectives
- Education
- Position and role

Individual Sources

- Culture
- Nationality
- Religion
- Class
- Economics
- Politics
- Society
- Resources
- Race

Source: Porter-O'Grady T., & Malloch, K. *Quantum Leadership: A Resource for Health Care Innovation*, 2nd ed. (2007). Sudbury, MA: Jones and Bartlett, p. 83.

Exhibit 2–12 Managing Conflict Effectively

Principle 1. Conflict is a natural occurrence and will always happen. We cannot avoid it.

Principle 2. Conflict reflects differences—different perspectives, different cultural backgrounds, different experiences, different knowledge bases, etc.

Principle 3. Conflict offers a rich source of possibilities. It can bring about better circumstances/ideas/ solutions/relationships—even changes in our own behavior.

Principle 4. In a healthy environment appropriate expression of conflict is encouraged.

Principle 5. It is not humanly possible to respond to all conflicts. It is best to respond to important conflicts so conditions do not escalate.

Principle 6. It is important to get to the *root cause* of the conflict, i.e., we may perceive that our conflict is with a person when instead it is with a difference in work styles, an organizational process, our expectations, or circumstances.

Principle 7. It is okay to disagree with the administrator. (This becomes easier when the administrator is at least at a Stage Four.)

Principle 8. Leadership competencies include self-control, developing consensus, and mitigating conflicts.

Principle 9. Conflict management involves
  * Respecting/valuing others
  * Dialogue with the person/people directly involved within an appropriate, safe environment
  * Staying in the *adult*
  * Using assertive ("I") objective statements
  * Being empathetic
  * Appropriate timing
  * Use the core value (i.e., *What is best for the patient?*) as the basis for discussion
  * Providing an appropriate, safe environment

Principle 10. Trying to force everyone to "get along" and brushing the conflict "under the carpet" is dangerous.

conflicts (discussed throughout this section) (Snow, 2001). Negotiating skills[6] can be helpful in conflict resolution. Developing consensus can be achieved when dialogue occurs between people who are experiencing a conflict. In fact, this can prevent war from occurring.

> The techniques for finding common ground, for sorting through the various landscapes representing the diversity inherent in each issue, are now required by every leader. Also required are consensus-building and group-process skills, because leaders have the job of getting people to come together around issues and helping them determine appropriate responses within the context of their own roles (Porter-O'Grady & Malloch, 2007, p. 27).

It is important to stay in the *adult*, being factual, and keeping emotion out of the conversation as much as possible. In fact, sometimes when we discuss the situation with the person involved, we find out reasons we had not considered pertaining to the situation being discussed. This can give us a better understanding of why the incident occurred. Aggression is in the *parent* or the *child* and emotion is involved—all signs that one is not reacting appropriately to conflict.

When we experience conflict, another emotional intelligence competency, *self-control*, is important. This is further defined as remaining poised even under pressure (Snow, 2001). Sometimes it helps to ask oneself, "Will I remember this five years from now?" If one finds it difficult to get into the *adult*, and it is not an emergency, it may be time to just exit the situation, regain balance, and then come back and deal with the situation.

---

[6] A helpful book on successful negotiating is *Getting to Yes: Negotiating Agreement Without Giving In*, by Fisher, Ury, and Patton (1991).

It can also help to phrase this statement in the context of a basic value, like *what is best for the patient*. This can help one more effectively deal with disagreements because it lifts the disagreement from a personal thing to something both people, hopefully, value.

This conflict resolution skill is something the administrators, as well as staff, needs to exhibit. It is behavior that everyone is encouraged to consistently use. It is hard because we are not taught in our society to honestly and respectfully discuss disagreements *directly* with the other person involved. Instead, we talk about the people we disagree with behind their backs, don't help them, get passive-aggressive, or even avoid the person. When this happens, nothing gets resolved. In fact, the problem can magnify. Too much of this in the workplace creates a toxic, dysfunctional work environment. People may leave. New staff will be eaten alive. It is an environment that we do not want to create or support.

In fact, it takes a lot of consistent effort for a nurse manager to overcome this toxic environment (it has probably occurred in Likert's System 2, discussed in Chapter 3). The nurse manager will need to directly confront this issue in a team meeting, discussing more healthy behavior that will be an expectation. Then the nurse manager will need to directly confront people who are perpetuating the toxic behavior. This is hard behavior to change, but it can be turned around. (Before the situation gets turned around, the *nurse manager* will be a topic of conversation with staff, behind the nurse manager's back.) Just be consistent and direct each time this behavior occurs.

The location for conflict resolution to take place is very important. Usually, it is best if dialogue can take place in a more private setting where all involved can be more relaxed, have privacy, and not be in the middle of many tasks.

Many times conflicts are caused by expectations. Think about this. If I have an expectation that you will (or should) respond a certain way, when you respond differently there is a conflict. This conflict could have been avoided if I had not had an expectation of how you should respond. This is why *dialogue* is so important—it gives us a chance to check out the other person's perceptions. The most effective leaders *let go of expectations of others*. After all, how a person responds is beyond our control.

We cannot respond to every conflict that exists. That is not humanly possible. Timing is important. It is important to know which situations to respond to immediately and which can wait. Some decisions are best made after input and dialogue has occurred between a number of people. Other times, when conflict is left unresolved, the situation escalates and interferes with the work getting completed effectively. This is when immediate intervention is needed. An administrator needs to know when it is important to get involved in a conflict, what the various viewpoints are in the conflict, and how to negotiate and resolve disagreements. Negotiating skills can be helpful in conflict resolution. Many times we cannot make decisions alone but must negotiate with others.

Conflict is a natural occurrence. It is up to us to set the environment to most effectively deal with the many conflicts that will occur. All the best!

DECISION MAKING

Effective decision making is an art (see **Exhibit 2–13**). It involves finding and selecting the best alternative and having the most appropriate person (or people) make and implement the decision at the right time. As one nurse executive said, "It is sifting out the new rules and building for an unknown tomorrow."

An effective leader possesses an ability to analyze difficult concepts, listen to and understand different perspectives, get appropriate facts needed to make a more appropriate decision, see the smaller picture and how it fits with the overall big picture, yet make a decision even when unknowns remain. Many times a leader does not know what to do. Some advocate that a leader

Exhibit 2–13 Decision-making Factors

- Communicate, dialogue, listen.
- Understand the different perspectives.
- Have people make decisions at the appropriate level in an organization.
- Encourage healthy disagreement.
- Have empathy for others.
- Use our intuition.
- Always support the core value(s).
- Timing of the decision is very important.
- One must prioritize—What decisions are really important?
- Tenacity or persistence may be necessary.
- Accountability—Where does it lie?
- Take risks.
- Experience successes and failures. Celebrate successes. Correct mistakes.
- Use effective negotiation skills.

bluff at such times, pretending to know the answer. The authors do not recommend this approach. Once people see through this (and they will), they lose trust in this leader. It is much more effective to admit one does not know what to do, to ask for others' ideas, and to say that one needs time to think on the situation. If something must be done right away, it is important to listen to one's "gut level" after hearing other ideas and take the action one intuitively chooses. We arrive at better decisions when we stay in touch with what feels right intuitively and encourage others to follow their intuition.

A number of factors can be helpful to determine the best way to handle a situation. Although many situations have similar themes, individual differences occur that can change the way something should be handled. Using these processes can aid one to make the most appropriate decision. First, go back to the core value of *what is best for the patient*. Decisions are best when the core value is supported. Second, decision making is tricky for another reason. There are times when it is best to leave the decision making to others (who are fully capable of making better decisions on the matter than we would make). For instance, in the work setting each staff member has the best understanding of his or her work. We do not know the nuances of their work. They are the experts. Each person is a capable adult. Who must make many decisions to appropriately do the needed work. This is also true for patients—patients need to make the decisions that they determine are best.

Letting others make the decisions—actually encouraging staff to do this—can be difficult. Many nurses and nurse managers do not delegate enough. They say, "I can do it better." In this case, they have not allowed others to make decisions. They have not treated others (this includes patients and families as well as other staff, physicians, and administrators) as capable people deserving respect. After all, if one person has to do it all because no one else can do it right, how does all the work get done? It is physically impossible for one person to do everything right. Meanwhile, patients suffer, staff members are unhappy and leave, physicians complain about staff, and so forth.

Instead, the workplace is most effective when all delegate effectively—this involves knowing, or learning about, others' capabilities, sharing information, and teaching others if they do not know how to do something and then letting the appropriate people do it at the most advantageous time. This means that others may go about accomplishing something very differently from us. Unless this is harming someone, let that person do it his or her way. Others' generally know more about themselves, or about doing their job, than we do.

When mistakes occur, help staff process what went wrong to prevent this from happening again. Perhaps the best question to ask when a mistake occurs is, "What did you learn from this?" We all make mistakes as we do our work. No one is perfect. Instead of punishing a person who has made a mistake (this is getting into the *parent* role), it is best to stay in the *adult* and factually find out what happened, listen to different perspectives, and try to help the person undo the damage that has been done. This is just as true for ourselves. Beating ourselves up for something does not help the situation. The situation does provide learning for us. It is important to go back and own up to the mistake and then go on from there, undoing the damage as much as we can.

Third, another issue is *prioritizing*. One cannot do it all. In this information age, there is so much paper and information one cannot know it all. Instead, we need to listen to our "gut level" and concentrate our time and decisions on important issues. As previously discussed, this can be difficult for some, because we need to delegate appropriately and then prioritize what we need to do. Certain things are very important, whereas other things can wait until tomorrow.

Fourth, *timing* is an issue. Knowing when to make the decision is another part of leadership effectiveness. Once again, it is important to stay in touch with one's intuition as well as with others in the environment. There are times when we must make the decision. But many times others need to make the decision. Knowing when to make the decision and when to leave the situation alone takes experience as well as being in touch with one's intuitive capabilities. Does it feel right to make the decision? If inexperienced, a good mentor can be very helpful in this area. At times it is important to have the courage to make a difficult, or an unpopular, decision, even though others may disagree with it.

Another aspect of decision making is *tenacity*. Sometimes if one really wants something to happen one must be persistent, as discussed earlier in this chapter. For example, a nurse manager wants to start a new service. The supervisor, the executive team, or the board turns it down. If this is really important, the nurse manager needs to bring it up again later.

Persistence is also needed in any change project. Just going through things once with everyone involved does not mean that the change will occur or that anyone will do it. Tenacity is important in its achievement. For example, a huge change occurs for the nursing staff when charting is computerized. At first, most staff will find that it takes more time as they are unfamiliar with it, as unexpected problems occur, or as the computer system goes down and nothing is available. With persistence, however (provided the computerized system was a good one), staff will love it and will find that it saves a lot of time.

With decision making comes accountability for the outcomes. As we lead, responsibilities follow. "The buck stops here." We are responsible for our decisions, as well as for the actions staff who report to us have taken. Were the outcomes what we expected? Was there an unexpected outcome? Should we have made the decision(s) or should others have been more involved? How could we have done it better? How can we fix something that happened due to our decision(s)? Or due to our staff's decisions? An effective leader does not blame oneself or others. A mistake was made. How can this mistake be rectified? What will we do differently next time? Did we learn from our mistake? These are better responses.

If we did not take risks, mistakes would not happen. Successes and growth would not happen either. An effective leader has to take risks, especially on important issues. Actually, any decision and any action are risky. What is important is the *value* of the issue. If the issue is important, the risk is probably greater but will result in more beneficial results. In fact, persistence may be necessary, involving additional risk. If the issue is *not* important, it is best not to take the risk.

Risk taking results in both successes and failures. Both success and mistakes are a natural result of change and of risk taking. Celebrate successes with everyone involved. Give credit where credit is due. If a staff member did something wonderful, give him or her the credit for the success.

Mistakes provide fodder for further learning. It can be easy to get bogged down when we know we have not been as effective in a situation or when a situation really bombs. However, beating ourselves up about it can actually keep us from being effective in the next situation that presents itself. Instead, we can admit that we made a mistake, work to repair damage if needed, and move on, learning from our mistakes. If it is others who have made the mistake, talk with them. Why did they do what they did? What would they do differently next time?

Because this is an imperfect world, we experience successes as well as make mistakes as we move through life. Part of effective leadership is realizing that often we have had some role or influence in others' successes and failures. Plus we can learn a lot from our own mistakes. In his consulting, Tom Peters talks about the person who tried a new venture, lost a million dollars, and, when the CEO asks to talk with the person, is afraid the CEO will fire him. Instead, the CEO says, "Why would I want to fire you so you can go on and give another company the benefit of your experience?" The manager stayed but had learned a valuable lesson.

> Mistakes are the portals of discovery.
>
> —*James Joyce*

So What Is Effective Leadership Anyway?

Effective leadership is a continuous learning process. It is a path of discovery.

> In this chaotic world, we need leaders. But we don't need bosses. We need leaders to help us develop the clear identity that lights the dark moments of confusion. We need leaders to support us as we learn how to live by our values. We need leaders to understand that we are best controlled by concepts that invite our participation, not policies and procedures that curtail our contribution (Wheatley, 2006, p. 131).

> Effective leadership, or *Love one another*, will continue to evolve. There is so much more to learn!

> The giving and receiving of love in whatever form it expresses itself can have a more lasting impact than any other single thing we do. All healing finds its roots in the expression of love.

> It can reach far deeper places than any pill can go.

> While it is imperative to give physical bodies the support they need, it is equally imperative to give spirits the love they need in order to access the tremendous healing power it carries (Joy, 2003, p. 26).

Discussion Questions

1. Give an example where poor leadership affects the bottom line. Describe the ineffective leadership, and place dollar amounts on the losses incurred.
2. Describe someone you have known who is an excellent leader. What was he or she like?
3. As you read this chapter, how do you rate yourself on each of the leadership components? How can you improve your leadership?
4. Give an example of poor leadership. Which fallacies apply to their leadership?
5. Are you an effective or a successful manager? Has your experience as a manager been like Luthans describes?

6. In your management role, how much are you able to lead versus how much do you have to manage? Do you want to change this ratio? If so, what actions will you take to change it?

7. Think of an example where you have effectively used first-order change. Then give an example where you have used second-order change. Were the situations appropriate for the level of change you used?

8. Go through each of the emotional intelligence components and rate your current level of leadership. What are your gifts? What do you want to improve? How will you improve them?

9. Describe an example where effective leadership has saved the organization money. If you had to describe this to a finance person, how would you most effectively present this information? Then if you had to describe this to a nurse, how would you describe it?

10. Nurse managers are caught in a squeeze between delivering quality care to patients, keeping patient satisfaction scores up, and meeting bottom line requirements. What advice would you give to a new nurse manager to help this person avoid some pitfalls that you have encountered because of this squeeze?

11. How do you achieve balance in your life?

12. What is wisdom? Humility? Integrity? Empathy? How can you tell if people have them?

13. Have you participated in any assessments of your leadership style? If so, what did the assessment(s) show?

14. Have you experienced intuition in your management role? In your nursing career?

15. How does the Pygmalion effect apply to effective leadership?

16. What is dialogue? How does a leader use this effectively?

17. Give an example of staying in the *adult* when in the midst of conflict?

18. Describe a conflict your work team has experienced. How did you all resolve it? Or was it not resolved? If it was not resolved, what would you do differently to more effectively deal with this situation if you were the nurse manager?

19. Have you experienced empowerment? Have you empowered others?

20. What is your usual stage of power, as Hagberg describes it, when at work?

21. What are some differences between having a supervisor who empowers others, and one who does not?

22. What are your gifts? Have you identified what gifts each member of the work team has?

23. Give an example of collaboration that has happened at work.

24. Describe a situation where it is best for the work group to make a decision about their work? Then describe a situation where it is best for the nurse manager to make a decision.

25. Have you thought about what your life purpose might be? What is it?

26. Have you experienced a crucible event that changed your approach to life?

References

Arbinger Institute. (2002). *Leadership and self-deception: Getting out of the box.* San Francisco: Berrett-Kohler.

Bass, B. (1998). *Transformational leadership: Industry, military, and educational impact.* Mahwah, NJ: Lawrence Erlbaum.

Benner, P. (1984). *From novice to expert: Excellence and power in clinical nursing practice.* Menlo Park, CA: Addison-Wesley.

Bennis, W., & Nanus, B. (1985). *Leaders: The strategies for taking charge.* New York: Harper & Row.

Bennis, W., & Thomas, R. (2002, September). Crucibles of leadership. *Harvard Business Review,* 39–45.

Bolman, L., & Deal, T. (2001). *Leading with soul: An uncommon journey of spirit.* San Francisco: Jossey-Bass.

Brooks, C. (1966). Report on work in sensory awareness and total functioning. In H. A. Otto (Ed.), *Explorations in human potentialities* (pp. 487–505). Springfield, IL: Charles C Thomas Publisher.

Buhler, C. (1966). In H.A. Otto (Ed), *Explorations in human potentialities* (pp. 19–26). Springfield, IL: Charles C Thomas Publisher.

Burns, J. (1978). *Leadership*. New York: Harper.

Byham, W., Cox, J., & Nelson, G. (1996). *Zapp! Empowerment in Health Care*. New York: Fawcett Columbine.

Collins, J., & Porras, J. (1994). *Built to last*. New York: HarperBusiness.

Distefano, S. & Nicholson Bledsoe, D. (2008). A balanced approach to leadership. *Nurse Leader 1*(5), 32–35.

Dunham-Taylor, J. (1995, July/August). Identifying the best in nurse executive leadership: Part 2, interview results. *The Journal of Nursing Administration*, *25*(7/8), 24–31.

Fisher, R., Ury, W., & Patton, B. (1991). *Getting to yes: Negotiating agreement without giving in*. New York: Houghton Mifflin.

Frankl, V. (1984). *Man's search for meaning*. New York: Washington Square Press.

Gergen, D. (2003, January). How presidents persuade. *Harvard Business Review*, 20–21.

Goleman, D. (1998). *Working with emotional intelligence*. New York: Bantam Books.

Hagberg, J. (2003). *Real power: Stages of personal power in organizations* (3rd ed.). Salem, WI: Sheffield.

Harvey, J. (1988). The Abilene paradox: The management of agreement. *Organizational Dynamics*, *17*(1), 16–43.

Johnson, S. (1998). *Who moved my cheese?* New York: Putnam's Sons.

Joy, S. (2003, March/April). Is there enough room in my job for love? *Nurse Leader*, 24–27.

Keirsey, D., & Bates, M. (1984). *Please understand me: Character & temperament types* (5th ed.). Del Mar, CA: Prometheus Nemesis.

Kerfoot, K. (1997). Leadership: When success leads to failure. *Nursing Economic$*, *15*(5), 275–276.

Khurana, R. (2002, September). The curse of the superstar CEO. *Harvard Business Review*, 60–66.

Kowalski, K., & Yoder-Wise, P. (2003, September/October). Five C's of leadership. *Nurse Leader*, *5*(1), 26–31.

Kuhnert, K., & Lewis, P. (1987). Transactional and transformational leadership: A constructive/developmental analysis. *Academy of Management Review*, *12*(4), 648–657.

Livingston, J. (2003, January). Pygmalion in management. *Harvard Business Review*, 121–130.

Luthans, F. (1988). Successful vs. effective real managers. *Academy of Management Executive*, *11*(2), 127–132.

McClelland, D. (1973). Testing for competence rather than intelligence. *American Psychologist*, *46*, 56–62.

Morris, T. (1994). *True success: A new philosophy of excellence*. New York: Berkley Books.

Nauright, L. (2003, January/February). Educating the nurse leader for today and tomorrow. *Nurse Leader*, 25–27.

Nightingale, F. (1869). *Notes on nursing*. New York: Dover.

Perra, B. (2000, Winter). Leadership: The key to quality outcomes. *Nursing Administration Quarterly*, *24*(2), 56.

Porter-O'Grady, R. (2003a, February). A different age for leadership, part 1: New context, new content. *The Journal of Nursing Administration*, *33*(2), 105–110.

Porter-O'Grady, T. (2003b, March–April). Of hubris and hope: Transforming nursing for a new age. *Nursing Economic$*, 59–64.

Porter-O'Grady, T., & Malloch, K. (2003). *Quantum leadership: A textbook of new leadership*. Sudbury, MA: Jones and Bartlett.

Porter-O'Grady, T., & Malloch, K. (2007). *Quantum leadership: A resource for health care innovation.* Sudbury, MA: Jones and Bartlett.

Schultz, M. (1965). *Awakening intuition: Using your mind-body network for insight and healing.* New York: Harmony Books.

Sharpe, R. (2000, November 20). As leaders, women rule. *Business Week*, 75–84.

Simons, T. (2002, September). The high cost of lost trust. *Harvard Business Review*, 18–19.

Snow, J. (2001, September). Looking beyond nursing for clues to effective leadership. *The Journal of Nursing Administration, 31*(9), 440–443.

Stein, N. (2000, October 2). The world's most admired companies. *Fortune*, 183–196.

Sundeen, S., Stuart, G., Rankin, E., & Cohen, S. (1985). *Nurse-client interaction: Implementing the nursing process.* St. Louis: Mosby.

Useem, M. (2001, October). The leadership lessons of Mount Everest. *Harvard Business Review*, 51–58.

Vitello-Cicciu, J. (2002, April). Exploring emotional intelligence: Implications for nursing leaders. *The Journal of Nursing Administration, 32*(4), 203–210.

Von Franz, M. (1980). *Alchemy: An introduction to the symbolism and the psychology.* Toronto: Inner City Books.

Watzlawick, P., Weakland, J., & Fisch, R. (1974). *Change: Principles of problem formation and problem resolution.* New York: Norton.

Wheatley, M. (2006). *Leadership and the new science: Discovering order in a chaotic world* (3rd ed.). San Francisco: Berrett-Koehler.

CHAPTER 3

Organizational Strategies

Janne Dunham-Taylor, PhD, RN
Tammy Samples, MSN, RN

If there is light in the soul, there will be beauty in the person.
If there is beauty in the person, there will be harmony in the house.
If there is harmony in the house, there will be order in the nation.
If there is order in the nation, there will be peace in the world.

—*Chinese Proverb*

Organizational Wholeness

Large health care organizations are changing and eroding. The monster brick and mortar hospitals are downsizing as more services are offered in outpatient settings like "doc in a box" facilities and doctors' offices and home care. In fact, at least 50% of health care services take place outside hospitals. (This is hard to estimate because so many people have turned to alternative medicine.) This percentage is constantly increasing as technology develops better noninvasive treatment modalities, as information is instantly available, and as health care workers have become more mobile. These organizations can survive but must adapt to this new environment, being constantly aware of possibilities and vastly different ways to better serve their clients. And although there are a lot of long-term care facilities, estimates of future needs indicate these numbers will be woefully inadequate. Meanwhile, insurance plans struggle with increasing payments for services, fewer people can pay for health care, and home-based caregivers have proliferated.

Much of the current work of health care leaders involves *de*constructing health services. The current infrastructure must be largely done away with so newer models of service and support can be implemented. Leaders need to perform a range of activities in reconfiguring health care to fit the coming age, when space and time will be further compressed, services will be more fluid and more highly mobilized, and the locus of control will shift from the provider to the user. These changes include the following:

- The hospital bed will cease to be the main point of service. During the next two decades, the number of hospital beds will decline by about 50%.
- The service structure will be decentralized. The health care system will deliver small, broadly dispersed units of service.
- Services will increasingly move out of the hospital. More than 70% of the medical services currently provided in hospitals will be provided in clinics and doctors' offices by the end of this decade.

- Core practices of the professions will be substantially altered. The institution-based, late-stage services that once predominated are being replaced by high-intensity interventions that do not require hospitalization, and these interventions will transform the roles of the various health professionals.
- Users of health services are becoming more accountable for their own health. Providers now have the major job of helping to transfer the locus of control for medical decision making and life management to individuals who have never had it and do not yet know what to do with it. Providers' work over the next two decades will include educating the users of health services and assisting users in acquiring the necessary skills.
- The users of health services and the technology of health care will progressively interface such that virtual and technical interaction and communication will become the norm of health service provision. Connection between providers and patients will increasingly be virtual, with supporting technology making clinical services possible without bringing patients to the provider to use these services (Porter-O'Grady & Malloch, 2007b, p. 34).

All this means that health care organizations must be able to change on a dime, and health care administrators need to constantly be able to invent newer, better ways to offer services to clients. Quantum leadership, discussed in Chapter 2, is absolutely imperative for survival. This needs to be coupled with major changes in the way health care organizations work. Actually, both administrators and staff will need to work to achieve the organizational mission, goals, and strategies as well as the core values. Everyone needs to know what the strategic plan specifies and how they can contribute to meeting this plan. It also means that they can adapt as problems occur, so that the goals can still be achieved, *or that they have the power to change the goals when something else seems to be more appropriate for patients.*

> A healthy work environment correlates to job satisfaction, primarily expressed as frequent and healthy communication with managers/leaders, recognition by direct managers and the organization, opportunities for professional growth and development, and support by peers. Organizational culture affects satisfaction, which affects retention and influences recruitment. Workplace culture is significant; yet few health care providers understand how to shape the environment for worker health and satisfaction.
>
> Job satisfaction is inversely related to centralized leadership, poor communication, powerlessness, alienation, reliance on policy and procedure, and stress. A positive work environment is essential for physical and mental well-being and for ensuring healthy outcomes for patients. Factors most favorably linked with job satisfaction are autonomy, communication with direct managers and peers, and recognition or feedback for good work (Sherwood, p. 37).

The old vertical authoritarian model is outmoded. Instead, health care workers need to be valued, need additional knowledge/abilities, and need to be empowered to make decisions at the point of care. It is important for all to see the organization as a whole—not just see their own department/unit silo (as discussed in the Introduction)—and see how this organizational whole fits into the community at large. Each small action affects the whole. If the action is positive, it is valuable. If the action is negative, it creates issues that if allowed to continue will bring about the organization's demise. This is the only way for health care organizations to survive and to achieve organizational success.

While looking at the interconnectedness of everyone in the organization, structure and design (we discuss both in more detail in a minute) are influenced by some new concepts that come from chaos theory and the science of complex systems. This is further explained in **Exhibit 3–1**. These dynamics are present in organizations and affect what happens in organizations. We weave in these

Exhibit 3–1 Ten Principles for Leaders

Principle 1. Wholes are made up of smaller units that are always interacting with each other to sustain the whole.

Principle 2. All health care is local. The integration and effectiveness of health services depend on local relationships not centralized authorities.

Principle 3. Anything that adds value to any part of a system adds value to the whole system.

Principle 4. Simple systems combine with other simple systems to form more complex systems. Complexity grows incrementally through the interconnecting of smaller, simpler systems (called "chunking").

Principle 5. Diversity is a necessity for life. Only where diversity is present can the ability to thrive be ensured. Diversity makes chaos visible, as it pushes systems to forever adapt to changes in their environment.

Principle 6. Error is essential to creation. Both random error and conscious error are essential to the process of creation. In fact, error underpins all change. Error contributes to adaptation and thriving.

Principle 7. Systems thrive when all their functions intersect and interact in a continual dance of relationship and transformation.

Principle 8. There is a constant and permanent tension between equilibrium (stabilizers) and disequilibrium (challenges). This tension is essential to life and reflects the fact that disequilibrium is the universe's natural state.

Principle 9. Change moves from the center of a system to all other parts, influencing everything else in the system. Because every system is part of a larger system, there is an ever-evolving dance of interchange between the activities inside the system and between the system and the larger system it is part of.

Principle 10. Revolution (hyper-evolution) occurs when the many local changes are aggregated to inexorably alter the prevailing reality (called the "paradigmatic moment"). A revolution is a dramatic, almost instantaneous, change in conditions, and it presents living creatures with the challenge of adjusting quickly enough. In a revolution, many events converge to create a situation in which life can no longer be lived in the same way.

Source: Adapted from Porter-O'Grady, T., & Malloch, K. (2007b). *Quantum leadership: A resource for health care innovation* (2nd ed.). Sudbury, MA: Jones & Bartlett.

concepts throughout this chapter—and, for that matter, throughout this book. Do you see how important each small work group actually is in achieving the whole?

This is further complicated in that time is getting more compressed. This time compression (for example, we see patients for a shorter amount of time now than in the past) is contributing further complications to work taking place within the organization. There just is not as much time to do all the things we might have done in the past. Although many mourn this, this change is happening—whether we want it to happen or not.

There is another big financial factor impacting health care. Health care organizations are part of the service industry in this country. People (health care workers) are serving other people (patients/residents/customers). However, our customers are generally *not* saving their money because they *want* our service. Instead, they often are very vulnerable when they need our services, are afraid of many of the services we offer, and dread that the illness event might deplete their life savings. Or, worse yet, they do not have money for the services they need, yet they are at our door needing care. In a store they would say, "No money. No merchandise." In health care, people are also being turned away in greater numbers. Yet hospital and long-term care providers are being forced by law to continue to treat people who cannot pay. This really impacts the bottom line.

This is coupled with insurance companies who continue to cut percentages given to providers for reimbursement, and Medicare, covering the majority of our population, continues to cut back payments to pennies on the dollar. In the midst of this environment, health care personnel grapple with giving quality service, yet making ends meet financially. It is a complicated dilemma fraught with many challenges.

This complicated group of factors is too much for the old, linear, authoritarian systems to deal with effectively. Our large buildings are expensive. Have you noticed how a bill for an operation performed in a hospital is more expensive than when it is performed in a stand-alone surgery center? And now insurance companies are sending patients to Thailand and other third world countries for surgery because it is so much cheaper. So what is happening here?

> Our concept of organizations is moving away from the mechanistic creations that flourished in the age of bureaucracy. We now speak in earnest of more fluid, organic structures, of boundaryless and seamless organizations. We are beginning to recognize organizations as whole systems, construing them as "learning organizations" or as "organic" and noticing that people exhibit self-organizing capacity. These are our first journeys that signal a growing appreciation for the changes required in today's organizations. My own experience suggests that we can forego the despair created by such common organizational events as change, chaos, information overload, and entrenched behaviors if we recognize that organizations are living systems, possessing the same capacity to adapt and grow that is common to all life.
>
> What is it that streams can teach me about organizations?... This stream has an impressive ability to adapt, to change the configurations, to let the power shift, to create new structures. But behind this adaptability, making it all happen, I think, is the water's need to flow. Water answers to gravity, to downhill, to the call of ocean. The forms change, but the mission remains clear. Structures emerge, but only as temporary solutions that facilitate rather than interfere. There is none of the rigid reliance that I have learned in organizations on single forms, on true answers, on past practices. Streams have more than one response to rocks; otherwise, there'd be no Grand Canyon. Or Grand Canyons everywhere. The Colorado river realized there were many ways to find ocean other than by staying broad and expansive....
>
> Organizations lack this kind of faith, faith that they can accomplish their purposes in varied ways and that they do best when they focus on intent and vision, letting forms emerge and disappear. We seem hypnotized by structures, and we build them strong and complex because they must, we believe, hold back the dark forces that threaten to destroy us.... Streams have a different relationship with natural forces. With sparkling confidence, they know that their intense yearning for ocean will be fulfilled, that nature creates not only the call, but the answer (Wheatley, 1999, pp. 15, 17–18).

Where Are We Headed? Determining Purpose

So what is a health care organization's ocean? Where are we headed? And, the greater question is, how do we get to that ocean? The ocean is the organization's primary purpose.

> Purpose = The organization's fundamental reasons for existence beyond just making money—a perpetual guiding star on the horizon; not to be confused with specific goals or business strategies (Collins & Porras, 1994, p. 73).

Purpose remains unchanged for years. It may be a similar purpose to other companies. For instance, Merck's purpose, "fighting disease, relieving suffering, and helping people" may be similar to other companies who manufacture medications or with a health care focus. Purpose is similar to quality where one is always working toward achieving it but never totally accomplishes it. Other examples of purpose are Marriott's "making people away from home feel that they're among friends and really wanted" or Disney's "bringing happiness to millions."

The purpose statements *do not* give a specific description of the products. Nor do they specifically define the customer. In fact, the purpose

> Get[s] at the deeper, more fundamental reasons for the organization's existence. An effective way to get at purpose is to pose the question, "Why not just shut this organization down, cash out, and sell off the assets?" and to push for an answer that would be equally valid both now and one hundred years into the future (Collins & Porras, 1994, p. 78).

Purpose helps to give clarity and direction to all in an organization.

> When leaders make their strategic intent abundantly clear—as Wal-Mart's management has in proclaiming its strategy of "low prices, every day"—employees know what to do without requiring myriad further instructions. Achieving that clarity, however, is often far more difficult than managers appreciate (Useem, 2001, p. 57).

We are mistaken if we believe that our ocean, our primary purpose, is making money. Many health care organizations are run by administrators who believe that the bottom line runs the organization, antithesis to the mission statement above their entrance that spells out various values. When we make the bottom line first, finances plummet, whereas *when service is the first priority with the bottom line in second place, finances are sustained or improved.*

This is not to say that revenue is unimportant. We still need money to operate. The money simply must remain *secondary* to the primary goal. Money is part of the meandering that the stream does while looking for the ocean. If revenues are unavailable from one source, there may be another source available. *The primary issue is, what services does the patient need or want?* Then we go from there to determine our actions. The research shows this to be true:

> Profitability is a necessary condition for existence and a means to more important ends, but it is not the end in itself.... Profit is like oxygen, food, water, and blood for the body; they are not the point of life, but without them, there is no life (Collins & Porras, 1994, p. 55).

If the chief financial officer, and perhaps most of the executive team, really believes that the bottom line is the ocean, conflict and frustration occur for others in the organization who believe the patient comes first. The issue then becomes how much we decide to confront this, whether we leave, whether we just work there and do nothing—or complain about it to the wrong people, or whether we continue there and work to fix the problems. The choice is ours.

There are two additional energies necessary to successfully navigate the meandering rivers heading to the ocean: *soul* and *spirit*. Understanding and believing in the ocean is the *soul*. It is the reason we are doing all this. It makes what we do meaningful. This is the most important part of our work. We feel it very deeply. Our relationships with each other reflect this soul. If relationships are not good, chances are we have lost touch with the soul part of our business. If the relationships are collaborative, chances are the soul part is present, alive, and well. The *spirit* is the energy that fuels getting to the ocean. It is the synergy that exists between team members, physicians, suppliers, patients, and families. It is the energy that works to achieve getting to the ocean. It is the "radical loving care" that is given. "The fruits of spirit are enthusiasm, motivation, and performance" (Nobre, 2001, p. 288). Nobre (2001) suggests that "Soul + Spirit + Resources + Leadership = Results" (p. 287).

Core Value(s): The Soul of the Organization

Let's start with defining how to create the soul part—understanding and believing in the ocean. This is where spirit gets its energy. Collins and Porras (1994) reported on an enormous research project with premier companies that have lasted 50 to 100 years, are known for excellence, yet have experienced multiple leaders and different product lines through the years. They report that:

> A visionary company almost religiously preserves its core ideology—changing it seldom, if ever. Core values in a visionary company form a rock-solid foundation and do not drift with the trends and fashions of the day; in some cases, the core values have remained intact for well over one hundred years. And the basic purpose of a visionary company—its reason for being—can serve as a guiding beacon for centuries, like an enduring star on the horizon. Yet, while keeping their core ideologies tightly fixed, visionary companies display a powerful drive for progress that enables them to change and adapt without compromising their cherished core ideals.
>
> There is no "right" set of core values.... Indeed, two companies can have radically different ideologies, yet both be visionary.... The crucial variable is not the content of a company's ideology, but how deeply it believes its ideology and how consistently it lives, breathes, and expresses it in all that it does. Visionary companies do not ask, "What should we value?" They ask, "What do we actually value deep down to our toes?" (pp. 8–9).

Core value(s), or belief(s), is a sentence or two that captures the general guiding principle of the organization. It can provide a common cause between people who work in the organization. When sound, *these beliefs provide the backbone of every policy or action people within the organization take*. The core values come first, before goals, policies, or procedures. If a goal, policy, or procedure violates a core value, then it must be changed. Generally, there is one, core value that remains unchanged for many years. An example of a core value is *We provide appropriate, safe care that our clients value*.

Examples of core values in other businesses are as follows:

- To "treat the patient the way we would want a family member to be treated."
- Sam Walton's value for Wal-Mart: "[We put] the customer ahead of everything else.... If you're not serving the customer, or supporting the folks who do, then we don't need you."
- John Young identified the Hewlett-Packard (HP) core value: "The HP Way basically means respect and concern for the individual; it says 'Do unto others as you would have them do unto you.' That's really what it's all about" (quoted material from Collins & Porras, 1994, p. 74).

When determining the core value, it needs to be authentically identified by people in the organization, not copied from some other organization, even though it is possible that a core value for one company is the same as for another. The core value does not have to be unique, but it is imperative that all within an organization support it with words, actions, and goals.

The core values are extremely important, and in the premier companies described in *Built to Last* (Collins & Porras, 1994), one becomes an outcast if one does not support the values:

> A visionary company creates a total environment that envelops employees, bombarding them with a set of signals so consistent and mutually reinforcing that it's virtually impossible to misunderstand the company's ideology and ambitions.... Because the visionary companies have such clarity about who they are, what they're all about, and what they're trying to achieve, they tend to not have much room for people unwilling or unsuited to their demanding standards, both in terms of performance and congruence (p. 121).

These companies promote from within, encouraging managers to immerse themselves in the company ideology for several years to make sure they understand what is expected from them, before being promoted.

We are most successful in defining our core values when they go *deeper* than just surface direction. Have you noticed how people accomplish the impossible for a cause?

> Ultimately the choice we make is between service and self-interest.... The antidote to self-interest is to commit and to find cause. To commit to something outside of ourselves. To be a part of creating something we care about so we can endure the sacrifice, risk, and adventure that commitment entails. This is the deeper meaning of service (Block, 1993, pp. 9–10).

When an organization derails and administrators want to fix the problems, it is important to start with the core values. Dialogue about the core values with all employees is very important. If all believe in the core value, *the belief will provide the energy, or spirit, for staff.* It is best if the change begins with the executive group, then with all the administrators, and then with staff. If anyone cannot support the core values in their words and actions, they may need to be dismissed.

There is a good book, written as a story, called *Walk the Talk... And Get the Results You Want* (Harvey and Lucia, n.d.), that portrays the importance, and the difficulties encountered, when a company president begins to realize that it is important to match his actions with the company values.

Several authors discuss the importance of core values in rallying staff but stress the difficulties of really living by the core values. For instance, Lencioni (2002) says that

> Coming up with strong values—and sticking to them—requires real guts. Indeed, an organization considering a values initiative must first come to terms with the fact that, when properly practiced, values inflict pain. They make some employees feel like outcasts. They limit an organization's strategic and operational freedom and constrain the behavior of its people. They leave executives open to heavy criticism for even minor violations. And they demand constant vigilance (p. 114).

This means that each person in the organization needs to provide the *radical loving care* described by Chapman (2004) and discussed in Chapter 4. What a powerful statement, steeped with meaning. Do you notice that money is not mentioned in this statement? The theme in Chapter 1 is that if we do what is right for the patient, the money will follow. We continue with that theme here.

When the bottom line has the greatest importance, facilities lose the *soul* of the organization (Bolman & Deal, 1997). Morale and job satisfaction of staff plunge. As budget cuts occur, workers feel depersonalized and suffer from battle fatigue. The problem is that staff do not feel valued. Problems spiral because clients coming for care sense that they are not important, that staff do not care. Staff members know this to be true because that is the way staff are treated. Any organization using this approach cannot survive in the long run.

The *value* part is really what patient satisfaction is all about. In "Serving Up Uncommon Service" Doucette (2003) points out the difference between quality, the "measurement of outcomes," and service, "a measure of perception or what matters to the patient." "Quality outcomes are a baseline. The one feature that units demonstrating consistently high-ranking customer satisfaction scores share is satisfied employees. The conclusion seems clear: To improve patient satisfaction, improve staff satisfaction" (pp. 26–27).

The key to this chapter is that *the goals and organizational strategies support the core value (going to the ocean)—and that all administrators and staff support this core value.* The processes, including the bottom line, are the meandering rivers heading to the ocean, and vary from organization to organization and from patient to patient. We provide some possible strategies, processes, or landmarks throughout this chapter, but in the case of each organization, there are differences in the strategies used as well as outcomes achieved. Just as no river is the same, no organization is the same. There are an infinite number of possibilities as to how to more effectively reach our ocean.

The Power of Meaningful Work

The core value(s) of the organization, or the *soul*, is the ocean toward which we are headed. *Spirit comes from our belief that we are doing meaningful work.* Work becomes meaningful when we strongly believe in, and are committed to, the core value(s). This intrinsic motivator is more important than pay. The research has, and continues, to show this. Still, we continue to get tripped up believing that paying bonuses, or some other payment scheme, will achieve success with employees, forgetting that *meaningful work comes first.* The pay helps but is not the most important factor.

Motivation comes from within. There is not a magic wand we can wave to achieve a motivated workforce. Instead, in the right environment, under the right conditions, the opportunity is there for personnel to be motivated about their work; whether they are motivated is their choice. Herzberg (2003) republished a classic that discusses motivation. In an early study he found that employee satisfaction was due to the following factors (in order of importance): achievement, recognition, the work itself, responsibility, advancement, and growth. Do you see the corollary this work has with Maslow's self-actualization need that we all have? For instance, if we love our work, chances are it is a match with our gifts and, chances are, we believe our work is meaningful because we are helping others. All this is related to the spirit part of the work we do. It is an intrinsic factor that comes from within.

Herzberg goes on with a list of dissatisfiers. These factors do not cause dissatisfaction, but if there is something wrong in the workplace, these can cause employees to feel dissatisfied and, if not resolved, could result in people leaving for greener pastures. The dissatisfiers, in order of importance, are company policy and administration, supervision, relationship with the supervisor, work conditions, salary, relationship with peers, personal life, relationship with staff colleagues, status, and security. Can you see how the dissatisfiers can erode *spirit*? It is a sad commentary on our present organizations that often company policy and administration, at the top of the list, are problematic.

Trust is an important factor that relates to our *spirit*. When employees trust the administrators and believe in the core value(s), any achievement is possible. Trust occurs when the administrator has integrity, exhibits consistent behaviors, and always strives to achieve the core values and purpose. When dissatisfiers are present, chances are someone is not trusted and does not have integrity. When nurses complain of feeling depersonalized, something is seriously wrong with the administrative leadership, and the leadership must be fixed before the *spirit* can come back into the organization. Listen to the Studer (2000) tape when he talks with nurse executives. He was a chief executive officer (CEO) of a hospital in serious trouble both financially and in *spirit*. He discusses how he had to fix himself, go within, before he could work on fixing the rest of the organization.

So when the administrator has integrity, employee trust follows. Staff support and make decisions when a trusted administrator empowers them, uses group process in decision making, and encourages all to support the core value(s). Trust is something to value very highly because it is not lightly given and, once lost, can probably never be regained.

This is the meaning that permeates our feelings of belonging and engagement. It is the heart of teamwork and connectedness within an organization. The *soul* provides meaning for the *spirit* to remain alive and well. "Courage comes from the French word which means *heart*. Once our heart is engaged, we operate with passion and not power and we can find ways to transform our world together" (Kerfoot, 2002, p. 298). Meaningful work feeds our soul.

When soul is there but the spirit is missing, we need to question within ourselves whether we are doing something to cause this problem. Curran (2000b) reports that the Gallop organization, after doing 25 years of research on 400 companies with 80,000 managers, concluded that one could measure the strength of the workplace with 12 simple questions:

1. Do I know what is expected of me at work?
2. Do I have the materials and equipment I need to do my work right?
3. At work, do I have the opportunity to do what I do best everyday?
4. In the last 7 days, have I received recognition or praise for doing good work?
5. Does my supervisor, or someone at work, care about me as a person?
6. Is there someone at work who encourages my development?
7. At work, do my opinions seem to count?
8. Does the mission/purpose of my company make me feel my job is important?
9. Are my co-workers committed to doing quality work?
10. Do I have a best friend at work?
11. In the last 6 months, has someone talked to me about my progress?
12. This last year, have I had opportunities at work to learn and grow?

Buckingham and Coffman (1999) demonstrated that these 12 questions separate great organizations from average ones.... Individuals may join organizations, but it is their immediate manager who directly influences how long they stay and how productive they are. Employees do not leave organizations, they leave managers (p. 277).

Spirit is more likely to be present when these 12 aspects are present in the workplace. Spirit comes from within each of us.

The condition of your employees' spirit is easily diagnosed. You can see spirit, or the lack of it, in their productivity. You can also see spirit in their eyes. You may see spirits overwhelmed and discouraged. And, in too many cases, you will see the depression of employees who have lost their spirit for healthcare work.... Employees want to be a part of an important work that is accomplished through collective effort.... Spirit and soul are not management techniques. They are available to us by personal commitment to their values. Soul and spirit are realities in us, as aspects of who we are. Soul and spirit are around us and available to energize our work relationships (Nobre, 2001, pp. 288–289).

Rounds

Another way to observe and exemplify *spirit* within an organization is to do frequent rounds and have regularly scheduled, round-the-clock meetings. These are times to share information, be open to questions and concerns of those attending, and have roundtable gatherings around issues. An open-door policy is also helpful. We can get a feel for the total organization, and an additional bonus is that many issues can be resolved on the spot. *It is critical that administrators at all levels of management do frequent rounds.*

Rounds are where the administrator is regularly out visiting with patients and families, as well as staff, at the points of service. This also means that when there is full census, or a unit or department needs help, the administrators are empathetic to the situation and pitch in.

Tom Peters coined the phrase "management by walking around," but nurses have been doing rounds for years before management by walking around became popular. One can find out all sorts of helpful information by visiting staff, physicians, patients and families, and other interdisciplinary staff while doing rounds. Rounds allow feedback from, and to, staff without having too many meetings. This is greatly facilitated when all administrators—from board members and the president on down to the nurse manager—are out doing rounds daily, being visible for the sake of more effective communication as well as giving support and living the core values.

The research supports this concept in so many different ways. There are fewer lawsuits when the patient and family perceive that the caregivers—and administrators—care. A health care administrator is always more effective when doing rounds because the real patient issues are more likely to be identified earlier and addressed.

While doing rounds, it is important to coach and mentor staff, rather than being too task oriented. One wants staff to think, not depend on someone else, such as the physician or nurse manager, for all the answers. We also want to encourage staff to use *systems thinking* because one action has a ripple effect and affects several other things. One can observe what organizational processes can be improved and what barriers exist that could be either eliminated or reduced.

There are some potential traps to avoid. First, the administrator needs to exhibit certain behaviors. While walking down the hall of an inpatient unit, if the administrator does not pay attention to call lights or patients/families who are having obvious problems, the message the administrator gives is that patient issues are not important. If the administrator does not greet staff but just goes to find the manager, staff gets the message they are not important. They can view the administrator as not caring about them.

Second, it is best not to become Attila the Hun. If one reacts to a situation and heads roll, everyone becomes afraid of the administrator, hides information from the administrator, resents the administrator, and does not actually change their behavior—unless the administrator is around. It is more advantageous to converse with staff and to help staff explore more effective options.

A third trap is to micro-manage. When an administrator micro-manages, the message is that staff members, or the manager, are not capable of doing the job right. However, the real problem is that the administrator has not learned to effectively delegate.

The most effective way to do rounds is to pay attention to everyone present, talk with people, demonstrate caring, and use rounds as a learning process. All actions support the core values and the purpose. As crises occur, remain calm and decisive and, when necessary, pitch in and help resolve the situation. As problems become evident, talk with those involved to explore how best to handle a situation or get into a dialogue about what happened and determine what could have been done to more effectively deal with the problem.

Round-the-clock meetings enable everyone, regardless of shift or work schedule, to learn what is important from other perspectives. This way the midnight or weekend personnel do not feel as isolated. Administrators at all levels should hold these meetings regularly.

Roundtable gatherings can be a helpful way to deal with the many issues that staff experience as they do their work. It is best if all attend a gathering based on interest in the topic to be discussed. It is especially helpful if those attending from administration represent various levels, and depending on the topic to be discussed, special invitations should go out to departments that deal with the issue being discussed.

An *open-door policy* means that someone who has an important issue is welcome to share it with us. An open door does not mean that a secretary intercedes for us, although, if the secretary is empowered, this person is invaluable to an administrator and actually deals with many issues directly, saving the administrator time.

Organizational Assessment: An Administrative Competency

Now let's look at administrative competencies that contribute to an energized work climate (the *spirit*). In administration, organizational assessment is a critical component necessary for role effectiveness. Organizational assessment is the ability to have a fairly accurate, dynamic picture of the *total* organization, such as how various people work together, which departments are more effective, how different departments have different cultures, how clients perceive the organization, and how the organization fits within the community that surrounds it. This picture is dynamic and changes as various components, relationships, and people change within the organization. What was true yesterday will be different today, and what is true today will change tomorrow. This organizational assessment capability helps the administrator to know, with fair accuracy, how different individuals and departments respond to situations. No matter how well we know an organization, we still experience surprises, but this organizational assessment capability is a key factor for effectiveness.

Assessment is *dynamic*, meaning that once one has assessed the current organization, the assessment changes as people and situations change. This is a lived experience that takes time and effort. Actually, one's picture never is totally accurate because there are always hidden factors that we do not know, both about ourselves and about others, and because everyone in the organization is constantly changing. Thus at times we can be surprised when someone else reacts in a way we had not anticipated.

Stewardship

Part of the organizational assessment has to include the facility obligations and interactions with the community. The organization is part of a community. If the community flounders, the organization could be at risk, or vice versa. Just as all departments need to be integrated and working together within an organization, all organizations are better off if they are integrated and working effectively with others in the community, helping the community to better serve its citizens. This is called *stewardship*.

Walter Gast, a former professor at Saint Louis University's John Cook School of Business, rightly claimed that to be successful in the long term, "a business had to follow six laws: 1) provide a just return on capital; 2) produce a useful commodity or service; 3) increase the wealth or quality of society; 4) provide productive employment opportunities; 5) help employees find satisfying work; and 6) pay fair wages" (O'Hallaron, 2002, p. 125).

Systems Thinking

Another word is useful here. Organizational systems describe how we accomplish the work. Senge (2006) coined the term "systems thinking," describing it as a framework for seeing wholes or seeing interrelationships rather than things. Using systems thinking, we are able to picture the entire organization and how it functions, not just our own department. As we assess organizations as a whole, they differ—many have a high ethic of collaboration, whereas others are heavily authoritarian where administrators have difficulty with systems thinking and are bottom-line oriented. And, of course, there are combinations of both in the same organization.

What do we mean by systems thinking? This type of thinking takes into account the overall, dynamic organizational picture. How will people across the organization, and even in the community, respond to a change? What outcomes might result if a decision is implemented? When decisions are made using systems thinking, the decisions are carefully crafted to include dialogue by all who would be affected by a change, incorporating issues they identify. This achieves the best result and avoids possible pitfalls that could actually worsen the situation. Without using systems thinking, it is easy to make quick-fix solutions that actually generate more problems and result in other unanticipated effects because solutions did not account for the entire system response to the change. This wholeness in systems thinking includes the way various departments work together within the organization. In today's complex organizations, systems thinking is a necessary administrative competency.

In fact, systems thinking is so important that it is helpful if other team members, not just administrators, also use systems thinking. Work teams are more effective when the entire team can view the organization as a whole. Unfortunately, team members' confidence and responsibility can be undermined by the complexity of a situation. How often do we hear team members and front-line leaders comment, "You can't change the system"? Systems thinking can drastically help to change this helpless feeling.

To accomplish systems thinking we must restructure the way we think. Senge (2006) states that systems thinking "lies in a shift of mind: seeing interrelationships rather than linear cause and effect and seeing processes of change rather than snapshots" (p. 73). As thinkers we often see things in straight lines, whereas reality is actually made up of circles.[1]

Understanding systems thinking begins with the concept of feedback. The word *feedback* can be used in many different ways. When we ask for feedback, we are often asking for someone's opinion, encouraging both positive and negative remarks. Systems thinkers use feedback as a broader concept. Senge (2006) describes feedback as any "reciprocal flow of influence," an "axiom that every influence is both cause and effect," and that "nothing is influenced in just one direction" (p. 75). So ongoing dialogue helps one better understand what is going on by providing feedback.

The issue of responsibility often complicates the concept of feedback. As linear thinkers we are always searching for someone or something to blame. For instance, this blame search occurs with patient safety. When we become accomplished systems thinkers, we renounce the idea that one individual is responsible. We begin to realize that responsibility is shared.

Likert's Authoritarian Versus Participative Model

To continue with the organizational assessment, think about an overall picture of the organization. Likert (1973) identifies a classic organizational model that shows how various organizational variables interact with one another (**Exhibit 3–2**). System 1 represents a very authoritarian model. Here there is little dialogue, communication occurs only in a downward direction (assuming the CEO is at the top—an authoritarian model), the informal rumor mill is rampant and needed because it is the best source of information for staff, decisions are made at the top, orders are given, no one dares to question the orders, often staff resist the orders covertly, and control is all important. Linear thinking is rampant here. Correspond this to a system 4 model, which is very participative. Here matrices exist where there is communication between and within all levels, communication is open and shared, dialogue occurs, decisions are made at the appropriate level, the organization consists of well-integrated staff, goals are determined by group action except in crisis, there is no need for an informal organization, because information is shared, and productivity is enhanced by each person, with everyone doing their own problem solving. Circular thinking exists here with people understanding the inner connectivity of everyone in the system.

---

[1] To explore thinking patterns, see DeBono (1976, 1994).

Exhibit 3–2 Likert's Organizational Systems

Organizational Variables	SYSTEM 1	SYSTEM 2	SYSTEM 3	SYSTEM 4
Leadership				
How much confidence and trust is shown in staff?	Virtually none	Some	Substantial amount	A great deal
How free do they feel to talk to supervisors about job?	Not very free	Somewhat free	Quite free	Very free
How often are staff's ideas sought and used constructively?	Seldom	Sometimes	Often	Very frequently
Motivation				
Is predominant use made of (1) fear, (2) threats, (3) punishment, (4) rewards, (5) involvement?	1, 2, 3, occasionally 4	4, some 3	4, some 3 and 5	5, 4, based on group
Where is responsibility felt for achieving the organization's goals?	Mostly at top	Top and middle	Fairly general	At all levels
How much cooperative teamwork exists?	Very little	Relatively little	Moderate amount	Great deal
Communications				
What is the usual direction of information flow?	Downward	Mostly downward	Down and up	Down, up, and sideways
How is downward communication accepted?	With suspicion	Possibly with suspicion	With caution	With a receptive mind
How accurate is upward communications?	Usually inaccurate	Often inaccurate	Often accurate	Almost always accurate

continued

Exhibit 3–2 Likert's Organizational Systems (continued)

Organizational Variables	SYSTEM 1	SYSTEM 2	SYSTEM 3	SYSTEM 4
Communications (continued)				
How well do administrators know the problems faced by staff?	Not very well	Rather well	Quite well	Very well
Decisions				
At what level are decisions made?	Mostly at top	Policy at top, some delegation	Broad policy at top, more delegation	Throughout but well-integrated
Are staff involved in decisions related to their work?	Almost never	Occasionally consulted	Generally consulted	Fully involved
What does the decision-making process contribute to motivation?	Not very much	Relatively little	Some contribution	Substantial contribution
Goals				
How are organizational goals established?	Orders issued	Orders, some comments invited	After discussion, by orders	By group action (except in crisis)
How much covert resistance to goals is present?	Strong resistance	Moderate resistance	Some resistance at times	Little or none
Evaluation				
How concentrated are review and evaluation functions?	Very highly at top	Quite highly at top	Moderate delegation to lower levels	Widely shared
Is there an informal organization resisting the formal one?	Yes	Usually	Sometimes	No—same goals as formal
What are cost, productivity, and other evaluation data used for?	Policing, punishment	Reward and punishment	Reward, some self-guidance	Self-guidance, problem solving

Source: Adapted from *The Human Organization: Its Management and Value* by Rensis Likert. Copyright 1967 by McGraw-Hill, Inc.

Systems 2 and 3 fall between these two extremes, with system 2 being slightly authoritarian whereas system 3 starts to become more participative.

Using Likert's model, we need to assess where our organization currently is and base our actions on this assessment. For instance, if we are a transformational leader, believing in a system 4 yet we are in a system 2, we become very frustrated, and staff do not understand our leadership style, if we interact with staff as though it is a system 4. Instead, we must start responding based on the system level. So in a staff meeting, (which staff may not be used to having until we came!), we want to get feedback from staff on an issue or on a potential piece of equipment. When we ask for feedback, we might get none. It is easy to wonder what we have done wrong. (This is internalizing the problem. Try not to do this.) Instead, realize that staff are suspicious of us, thinking, "What does she or he want from me? I'm not going to stick my neck out." Repeated meetings where we ask for feedback are necessary, before staff begin to trust us enough to start offering suggestions. Even then, it occurs only on issues that are perceived to be safe or not as emotionally laden. When this breakthrough happens, the group starts to move to a more participative model.

When we want to move an organization, department, or floor staff from a system 2 to a system 3, it takes repeated efforts for a couple of years before one begins to see movement in this direction. This cultural change is an enormous one and is particularly hard if a number of administrators at the executive level are still authoritarian. So it is important not to get impatient. The best place to begin is to look for small changes. Maybe a staff member starts to give honest feedback when alone with you, even though in meetings this person remains silent. This is an important breakthrough; it means that this staff member is starting to trust you and starting to move to the next level.

When looking for a job, identification of the system level is an important factor to assess in the interview process. For instance, if one is used to a system 2 and is comfortable there, moving to a system 4 department or organization may not be one's choice. In fact, the system 4 characteristics may seem like a foreign language that one does not know.

The author has seen nurse executives operating at a system 4 level move to a system 2 organization. This can work, but often it presents many problems. It is especially important to know what the nurse executive's boss is like. If the new boss functions as a system 2 administrator and likes this system, this new boss will not understand the nurse executive's leadership style and might even believe that the nurse executive is not competent. After all, from the boss' perspective, when the new nurse executive asks staff what they think about issues, the boss might think, "Isn't the new nurse executive able to make his/her own decisions?" In other words, "Doesn't this nurse executive know what to do? Is this person incompetent?" The boss operates in a system 2 mode by giving edicts. Staff members are to follow the edicts. No reasons for questions or dialogue. This approach could be very frustrating for the system 4 nurse executive unless the executive understands this and deals with the boss on a system 2 level.

In fact, in some previous research the author found that when system 4 nurse executives had bosses who were in a system 1 or 2, often the nurse executive lost his or her job within the first year or two. In one case where this did not happen, the system 2 boss had hired the system 4 nurse executive to change the system because the boss knew it needed to be changed. In fact, the boss said that sometimes he did not understand the nurse executive but knew she was leading her departments, and the hospital, in a needed direction. The system 4 nurse executive was effective, stayed, and helped to move the organization to a system 3. The result was an increase in staff pride in the organization and in their work.

The systems model can also help explain why a successful program in one facility will not work in another. Perhaps the successful strategy worked in a system 3 environment. Is it any wonder that it will not work in a system 2 setting?

Organizing the Assessment Data

As part of the organizational assessment process, it is important to discuss various components of an organization. If we use linear thinking, we can look at each aspect as separate entities. *Please remember that actually all these components are intertwined and connected to make the whole.* Collins and Porras (1994) suggest a way to organize the organizational assessment data one needs to know as an administrator. All the components, when integrated together, give us a more complete organizational assessment. As we think of the organizational assessment, it is like describing a person. We cannot take a person apart and look at each component of the person to get a true description of that person. We can only describe how the whole person seems to operate. And each moment this whole person is changing as events happen and the person responds to the events. So although we describe the components to help get a better handle on this whole, it is necessary to go beyond linear thinking and see the organization as a *whole, ever-changing, dynamic entity.*

As we assess an organization, we need to define not only our own department but the overall organization (this could be a single facility but could include a larger corporate health care system). If there is a large corporate system, this will have its own dynamic, as will the individual facility where one works. (For instance, the system might have one culture, the facility another, and the department or unit yet another.)

Organizing Arrangements

Collins and Porras (1994, pp. 259–260) defined nine organizational assessment categories that are helpful to use when assessing an organization.

- Category 1: Organizing Arrangements. 'Hard' items, such as organization structure, policies and procedures, systems, rewards and incentives, ownership structure, and general business strategies and activities of the company (e.g., acquisitions, significant changes in strategy, going public).
- Category 2: Social Factors. 'Soft' items, such as the company's cultural practices, atmosphere, norms rituals, mythology and stories, group dynamics, and management style.
- Category 3: Physical Setting. Significant aspects of the way the company handled physical space, such as plant and office layout or new facilities. This included any significant decisions regarding the geographic location of key parts of the company.
- Category 4: Technology. How the company used technology: information technology, state-of-the-art processes and equipment, advanced job configurations, and related items.
- Category 5: Leadership. Leadership of the firm since its inception: the transition between key early shapers of the organization and later generations, leadership tenure, the length of time the leaders were with the organization before becoming CEO (Were they brought in from the outside or grown from within? When did they join?), leadership selection processes and criteria.
- Category 6: Products and Services. Significant products and services in the company's history. How did the product or service ideas come about? What guided their selection and development? Did the company have any product failures, and how did it deal with them? Did the company lead with new products or follow in the marketplace?
- Category 7: Vision: Core Values, Purpose, and Visionary Goals. Were these variables present? If yes, how did they come into being: Did the organization have them at certain points in its history and not others? What role did they play? If it had strong values and purpose, did they remain intact or become diluted? Why?
- Category 8: Financial Analysis. Ratio and spreadsheet analysis of all income statements and balance sheets for every year going back to the date when the company became public: sales

and profit growth, gross margins, return on assets, return on sales, return on equity, debt to equity ratio, cash flow and working capital, liquidity ratios, dividend payout ratio, increase in gross property plant and equipment as a percentage of sales, asset turnover. Also examine stock returns and overall stock performance relative to the market (if applicable).

- Category 9: Markets/Environment. Significant aspects of the company's external environment: major market shifts, dramatic national or international events, government regulatons, industry structural issues, dramatic technology changes, and related items.

Following Collins and Porras' organizational assessment components, or categories, in Exhibit 3–3, we now turn to the various categories within the organization. The first organizational assessment category describes the *organizing arrangements*. This includes structure and design elements.

Structure in linear language refers to the way an organization delineates jobs and reporting relationships, or the arrangement of roles within an organization (Gordon, 2002). "Advances are being made at an astounding rate in the medical, biological, and pharmaceutical fields, yet the structure of the health care delivery system in many places operates as it did decades ago" (McDonagh, 2003, p. 46). Although an organizational chart begins to define structure, it does not capture the various relationships between people on the chart or the resulting effectiveness of a group. We are all interconnected with each other to accomplish our work. The design of an organization describes the process of "setting up" or the "appearance" of the organization. Though the terms "structure" and "design" are closely related, there is a lack of consistency and clarity in the use of these words. Many times these terms are used interchangeably. We use design as also having a broader definition that reflects the relationships and processes used within an organization.

Within the organizational structure and design, two forms are usually described: formal and informal. The *formal* organization, or "official" structure, is described within the organizational chart. The organizational chart displays the chain of command or the relationship of authority. The solid lines that connect the boxes show the formal channels of communication and reporting relationships; the dotted lines show an informal reporting relationship. Doesn't this sound linear?

Most often the organizational chart has the board and the CEO, or president, at the top of the chart. Some would suggest that this chart should be inverted, with the customer at the top and the president at the bottom. The organizational chart provides clarity and specifies areas of responsibility. However, it is a very imperfect picture because it does not capture the relationships that exist. The relationships are more important with getting the work accomplished than knowing areas of responsibility. Therefore the chart must be taken in context with the actual workings of the organization.

The formal structure also includes the regularly scheduled meetings that take place within the organization. Hopefully, these meetings aid those in the organization to function more effectively. However, there is a great divergence in actual meeting effectiveness—some being very helpful, some being ponderous, and some being a total waste of time. Some organizations have so many meetings the administrators cannot get their work done! Which comes first—the patient or the meeting? And, often, rounds would provide much better information for everyone that many ponderous meetings.

One issue that can happen in nursing is that staff are generally expected to attend and participate in certain meetings. The problem becomes how do we relieve staff of patient care responsibilities long enough to attend and participate in these meetings? In an authoritarian environment, these meetings are not considered as important, and there could easily be other issues interfering with staff being able to attend these meetings. In a participative environment, these meetings generally have more importance as administration realize that they accomplish many important functions. These meetings, when functioning well, more than pay for the release time needed. It is important to find ways to release staff to attend the meetings.

The *informal*, or the "unofficial," structure of an organization includes all the relationships and people's personal characteristics. For example, if one department head is very difficult to work with, others in the organization know this and try to work around this person, or if the director's secretary is married to a board member, this needs to be taken into consideration.

The informal organization reflects all the interpersonal relationships between people that are not reflected on the organizational chart but that affect operations. For instance, a nurse manager may realize that the unit secretary's informal leadership can really enhance the nurse manager's effectiveness and helps the unit to function much more efficiently. If the nurse manager chooses to ignore or suppress this person's leadership capabilities, unnecessary conflicts can result, patient care may suffer, and the dysfunctional situation spirals downward from there.

When there are flaws or inefficiencies in the administrative leadership, such as being secretive and not sharing information, the informal information network becomes rampant. When most information is shared and there is trust in the leadership, the informal network becomes fairly inactive. Everything and everyone in an organization is interconnected.

In the informal organizational structure, the free-flowing exchange of communication is known as "the grapevine." This type of communication reaches every corner and level within the organization. When team members do not receive credible information, the grapevine takes over. Generally, information spread through the grapevine is about 75% correct. Leadership can use the grapevine to gauge employee responses by allowing new ideas and policies to be spread through the grapevine. Although it is critical for nurses to learn formal channels of communication, the informal communication networks cannot be ignored.

In the past, there have been three common types of formal communication patterns defined in a formal organization: downward, upward, and lateral. Presently, we realize there is another communication pattern that is most effective: It is *circular and messy*. It is people at all levels talking with one another. It is talking with those within and those that touch our organization. For instance, as we do rounds we come in contact with people from across the organization, with patients and families, with physicians, with suppliers, and with anyone present. (Rounds break the rigid barriers of the protected office with a secretary out front to prevent others reaching the administrator.)

This circular communication pattern is messy because it opens up the realization that we may have misperceptions about a situation (in an authoritarian system we were not aware of this). It changes our judgmental attitude to one of curiosity (yeah!). At the same time it creates synergy and belonging.

> The most powerful way to make a significant change is to convene a conversation. But we know that often that is the most difficult thing to do. It is easier to talk about the person than to the person, but no progress is made toward solving a particular problem or learning about new ways to interact to make a real change....
>
> A sign of professional maturity is a person's capacity and appreciation for conversation. Our world and our organization's world would be in a much more peaceful state if the capacity for conversation between the parts were more mature.
>
> The art and science of focused conversation [is]... a collaborative dialogue of discovery where you invite others to share differing views and you test your thinking and understanding in the context of this dialogue so you can hear in a different manner... trusting the wisdom of the person or group and believing that this is the right person or group to solve the problem.... The leader will only succeed if he/she truly believes in the group's wisdom and does not come armed with solutions....
>
> We must be open to seeing the issues in a much more messy context than our little world of making judgments has allowed us. When you open yourself to a conversation among equals, you open yourself to the necessity of questioning your positions and the "truths" from which you operate. The only way to enter a productive conversation is to give yourself

> permission and willingness to be disturbed.... Real conversations change you and the people/groups you are talking to. That is the whole point: to make new relationships and synergies out of old dysfunctional patterns of parts interacting with each other. To have a conversation, you must allow for messiness and for being disturbed and confused as a way to make new growth.
>
> The only way to improve the world is through relationships, and conversations are the prelude to creating that change (Kerfoot, 2002, pp. 298–299).

In today's explosion of information technology, communication has become even more complex. Misunderstandings, misreadings, and unclear or selective hearing all play into faulty communication exchanges within an organization.

Communication is also messy because of gender differences and the ways men and women do work. Rutan (2003) reports that female nurse managers discuss "domestic, family, personal, and social issues before the meetings" and sometimes these issues are interwoven in meeting discussions, whereas male leaders stick to business and work-related subjects. He describes the female leader as follows:

> [She] projected a warm demeanor and took a personal as well as professional interest in members of the group. The social dimensions of her behavior, when contrasted with those of the male… in the group who assumed leadership in her absence, did not clearly identify why she was an effective and respected leader. But a close analysis of the data revealed that her personal style facilitated a rotation of leadership and promoted the professional growth of individual team members (p. 181).

Another thing that occurred was that male leaders discussed meeting agenda items before the meeting in various locations, and once a meeting started,

> The male who began the discussion acted as a coach in charge of a team, with the other males helping him carry out the play. Female team members were never part of this "meeting before the meeting."… [During the meeting] the male participants communicated more actively, asking more questions, contributing information and data, and making frequent recommendations and suggestions. Males avoided both eye contact and exchanging personal thoughts and feelings. They were interested in getting to the point of issues by being assertive, dominant, competitive, independent, and aggressive (p. 184).

Females usually did not understand this dynamic and, instead, would bring ideas up in the meeting:

> Women see the leader's competence, respect, and fairness as significantly more important to team effectiveness than men do. Women see the team members' knowledge of their jobs as significantly more important to team effectiveness than men do. Women see the team members' liking, trusting, and helping each other as significantly more important to team effectiveness than men do (p. 184).

A nurse manager is more effective if he or she understands these differences. For women, it is important to not only be attentive to nurturing and socializing roles but to be task oriented with well-developed business and financial skills. For men, it is important to incorporate more of the interpersonal skills and be open to changes occurring during the meeting. Rutan (2003) suggests that the following learning needs to take place:

> Females must understand that males do not share personal experiences primarily because they do not want to appear vulnerable. Nurse leaders should… devote time prior to a formal

meeting for idea generation, problem solving, and information sharing, just as the… male administrators… need to concentrate on being more open to new ideas as they are proposed or be prepared to present ideas and work out solutions while team meetings are in session (p. 185).

Staff development activities that identify gender differences but also encourage everyone regardless of gender to understand and use the positive aspects of both perspectives go a long way to achieve better teamwork. We recommend the Pat Heim tapes (1996) as a helpful tool to accomplish this goal.

One current flaw in health care is that often we have notebooks full of policies and procedures for registered nurses, the professionals, and few policies and procedures for nurse aides, the nonprofessionals. As a rule of thumb, more policies and procedures are needed for the nonprofessional group. So why do we have more for professional staff? For instance, doesn't *love one another* say it all? Look at what Nordstrom's set up for their policies:

Nordstrom Rules:

Rule #1: Use your good judgment in all situations.

There will be no additional rules.

Please feel free to ask your department manager, store manager or division manager any question at any time (Collins & Porras, 1994).

Don't we want nurses to be professionals? Isn't it better to have references for them to refer to when they do not know what to do? Does anyone really pay attention to all the policies and procedures anyway? Legally, don't we leave ourselves open for additional problems with all this volume if a nurse does not follow some procedure somewhere and something happens?

Paige (2003) advocates taking a multidisciplinary approach to policies and procedures. This is because policies and procedures often apply to more than one department, so each department having a separate policy is redundant. Or worse yet, they may be different. It is possible that combining efforts can produce a better one. It can also help ensure that departments are consistent and that legal problems do not result due to the inconsistencies.

In the organizational assessment, one must also consider rewards and incentives. If not carefully thought out, rewards and incentives can produce very negative results. For example, one incentive for an executive team might be a bonus if they can keep costs below a certain amount for the quarter or for the year. But this can have downsides. First, this is not linked with a quality dimension and so encourages executives to save money even when it is at the cost of the patient, and patient outcomes may be worsened as a result of these decisions—in the long run costing more money not to mention patients' lives. Second, these bonuses reward only executive-level administrators for meeting standards, yet the people doing the everyday work with patients are not given bonuses.

Another disincentive for nurses is that they are professionals, yet we make them use timecards to clock in and out. What if their patient(s) needed something beyond the shift time that the nurse wanted to provide? Some organizations have chosen to put nurses on annual salaries rather than hourly pay. (Sometimes the salary issue has been abused by administrators as a way to avoid overtime. This is not the intent here. It should be a fair wage.) This is positive *when nurses are given the freedom to come in as their patients need them*. If this is an inpatient setting, some nurses could choose their hours while others cover actual shift times. The main thing is that nurses have meaningful work—satisfying experiences with patients and families that enhance nurse retention and better serve the patients.

Another disincentive presently is the high amount of money paid for traveler nurses or sign-on bonuses, ignoring our best loyal workforce already present day after day working for us. Our message is that this loyal group is not as important as the traveler nurses. Who deserves the higher salary? Surely it is the loyal workforce!

It is important to give careful thought to the rewards and incentives provided because these should support desired behaviors. For instance, employee performance evaluations have no clout if they are not used to determine merit increases. Or, organizational performance evaluations are worthless if not everyone in the workplace is rewarded for meeting performance standards.

When incentives are used to reward certain behaviors, it is important to provide the staff with development activities that teach them the specific behaviors. For instance, if all are rewarded for being patient centered, it is important to have educational activities available to teach all staff what patient centered actually means in daily behaviors, including the thinking and decision-making process to be used. In addition, it is helpful if all, including top-level administrators, model and support the desired behaviors.

Another important incentive is to pay for staff to attend conferences. During budget cuts, conference monies are often cut, a short-sighted decision. It is important that all staff, including aides and housekeeping staff, are up to date doing meaningful work. (In fact, right now the research shows that these two groups spend the most time with patients in inpatient facilities.) Budget cuts also often affect staff education monies, yet the executive group continues to attend national conferences with travel costs fully paid. This gets back to the fact that our actions speak louder than our words.

DECISION-MAKING MODELS AT THE POINT OF SERVICE

We are presently at an interesting juncture in time because the organizational structure is changing very significantly. The old model was either based on who had authority (physicians or executive group) or the location of the service (nursing, laboratory, radiology). A wonderful book about tearing down silos, Lencioni's *Silos, Politics and Turf Wars: A Leadership Fable About Destroying the Barriers That Turn Colleagues Into Competitors* (2006), is written as a story.

As this old model crumbles, health care leaders need to focus on interpreting external realities that are changing, translating these changes into internal actions. Leaders are being called into the chaos of creativity to produce a good fit between the new framework demanded and the infrastructure that needs to be constructed to support it. It is important to replace it with decision-making models at the point of service, such as shared governance, discussed later in this chapter.

Work teams are a part of organizational work life. *Group dynamics* can be very positive and helpful where team members support each other and do what is best for the patients. It can alternately become destructive if individuals are allowed to continue with more selfish behaviors, such as never helping someone else, making their personal life and personal problems permeate their work, being negative about everything that happens, or complaining all the time. The nurse manager has an important role in this situation, because it may be necessary to build teams, and when there are problems to deal with them. This includes counseling individuals exhibiting negative behaviors. It takes time to fix something that is broken, and there will probably be additional turnover as one is fixing the problem(s).

The leader is only as effective as the team. Part of leadership effectiveness is recognizing the individual differences in team members:

> Some people work best as team members. Others work best alone. Some are exceptionally talented as coaches and mentors; others are simply incompetent as mentors.... A great many people perform best as advisers but cannot take the burden and pressure of making the decision. A good many other people, by contrast, need an adviser to force themselves to think; then they can make decisions and act on them with speed, self-confidence, and courage. This is the reason, by the way, that the number two person in an organization often fails when promoted to the number one position. The top spot requires a decision maker.

Strong decision makers often put somebody they trust into the number two spot as their adviser—and in that position the person is outstanding. But in the number one spot, the same person fails. He or she knows what the decision should be but cannot accept the responsibility of actually making it (Drucker, 1999, pp. 68–69).

The groups, or work teams, function using the core values as the reason for their actions and are working to constantly improve outcomes. Outcomes can be phenomenal. The sum of their involvement is greater than the whole. The converse is also true; if the team is not functioning properly, the sum is lesser than the whole. For instance, the Washington Redskins paid tens of millions to lure top football players to their team and then the team went nowhere. Teamwork was lacking. A lot of egos got in the way of success.

So group energy can increase, or decrease, what is accomplished. When teamwork is excellent, outcomes are very positive. Magic happens. We advocate self-managed teams be used as much as possible because generally *90% of the decisions need to be made at the point of service*. Generally, certain people within a team are better at certain team functions. Using sports as an example, a quarterback cannot win games alone; it takes a *team* working toward the same goal, with certain people more effective in certain positions within the team.

There are several reasons why using the team approach to decision making is more advantageous in organizations. First, synergy occurs with the knowledge and skills that each individual brings to the group. Second, we see an increase in creativity among team members, often due to the diversity seen in multidisciplinary teams and the different world views that each brings to the group. Finally, because team decisions usually reflect a consensus, decisions are more readily accepted.

According to Orsburn and colleagues (1990), *most organizations experience a 20 to 40 percent increase in productivity when employees are deeply involved in their work* (Porter-O'Grady & Malloch, 2007, p. 278) [emphasis added].

To achieve effective teamwork, trained group facilitators can work with a team to help the team members achieve better working relationships and more effective teamwork. Once the team functions effectively, the group facilitator may no longer be needed. When one examines the costs of effective teamwork, further education and facilitation for the team can save countless hours of wasted time and will enhance successful completion of the goal.

According to Wellins, Byham, and Wilson (1991), there are six key factors in team development: commitment, trust, purpose, communication, involvement, and process orientation. All these occur as a team evolves. In the first stage, *getting started*, the purpose, or goal, of the group needs to be clearly defined, and all members need to get acquainted.

The second stage, *going in circles*, deals with the question of now that we know who we are and where we are going, how do we get there? There is often an urge to pull out of the team and work alone or to work in subgroups. Members are sorting out those they trust, don't trust, and those they are not sure of at this point. There is a better understanding of purpose, but the team still requires reassurance and guidance. Often, much time is spent on how the meeting will be conducted, setting agendas, and setting up ground rules. Task completion is the goal.

In this stage we see conflict begin to arise, especially if certain members attempt to dominate the team. This conflict is disturbing to members who want the team to succeed. It is important to keep coming back to the group goal. Power moves will tend to decline as more effective group process develops, feedback occurs, and members begin to identify specific gifts each member brings to the table. However, if this does not occur, the team will be stuck and probably not accomplish the original purpose.

The third stage, *getting on* course, is exactly what it implies. The team is more comfortable with each other, more comfortable about their roles within the group, and they are committed to getting the job done. The purpose is now focused on achieving the goal. The group process is more natural because members now understand the purpose, are beginning to know and appreciate each other, and can begin to explore different solutions that may not be status quo.

The final stage, *full speed ahead*, is when teams are more comfortable with the benefits of being empowered. They are committed to both the team and the organization at this stage. Trust is a stable commodity and extended openly. There is a clear sense of mission and vision that is maintained, and the team becomes more flexible. Changes in meeting frequency and communication occur at this level. There is constant involvement and the acceptance of new roles and responsibilities by members. The team focus is centered on quality and continuous improvement. This becomes a system 4 environment.

Porter-O'Grady and Malloch (2007) have divided this stage into three more levels: competent, proficient, and expert. At the *competent* stage, team members want to hear each other's concerns and ideas and integrate this information into a cohesive group collective. The members have established an effective set of ground rules. They may mentor and coach each other for increased effectiveness. They may find solutions that challenge the status quo.

> Teams at the competent stage can meet the requirements for standard success but find it impossible to become passionately optimistic while recreating the future or to maintain resilience in the face of negative events. They accomplish the assigned work but seldom move beyond the assigned boundaries (p. 286).

At the *proficient* stage team members are more likely to have a total organizational assessment, be passionately optimistic, be aware of individual differences, but able to arrive at consensus decisions, not just saying that the majority rules. They honestly recognize team member failings but give emotional support to help the person deal with personal failings. They consider the emotional components of the conflicts and work through these conflicts, supporting both the emotions and the actual work that needs to be accomplished. Relationships stay intact and are based on honesty.

At the *expert* stage, all the healthy internal group work is occurring, but the group is also recognizing the organizational issues and culture and will make sure that the proposed solutions fit within the existing organizational components. The group is proactive and affirmative with one another, recognizing and dealing effectively with each member's emotional needs and undercurrents yet arriving at effective solutions for the individuals, the group, and the organization. At times this could extend to the community as well.

Teams develop over time, often composed of very diverse members, with a variety of values and backgrounds. Teams progress at different rates depending on internal and external influences. In fact, if membership changes or goals are not well defined or change, the group may revert back to previous stages or may never resolve the ensuing conflicts and thus never achieve the goal.

Team development is not a linear process. Teams are often composed of very diverse members, with a variety of values and backgrounds. Some members may be into negative, selfish behaviors. The team will probably fail unless the team can reach such individuals and pull them into the team or unless these individuals are effectively dealt with, or asked to leave the team, or even to leave the organization. Team development takes time, patience, and effort.

Other issues that surface are identified by Lencioni in *The Five Dysfunctions of a Team* (2002). This is written as a novel, presents some individual issues that can lead a team astray, and presents how to fix these problems: invulnerability (absence of trust), artificial harmony (fear of conflict), ambiguity (lack of commitment), low standards (avoidance of accountability), and status and ego (inattention to results). These barriers create a tremendous cost to the organization. First, there is the cost of everyone's salaries that are wasted, but there are many larger costs—this lack of team-work will occur in other work areas, conflicts not resolved will resurface, administration will be viewed as ineffective, patient care and patient outcomes will suffer, physicians will prefer to be somewhere else, and legal issues will result. The higher the level of dysfunction, the more it per-meates the entire organization.

As conflicts occur, if the team is able to resolve the conflict without decimating members and use the situation as an opportunity for learning, the team is more likely to make good progress with group development. They begin to develop a group identity and a feeling that they are making a dif-ference. The *spirit* increases because of each person's involvement and commitment to the goals of the group. The team can become self-actualized and believe they can make things happen.

> Self-actualized teams... use the whole potential of each team member to remain incredi-bly focused on "their" work, and they use skepticism in a healthy and productive way. They are willing to live at the border and do not eliminate ideas, no matter how outrageous. All ideas are reviewed with the typical constraints of finance, practicality, time, and ethics. More importantly, self-actualized teams effectively deal with members who are congenital victims and continually tell us that this and that will not work now because it didn't work in 1947. Self-actualized teams regulate behavior and focus it toward innovation and away from the troubles of the day. They are able to be in the moment and image the future simul-taneously, rearranging existing patterns into new and innovative strategies that will solve problems (Crow, 2003, p. 35).

Social Factors

Social factors include the way people work together. It reflects the *spirit* aspect. It speaks to the *rad-ical loving care*, discussed in Chapter 4, as well as effective leadership, or *love one another*, as dis-cussed in Chapter 2. Perhaps these are the most important factors within an organization because these social factors are what achieve the patient outcomes. Ideally, one hopes to achieve a culture of participation and teamwork around the core values.

With these new decision-making models at the point of service, team effectiveness or relation-ship building is enhanced when *collaboration* occurs. When we collaborate, we are working with others to achieve shared goals. We are proactive, that is, a person does not just complain about problems but thinks of ways to solve them. We cooperate and share knowledge with each other. There is an element of shared meaning within the group. We create group synergy in the pursuit of collective goals. We make sacrifices to achieve the group goals. Group energy is harnessed. Different views are encouraged and it is safe to express these views. (See the section on *Conflict: A Rich Resource!* in Chapter 2, which describes how to effectively manage conflicts.)

Collaboration occurs when we realize that we need to be true to ourselves and to others equally. This is also a current societal dilemma:

> Very few people work by themselves and achieve results by themselves.... Most people work with others and are effective with other people.... Managing yourself requires taking responsibility for relationships. This has two parts. The first is to accept the fact that other people are as much individuals as you yourself are. They perversely insist on behaving like human beings. This means that they too have their strengths; they too have their ways of getting things done; they too have their values. To be effective, therefore, you have to know

the strengths, the performance modes, and the values of your coworkers.... Each [coworker] works his or her way, not your way. And each is entitled to work in his or her way. What matters is whether they perform and what their values are.... The first secret of effectiveness is to understand the people you work with and depend on so that you can make use of their strengths, their ways of working, and their values. Working relationships are as much based on the people as they are on the work.

The second part of relationship responsibility is taking responsibility for communication.... Personality conflicts... arise from the fact that people do not know what other people are doing and how they do their work, or what contribution the other people are concentrating on and what results they expect. And the reason they do not know is that they have not been asked and therefore have not been told.... Even people who understand the importance of taking responsibility for relationships often do not communicate sufficiently with their associates. They are afraid of being thought presumptuous or inquisitive or stupid. They are wrong. Whenever someone goes to his or her associates and says, "This is what I am good at. This is how I work. These are my values. This is the contribution I plan to concentrate on and the results I should be expected to deliver," the response is always, "This is most helpful. But why didn't you tell me earlier?" [It is important for the leader to ask,] "What do I need to know about your strengths, how you perform, your values, and your proposed contribution?"... Trust... means that they understand one another (Drucker, 1999, pp. 71–72).

Porter-O'Grady and Malloch, in their award winning book, *Managing for Success in Health Care* (2007a), discuss working toward better collaboration with teams of health care personnel.

CULTURE REFLECTS SPIRIT

A large portion of the social factor is *culture*. Culture has a lot of power. "Culture can kill the best strategic plan" (Curran, 2002a, p. 257). That is because culture reflects spirit. It is spirit that moves the organization forward. Although there are many definitions of culture, according to Gordon (2002), an organization's culture "describes the part of its internal environment that incorporates a set of assumptions, beliefs, and values that organizational members share and use to guide their functioning" (p. 374). A strong culture (such as the expectation that all will give 200% effort) has great impact on team members and results in effective teams, goal fulfillment, innovations, and a strategic capacity (Gordon, 2002).

As organizations grow and diversify, changes in culture also occur. In every organization there is a particular culture of learned patterns, norms, values, beliefs, and customs. Culture is a pattern of assumptions or behaviors, often implied and not formally recognized, that are indirectly taught to new members as they enter an organization. For example, perhaps most nurses prefer to wear scrubs or there is a taboo about wearing turtleneck garments. This is not written anywhere, but everyone *knows it* and dresses accordingly. Perhaps there is a pattern that staff consistently takes for lunch breaks, with certain people always going together. Maybe each staff member helps other staff complete the work when help is needed.

To assess the culture, Curran (2002a) suggests answering the following question:

Where does your organization [nursing department/unit] spend its time and money?... When I see a physician's parking lot, a physician's lounge, and a physician's dining room, I conclude, "this place values physicians." I have never seen a nurse's parking lot or a nurse's dining room.... Things like meeting agendas and minutes tell a great deal about values. Most health care "board packers" that I have seen are filled with financial information, and a long list of physician names for credentialing, but there is little about human resources and patient care (p. 257).

A weak culture has more inconsistencies, having a negative impact on members. For example, nurses might be very task oriented. We forget the importance of relationships with this culture. This can be fixed but takes a lot of time. Relationships and organizational processes are as important as getting the work done.

Within the empowering culture that we want to achieve, there will be individuals who do not fit. Sometimes this can just be a style difference or an example of the Pygmalion effect discussed in Chapter 2. Moving to another work area with a different supervisor may better suit this individual.

If the individual is having a negative effect on the culture and needs to be counseled, the best way to counsel is to recognize that individual's personal responsibility for changing negative behavior(s). Campbell, Fleming, and Grote (1985) published a classic on disciplinary action that *involves the employee in solving the problem*. This includes the use of reminders rather than warnings, and in the third step actually gives the employee a paid leave day to decide whether to change, specifying how behaviors will change, or to quit. This method of disciplinary action is preferable to action where the supervisor *tells* the employee.

Another factor with culture is that as we have become global; cultures are melding as East meets West. In the West we overemphasize individuality, whereas in the East group collectivity—doing what is best for the group at personal sacrifice—is the mode. Each taken too far to the extreme ignores the other. For instance, individuality can support competition, and conflicting people never enter into a dialogue with each other. Therefore, a better result is never achieved. Everyone is too busy trying to win, even if the opposition loses. On the other hand, if all decisions are made based on what is best for the group as a whole, someone's gifts may not be able to blossom. Bringing about a synergy between these two opposites, individuality and group collectivity, may be part of our collective societal purpose presently. It may also help us to achieve better collaboration with conflicting viewpoints. Presently, our test seems to be remaining true to ourselves while doing what is best for everyone concerned. Doesn't this sound like we are synergizing the East and West philosophies?

Authoritarian cultures, in this new context, are weak cultures. This can produce a culture of silence within the organization. Employees do not speak up about ideas and do not disagree with anyone openly. This culture quickly erodes spirit. It creates a "we/they" mentality. In Chapter 2 we discussed the road to Abilene situation where no one spoke out and everyone did something no one wanted to do. In organizations, if no one shares differences decisions can be erroneous, products can fail, and processes can remain problematic with deleterious side effects. Along with silence, there often is a culture of secrecy, especially when the finances, revenues, or even vision are discussed at the executive level in an organization and are not shared with those at other levels in the organization.

Breaking this cycle is possible but requires much work because the culture must change to one where people feel free, and are expected, to speak up. In administrative roles, this means that we never are directly or indirectly punitive to others when they do speak up. This takes years of consistent work. And if we really achieve this culture, they may be speaking up about not agreeing with us. The administrator must also encourage, and help, others when they disagree to learn how to express themselves in a way that explores differences rather than blast each other with built-up anger. Conflict can actually lead us to better decisions, as long as the conflicts are honest, never put others down, and are resolved in a trusting environment. Haven't you known others who are just considered eccentric around certain issues? Everyone says "that is just the way they are."

Bohn (2000, p. 84) warns that if at least three of the following symptoms are present, the organization is in trouble, productivity will suffer, and everyone will be burned out rushing from crisis to crisis:

1. There isn't enough time to solve all the problems. [We do not have enough nurses present for the current number of patients.]
2. Solutions are incomplete. [As nurses try to deal with everything, they patch the present problem but do not fix it.]
3. Problems recur and cascade. [So the same problems come up again, or are even worse because they were not dealt with properly in the first place.]
4. Urgency supersedes importance. [There is never any time to examine processes or work on improvements because of all the crises the nurses are dealing with.]
5. Many problems become crises. [Smaller problems flare up to larger ones that may require heroic efforts on the part of the nurses.]
6. Performance drops.

> Failure to purposely lead the workplace for growth and individual development allows contradictory paradigms of behavior and conflict. Shared values and group behavior norms are building blocks of corporate culture.... [For example,] does the group reward tardiness or positively reinforce timeliness?... The organization's culture is learned through the connection between behaviors and their consequences. Changing the culture means changing behaviors. Behaviors must match values. For instance, a hospital that values career progression, quality, and excellence will shift cultures from pay by seniority to pay according to performance and development (Sherwood, p. 37).

Think about this. We have people's lives at stake. This is where empowering nurses, such as giving the nurses options to close units to new patients with physicians and administrators *not being able to override this decision*, becomes a necessity.

We have spent the previous chapter describing the new paradigm of leadership needed to achieve a deeply satisfying work culture. The nurse administrator, using this kind of leadership paired with continued emphasis on the core value (doing what the patient values), creates a healthy work environment.

> Two factors contribute to a deeply satisfying work culture. The quality of worker engagement at the point of service, the first factor, is similar to the caring concept of presence with the patient, which nurses find deeply satisfying. The second factor is the ability of front-line leaders to move out of supervision to focus on motivating and enabling workers to do their work effectively. These factors are challenged by emphases on efficiency and economics, such that employees often feel depersonalized as an expense item (Sherwood, p. 37).

In building a credible culture, the most important thing to remember is to model the behavior that one wants to promote. Actions speak louder than words. Building trust and keeping it is the key to the success of any organization. Bates (2003, p. 38) gives us five tips for building a credible culture:

- Reward people who communicate openly and build trust in the workplace; counsel those who don't.
- Talk about the values of your organization from the top down and encourage conversation about issues.
- Build your own credibility bank by practicing open communication; if you make a mistake, you will get the benefit of the doubt.

- Encourage questions. Trust thrives on open lines of communication. The people who work for you know it's okay to question a decision or priority.
- Don't assume people know what is expected; be clear about the kind of behavior and communication you expect and find acceptable.

What we are striving for is to establish a culture of teamwork and collegiality, a culture that is capable of making rapid changes, and a culture where the expectation is that everyone gives their best. The problem with changing culture is that often we are trying to meld two opposing concepts or paradoxes. Consider some examples:

- We want to be able to change instantly, try things, improvise, experiment. Yet at the same time we want order, neatness, and consistency following procedures for patient safety.
- We want to change something, be a risk taker, and push beyond the limits of our comfort zone. We have trouble enough with ourselves on these issues, but we also need to encourage staff to be that way. Yet we continue to need status quo for comfort and stability.
- We experience conflict yet want only peace.
- We want things to be simple yet experience complexity.
- We need to balance data and intuition.
- We need to balance planning and action.
- We need to balance cooperation with competition.

It is precisely these opposing concepts that provide us with grist for the mill. Because these are seemingly opposing concepts if we think *linearly*, they present sources of conflict for us. However, if we can realize that our responsibility is to rise above the seeming differences and find ways to combine the opposing forces, we can resolve these conflicts and create a better workplace. New tensions that need resolution always exist. It is like the piece of sand in the oyster causing friction that eventually results in a perfect pearl. Right now we cannot see the pearl, but it is there, and as we work through the tensions, the pearl manifests itself. We can choose to remain in our linear world with the pearl never manifesting and feel the continuing frustrations—or build toward a better future.

Currently, we grapple with these issues, hoping to resolve them. This issue permeates our society. We all are working out these paradoxes. Exploration and tension come before resolution. That is to be expected. Our explorations eventually find solutions. For instance, we begin to realize that conflicts can bring about a better peace. Or that we begin to sense what is right at a moment in time while something else is right for a different moment. Many times the answers come from unexpected sources or happenings. Some people, or workgroups, or organizations are further along in this quest than others.

It is important to change the culture so everyone is encouraged to *think* and *sense*. Each person needs to be able to use his or her knowledge and/or judgment and/or intuition on issues because no issue is ever exactly the same, nor will it get resolved the same way.

What conditions are present when we think or sense best? Isn't it when we are taking a shower, driving the car, exercising, or even sleeping on it? Do we provide time for staff, or ourselves, to think or sense? As an administrator, it is important to set aside 2 days a week with no meetings. This provides catch-up time and time to think or sense. Sometimes meetings can be more effective over lunch, or while taking a walk, or while riding to another location. Men have been doing this for years while playing golf.

So thinking and questioning everything is where we want to go with cultural change. This begins with us. It is so easy to get in a rut and do the job the same way every day (status quo), yet the answers for needed changes are all around us. We just need to be open to them and know that they are there.

Physical Setting

The physical setting can be a significant factor and can use many budget dollars. For instance, as more elderly people navigate our health systems, it is important for them to have easy access to services (i.e., not having to walk long distances). The physical setting can also affect how well we can accomplish our work. If the environment is always too hot or too cold, or we have only double rooms available, or we have to go to different locations for equipment, supplies, and so forth, we are less effective. As we have added increased technology, many work settings, if older, are really not adequate to handle the newer technology necessary for care. One goal in many health care organizations is to have everything the health care worker needs present at the point of care. Fixing physical setting factors can create considerable expense, but these factors are very important.

Technology

We are in the Information Age. Technology has exploded across the health care landscape. (We devote Chapter 5 to this aspect.) Health care organizations, if they are not keeping up with state-of-the-art processes and equipment, are becoming obsolete. At the same time, organizations are faced with how to keep confidential information safe, resulting in, for instance, Health Insurance Portability and Accountability Act laws. The result is new ethical dilemmas.

Leadership

Leadership, discussed in Chapter 2, can make or break organizational effectiveness. It is so important that when a work group is dysfunctional, the first place to look is the leadership. Most likely the leader is ineffective, which leads to more and more dysfunction in a group.

Currently, there is a high level of turnover in the nurse manager group. Many experience overwhelming feelings about their role. They are caught in the middle: expected to "keep staff happy," do what the administration wants them to do even when administrators do not understand how their decisions impact staff, keep patient satisfaction scores up, maintain a safe environment, keep budgets under control, and keep up with current technology, not only for patient treatments, administering medications, or documentation but to understand administrative systems and respond to data using these systems. A big issue is that the administrators they report to may need to grow themselves. We are all in this dance together. As we ponder this, one helpful book is Wheatley's *Turning to One Another: Simple Conversations to Restore Hope to the Future* (2002). The answers are all around us. We just need to open ourselves to them. Hope and healing are there too. All the best on this quest!

Products and Services

Products, such as oncology or cardiology services, are a key factor to organizational success. As we serve clients, it is important to pay attention to what our health care clients need and value. This is what we need to provide rather than what we personally might like if we were the patients. All this is outlined in Chapter 4, including quality and safety concerns. As services are delivered, an organization needs to pay attention to ethical (see Chapter 7) and legal issues (see Chapter 8) as well.

As organizations examine which services to offer, it is important to look around the local community to identify what is already available and what is needed. Chapter 16 outlines strategic management strategies. As health care services are delivered, case management is necessary, covered in Chapter 18, and workload management is discussed in Chapter 6.

Vision: Core Values, Purpose, and Visionary Goals

The first part of this chapter is devoted to core values and organizational purpose. These are so important that we started the chapter discussing them. Vision and goals are outlined in Chapter 16 on strategic management.

Financial Analysis

We have devoted two chapters that provide ratio and spreadsheet analysis data in organizations. Chapter 19 outlines accounting principles, whereas Chapter 20 discusses ratios that are useful. Nursing personnel are most concerned with budgets; Chapters 12, 13, and 14 cover developing and analyzing budgets, and Chapter 15 covers understanding how to compare reimbursements with the costs of services provided.

Markets and Environment

Significant national events that have resulted in our present illness care system are outlined in Chapters 9 and 10. The micro- and macroeconomics are then discussed in Chapter 11.

Designing the Organization

Once we have a fairly accurate organizational assessment, we can use this information to determine what organizational strategies are best suited to our organization. This is called organizational design. *Design* goes beyond assessment, not only looking at the parts (such as the assessment categories or department work units) but at how they are interconnected both internally and externally.

Using the quantum view of leadership, Senge (2006) tells us that leaders (leaders refers to both administrators and staff—in Chapter 2 the message is that our administrative aim is to have everyone be leaders in their areas of work) are designers, stewards, and teachers. Administrator responsibilities lie in building organizations where people can expand their capabilities, clarify visions, and improve shared mental models. Designing an organization starts with the purpose and core values, or mission statement, used to build a shared vision but also includes all organizational processes. Design goes beyond assessment, not only looking at the parts (such as the assessment categories or department work units) but at how they are interconnected both internally and externally. Senge (2006) stresses that trying to understand *wholes* by using systems thinking is the job of a true designer.

As designers, we must constantly think about, and implement, change. Status quo, although more comfortable because we are used to it, is actually the kiss of death. We cannot escape change. Change happens even when we cling tenaciously to the status quo, so our choice is whether we try to influence the changes in a certain direction. It's like they say in *Who Moved My Cheese*, we "need flexible people who are not possessive about 'the way things are done around here'" (Johnson, 1998, p. 17).

In the administrative role we want to promote future-oriented system changes. After all, we are on a constant quest to improve clinical quality and safety, to enhance customer satisfaction, and to stay viable with costs. We need to redesign systems so they are more efficient and effective, to improve each staff member's performance, to increase the teamwork between workers, and to stay updated on the latest outcomes research and technological advances. And if we are effective administrators, we are encouraging each person in the organization to improve organizational systems. This may mean redefining roles, improving processes, adding equipment, dealing with challenges, redesigning buildings, discussing issues with customers, and so on. Sometimes we experience successes, and sometimes we fail and have to figure out some other way.

One fallacy that many of us hold is that as we develop strategies, the strategies are perfect from the get-go. The rule of thumb is that when the strategy is first implemented, it is full of problematic issues that need to be resolved—even when we have used systems thinking and have involved inter-disciplinary groups to design it. Expect that more changes will be necessary after implementation. It is best to pilot a new strategy with a small group first. At least some of the problems can be worked out before a large group is involved. But even when the pilot occurs, more changes will be necessary as different groups or departments use the strategy.

The main theme with designing the organization and selecting organizational strategies is our thinking, our perceptions, and what we do with this information. So often our picture of where we are going with the strategies is flawed in that we ourselves, as well as others in the organization, have too limited a picture of what we want to achieve.

Peter Senge (2006) has dealt with this issue in his book, *The Fifth Discipline: The Art and Practice of the Learning Organization*. This book has become a classic for administrators. He sug-gests that what we want to achieve is a *learning organization*. This title is, in a way, a misnomer. An organization is not a person and therefore is incapable of learning. Yet people within an organiza-tion can change their picture of what they want the organization to be and change the way they think by using *systems thinking*.

The name of Senge's book refers to the five disciplines that create the learning organization:

1. *Building shared vision*—the practice of unearthing shared "pictures of the future" that fos-ter genuine commitment.
2. *Personal mastery*—the skill of continually clarifying and deepening our personal vision.
3. *Mental models*—the ability to unearth our internal pictures of the world, to scrutinize them, and to make them open to the influence of others.
4. *Team learning*—the capacity to "think together" that is gained by mastering the practice of dialogue and discussion.
5. *Systems thinking*—the discipline that integrates the others, fusing them into a coherent body of theory and practice (Fulmer & Keys, 1998, p. 34).

Feedback Issues

To be a more effective designer and to get at our mental models, we must understand feedback issues. According to Senge (2006), there are two types of feedback: reinforcing and balancing. *Reinforcement feedback* (the "engine of growth") occurs in many ways throughout the organization, such as when leaders/team members praise those who have done well and ignore or "label" low per-formers. Reinforcing processes may become vicious cycles. For example, if a person is interfering with other team members' work and this behavior is allowed to continue, another more positive team member may leave for a healthier work environment.

The second principle in systems thinking is that of *balancing feedback* (or "goal-oriented behav-ior"). This occurs as we encounter limits or boundaries. A classic example is when managers, under budgetary constraints, cut team members to help meet or decrease the budget. In turn, the remain-ing team members are now overworked, and the budget does not improve due to an increase in turnover and required overtime. If the managers had used systems thinking, they would have antic-ipated this result and would have met the budget constraints in another way.

Balancing feedback is often difficult to manage because the goals are implicit, the goals go unrecognized, and no one realizes that they even exist. One example that Senge gives us is the leader who tried relentlessly to decrease burnout among professionals by decreasing work hours and locking offices so that people stopped working late. This backfired, with people taking work home because the offices were locked. Balancing processes are more difficult to handle than reinforcing processes; we often do not see change occurring because of the actual balancing process.

Senge (2006) describes 11 laws of the fifth discipline, or *systems thinking*.

1. *"Today's problems can come from yesterday's solutions"* describes what it is like when one has to deal with a quick-fix solution that was made in the past but did not work in the long run. Quick-fix solutions may seem best at the time but can actually create more problems and may not even fix the original problem. For instance, a nursing shortage strategy has been to entice nurses with large "sign-on" bonuses and "crisis pay," only to find that once the time commitments are met for sign-on bonuses, staff move on to other positions. And crisis pay for one group can result in other staff groups feeling that they are disenfranchised and not valued. So yesterday's solution did not work in the long run. Instead, if administrators could look beyond these strategies by first examining the real problems, then these expensive quick fixes could have been avoided.

2. *"The harder you push, the harder the system pushes back"* discusses the phenomenon "compensating feedback." This occurs when the more personal effort you exert to improve or change matters, the more effort seems to be required. Instead, it is better when a larger group has been involved and has decided to make the change.

3. *"Behavior grows better before it grows worse"* talks about systems that may make things look better in the short run, only to return in 2 or 3 years to haunt you. The sign-on bonuses worked at first.

4. *"The easy way out usually leads back in"* discusses how we often apply familiar solutions to problems. This idea of sticking to what we know best is comforting, but very often the real solution is not obvious and the answer is hiding somewhere in the darkness.

5. *"The cure can be worse than the disease"* is seen when familiar solutions are not only ineffective but sometimes addictive and dangerous. For instance, many organizations become dependent on consultants, instead of training their own staff and solving problems themselves.

6. *"Faster is slower"* comes from the old story of the tortoise and the hare. Making a change quickly without involving all the players results in many unanticipated problems that could have been avoided with more dialogue between all the players in the first place.

7. *"Cause and effect are not closely related in time and space"* uses the example where there are sagging profits and unemployment in this country. The "cause" is the underlying reason that companies have moved beyond our borders for cheaper labor.

8. *"Small changes can produce big results—but the areas of highest leverage are often the least obvious."* Senge explains that large changes often have the least effect. Have you noticed how easy it is for people to go back to the status quo after a large change, especially when they were not involved in planning it?

9. *"You can have your cake and eat it too—but not at once."* For instance, organizations can improve on processes and achieve better quality (the cake) that in the long run result in lower costs (eat it too).

10. *"Dividing an elephant in half does not produce two small elephants"* describes how many organizations can see problems within individual departments but do not realize how they interconnect with the "whole" organization.

11. *"There is no blame"* indicates that the real problem is probably a complicated group of processes that occurred.

Many of the 11 laws that Senge describes can be applied to the quick fixes we have experienced in many organizations. Can you see how important it is to have dialogue with all those involved in the change before implementation?

So What Works?

Once we are aware of the 11 laws, we then need to more effectively change events using systems thinking. Time, energy, and resources need to be invested for change to occur. Senge and colleagues (1999) list several qualities that are seen in most successful change initiatives:

- They are connected with real work goals and processes.
- They are connected with improving performance.
- They involve people who have the power to take action regarding these goals.
- They seek to balance action and reflection, connecting inquiry and experimentation.
- They afford people an increased amount of "white space," opportunities for people to think and reflect without pressure to make decisions.
- They are intended to increase people's capacity, individually and collectively.
- They focus on learning about learning in settings that matter (p. 43).

Change initiatives can take on many different masks. They can be as simple as a series of meetings or as large as an organizational transformation. Effective leaders do not tell everyone what to do. The authoritarian model does not work. It is more important to encourage people to use their best judgment in situations and make their own decisions. The administrator's role is to provide ways that people can enhance their learning.

> The wise agent of change must know at the outset that there are people who have devoted their lives to preserving and assuring that change does not operate in their lives and, by reflection, in the lives of anyone around them.... These people are often addicted to negation. However, one blocking person can bring the entire change process to a grinding halt. The leader must name, identify, challenge, work with, and, if necessary, shift people who can't adapt. Staff must be empowered and inculcated in the process of their own transformation so they do not themselves become stuck in effectively forestalling what is necessary to assure the organization thrives in its new reality. Group barrier identification and strategic efforts to address them is a critical first stage in engaging staff in meaningful work (Porter-O'Grady, 2003, pp. 63–64).

Change is not just a one-time event; it is a journey. We must first consider whether the present culture can even support the change. As a change occurs, it is better to think of it as a spiral that starts, touches many different people as it circles around, and, hopefully, leads upward toward improved processes and relationships. The change may start with us or with someone else, especially in an empowering environment. Even when we are masters at organizational assessment, there are always surprises that we did not anticipate that may need our response. Some of the surprises may be about ourselves needing to change; change can expose our own vulnerabilities, as well as those of others. It also means that we are doing rounds, talking with others, and are available and that our actions agree with, and support, the change.

> The clinical leader must look at change as a journey not an event.... It is premature to claim victory or arrival. Every arrival point is also a debarking point. There really is no permanent point of respite from change. Since everything in life is a journey, it is important for the nurse leader to keep an honest perspective. The arrival points are merely points of demarcation, of momentary rest. The wise clinical leader carefully balances the moments of rest and celebration with those of effort and action. Depending upon the demand, the timeframe, and the circumstances, leaders choose the moments of marking success carefully so that they can serve to reenergize when necessary, refresh when possible, and challenge when appropriate (Porter-O'Grady, 2003. p. 64).

Shared Governance

Shared governance is a structural framework that affords nursing—and all other organizational members—professional autonomy at the point of care. This is where staff members make decisions about their work. "Shared governance is not a democracy. It is an accountability-based approach to structure in which there is a clear expectation that all members of a system participate in its work" (Porter-O'Grady, 2009, p. 45).

Shared governance operates in a true environment of empowerment. Remember in Chapter 2 how empowerment does not even happen until a leader is at least at stage 4 of Hagberg's power model? With shared governance, staff and leaders are empowered to contribute collectively to the decision-making process related to clinical practice, standards, and procedures. Shared governance also provides the organization with a mechanism to make decisions that improve patient care and the workplace environment. For example, nurses know how processes can be improved, so the decisions can be made directly by the nurses that deliver the care.

Shared governance benefits an organization because staff members (all staff members, not just nurses) are involved in the design of their work. In our current organizational environment, nurses can leave if they believe they are not valued. Authoritarian environments are not effective. There are more jobs available than there are nurses to fill them. If there is an ideal time for shared governance and true empowerment, it is now. This is the only way to achieve retention, and, for that matter, organizational longevity. The research supports this (Erickson, Hamilton, Jones, & Ditomassi, 2003; Kuokkanen & Katajisto, 2003; Laschinger, Finegan, Shamian, & Almost, 2001).

Creating an empowering environment is hard work, meaning that decision making is increased at the point of service. It takes constant effort. It can be painful. It means staff should be making 90% of the decisions and may choose directions that never occurred to us. Staff need to be involved in the decision making with hiring, budgeting, allocating, discipline, and policy. Porter-O'Grady (2001) describes the leader's perspective of an empowering environment as "overwhelming, treacherous, noisy, slow, and time-consuming. It often is tedious, not glamorous, and painful to make the required changes in the system for real empowerment to become the modus operandi for an organization" (p. 471). Today, many nurse managers feel overwhelmed, especially when they are in environments where they are not empowered and not supported by supervisors. This leads to higher nurse manager (and nurse executive) turnover. So in this chaotic time, it is time to support each other as we create this new reality.

In a whole-systems shared governance model, each member has equal power and responsibilities in the decision-making process, putting what the patient values and wants first. Porter-O'Grady (2009) advocates having an operations council (concerned with resources, linkage, planning, market strategy, implementation, and compliance), a patient care council (concerned with service delivery, system models, disciplines, service design, roles, quality, and process), and a governance council (concerned with mission, strategy, priorities, policy, and integration).

The physicians have had a medical staff organization historically, but Porter-O'Grady (2009) advocate that "many of the current separate functions of the medical staff will disappear as they become more integrated within the system.... The real struggle for physicians is seeing themselves as partners in the health system rather than the controllers of it" (pp. 264–265).

Using this model, there is a shared governance steering group that shares information and integrates decisions between and among the three councils. It is important that "every key role in the system, staff or management, should be represented in the steering group. The majority of planners, however, should be from the staff, not from management" (Porter-O'Grady, 2009, p. 80). "Integration is evidence of the attempt to configure services around the point of care and to bring providers together in a service partnership.... Compartmentalization is the death of integration" (Porter-O'Grady, 2009, p. 40).

Exhibit 3–3 Principles of Shared Governance

Partnership
- Role expectations are negotiated.
- Equality exists between the players.
- Relationships are founded upon shared risk.
- Expectations and contributions are clear.
- Solid measure of contribution to outcomes is established.
- Horizontal linkages are well defined.

Equity
- Each player's contribution is understood.
- Payment reflects value of contribution to outcomes.
- Role is based on relationship, not status.
- Team defines service roles, relationships, and outcomes.
- Methodology is defined for team conflict and service issues.
- Evaluation assesses team's outcomes and contributions.

Accountability
- Accountability is internally defined by person in the role.
- Accountability defines roles, not jobs.
- Accountability is based on outcomes, not process.
- Accountability is defined in advance of performance.
- Accountability leads to desired and defined results.
- Performance is validated by the results achieved.
- Processes are generally loud and noisy.

Ownership
- All workers are invested in the enterprise.
- Every role has a stake in the outcome.
- Rewards are directly related to outcomes.
- All members are associated with a team.
- Processes support relationships.
- Opportunity is based on competence.

Source: Porter-O'Grady, T. (2009). *Interdisciplinary shared governance: Integrating practice, transforming health care.* Sudbury, MA: Jones and Bartlett.

To make all this work effectively, caregivers who are at the point of service need access to accurate information, need to tune in to what the patient values, need administrative support from the top down to make these decisions, and need to feel accountable for their decisions. Shared governance structure ensures "that the decisions made there are correct, 'implementable,' and do not require broad organizational approval or a long decision making process (which might reduce the efficiency and effectiveness of the clinical delivery system)" (Porter-O'Grady, 2009, pp. 77–78). It is a system based on accountability coming internally from staff who want to give their best effort to their work. The principles of shared governance can be found in **Exhibit 3–3**.

Regular Identification and Implementation of Major Issues

Consider the following excerpts from various sources:

> Half the decisions in organizations fail. Studies of 356 decisions in medium to large organizations in the U.S., and Canada reveal that these failures can be traced to managers who impose solutions, limit the search for alternatives, and use power to implement their plans.

> Managers who make the need for action clear at the outset, set objectives, carry out an unrestricted search for solutions, and get key people to participate are more apt to be successful. Tactics prone to fail were used in two of every three decisions that were studied (Nutt, 1999, p. 75).

> Even the best concepts or strategies tend to develop incrementally. They rarely ever work the first time out or unfold just as they were planned (*HBR*, August 2002, p. 122).

> The real voyage of discovery is not in seeking new landscapes but in having new eyes (M. Proust).

> In Honda plants,… even relatively routine… problems are solved by rapidly created, temporary teams assembled when needed from people who come from throughout the [facility]—not just from the specific area where the problem was first observed. The roots of even seemingly straightforward problems can be far-flung and thus require a surprisingly broad range of institutional knowledge to be resolved (Watts, 2003, p. 17).

We have already discussed the importance of the administrator regularly doing rounds. Rounds aid administrators to have a more accurate organizational assessment, observe broken organizational processes, establish better relationships with staff, help out with the work, and help work through problems with new implementations. However, rounds have an additional benefit with organizational design—rounds provide regular dialogue with the work group about major issues that need to be fixed, involve appropriate people to work on and identify solutions to fix the problem issues and then continue to involve appropriate people to implement the chosen solution, to tweak it when needed, and to evaluate the effectiveness of what occurred to make sure the desired outcomes were achieved.

This sounds fairly simple, but it is really very complex. Because 90% of decisions need to be made at the point of service, this process must be understood and used by staff teams to improve their outcomes. If each team leader, as well as each administrator, is using this process, it is easier to fix problems. However, if there are any flies in the ointment, effectiveness may not be achieved. Many problems need interdisciplinary involvement before they can be solved. Often, more than one department identifies a problem, but each will have a different perspective (they each have different functions) and each may want a different solution. Establishing a dialogue with all involved can help alter perspectives for a broader organizational picture. Then more effective long-term solutions can be tried with the additional bonus that all are more committed to try the change. After the work group(s) decides on a change, the implementation takes consistent follow-up before it can be successfully realized. This takes a lot of time and constant effort.

Helpful principles for change projects are as follows:

- New projects or improvements have a better chance for success when the person assigned to the project believes in it. When the implementer burns with the issue, his or her belief in it helps the project to succeed.
- An effective leader knows that when entering a new administrative role it is best not to make a lot of changes in the beginning. Instead, it is better to get to know people, build relationships, and get an accurate organizational assessment. Thus it is important to talk to staff both in groups and individually, make rounds, and come in at different times. This way the administrator has a chance to see how care is being delivered, to begin to understand processes, to identify systems problems, to ask questions, and to find out what improvements staff suggest. After all this has occurred, then one can begin to plan and discuss changes with the work group.
- Keep one's boss informed about what is going on and what you plan to do. Or, if you are unsure what to do, ask for help, thinking of ways you might deal with a particular situation.

Having good chemistry with one's boss is important. The hardest issue with one's boss is when you do not agree with how he or she is handling something. Often, in this case the boss has not realized a significant factor, but it can also be that the person has a blind spot about something. It requires tremendous diplomacy and tact to avoid a political blunder that can derail or end a promising career. At the same time, many great companies have floundered because of faulty decisions made at the top while middle managers sat on their hands. In effect, we all need to be ready to lead even when we are not in charge (Useem, 2001).

- Conflict can help to identify issues and different perspectives and can provide better ways to resolve issues.

There are an infinite number of actions, improvements, and strategies that are possible. We need to use systems thinking and empower the appropriate people to make decisions. Some of these strategies enhance certain organizations, whereas they may not work, or be as effective, in others. Take self-scheduling, for example. If a unit is in a system 4, this can work very well. However, if this is introduced in a system 2 environment, it will inevitably fail. A nurse administrator must keep in mind the total organizational assessment, (i.e., such factors as staff personalities, the unit culture, the hierarchy, cost constraints, and the patients served). Then it is important the appropriate person chooses what seems to be best for the present moment under the current circumstances. Tall order!

Connectedness: The Best Way to Deal with Conflict

Because we are not taught to *value* conflict and see its many benefits in our society, most of us can do a better job with managing conflict, both within ourselves and within our work group. In fact, chances are, we have way more to learn. Conflict (discussed in Chapter 2) is like gold—it can be very valuable and lead us to new avenues in our life and at work. Exploration using dialogue is the method that leads us to these new avenues. It is not about winning and losing. It is about what we value, and how we can best achieve that. Conflict can strengthen relationships, or it can tear us apart. When the culture, or climate, encourages different views, and expressing those views, more positive outcomes result. Teamwork, collaboration, and connectedness occur.

Connectedness is part of "love one another"—leadership effectiveness, discussed in Chapter 2. This is hardest to do when there are differences between us. A common response is to hate the whole person when we disagree with him or her. Instead, it is not the whole person but someone's actions or opinions with which we disagree. And if it is a patient, we have to be very careful not to superimpose our set of "shoulds" on the patient. Instead, we need to help the patient explore what is needed and find out what the patient needs from us. This is what "radical loving care" is about (discussed in Chapter 4).

Regardless of with whom our conflict exists, it is not right to superimpose our beliefs on someone else. It is up to the other person to decide what is best to do. If this action does not meet the standards set within the organization, this may need to result in counseling, but every person always is given respect for his or her differences. In fact, in an effective team, members celebrate their differences, knowing that it is these differences that make the team more effective.

Connectedness means that we have shared goals. For instance, what is best for the patient? We are cooperating. We help each other. We share knowledge with each other. There is an element of shared meaning with the group. We are creating group synergy in the pursuit of collective goals. We are making sacrifices to achieve these goals.

Connectedness means that we do not judge. Remember the saying about walking in another's shoes? We might be right where that person is if we had done that.

Past research indicates five ways that people deal with conflicts. *Collaboration* is most effective. Here individuals work together to come up with a mutually acceptable solution. Although this takes more time, no one loses. Other approaches that are not as effective can occur. For instance, some use *competition* where it is all important to win, regardless of the cost; one might *compromise*, where each person gives up something but agrees on the best alternative; one could *accommodate* where one concedes to others, letting them get their way; and finally one could *avoid* situations and not take any action.

> Collaboration focuses on trying to reach agreement among divergent opinions to accomplish mutual goals. Weiss suggests that the conflicts between nurses and physicians are due to the overlapping nature of their domains and the lack of clarification between their roles. Adding to the difficulty of achieving agreement, doctors and nurses use different methods of conflict resolution. When resolving differences, physicians tend to bargain or negotiate while nurses avoid, accommodate, or compete.
>
> Collaboration... involves a high level of concern for others (cooperativeness), as well as a high concern for self (assertiveness).... Dechairo... found that self-confidence was a predictor of nurse case manager satisfaction with nurse/physician collaboration.
>
> The Thomas and Kilman model of conflict resolution is one of problem solving, and it is useful in complex situations where parties have common interests and the stakes are high. Inherent in this model is the assumption that conflict resolution [and mediation tools] can be taught and that effective collaboration will be the outcome. Using this model, willing participants can overcome the handicaps of a history of competition and style of avoidance or dominance (Dechairo-Marino, Jordan-Marsh, Traiger, & Saulo, 2001, p. 225).

Fisher, Ury, and Patton (1991) published a classic that is very helpful on negotiation, *Getting to Yes: Negotiating Agreement Without Giving In*. This can be used in any setting and is so successful that the American Nurses Association started using it to negotiate collective bargaining agreements. Fisher et al. (1991) advocate that it is best to "separate the people from the problem; focus on interests, not positions; generate a variety of possibilities before deciding what to do; and insist that the result be based on some objective standard" (p. 11). This is a must read for administrators.

Collaboration is the glue that holds together the relationships, teamwork between people, and the communication that occurs between everyone involved in the organization. The better the glue, the more effective the organization. This glue is not what we think of as permanently adhesive, nor is it removable. Instead, this is a magic, dynamic glue. The bond is strong, yet ever-changing. The bond is between people who know and trust each other. Magic happens when people work effectively together. Everyone, including the patients (residents, clients), staff, and physicians, fares better when this glue is present. This is where the spirit, or love, comes in.

Collegiality or collaboration between nurses and physicians, when effective, can affect patient outcomes. Kramer and Schmalenberg (2003) cite lower mortality rates in intensive care units when this is achieved. In their research they came up with a five-category scale describing this relationship:

- Category 1: Collegial. Described as excellent, the essential ingredient in these relationships is equality based on "different but equal" power and knowledge.
- Category 2: Collaborative. In these "good" or "great" relationships, staff work together very well. Nurses describe mutuality but not equality of power.
- Category 3: Student-Teacher. Physicians are willing to discuss, explain, and teach. Power is unequal, but outcomes are beneficial. Either nurse or physician acts as the teacher.
- Category 4: Neutral. A near absence of feeling marks this relationship. Often, there's only information exchange. But, physicians frequently fail to acknowledge receiving the information, which leaves the nurses feeling they aren't contributing much.

- Category 5: Negative. Frustration, hostility, and resignation characterize this relationship. Power is unequal and outcomes are negative because of their reactions to power plays (pp. 36–37).

From this research, they suggest it is important to plant and nurture the "equal but different" seed; create a culture that values, expects, and rewards collegial nurse–physician relationships; and fosters, supports, and encourages education programs of all types (so all stay clinically competent). This collegiality improves with ongoing relationships over time.

Collaboration must happen in different ways now that we are in the information age. Richards (2001) suggests that "collaborative practice involves a community of electronically connected practitioners providing a richer and more scientific foundation for practice" (p. 6).

Staff Development

Staff education/development is an important organizational strategy that enhances staff capabilities to better see what is coming in the future. It helps everyone to stretch and grow. By staff development, we mean that every member of the organization—from the board member to the housekeeping person cleaning the bathrooms—can benefit from additional learning opportunities. Opportunities can occur anywhere and in many different environments. In fact, we probably could really help one another do better on the love aspect when differences occur. Generally, every staff member should experience learning opportunities both within and outside the organization. Because we learn differently—some by seeing, some by hearing, some by experiencing—we need to provide various opportunities that correspond to a person's learning style. And sometimes we learn best when we have to teach someone else. The sky is the limit here, because there are an infinite number of possibilities.

Unfortunately, it is often the education budget that gets cut. This is a major error. In the current environment that is constantly changing, educational offerings provide effective strategies for remaining viable. If no educational opportunities are available, this ignores the fact that we all need to do meaningful work and have opportunities to continue to grow. Scott (2002) makes the following observation:

> When learning and professional development are viewed only in terms of an optional opportunity for improvement—*rather than as a threat* to your organization's survival if ignored—the commitment to sustain successful change will be missing. Thus, look at professional development from two angles: what you and your team will gain if everyone worked differently, and what you and your team will lose by simply maintaining the status quo. Bottom line, will you achieve your strategic goals if you and your staff continue to lead the way you are leading today (p. 17)?

We have discussed the shifts that all of us need to be living in this new information age. Scott (2002) names 10:

> From a provider orientation to customer obsession; from silo thinking to an organizational perspective; from directing to coaching; from status quo to courage, risk, and change; from busyness to results; from telling to facilitating dialogue; from protecting turf to building relationships; from a function manager to a business leader; from the employee as expendable to the employee as precious; and from pressure and overwork to perspective and balance (p. 18).

There are many more examples sprinkled throughout this book. The exciting thing is that there is so much more to learn, which is true for the nurse aide all the way through to the board.

Conclusion

This chapter is only the beginning. As we head toward the ocean, we take various paths. Some meander here and there. Some get there successfully despite many obstacles. Many experience temporary setbacks but know that sometimes it is these setbacks that lead us into a better direction. The charted course is different for each organization. Money can continue to be adequate or, if bottom line thinking prevails, will be scarce. We always continue to evolve, either into better systems that run closer to the mission or as antiquated relics of days gone by, floundering and disappearing midstream. The choice is ours.

Discussion Questions

1. From your perspective, what is the most important core value in a health care organization? What are the core values at work?
2. As a nurse manager, what actions can you take to facilitate more meaningful work for each staff member?
3. Assess your organization using the information given under the section "Organizing Arrangements". As you assess each category, start with the corporate organization, then the facility, and then the unit/department where you work.
4. Why is it so important for everyone from the CEO to the nurse manager to do rounds? Give examples of what can be accomplished during rounds?
5. Assess the meetings you attend or lead. Are they necessary? Is there a better way to achieve the goal(s) of each meeting? Is a different meeting with different participants needed for a specific purpose? How could the meetings be more meaningful?
6. How can a nurse manager increase staff decision making at the point of service?
7. Give an example of effective collaboration in the workplace.
8. What measures can a nurse manager take to increase team effectiveness?
9. Choose 1 of the 11 laws of the fifth discipline and give an example where this might occur.
10. Give an example of a systems problem. Discuss the process a nurse administrator could take to resolve the problem.
11. Give an example where shared governance could improve the work setting.
12. What are five major issues that need to be resolved in your organization?

References

Bates, S. (2003, January/February). Creating a credible culture. *Nurse Leader*, 37–38.

Block, P. (1993). *Stewardship*. San Francisco: Berrett Koehler.

Bohn, R. (2000). Stop fighting fires. *Harvard Business Review, 74*(4), 82–91.

Bolman, L., & Deal, T. (1997). *Reframing organizations: Artistry, choice, and leadership* (2nd ed.). San Francisco: Jossey-Bass.

Campbell, D., Fleming, R., & Grote, R. (1985, July–August). Discipline without punishment—at last. *Harvard Business Review*, 162–178.

Chapman, E. (2004). *Radical loving care: Building the healing hospital in America*. Nashville, TN: Baptist Healing Hospital Trust.

Collins, J., & Porras, J. (1994). *Built to last: Successful habits of visionary companies*. New York: Harper Business.

Crow, G. (2003, March/April). Creativity and management in the 21st century. *Nurse Leader*, 32–35.

Curran, C. (2002a). Culture eats strategy for lunch every time. *Nursing Economic$, 20*(6), 257.

Curran, C. (2000b). Musings on managerial excellence. *Nursing Economic$, 18*(6), 277, 322.

DeBono, E. (1976). *Teaching thinking*. New York: Penguin.

DeBono, E. (1994). *DeBono's thinking course* (revised ed.). New York: Facts on File, Inc.

Dechairo-Marino, A., Jordan-Marsh, M., Traiger, G., & Saulo, M. (2001). Nurse/physician collaboration: Action research and the lessons learned. *Journal of Nursing Administration, 31*(5), 223–232.

Doucette, J. (2003, November). Serving up uncommon service. *Nursing Management, 34*, 26–29.

Drucker, P. (1999). Managing oneself. *Harvard Business Review, 77*(2), 65.

Erickson, J., Hamilton, G., Jones, D., & Ditomassi, M. (2003). The value of collaborative governance/staff empowerment. *Journal of Nursing Administration, 33*(2), 96–104.

Fisher, R., Ury, W., & Patton, B. (1991). *Getting to yes: Negotiating agreement without giving in*. New York: Penguin.

Fulmer, R., & Keys, J. (1998, Autumn). A conversation with Peter Senge: New developments in organizational learning. *Organizational Dynamics, 27*(2), 33–41.

Gordon, J. (2002). *Organizational behavior: A diagnostic approach* (7th ed.). Upper Saddle River, NJ: Prentice Hall.

Harvey, E., & Lucia, A. (n.d.). *Walk the talk... And get the results you want* (2nd ed.). Dallas: WALK THE TALK Company, Copyright by Performance Systems Corporation.

Harvard Business Review (2002). *80*(8), 117.

Heim, P. (1996). *Gender differences in the workplace series*. Videotapes produced by Cynosure productions, LTD. And KTEH, Channel 54, San Jose, California.

Herzberg, F. (2003, January). One more time: How do you motivate employees? *Harvard Business Review*, (1), 87–96.

Johnson, S. (1998). *Who moved my cheese?* New York: Penguin Putman.

Kerfoot, K. (2002). Messy conversations and the willingness to be disturbed. *Nursing Economic$, 10*(6), 297–299.

Kramer, M., & Schmalenberg, C. (2003, July). Securing "good" nurse/physician relationships. *Nursing Management, 34*(7), 34–38.

Kuokkanen, L., & Katajisto, J. (2003). Promoting or impeding empowerment? Nurses' assessments of their work environment. *Journal of Nursing Administration, 33*(4), 209–215.

Laschinger, H., Finegan, J., Shamian, J., & Almost, J. (2001). Testing karasek's demands—control model in restructured healthcare settings: Effects of job strain on staff nurses' quality of work life. *Journal of Nursing Administration, 31*(3), 233–243.

Lencioni, P. (2002). *The five dysfunctions of a team*. San Francisco: Jossey-Bass.

Lencioni, P. (2002, July). Make your values mean something. *Harvard Business Review*, 113–117.

Lencioni, P. (2006). *Silos, politics and turf wars: A leadership fable about destroying the barriers that turn colleagues into competitors*. San Francisco: Jossey-Bass.

McDonagh, K. (2003, January/February). Reaching for a dream: Challenges for the innovative nurse leader. *Nurse Leader*, 46–48.

Nobre, A. (2001). Soul + spirit + resources + leadership = results. *Journal of Nursing Administration, 31*(6), 287–289.

Nutt, P. (1999). Surprising but true: Half the decisions in organizations fail. *Academy of Management Review, 13*(4), 75–90.

O'Hallaron, R. (2002, October). Letter to the editor: Corporate values. *Harvard Business Review*, 125.

Paige, J. (2003, March). Solve the policy and procedure puzzle. *Nursing Management*, 45–48.

Porter-O'Grady, T. (2001). Is shared governance still relevant? *Journal of Nursing Administration, 31*(10), 468–473.

Porter-O'Grady, T. (2003). Of hubris and hope: Transforming nursing for a new age. *Nursing Economic$, 21*(2), 59–64.

Porter-O'Grady, (2009). *Interdisciplinary shared governance: Integrating practice, transforming health care.* Sudbury, MA: Jones and Bartlett.

Porter-O'Grady, T., & Malloch, K. (2007a). *Managing for success in health care.* St. Louis, MO: Mosby/Elsevier.

Porter-O'Grady, T., & Malloch, K. (2007b). *Quantum leadership: A resource for health care innovation.* Sudbury, MA: Jones and Bartlett.

Richards, J. (2001). Nursing in a digital age. *Nursing Economic$, 19*(1), 6–11, 34.

Rutan, V. (2003). The best of both worlds: A consideration of gender in team building. *Journal of Nursing Administration, 33*(3), 179–186.

Scott, G. (2002, November/December). Coach, challenge, lead: Developing an indispensable management team. *Healthcare Executive*, 16–20.

Senge, P. (2006). *The fifth discipline: The art and practice of the learning organization.* New York: Doubleday/Currency.

Senge, P., Roberts, C., Ross, R., Smith, B., & Kleinor, A. (1999). *The dance of change: The challenges of sustaining momentum in learning organizations.* New York: Currency.

Sherwood, G. (2003). Leadership for a healthy work environment: Caring for the human spirit. *Nurse Leader 1*(5), 36–40.

Studer, Q. (2000). *Taking your organization to the next level.* Presented at the annual meeting of the American Organization of Nurse Executives, March 26. National Nursing Network Inc., 4465 Washington St., Denver, CO 80216 or www.studergroup.com.

Useem, M. (2001, October). The leadership lessons of Mount Everest. *Harvard Business Review*, 51–58.

Watts, D. (2003, February). The science behind six degrees. *Harvard Business Review*, 16–17.

Wellins, R., Byham, W., & Wilson, J. (1991). *Empowered teams: Creating self-directed work groups that improve quality, productivity and participation.* San Francisco: Jossey-Bass.

Wheatley, M. (1999). *Leadership and the new science: Discovering order in a chaotic world.* San Francisco: Berrett-Koehler.

Wheatley, M. (2002). *Turning to one another: Simple conversations to restore hope to the future.* San Francisco: Berrett-Koehler.

PART II

Providing Value-Based Service

Now that we have discussed the importance of both good leadership and achieving change in organizations along with the importance of working as part of a team, we need to get to the basics—the main reason we are here. We have discussed the importance of placing the patient as top priority. This is so important that we made a separate section just to discuss providing value-based services. As we said previously, this is first priority, not the bottom line.

Chapter 4 is concerned with how to best provide value-based services to our patients/residents/customers. In health care settings, we have not always stressed the importance of listening to our patient/resident/customer to find out what he or she wants and needs. Also, we must give our patient/resident/customer information so he or she can decide on what happens next. It is a constant process of keeping the patient informed and involving him or her in making the care decisions. The old patriarchal system where we made decisions for the patient is outdated and perhaps did not tell our patients what would happen. We, as nurses, are often stuck in our "task" box, not even thinking of how the patient may be responding to our services. So this new perspective—listening to the patient, providing information, and having the patient make the care decisions—is so important.

Chapter 4 also includes information on both quality and patient safety. This is more familiar territory to a nurse. We understand more about quality and the need to provide patient safety. We may believe we are providing a quality service, but if it is not what the patient wants, we have entirely missed the boat! In addition, there is so much more we need to be doing to provide patient safety. We are still harming too many patients in our health care systems. We would never choose an airline with that kind of record! So why should patients choose our services? In fact, many patient safety issues are caused by a series of events or organizational processes that are broken. It is time to fix this problem, to leave blame behind (after all, we are all human and, chances are, one person did not cause the problem alone). Every single one of us needs to do everything in our power to ensure patient safety.

As we provide quality care and patient safety, chances are we health care providers have a knowledge deficit—it is not possible to keep up with all the current treatments, drugs, and research results that could improve our practice. There is so much information that no one can keep track of it all. Information is not a big secret anymore. It is easy to access a lot of information, and our clients have become better informed. At times, they are better informed about their illness than we are. Research indicates that caregivers—both physicians and nurses—tend to go on doing what we were taught in school, even though there is current practice, or evidence-based, information that indicates a better way to give care. This is where Chapter 5 comes to the rescue via some very dedicated librarians, using the just-in-time concept to provide us with evidence-based information as we need it.

Chapter 5 has a much broader focus than just identifying the best clinical care for our patients. Evidence-based information is available to help us, as administrators, to better manage and lead the health care team. Finding information on the latest administrative/educational evidence can be very helpful as we work on various issues each day. Chapter 5 is packed with information to help the nurse manager be more effective in the role. And, because many of us are not terribly computer literate, the librarians in Chapter 5 take us through the process step by step so we can successfully navigate the information highway.

CHAPTER 4

Providing Value-Based Services While Achieving Quality, Safety, and Financial Accountability

Janne Dunham-Taylor, PhD, RN

Dru Malcolm, MSN, RN, CNAA-BC, CPHRM

Karen W. Snyder, MSN, RN

Sandy K. Calhoun, PhD(c), MSN, RN, CPHQ

The top priority in any health care setting is to find out what the patient values; to provide that care in a loving, safe, excellent way when possible, to strive to constantly improve our care delivery, and to accomplish all this in a cost-effective way. This is true for both staff and physicians at the point of care, and for us as administrators in all our decisions and actions.

Introduction

What a tall order!! Thankfully, at times this is achieved. At this point both patient and caregivers feel like it has all been worthwhile. If you need an uplifting experience, read Bargmann's, *The Top Hospital in America: The Heart and Soul of a Great Medical Center* (2002). Additionally, a few health care organizations have been awarded the Malcolm Baldrige National Quality Award. A compelling book, *Radical Loving Care: Building the Healing Hospital in America* (Chapman, 2004), provides some answers on ways to achieve this goal. Although the above-mentioned are about hospitals, they could just as easily describe long-term care, home care, ambulatory care, and primary care settings. We will return to achieve this goal after discussing the present situation and some of the problems that have surfaced.

There are four enormous challenges confronting us in health care today (**Exhibit 4–1**):

1. *To regularly determine what our patient/client/resident wants and values.* We often have totally missed the mark on this challenge. Many of us do not know how to find this information. We have not been good listeners—and that starts with those of us in administrative roles. The way we treat employees is the way the employees will treat patients. Quality boils down to what the patient values and wants. Because this is such a misunderstood concept, we devote a section of this chapter to patient values (see Our First Priority—What Does the Patient Want and Value Anyway?, below).

2. *To provide the very best quality care, once we know what the patient values.* The quality of the care must take what the patient values into account in combination with safe, evidence-based

---

Exhibit 4–1   Four Enormous Challenges in Health Care

1. To regularly determine what our patient/client/resident wants and values
2. To provide the very best quality care, once we know what the patient values
3. To keep our patient/client/resident safe
4. To accomplish the first three items in a cost-effective way

---

care. Otherwise, it is possible that what we believe is quality actually goes against what the patient wants. Quality, as measured by the patient perception, is what we stress here in this chapter, keeping in mind that the patient may not always realize what is the best quality.

3. *To keep our patient/client/resident safe.* To accomplish this, every one of us in health care needs to constantly strive to think of ways to improve safety. This means the small things from wiping up a water spill someone has left, to purchasing technology, to implementing systems or processes that all of us need to follow to the letter.
4. *To accomplish the first three items in a cost-effective way.* Cost-effectiveness is listed fourth because it should never be given higher priority than the previous three items. As stated in Chapter 1, "If we do what is right for the patients, financial well-being will follow." The bottom line is *never* the first priority.

We Have a L-O-N-G Way to Go to Fix Our Healthcare System

There are big problems in health care. Care is often fragmented and depersonalized. We may unwittingly do harm. At times, patients become worse rather than better when they come in contact with us. At times, we even do things that are against the patient's wishes. This is coupled with 15% of the population being uninsured. Is there ever a need for change! Statistics show that the United States ranks 37th in overall quality of health care, according to the World Health Organization, but spends more per person on health care than any other country. More recently, the Common Wealth Fund (Cantor, Schoen, Belloff, How, & McCarthy, 2007) ranked health systems using state scorecards based on five performance dimensions: access to care, quality, avoidable hospital use and costs, equity, and healthy lives. The result points out that some states are doing better than others, but there is room for improvement all around.

Patient Safety Issues

In a groundbreaking report, the Institute of Medicine (IOM, 2000) estimated that there were up to 98,000 hospital deaths per year from avoidable hospital errors, not to mention errors occurring in other health care settings. This report startled the health care community and consumers into action, yet that action has been slow to create change. In 2007, the IOM published findings from a workshop, *Creating a Business Case for Quality Improvement Research.* This report acknowledges a "reluctance to invest in quality improvement" (p. 1) throughout the country. Resources are limited and tend to be spent on "highly visible technology-driven programs" (p. 1). Sure, technology can improve systems, but it is not the single answer to providing a safer health care system.

In *The Fifth Annual HealthGrades on Patient Safety in American Hospitals Study* (National Center for Patient Safety, 2008), researchers report that over 200,000 deaths occurred among Medicare patients from potentially preventable causes. The same study revealed the following:

- Patients who experienced a patient safety incident had a 20% chance of dying as a result of the incident.
- The overall death rate among patients who experienced one or more patient safety incidents fell by almost 5% between 2004 and 2006.
- However, over that time, there were increases in postoperative respiratory failure, postoperative pulmonary embolism or deep vein thrombosis, postoperative sepsis (blood infection), and postoperative abdominal wound separation/splitting.
- The most common types of medical errors were bed sores, failure to rescue, and postoperative respiratory failure. Together, they accounted for 63.4% of incidents. Failure to rescue improved 11.1% from 2004 to 2006, whereas both bed sores and postoperative respiratory failure worsened during that time.
- Of the 270,491 deaths that occurred among patients who experienced one or more patient safety incidents, 238,337 were potentially preventable, the researchers said.
- If all hospitals performed at the level of the top-ranked hospitals, about 220,106 patient safety incidents and 37,214 patient deaths could have been avoided, and about $2 billion could have been saved (www.ncpa.org/sub/dpd/index.php?Article_ID=16556).

MEDICATION ERRORS

The IOM released a new report in 2006 on prevention of medication errors. Their research discovered that "a hospital patient can expect on average to be subjected to more than one medication error each day" (p. 1). This is a frightening statistic. Errors occurred in every step of the medication process but more during prescribing and administration. Experts estimate that error rates are actually *higher* than the numbers reported. One of the studies cited in the report documented an additional cost of $8,750 per hospital stay for each adverse drug event. IOM (2004a) reported in an earlier study "in two hospitals over a 6-month period found that nurses were responsible for intercepting 86 percent of all medication errors made by physicians, pharmacists, and others involved in providing medications for patients before the error reached the patient" (p. 3). The IOM (2006) believes that *most* of the errors and the additional costs are preventable.

The risks of adverse drug events are higher for nursing home patients. Garcia (2006) predicts that nearly "two thirds of nursing facility residents will experience an adverse drug event over a 4-year period of time, with 1 in 7 of these residents requiring hospitalization" (p. 306). Simonson and Feinberg (2005), in extensive work reviewing the medication issues in the elderly, identified that *one half* of adverse drug events in nursing home facilities are preventable.

NOSOCOMIAL INFECTIONS

Hospital-acquired infections continue to be an issue in organizations across the country. "In American hospitals alone, healthcare-associated infections account for an estimated 1.7 million infections and 99,000 associated deaths each year" (Centers for Disease Control and Prevention, 2007). Methicillin-resistant *Staphylococcus aureus*, or MRSA, has reached endemic levels in hospitals and long-term care facilities, and rates continue to rise. The increasing numbers of patients with health care–acquired infections is evidence that we are not following the basic preventive measures of *good hand hygiene*.

FALLS

Falls among the elderly continue to be a safety issue. "In 2005, 15,800 people 65 and older died from injuries related to unintentional falls; about 1.8 million people 65 and older were treated in emergency departments for nonfatal injuries from falls, and more than 433,000 of these patients were hospitalized" (Centers for Disease Control and Prevention, 2008). One study estimated the direct medical costs to be $19.2 billion for 1 year (Stevens, Corso, Finkelstein, & Miller, 2006). This did not include subsequent long-term care costs or loss of quality of life. The National Center for Patient Safety (2006) estimates that the annual costs of falls might exceed $32 billion by 2020. Falls occur across health care settings. The Institute for Healthcare Improvement (IHI) reports that 10% of all falls among the elderly occur in the hospital setting. The National Center for Patient Safety (2006) reported higher numbers, with 14.8% in acute care and 20.4% in the nursing home units. Research suggests an increasing risk of falls with lower nurse staffing levels (Whitman, Kim, Davidson, Wolf, & Wang, 2002).

These are just a few of the safety issues facing today's health care system. In our role as administrators, we must find ways to create a culture of safety that does not tolerate continuation of these problems. Doesn't it appeal to our ethical duty and responsibility?

Disparities Issues

Besides all the safety issues, major access issues continue. The fifth *National Healthcare Disparities Report* (Agency for Healthcare Research and Quality, 2008) describes disparities related to the quality of and access to health care (discussed in Chapter 9). Although some progress is being made, they report that many gaps have not become smaller (**Exhibit 4–2**.) The primary problem in decreasing gaps is related to lack of insurance.

According to the Kaiser Family Foundation (Kaiser Commission, 2006), 18% of the U.S. population is uninsured. In a statistical brief for the Agency for Healthcare Research and Quality, Rhoades (2005) presents data showing that the percentage of uninsured varies throughout the year but up to 13.6% are uninsured for the entire year. Those without insurance do not get needed medical care. The good news is that almost "seven out of every ten Americans under age 65 years are covered by employment-based health insurance" (Committee on the Consequences of Uninsurance, 2001, p. 4).

Miller, Vigdor, and Manning (2004) claim that lack of insurance creates hidden costs for society. They base this claim on data from the IOM report that estimated the cost in terms of foregone health, shorter lives, and demands on the health care infrastructure at $65 to $130 billion a year. Why not take this hidden cost and convert it to insurance coverage for those who cannot afford it on their own?

Currently, the health care "safety net" is providing care to the uninsured or underinsured for 44 million low-income Americans. The biggest provider in this safety net is hospital emergency departments. Community clinics, public health departments, and hospital-based clinics, created to provide this care, are not able to handle the load. Hospital emergency department visits classified as nonurgent are continuing to increase, totaling 14% of total visits in 2005. Key reasons for this

---

Exhibit 4–2 Disparities Among Races

- Blacks had a rate of new AIDS cases 10 times higher than Whites.
- Asian adults aged 65 and over were 50% more likely than Whites to lack immunization against pneumonia.
- Native Americans and Alaska Natives were twice as likely to lack prenatal care in the first trimester as Whites.
- Hispanics had a rate of new AIDS cases over 3.5 times higher than that of non-Hispanic Whites.
- Poor children were over 28% more likely than high-income children to experience poor communication with their health care providers.

Source: Agency for Healthcare Research and Quality. (2008). *National Healthcare Disparities Report: 2007.* AHRQ Pub. No. 08-0041. Rockville, MD: U.S. Department of Health and Human Services.

include difficulty getting timely appointments with a primary care provider, the lack of affordable transportation, and the lack of insurance. Much of this is not reimbursed so hospitals incur more and more expense providing this care.

Regulatory Response: Restricting or Eliminating Reimbursement for Facility-Acquired Conditions

The Centers for Medicare and Medicaid Services (CMS), which has taken over much of the health insurance system in this country, responded to all this. In addition, as health care expenses rise and the elderly group eligible for Medicare grows, federal and state governments are faced with finding the money to cover the expenses these large systems have incurred. In their adjusted rate prospective payment system, implemented to curtail costs, health care facilities must show how they meet CMS quality indicators as part of the Medicare Quality Monitoring System. This program was developed to "assure quality health care for all Americans through accountability and public disclosure" (CMS, 2008b). Basically, facilities must demonstrate meeting the guidelines for care of certain conditions to receive the highest possible reimbursement.

For instance, a payer might specify a care path to obtain reimbursement. If the care path is not followed as specified, the health care organization does not receive reimbursement for the care. So, for example, if antibiotics are not given within 2 hours of a pneumonia diagnosis (the care path specification), the payer will not reimburse the hospital. In this case, the clinician needs to be timely in treating the patient or everyone loses, including the patient.

In 2008, additional indicators were put in place restricting or eliminating reimbursement for certain hospital-acquired conditions that could "reasonably have been prevented through the application of evidence-based guidelines" (CMS, 2008a) (**Exhibit 4–3**.) These have been nicknamed "never events." CMS also has initiatives underway for home health, nursing home, and physician-focused quality improvement. There are new outpatient measures focusing on emergency departments and surgical care. There are currently 41 measures related to home health and 19 for long-term care. Visit the CMS website (www.cms.hhs.gov/center/quality.asp) for more information and to compare results.

Exhibit 4–3 2008 CMS Hospital-Acquired Conditions Selected for Payment Restriction or Elimination

1. Foreign object retained after surgery
2. Air embolism
3. Blood incompatibility
4. Stage III and IV pressure ulcers
5. Falls and trauma
   - Fractures
   - Dislocations
   - Intracranial injuries
   - Crushing injuries
   - Burns
6. Catheter-associated urinary tract infection
7. Vascular catheter-associated infection
8. Surgical site infection-mediastinitis after coronary artery bypass graft
9. Pressure ulcers.

Source: Centers for Medicare and Medicaid. (2008). Hospital-acquired conditions (present on admission indicator). Retrieved June 1, 2008 from http://www.cms.hhs.gov/HospitalAcqCond/06_Hospital-Acquired%20Conditions.asp

---

Because Medicaid programs are funded at both state and federal levels, these restrictions on reimbursement are being linked to Medicaid payments as well. Then the American Hospital Association developed guiding principles for nonpayment with patients and all insurance companies for certain serious adverse events (that are preventable, may indicate a hospital system error, and where there are published guidelines for prevention of these errors if the hospital deems the event was preventable) from the National Quality Forum's list of 28 serious reportable events (Tennessee Hospitals & Health Systems, 2008) (**Exhibit 4–4**).

Patient safety is of such concern to the public that the Joint Commission on Accreditation of Healthcare Organizations (JCAHO, 2008) implemented patient safety goals. Accredited facilities must demonstrate meeting the intent of these goals to maintain accreditation status.

Other organizations have implemented voluntary programs that measure and report safety data and outcomes. One of these is the LeapFrog Group that supports pay for performance. The Leapfrog Group is a "consortium of major companies and other large private and public healthcare purchasers... members and their employees spend tens of billions of dollars on health care annually. Leapfrog members have agreed to base their purchase of health care on principles that encourage quality improvement among providers and consumer involvement" (Leapfrog Group, n.d.). Their primary focus is on improving and implementing best practice.

Finally, The National Database of Nursing Quality Indicators was developed by the American Nurses Association to collect and report nurse-sensitive outcomes data in an effort to show how nursing care promotes quality and patient safety. It is also based on voluntary participation and thus may not provide a truly accurate picture of nursing care across the nation, but it has given nurse administrators a tool to help compare outcomes, staffing, and other nursing factors. Some of the data measured are incidents of hospital-acquired pressure ulcers, fall rates, and restraint use in relation to nursing hours per patient day and skill mix.

Exhibit 4–4 The American Hospital Association Guidelines for Reimbursement Restriction

The American Hospital Association recommends that hospitals not seek payment from patients or their insurance companies for the following serious preventable adverse events if the hospital deems the event was preventable:
- Surgery on a wrong body part
- Surgery on the wrong patient
- Wrong surgical procedure
- Unintended retention of a foreign object
- Patient death or serious disability associated with an air embolism that occurs while being treated in a health care facility
- Patient death or serious disability associated with a medication error
- Patient death or serious disability associated with a hemolytic reaction due to administration of ABO/HLA incompatible blood or blood products
- Artificial insemination with the wrong donor sperm or wrong egg
- Infant discharged to the wrong person
- Death or serious disability (kernicterus) associated with failure to identify and treat hyperbilirubinemia in neonates
- Patient death or serious disability associated with a burn incurred from any source while being cared for in a health care facility

Source: Data from Tennessee Hospitals & Health Systems. (2008). *THA develops nonpayment policy on serious adverse events*. Nashville, TN: Tennessee Hospital Association.

Our Reality Is Changing Whether We Want It To or Not!

Safety and access to health care are two enormous issues our country is facing. Yet another enormous change is occurring throughout society as we move from the Industrial Age into the Information Age. In fact, the Information Age has arrived and the Industrial Age is quickly dying.

Many of us are still stuck in the Industrial Age that is replete with patriarchal systems and huge health care system dinosaurs dominated by administrators heavily committed to the bottom line as first priority with no understanding of the care side (patients and what patients need) of health care. These administrators think nothing of cutting costs by cutting nursing budgets (they are the largest budget in most facilities) and by cutting registered nurses (RNs). These administrators do not have a clue what they have done. When the bottom line is the first priority, the organization will eventually fail and go out of business. This is happening.

Let's examine what happens when RNs or nursing budgets are cut. Presently, nurses are dissatisfied with their work. Studies have shown that the dissatisfaction rate is *four times greater* for hospital nurses than all other U.S. workers (Aiken, Clarke, Sloane, Sochalski, & Silber, 2002). Dissatisfaction is related to the high patient-to-nurse ratios. A poll of RNs by the American Nurses Association (ANA, 2008) revealed that *close to half* of the respondents are considering leaving their job due to inadequate staffing.

- 73% of nurses asked don't believe the staffing on their unit or shift is sufficient.
- 59.8% of those asked said they knew of someone who left direct care nursing due to concerns about safe staffing.
- Of the 51.9% of respondents who are considering leaving their current position, 46% cite inadequate staffing as the reason.
- 51.7% of respondents said they thought the quality of nursing care on their unit has declined in the last year.
- 48.2% would not feel confident having someone close to them receiving care in the facility where they work (American Nurse Association, 2008).

Others have shown that improving the work environment for nurses can lead to improved job satisfaction and increased patient satisfaction as well as enhanced patient safety (Dunton, Gajewski, Klaus, & Pierson, 2007; Vanhey, Aiken, Sloane, Clarke, & Vargas, 2004).

Research supports the issue of inadequate staffing. Aiken et al. (2002) showed that *nurse staffing ratios are linked to quality of care and patient outcomes*. Adding one additional patient to the nurse assignment increases the likelihood by 7% for patient death within 30 days of hospital admission.

Research compiled from the National Database of Nursing Quality Indicators looked at the nursing environment and characteristics in relation to patient outcomes. This research concluded that multiple factors, including nurse staffing, percentage of RN staff, and RN years of experience, impact patient safety and nurse-sensitive outcomes. For instance, the incidence of hospital-acquired pressure ulcers *decreased* with a more experienced staff along with having a higher percent of RNs caring for the patient (Dunton et al., 2007).

IOM (2004b) supports the following data in their report *Keeping Patients Safe: Transforming the Work Environment of Nurses*:

> Leaner nurse staffing is associated with increased length of stay, nosocomial infection (urinary tract infection, postoperative infection, and pneumonia), and pressure ulcers. …
> These studies… taken together, provide substantial evidence that richer nurse staffing is associated with better patient outcomes.… Greater numbers of patient deaths are associated with fewer nurses to provide care.… and less nursing time provided to patients is

associated with higher rates of infection, gastrointestinal bleeding, pneumonia, cardiac arrest, and death from these and other causes.... In caring for us all, nurses are indispensable to our safety (p. 3).

Other supporting studies are finding similar outcomes. One meta-analysis worth reviewing was published by the Agency for Healthcare Research and Quality (Kane, Shamliyan, Mueller, Duvai, & Witt, 2007), finding strong evidence that higher RN hours per patient day related to lower complication rates and lower mortality.

Based on these data, the ANA is calling for support of the Registered Nurse Safe Staffing Act that would create reliable nurse staffing levels. The ANA believes that managing the RN-to-patient ratio improves job satisfaction and patient outcomes. Nurses' dissatisfaction claiming that staffing is often inadequate is supported by the research and is linked to less than satisfactory patient outcomes. Yet this is only the tip of the iceberg. IOM (2004b) in *Keeping Patients Safe: Transforming the Work Environment of Nurses* notes the following (**Exhibit 4–5**):

- **Loss of trust in hospital administration is widespread among nursing staff.**... This loss of trust stems in part from a perception that initiatives in patient care and nursing work redesign have emphasized efficiency over patient safety.... Poor communication practices have also led to mistrust.
- **Clinical nursing leadership has been reduced at multiple levels, and the voice of nurses in patient care has diminished.** Hospital reengineering initiatives often have resulted in the loss of a separate department of nursing.... At the same time, nursing staff have perceived a decline in chief nursing executives with power and authority equal to that of other top hospital officials, as well as in directors of nursing who are highly visible and accessible to staff.... These changes— along with losses of chief nursing officers without replacement; decreases in the numbers of nurse managers; and increased responsibilities for remaining nurse managers for more than one patient care unit, as well as for supervising personnel other than nursing staff...—have had the cumulative effect of reducing direct management support available to patient care staff. This situation hampers nurses' ability to fix problems in their work environments that threaten patient safety (p. 4).

We have a LOT of work to do!!

There are additional complications caused by this new reality, the Information Age. In the midst of not having enough staff, time has become more compressed, so time passes more quickly. Have you noticed that you do not seem to have as much time? This just exacerbates the staffing issues.

Exhibit 4–5 IOM Notes Negative Quality/Patient Safety Effects of Work Redesign

- Loss of trust in hospital administration
- Work redesign emphasized efficiency over patient safety
- Loss of a separate department of nursing
- Decline in nurse executives with the power and authority equal to the rest of the executive team
- Decrease in the number of nurse managers
- Remaining nurse managers have responsibility for more than one unit

Source: Data from Institute of Medicine. (2004). *Keeping patients safe: Transforming the work environment of nurses.* Washington, DC: The National Academies Press.

Along with not having enough time, suddenly there is too much information in our reality, and the way we perceive information has changed. The question is not necessarily how much information we can learn, retain, and use. Instead, it is how well we can access the needed information. Baby boomers are having difficulty with this reality, but the newer generations are already experiencing and living it. Health care systems are moving to highly integrated computer systems, a costly venture.

So the Information Age has brought about more technology to purchase and to learn how to use. As health care monies are curtailed or cut, we have computer systems that cannot talk to one another (they are not integrated), purchased information systems quickly become obsolete, and information system companies fold and leave us holding the bag. Yet, if we want prompt payment, we must use a computerized system to report care given, and the current movement for patient safety involves many necessary technological purchases. Then, to add insult to injury, the government insisted that we meet Health Insurance Portability and Accountability Act of 1996 (explained in Chapter 9) requirements while keeping down health care costs with the Balanced Budget Act. The dilemma is that all these technology purchases need to be made at a time when reimbursements are curtailed.

Technology has brought about other significant care changes. Porter-O'Grady (2003) observes the following:

> The technology of the time is quickly moving the health professions into a context where the kind of therapies that will be used require less mechanical and manual intervention and a greater use of other innovative approaches. This transition makes it possible to treat illness at an earlier stage and either eliminate or alter the need for more mechanical (surgical) interventions that are more intensive and costly. It is quickly becoming a time of ending for the health care system as we know it. Furthermore, it is the end of the Newtonian, 20th century medical and nursing practice, and other health-related practices, as those disciplines have historically understood them (p. 62).

All of us in the health professions are facing new realities. Health care administrators can choose whether to respond to this new reality, working to change behaviors and practices, or can choose to continue with the same patriarchal practices of old. The former results in an enhanced, more satisfying health care environment for both patients and for health care workers. The latter is outdated, and eventually the organization will dissolve.

Porter-O'Grady and Malloch (2007) stated as follows:

> What one does and what difference it makes are the key issues for all providers. If an organization provides 1,000 services and only 25 make a difference, then the other 975 services must be considered for elimination—even if the 975 services have billing codes that render them reimbursable.
>
> Provider accountability for contributions to patient care outcomes is a missing piece of health care. All professional care providers must focus their actions on achieving desired outcomes and implement only interventions that have a basis in science or a realistic chance of benefiting patients.
>
> The measurement of health care outcomes is gradually becoming more meaningful and reflective of patient needs. Unfortunately, indicators are often looked at in an order that fails to take into account the basic goal of health care—health improvement. For example, productivity measures are typically examined prior to clinical outcomes. If productivity targets are exceeded, increases in productivity are mandated without consideration of their potential impact on care provision (p. 387).

The new information age requires different approaches and perspectives:

> Moving into a new age does not mean leaving everything behind. It does mean thinking
> about what needs to be left behind and reflecting on what does go with us as we move into
> an age with a different set of parameters (Porter-O'Grady & Malloch, 2003, p. 10).

We are facing many significant changes that affect the care we give, the systems that are in place to deliver care, and even the present perspectives we have on the world in general. It is easy to be complacent and not pay attention to the changes. However, they are all around us:

> This is the beginning of the end of nursing care as we have all become accustomed to provid-
> ing and using.... The hospital-based, sickness-oriented, late-stage model of nursing service
> delivery is no longer either appropriate or prevailing. Nurses now must determine what tradi-
> tional practices and functions are no longer relevant or sustainable and let them go. At the
> same time, nurses must discern what is emerging on the practice horizon that must now
> become increasingly a part of nursing practice. Influences like genomics, nano-therapy,
> fiberoptics, pharmacotherapeutics, virtual care models, early-stage interventions, patient man-
> aged delivery, [alternative therapies], etc. are now pressing on the periphery of the profession
> and will dominate nursing adaptation for the next 2 decades (Porter-O'Grady, 2003, p. 62).

The only constant in our present reality is that it will change. We are at a crossroads. We can lament what we are losing, or have lost, or we can look around us for clues as to what we might expect and begin to design where we need to go next. Because we are all in the health care box, some of these changes are hard to perceive because they are outside our view of reality.

In addition to the traditional nursing role changing, our leadership roles are changing. The choice is, do we remain stuck in our past or can we move into an exciting, more fulfilling, unknown future? We have an opportunity to create our new reality. It is up to us as we respond to each situation as we go through the day. This is an exciting, challenging time when we, as nurse professionals and as nurse (or health care) administrators, can be forging new roles that better fit the new realities, encouraging staff to do the same.

Last, but perhaps most important, the new reality is that the relationship is very important— starting with listening to our patients and involving them in their care (see below), talking with each other about this change, mourning the loss of the familiar environment but welcoming the opportunity to get closer to the patient (our present system has pulled the nurse from the bedside where housekeeping staff see the patient more than the nurse), and where we will thrive only if we are able to constantly value the people we serve *and* the people on our team.

> The work of the time for the clinical leader is helping colleagues and patients end their
> attachment to the kind of health care system they have grown comfortable with. So many
> nurses are mourning the loss of something they think should not have passed or should be
> retained. Many nurses are mourning the loss of those very practices, sentiments, or roles
> that brought them to nursing in the first place. Some even wish those traditions would
> return. The truth is that most of what is being mourned should neither be retained nor pro-
> tected. Neither the times nor yesterday's circumstances will return, nor should they....
> Those ideals that brought many of us to nursing (enough time for good care, long stays,
> detailed care processes, residential models of care, heavy emphasis on manual procedures,
> compliant and passive patient roles, etc.) no longer exist. The question is not will these
> processes return but instead: *what is nursing now becoming and how must I adapt?*

> A major role of the clinical leader in this day and time is engaging others around the real-
> ity of their own change. Complacency at this time of radical shifting is a strategy that

guarantees failure. The leader must take whatever action is necessary to impress upon those he or she leads that this is a time of great mobility and shifting foundations (Porter-O'Grady, 2003, p. 62).

So Where Do We Start?

> No problem can be solved from the same consciousness that created it. We must learn to see the world anew.
>
> *—Albert Einstein*

Reframing Our View of the World

In the Information Age, the locus of control is shifting from the provider to the patient. Yet many of us still act as though we, the provider, have the locus of control. We do things to patients without consulting them. Many of us do not take the time to find out what our patients want and expect. Yet the Information Age is here, and our old world is disintegrating and, if we cling to it, will lead to obsolescence. It will disappear. We can mourn and moan and complain, but this will not change reality. Our world has changed.

Perhaps a better response is to look around and observe what is happening so quickly. There are opportunities all around us. Patients have access to more information about their care yet need our help in translating the meaning of various options available to them when they experience dis-ease. At the same time they are turning to health and healthier lifestyles so they can live longer and avoid disease. Treatments are less invasive. Nurses have an advantage in this environment because, although we learn about disease and how it is treated, we also learn about prevention and health. And in health care organizations, we are with patients/residents far more than the physician, who quickly comes by to see patients and then is gone. Our interpersonal skills are valued by these patients because we are more likely to listen and to help. So, for us, moving into this new age is not as difficult as it is for the physician who is mainly into disease and what medications to prescribe to deal with disease.

Nurses also have a lot to offer to bottom-line health care administrators who do not understand the care side unless they experience disease, at which point their perspective often dramatically shifts to a new appreciation of the care side and of what nurses have to offer. We can help them in this shift, because we are closer to the patient and can bring that perspective to the table now that the locus of control is shifting from the provider to the patient. One purpose of this book is to aid nurse administrators to express what is needed, using more numbers so linear administrators will be more likely to listen.

Porter-O'Grady and Malloch (2007) stress the importance of increasing the focus on patients:

> It is no secret that the locus of control for health care services should be the patient, not the provider. Yet in spite of all the efforts to create patient-focused care delivery systems, few patients would agree that they are in fact the focus of services or in control of anything. In explanation, they could cite facts such as these:
>
> - Providers continue to prescribe treatments without discussion with the patients.
> - Visiting hours are still in effect.
> - Appointment times for services are based on Monday through Friday schedules.
> - Patient procedures and their scheduled times are determined by providers without input from patients or families (p. 393).

Hopefully, as you read this you can begin to think of the many ways that we can change how health care services are provided—ways that are much more effective and that involve the patient in all the care decisions. This leads us to something that we need to make the top priority as we give care: *finding out what the patient wants and what the patient values.*

Our First Priority: What Does the *Patient* Want and Value Anyway?

Value, from the patient's perspective, is a very important issue. Sometimes patients believe that the health care provider does not listen, nor care about listening to, what the patient actually wants or needs. The old paternalistic medical model—we'll just tell you what is best for you—is outdated, is resented, and no longer applies to most patients. Patients often feel depersonalized, experience long waits, and, worse yet, receive substandard care, as already discussed in Exhibit 4–2—especially if they are in a lower socioeconomic group or if they are a racial or ethnic minority.

Porter-O'Grady and Malloch (2007) discuss the change in the patient–provider relationship:

- Patients now determine the parameters of the patient-provider relationship, setting the stage for a different kind of interaction than has historically occurred.

- Patients need to develop partnerships with providers to sort through the available choices and pick the best. They need providers to act as educators who are willing to assist them in making health care decisions.

- Patients need help from providers both in verifying the accuracy of the data they have independently garnered from a host of sources and in interpreting the data.

- Patients are interested in options, not an order to undergo a particular treatment. They want to be able to consider a range of options within the context of their own personal values and priorities and choose the one option that best fits these.

- Providers now need to be concerned with what patients know and can do with regard to controlling their own health decisions in a "user-driven" world. Providers must now transfer skills to others and surrender ownership of care to others (p. 17).

It is important for the nurse manager to constantly be thinking, "*What does the patient want and value?*"— along with "*safety, safety, safety,*" "*quality, quality, quality,*" yet "*cost effectiveness, cost effectiveness, cost effectiveness.*" The nurse manager can help to make sure the services provided are only the ones that are valuable to the patients. And the expectation is that staff at the point of care are thinking the same thing. This is a change for most of us who are used to providing care with no thought given to consider the *patient's* perspective.

So far **we have not found what the patient wants and values, and there are no outcome measurements that can tell us how successfully we have accomplished this goal**. Instead, our measurements are patient satisfaction scores, complications that may have occurred, financial ratios, and/or staffing or turnover numbers—none of which tells us what the patient wanted and if the patient got it.

We administrators are not alone in needing to make this change in perspective. All staff, the board, the executive team, and physicians need to learn to think this way. Everyone has to get into the act of talking with each patient and listening to what he or she has to say. After all, everyone contributes to achieving this goal, and we can always do better. Paying attention to what the patient values as *first priority*, with safety and quality second, helps us to make better decisions, be more effective, and save a lot of money and risk to the patient. It will have a positive impact on the bottom line as well. Everyone wins!

Values pivot on the circumstances at hand and whose point of view is considered. Patient perceptions, and what the patient wants, are more important than what we believe the patient *should* want when determining quality indicators. Once we have determined what evidence-based care (see Chapter 5) might be necessary for a specific patient (after we have found out this is what the patient wants), there is still more to do. We need to then offer the patient choices in specific remedies and therapies that fall under that evidence-based care rubric, being sure he or she is fully informed. We presently fail in health care delivery because we often consider what we would want instead of consulting the patient and finding out the patient's wishes.

Value has another implication. We all must understand the importance of including our patients in the decision-making process. The patient has to be involved in deciding what services will be provided. Such a challenge! Or, let's change the way we think about this. Such an opportunity! It is exciting to be part of the cutting edge of true health care, based on what has value for the patient. This is a pivotal point that will change health care as we know it.

The Consumer-Driven Health Care Institute (n.d.) is working to promote policy that empowers individuals to make decisions about their health care, advocating the following:

- Consumers will work with their physicians and health care providers to create a better health care outcome for themselves and their families.
- Health care usage is more cost efficient with empowered and knowledgeable consumers who use information tools.
- Price and quality transparency about health care professionals is a key method for effective consumer health care choices.

Transparency means that we share everything. (And even if we did not share, the Internet provides all sorts of information, and CMS provides information available to the general public, including facility quality ratings.) We cannot stop the tide—information is out there. Some of the information is helpful and excellent; some is erroneous and misleading. We can help patients appropriately sift through this so they can make the best decisions. (Chapter 5 discusses how to find health care information and how to evaluate it.)

So the first issue is to find out what the patient values, or really wants, and then provide this service in a loving, patient-centered way. An important part of our administrative role is to pay attention to, and promote, ways the health care team can *reframe* their work to better achieve each patient's goals. This is complicated because it is a new concept for all of us in health care.

Paying attention to value (and quality and safety) puts us in an interesting dilemma. Value, quality, and safety are those elusive things that we never totally achieve. Yet we need to constantly improve what we do. Why should we spend so much time and effort striving to achieve them? When we believe that we have done our best, we achieve our most satisfying work experiences. When excellent, safe care is delivered, and the patient has valued the service, everyone on the health care team feels good about his or her work, and, most importantly, the patient benefits by experiencing the best we can offer.

Another trap we can get into is to say that because we have inadequate resources, there is no way we can make improvements. Nurses cannot be assigned to as many patients if they have to be listening to what the patients want and value, and there is a nursing shortage. If we say this, and do not even try to do anything, bemoaning the fact that with shortages and with reimbursements not being as high as they should be that we cannot do anything, then nothing happens. We need to throw away this crutch (the excuse of inadequate resources) and instead *ask* how we can make a difference. Then we must go about figuring out how to accomplish it.

After all, if we cannot figure out a way to do things better, someone else will. Take the freestanding surgery centers, for example. They can do some of the same surgery procedures at less cost than the hospital. Yes, it is partly because the overhead is cheaper in a surgery center. So why does overhead in a hospital have to be so much higher??

We need to be creative and encourage all staff and physicians to be creative, thinking about our present practices and evaluating which ones we need to change. Are limited visiting hours really necessary? Why are all procedures scheduled Monday through Friday? In fact, consumer groups are advocating *not* having procedures scheduled on Friday because if anything happens staff are limited over the weekend to deal with patient complications. If a patient has an acute episode on Friday evening, why does the patient have to wait for most services until Monday? Question, question, question everything we are doing!

Have you noticed that we have not said much about quality and safety in this section? We get to these issues because they are very important as we deliver services the patient values. But first we wanted to emphasize listening to the patient and supporting the patient to make the treatment decisions, once he or she has all the information.

The Healing Relationship

The IOM advocates, "Care is based on continuous healing relationships" (2001, p. 3). At times in this chapter we have mentioned "loving" care. Love is necessary for healing. By love, we mean a caring relationship. Jean Watson examined the relationship between caring and curing in her book, *Postmodern Nursing and Beyond* (2004). Here she examines both the technical side of nursing and the holistic side more traditionally associated with caring. Over the years there has been a lot of emphasis on the caring component of nursing practice.

Another excellent resource is *Radical Loving Care: Building the Healing Hospital in America* by Erie Chapman (2004). He makes the connection between loving and healing, stressing the importance of listening to the patient. This means that as we listen to each patient, we read between the lines. The physical diagnosis may not be the most important issue for the patient. Instead, we should find out what the patient values and provide this when possible.

He emphasizes not seeing a patient as a stranger but as a brother or sister. He encourages us to see that what the patient needs goes beyond the physical needs to the emotions behind it. Significant life changes may be thrust upon a patient. Pain may be occurring, and pain is a lonely experience. "Radical loving care" is about making a significant connection with each patient. It is a trinity that one wants to have present in a health care organization: The Golden Thread (the loving thread that connects us), The Sacred Encounter (each time we interact with a patient), and The Servant's Heart (we are serving others). It is so important that we included *heart* in the title of this book!

> Loving care has a long and beautiful tradition in human history. In these pages the heritage of loving care is symbolized by the image of a Golden Thread, which is also a symbol of faith in God. It represents the positive tradition of healing versus the negative tradition of transaction-based behavior (Chapman, 2004, p. 10).

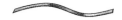

> A second symbol, a pair of intersecting circles, signifies the merging of love and need in the Sacred Encounter, which is the fundamental relationship between caregiver and patient. This symbol also signifies hope—the hope that comes into our hearts when we experience loving encounters (Chapman, 2004, p. 10).

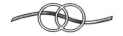

The third symbol, a red heart, signifies the nature of the Servant's Heart. It also symbolizes love and is love's greatest expression. This expression, although it specifically references the heart, assumes the full involvement of our best thought processes. Loving care is not loving if it fails to engage the best skills and competency of caregivers (Chapman, 2004, p. 10).

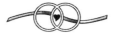

Cultural Diversity

Another value factor is cultural diversity. We are increasingly seeing a worldwide crossover of people and cultures. Here in the United States, "the non-Hispanic, white population...would comprise just 50.1 percent of the total population in 2050, compared with 69.4 percent in 2000" (U.S. Census Bureau, 2007). It is not uncommon to see Spanish-speaking television stations or to buy something and have the instructions be given in several languages.

This diversity constitutes a new perspective toward not only culturally diverse patients, but also toward culturally diverse staff. We are often unaware of specific cultural beliefs, values, and life ways and may, inadvertently, tread on those beliefs and practices. Like patient safety, there is room for improvement.

As health care professionals, it is important to recognize the wonderful differences that exist between different cultures, and we support these cultural beliefs. It is important to educate all staff about cultural differences and have systems in place that encourage everyone to respect and give radical loving care to each person based on that person's cultural beliefs. Alexander (2002) recommends that this needs to "include the following core components: cultural/racial/ethnic identity, language/communication ability and style, religious beliefs and practices, illness and wellness behaviors, and healing beliefs and practices" (p. 32).

We have a lot of work to do to achieve better cultural understanding. There are some good references available. The following describe different cultures and give a description of how nursing care needs to differ depending on a person's ethnic, cultural, or regional background:

- Giger and Davidhizar's book, *Transcultural Nursing: Assessment and Intervention*
- St. Hill, Lipson, and Meleis's book, *Caring for Women Cross-Culturally*
- Purnell and Paulanka's book, *Transcultural Health Care: A Culturally Competent Approach*
- Culhane-Pera, Vawter, Xiong, Babbitt, and Solberg's book, *Healing by Heart: Clinical and Ethical Case Stories of Hmong Families and Western Providers*

These books are a must read. They provide information that is unknown to many health care providers.

Can you see how many of us are ethnocentric in giving care to clients when we do not find out what clients value? And when we do not take the time to learn about their cultural or ethnic differences? As we give care based on cultural differences, it affects nutrition, family functioning, lifestyle differences, spiritual or religious differences, biological variations, the way one relates to both health and disease, communication issues, differences in locus of control, differences in views about independence versus collectivism, and socioeconomic realities.

Another cultural difference is between physicians, nurses, and nonclinical administrators. Physicians learn right from medical school that they are autonomous, independent (although this is changing with group practices), and it is easy for some to be autocratic and domineering because they never learned about teamwork and collaboration. Nurses can often feel they are in a one-down position in a hierarchy of importance, because administrators tend to give more importance to the physicians and tend to give physicians more of what they want. When all come from the same core values and work together to provide care for patients (see Chapter 3), these differences can be overcome. When the administration does not support core values and gives too much autonomy to physicians, disruptive physician behaviors may be allowed to continue, creating a less effective work environment. Care can be compromised when this occurs.

Gender cultural differences are discussed in Chapter 3.

This cultural diversity section, obviously, could be a whole book, because there are so many cultural differences surrounding us every day. It is of the utmost importance that cultural differences are recognized and respected within our health care system and that each person receives loving care specific to his or her expectations.

Patient and Family Advisory Councils

One way to find out what patients want and need is to have focus groups with patients and families. For example, Pointe et al. (2003) established two Patient and Family Advisory Councils, one for pediatrics and one for adults. It probably would be helpful to establish one for the elderly as well.

> At Dana-Farber Cancer Institute in Boston, we have been engaged for more than 5 years in a process of rethinking and redesigning many of our most critical operations in order to integrate the voices of patients and families into virtually everything we do. Although this work is far from complete, we believe we have made significant progress in crafting a new paradigm of care: one that places the patient and family in an entirely new position within the organization's operational and care structures.... By working through the councils, the voices of patients and families are blended with those of clinicians, administrators, and other staff as the processes and systems of care are designed and delivered. Patients provide input on organizational policies, are placed on continuous improvement teams, and are invited to join search committees and develop educational programming for staff. Members of the councils also sit on the Joint Committee on Quality Improvement and Risk Management, a board-level committee that approves the institute's quality improvement plan, evaluates outcomes of quality improvement activities, and reviews reports regarding sentinel events.

> Creating this level of integration requires important preliminary work within the organization. There must be a shared understanding of the critical components of patient-centered care. There must be strong advocacy for the concept at the highest levels of the administrative leadership team. And there must be in place a strong, interdisciplinary work team, for it is premature to think about integrating patients and families into a team if the underpinnings of effective teamwork are not yet in place (pp. 82–83).

Focus groups or patient advisory councils can be very beneficial in determining what the patients and families value related to health care. Many organizations find focus groups to be valuable in addition to other forms of feedback. Consumers Advancing Patient Safety has a step-by-step guide with examples on how to partner with patient groups to enhance value and safety (Leonhardt, Bonin, & Pagel, 2007). Go to http://www.patientsafety.org for more information.

Replace Patient Compliance with What the Patient Wants and Values

Because we have been defining what has value to the patient, the phrase "patient compliance" must be eliminated from our health care dictionary The term is a throwback to the patriarchal medical system. It assumes that we know better than the patient what is good for the patient. Because of the negative connotation, many now use the term "adherence" instead of compliance. In fact, the patient has a choice and may be making the "noncompliant" decisions for good reasons or may lack the knowledge needed to make good decisions. Consider these findings:

- Only 73% of patients filled their prescriptions within 1 week of leaving the hospital. Patients filled 82% of their heart-related prescriptions and only 35% of those not related to the heart (Jackevicius, Li, & Tu, 2008).
- Only 60% of patients discharged from the hospital filled their prescriptions within 2 days. Patients reported difficulties in understanding why they needed the medications, concerns about costs, transportation challenges, and wait times as reasons for noncompliance (Kripalani, Henderson, Jacobson, & Vaccarino, 2008).
- The Mayo Clinical published a study finding that only 86% of patients recently discharged from the hospital realized they had been prescribed new medications. Of those, only 22% could name at least one adverse effect (Maniaci, Heckman, & Dawson, 2008).

Why are patients noncompliant? Think of all the side effects that can occur with medications. Some say that their doctors have ordered a drug—for instance, a steroid—and they know that they have such bad side effects they don't want to take the medication. Maybe being "noncompliant" is smart and safer!

Health literacy has come to light as a problem that influences patient adherence to recommended treatment. The U.S. Department of Health and Human Services (n.d.) defines health literacy as the "degree to which individuals have the capacity to obtain, process, and understand basic health information and services needed to make appropriate health decisions." This includes their basic reading levels. Poor health literacy is associated with poor health outcomes. The IOM reported that 90 million people in America "have difficulty understanding and acting upon health information" (2004a, p. 1). Inability to understand medical language and printed instructions certainly impacts ability to follow recommended treatments. Clear communication in plain language is imperative. How do we know when our patient education is understood?

Another noncompliance issue is the cost of our services. Still using medications as an example, I can't help but think of a scenario recently observed in the local pharmacy. An elderly woman was talking to the pharmacist. He had just told her that her medications were $568. She said, "I am on a fixed income. I don't have that much money." He said, "Well, your doctor insists on not using generic medications so there is nothing I can do to bring the cost down." What they finally agreed to do was for her to pay for a week's worth of medications and wait for her next Social Security check. I wondered, if she used the Social Security check for the medications, how she was going to pay for the other necessities, such as eating for the month. I'm sure the physician thought that the generic medications were not as effective. However, was the physician really taking into account the value question, that is, this woman's situation? Should the pharmacist have called the physician to discuss the possibility of using generic drugs to save costs for the client? And even if generic drugs were used, can this woman afford to buy the medications and still have food and a roof over her head? Were *all* these drugs necessary? Do the drugs really have to cost so much?

There are larger societal issues adding to the problem of noncompliance. Think of how difficult it is for many patients to get back in to see their doctors when they experience problems. Additionally, they are charged for another office visit. If they need to be transferred to a specialist, in a health maintenance organization system they may or may not be able to get beyond the gatekeeper to get the care they need. So the public deals with these issues by being noncompliant by reading the Internet and other literature on health and on their illnesses—sometimes being better informed than we are—and by turning to alternative medicine. Perhaps the most important adherence issue is that we forget that patients have the right to make choices.

It is so important to discuss treatments, including medications, with patients. We need to do a better job of patient (and family) education. We must encourage the patient (and family) to ask questions and to understand how to best deal with health problems. Nurses need to have time to do this activity and to be expected to teach patients in ways the patients understand. Once we have thrown out the patient compliance patriarchal system, we need to replace it with what the patient wants and values.

The Quality Dimension

Now let's turn to quality (but please remember that what the patient wants and values comes first!). Aside from listening to the patient and involving the patient in making the decisions about treatments and care, from the patient value perspective, quality (including safety) is very important. When we are effective in the quality arena, our every decision and every action strive to provide the care that is needed in the safest, most effective way. But what exactly is quality?

In this chapter, we take a fundamentally different perspective in defining quality and what quality is really all about. Quality has many definitions. Quality can mean different things to different people. The IHI defines quality care in terms of meeting each of the IOM's 10 rules. The Joint Commission defines quality in terms of meeting prescribed standards. Standards and scope of practice legally define our practice as well (see Chapter 8 on Legal Issues). CMS defines quality as the percentage of patients that receive the recommended interventions defined in the guidelines. Many organizations have chosen to identify quality indicators that can be measured and compared. Chapter 16 defines how to actually measure quality where metrics capture how well these measures have been achieved. This provides an overall balanced scorecard approach organizationally.

The definition of quality has been inadequate. In fact, most of it has not considered the patient's perspective but relies heavily on the health care professional's perspective, or that of the payer or regulator. We have forgotten the most important person in the equation—our *patient*, our *client*, our *resident*. Frequently, the health care professional never consulted the patient to find out what the patient wanted, needed, or valued. Perhaps this is captured in the definition in the book, *Through the Patients' Eyes* (Gerteis, Edgman-Levitan, Daley, & Delbanco, 1993):

> Quality…has two dimensions. One has to do with technical excellence: the skill and competence of professionals and the ability of diagnostic or therapeutic equipment, procedures, and systems to accomplish what they are meant to accomplish, reliably and effectively. Borrowing the language and conceptual models of industrial engineering, we speak in this sense of "quality control," "quality assurance," and "quality improvement."
>
> The other dimension is related to subjective experience—its texture and substance, its sentient quality. In this sense, we speak of the quality of a sensation or experience or the quality of human relationships. In health care, it is quality in this subjective dimension that patients experience most directly—in their perception of illness or well-being and in their encounters with health care professionals and institutions (p. xi).

The IOM (2001) has recommended that for this new century we commit to six goals for improvement that will change this perspective to what the patient wants and values:

> Advances must begin with all health care constituencies—health professionals, federal and state policy makers, public and private purchasers of care, regulators, organization managers and governing boards, and consumers—committing to a national statement of

purpose for the health care system as a whole. In making this commitment, the parties would accept as their explicit purpose "to continually reduce the burden of illness, injury, and disability, and to improve the health and functioning of the people of the United States." The parties also would adopt a shared vision of six specific aims for improvement. These aims are built around the core need for health care to be:

- Safe: avoiding injuries to patients from the care that is intended to help them.
- Effective: providing services based on scientific knowledge to all who could benefit, and reframing from providing services to those not likely to benefit.
- Patient-centered: providing care that is respectful of and responsive to individual patient preferences, needs, and values, and ensuring that patient values guide all clinical decisions.
- Timely: reducing waits and sometimes harmful delays for both those who receive and those who give care.
- Efficient: avoiding waste, including waste of equipment, supplies, ideas, and energy. [Efficiency is discussed in Chapter 6, Workload Management, with additional information in Chapter 17, Budget Strategies.]
- Equitable: providing care that does not vary in quality because of personal characteristics such as gender, ethnicity, geographic location, and socioeconomic status.

A health care system that achieves major gains in these six areas would be far better at meeting patient needs. Patients would experience care that is safer, more reliable, more responsible to their needs, more integrated, and more available, and they could count on receiving the full array of preventive, acute, and chronic services that are likely to prove beneficial. Clinicians and other health workers also would benefit through their increased satisfaction at being better able to do their jobs and thereby bring improved health, greater longevity, less pain and suffering, and increased personal productivity to those who receive their care (pp. 2–3).

Patient-*centered* means listening to each patient. The patient might value something entirely different from the care we are providing. What do patients value? It is best to ask them. Often, patients value different things at different times. For instance, when a patient is in critical condition, the patient wants a highly skilled, prompt, technologically advanced, yet kind caregiver, whereas a nonacute patient wants a rapid turnaround with a kind, personable caregiver. But it is more than that. The answer to the value question depends on how the patient defines quality of life.

Evidence-Based Practice

When examining quality, one must ask if we are giving the most appropriate, up-to-date care. Research has shown that both physicians and nurses plan care and treatment based on what was done when they graduated from school, even if that was 20 years ago. In addition, we may not know what is best for a certain individual with a particular need. We need to have access to the latest research on that problem, and/or treatment of the problem, and use that information to determine the most appropriate treatment approach. Evidence-based practice is a synthesis of research and clinical expertise demonstrated to be successful that result in a plan of care specific to particular conditions. This is where the information highway is important. However, there is so much information that knowing where to find it, evaluating what is found so that we are taking the best, or most appropriate, research, and applying it in practice is more challenging than it sounds. That is why we devoted Chapter 5 to finding and evaluating information.

The Internet and technology systems are wonderful resources. For instance, there is a lot of research currently available on patient outcomes. As a physician or nurse practitioner writes a medication order, he or she may not know which of several drugs might be most effective. Evidence-based decision support systems are now available that quickly point to the best available research for specific topics. These systems also provide evidence-based plans of care and therapy recommendations. Zynx Health is one system that distributes this service.

Why is evidence-based practice so important? Only 15% of the nursing workforce consistently implements practice based on evidence (Shirey, 2006). One big problem is that nurses and providers do not realize how easily information can be accessed or do not take the time to look up the current research results. Many lack the skills to translate research knowledge into practice. Getting the information is just the first step.

Administratively, we must encourage evidence-based practice by removing barriers to access and by setting the expectation that practice must be based on current evidence. To help close the gap between what is known as evidence and what is practiced, a national consensus committee has convened, identifying appropriate competencies for basic, advanced, and doctoral level nursing education. Use of competencies to evaluate and build nursing skills is essential in promoting practice based on evidence. Kathleen Stevens and team developed the ACE Star Model of Knowledge Transformation that provides a framework for moving research study findings to bedside practice, creating a positive impact on health outcomes. Check out the model and find more about evidence-based competencies at Academic Center for Evidence-Based Practice (2007) website (http://www.acestar.uthscsa.edu).

Additionally, as administrators and leaders, we must use evidence to guide our leadership and management practices. This is why Chapter 5 is named Pinpointing Evidence-Based Information, because it has included many additional websites that provide good resources for the nurse administrator as well as the best sites for clinical information.

CLINICAL PATHWAYS/PROTOCOLS

Evidence-based practice can be achieved by using clinical pathways, order sets, or clinical protocols when delivering care, as long as the pathways or protocols are kept up to date. An effective clinical pathway is the result of interdisciplinary teamwork; the team includes the physician, nurse, social worker, dietitian, and patient and may include other members such as chaplain or nurse aide or significant family members. Protocols that physicians have agreed on can automatically be implemented without an order. The only caution to clinical pathways is that all caregivers continue to take into account patient idiosyncrasies or differences that might change the pathway.

Performance Improvement

The question is always are we doing our best as a total organization in achieving quality? Of course, the answer is always that we could do better. All organizations need performance improvement to examine current quality and safety issues as well as to identify opportunities to enhance quality. It is a proactive process, meaning that everyone not only identifies problems but has suggestions for improvements. Performance improvement may have been implemented with varying success by many health care organizations and businesses.

Performance improvement is referred to by various names, such as continuous improvement, continuous quality improvement, and total quality measurement, to name a few. Different methodologies may be used to initiate performance improvement, but many health care organizations use some form of "plan, do, study, act," or PDSA, to address quality improvement. The IHI (n.d., b) outlined a two-part model including a set of questions the organization must answer followed by the PDSA cycle to test the change to determine if improvement was made (**Exhibit 4–6**).

Exhibit 4–6 PDSA Model for Improvement

Questions to answer:

- *What are we trying to accomplish?* Set aims and time specific measurable goals.
- *How will we know that a change is an improvement?* Establish measures, compare with a baseline measure for evaluating results.
- *What changes can we make that will result in improvement?* Brainstorm ideas and test one at a time in a pilot setting. The idea is to fine-tune the process before fully implementing it across the organization. Prioritize which change should be tried first.

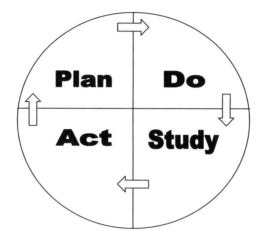

Plan the test of change. Activities, actions, task, or process step.
Do implement the change.
Study the change results. Is the result or outcome better? Was the defined goal met?
Act keep the change or go back to planning. Is fine-tuning needed or start from scratch? Revisit the fundamental questions.

Source: Adapted from the Institute for Healthcare Improvement. (n.d., b). *How to improve.* Retrieved June 3, 2008 from http://www.ihi.org/IHI/Topics/ChronicConditions/AllConditions/HowToImprove/.

Interestingly, *when performance improvement is effective, it often decreases expenses as well.* Additionally, it produces a more efficient practice that results in increased patient satisfaction and quality.

Changing Our Administrative Practices

The reason for variance in the success of performance improvement programs is that many times there are administrative leadership problems that are not being fixed, that many organizational processes need to be fixed and may negatively impact the success of the performance improvement plan, and that performance improvement is not perceived as being important. This entire book provides solutions to more effectively do our administrative work. For example, first, we need to examine our leadership (see Chapter 2). If that is broken, everything else is too. The IHI put together a free *Leadership Guide to Patient Safety* (2006) that can be downloaded from their website (http://www.ihi.org; you must register to download, but it is free). This is a marvelous resource addressing the top safety issues in health care along with links to resources and tools for improvement (**Exhibit 4–7**).

Second, we need to make sure we do an organizational assessment and learn how to identify and make systems changes effectively (see Chapter 3). Third, we need to know how to find information relating to our administrative work so we remain updated in our administrative practice, as well as encouraging staff and physicians to use these resources (see Chapter 5).

As we are moving into the Information Age, there are many administrative practices that need to be left behind, and there are others that we need to pursue that traditionally have not been part of our role. Porter-O'Grady and Malloch (2007) define what they see as our major administrative tasks in the 21st century:

- Deconstructing the barriers and structures of the 20th Century,
- Alerting staff about the implications of changing what they do,
- Establishing safety around taking risks and experimenting,
- Embracing new technologies as a way of doing work,
- Reading the signposts along the road to the future,
- Translating the emerging reality into language the staff can use,
- Demonstrating personal engagement with the change effort,
- Helping others adapt to the demands of a changing health system,
- Creating a safe milieu for the struggles and pain of change,
- Enumerating small successes as a basis for supporting staff, and
- Celebrating the journey and all progress made (p. 19).

We add the following to this list:

- Are we giving the most appropriate up-to-date care?
- Do our administrative practices reflect the Information Age? Or are we still stuck in the Industrial Age?
- Are we consistently listening to the patient, sharing information with patients, and involving the patient in treatment decisions?

As we really work on accomplishing this list, it is important to always work toward a goal. The importance behind all this gets back to listening to our patients and involving them in their treatment decisions. Perhaps the IOM (2001) provided the best signpost, to date, for us to use as our

---

Exhibit 4–7 Process for Achieving Patient Safety and High Reliability

1. Address strategic priorities, culture, and infrastructure.
2. Engage key stakeholders.
3. Communicate and build awareness.
4. Establish, oversee, and communicate system-level aims.
5. Track/measure performance over time, strengthen analysis.
6. Support staff and patient/families impacted by medical errors.
7. Align system-wide activities and incentives.
8. Redesign systems and improve reliability.

Source: Adapted from the Institute for Healthcare Improvement. (2006). *Leadership guide to patient safety.* Retrieved from http://www.ihi.org/IHI/Results/WhitePapers/LeadershipGuidetoPatientSafetyWhitePaper.htm

ultimate goal. They advocate that we need to redesign our health care delivery systems and recommend 10 rules to achieve this redesign (Please read on and bear with us here. *Redesign* has been so mismanaged in the past we hate to even use the word. The difference here is that this redesign uses all the administrative practices we have been discussing in this book. It is *not* a bottom-line approach to downsize.):

1. *Care is based on continuous healing relationships.* Patients should receive care whenever they need it and in many forms, not just face-to-face visits. This implies that the health care system must be responsive at all times, and access to care should be provided over the Internet, by telephone, and by other means in addition to in-person visits.
2. *Care is customized according to patient needs and values.* The system should be designed to meet the most common types of needs but should have the capability to respond to individual patient choices and preferences.
3. *The patient is the source of control.* Patients should be given the necessary information and opportunity to exercise the degree of control they choose over health care decisions that affect them. The system should be able to accommodate differences in patient preferences and encourage shared decision making.
4. *Knowledge is shared and information flows freely.* Patients should have unfettered access to their own medical information and to clinical knowledge. Clinicians and patients should communicate effectively and share information.
5. *Decision making is evidence-based.* Patients should receive care based on the best available scientific knowledge. Care should not vary illogically from clinician to clinician or from place to place.
6. *Safety is a system property.* Patients should be safe from injury caused by the care system. Reducing risk and ensuring safety require greater attention to systems that help prevent and mitigate errors.
7. *Transparency is necessary.* The system should make available to patients and their families information that enables them to make informed decisions when selecting a health plan, hospital, or clinical practice, or when choosing among alternative treatments. This should include information describing the system's performance on safety, evidence-based practice, and patient satisfaction.
8. *Needs are anticipated.* The system should anticipate patient needs rather than simply react to events.
9. *Waste is continuously decreased.* The system should not waste resources or patient time.
10. *Cooperation among clinicians is a priority.* Clinicians and institutions should actively collaborate and communicate to ensure an appropriate exchange of information and coordination of care (pp. 3–4).

Provider Accountability in the Cost-Quality Dilemma

Can't you hear the linear health care administrator, heavily committed to the bottom line, saying, "Where is the money coming from for all this?" We suggest a couple reframing options. (Remember that we are now in the Information Age and the rules have changed. This bottom-line oriented administrator may not have realized this presently so be patient, but keep on persistently creating the new health care environment.) First, Porter-O'Grady and Malloch (2007) suggest that we should reframe the cost–quality dilemma by asking a value question. "The problem... is how to provide value-based, high-quality care that is affordable and at the same time make money. (This is different from making as much money as possible)" (p. 387).

Given the constraints caused by balanced budget initiatives, leaders are often caught in a cost-quality balancing act and are not always sure how to achieve value-based care.... Perhaps it would be helpful to reframe the quality question as a value question. Value is determined by the three elements of cost, quality, and service. Cost is driven by the available resources....Quality is partly determined by the outcomes of care. Service is a matter of the time and type of care provided. Thus the question becomes: Are health care leaders obligated to provide value-based services to patients and family members? The issue of spending money on quality is now linked to both cost and service.

Achieving value-based health care faces an additional challenge: drawing conclusions about quality initiatives and return on investment when there are multiple factors involved. A further complication is the extensive use of a type of cost-benefit analysis that is not sensitive to health care objectives. If the benefits of a program can be priced in dollars, then a cost-benefit analysis will be able to identify the alternative with the largest benefit-to-cost ratio. However, many decisions involve benefits that are not easily quantifiable in monetary terms or otherwise, such as psychological benefits and environmental benefits (clean air and water).

Health care leaders and providers are now required to examine services using the value equation and make decisions accordingly. If resources are limited, leaders must ask whether every patient sign and symptom require intervention, particularly if minimal or no improvement in the patient's clinical condition is the likely outcome. Paying close attention to the health improvement value of health care services is an incredibly difficult challenge for providers and leaders schooled in the doctrine that increasing access to health care and growth in the health care system were absolute goods. Unfortunately, accountability and control were absent from the cost-based payment system, and the results are well known—exhaustion of resources. Health professionals are currently challenged to move from "rich" care to "wise" care (pp. 387–388).

So what has value that will make a difference? The nurse manager has a tremendous impact with this "wise" patient care issue, can teach this concept to staff, and, as treatments are being considered, can question what is wise versus what probably will not make a difference. This may be a new concept for patients/families involved as well. In reality it is far more accountable.

Now let's move to a second observation about cost. *Are RNs really more expensive?* Our bottom-line administrator would answer, "Of course. That is a no brainer. Their salaries are higher than LPNs [licensed practical nurses] and nurse aides. Just decrease RNs and add another LPN or aide to the budget and save money."

Reality does not prove this however. It is a fallacy that RNs are more expensive. Melberg (1997) examined budgets and staffing at five hospitals, documenting that a hospital budget with a 96% RN staff mix is *less expensive* than another hospital budget with a 64% RN mix. In fact, the hospital with the highest costs had the *lowest* RN skill mix (64%).

A high RN mix [96 percent] does not correlate with higher nursing costs per patient day in acute or critical care. Diluting the RN mix does not always reduce staffing costs. Although hospital A has a 96 percent RN-skill mix, the highest in the system, total nursing salary per patient day falls exactly in the middle. The highest costs occurred at hospital C where, in fact, the 64 percent RN mix is the lowest in the system. This finding is consistent in acute care, in critical care and on the orthopedic units—specialty nursing areas found in all five hospitals and therefore used for comparison. This difference is not explained by regional variations in RN salary, since RN salary at hospital A during the period of study was higher than at any hospital in the system except hospital E (p. 48).

So cost can actually be *higher* with a higher ratio of LPNs and nurse aides.

However, that is only the tip of the iceberg. RNs save on other costs besides just the salaries. One must go beyond the salary costs to patient outcomes—costs of adverse reactions. Remember the IOM statement that each adverse reaction costs an additional $8,750 per hospital stay? Remember all the data we have previously discussed on how higher RN ratios were linked to better patient outcomes? From the patient perspective when the result of lower RN staffing is death or permanent injury, this is a *very high* cost. And this cost could result in a lawsuit against the health care facility that could get even more expensive. A study by Lindrooth, Bazzoli, Needleman, and Hasnain-Wynia (2006) corroborated that it was more cost effective to provide a higher RN ratio.

As administrators it would behoove us to take a look at staffing and the percentage of staffing supplied by experienced RNs. The research is fairly clear on the impact RN staffing has on patient safety. This should provide impetus for us to come up with ways to attract and retain seasoned RNs at the bedside.

An important factor in determining appropriate staffing is the *nursing staff skill mix*, the various types of nursing staff by job classification necessary to care for the patient population being served. To determine the skill mix one should ask several questions: How do we deliver the care? Who is best to deliver the care? How is the care divided among the various caregivers? What skill mix provides the safest care? Which is cost effective? Unfortunately, there are no ideal answers. What works best in one setting (i.e., in a stepdown unit) may not be best in another (i.e., a skilled unit). And the answer to any one of these questions may depend on current circumstances, such as patient acuity, turnover of patients, discharges pushed to Fridays, admissions arriving on the evening shift, staff competencies or availability, or budget deficits. So skill mix is partially determined by current circumstances and must change to meet new situations as they occur.

Providing Patient Safety

Another very important mandate with quality improvement is *always* to provide a safe environment. The question is how can we set up systems to prevent mistakes from occurring? Mechanisms to bring about patient safety are being published daily. For instance, the Leapfrog Group, mentioned earlier, published recommended "leaps" organizations should take that promote quality. The recommendations included implementing computerized physician order entry, evidence-based hospital referral, intensive care unit staffing by physicians experienced in critical care medicine, and attaining a high Leapfrog Safe Practices score. The safe practices score measures the organization progress in meeting and implementing the safe practices endorsed by the national quality forum that would reduce the risk of harm in certain processes, systems, or environments of care (Leapfrog Group, n.d.).

Another approach to performance improvement is called *Six Sigma*, previously used in other non-health care businesses. Six Sigma provides a systematic approach used to improve patient outcomes. It is now being implemented in many hospitals to reduce errors by decreasing variation in process and outcomes. This performance improvement tool incorporates data analysis to identify and reduce variation. By reducing variability and promoting standardization, the potential for errors is greatly decreased, resulting in increased patient safety and a better product. Standardization is an important concept here. For instance, because we have different people interacting with patients in our service industry, we want all staff to be cognizant of, and use, certain customer service behaviors and scripting responses. This means that customer service is standardized so that no matter who the patient comes in contact with, the customer service behaviors are present (**Exhibit 4–8**).

The idea behind performance improvement is that it results in changes in practice that provide better quality or value to the patient. An excellent example of a performance improvement project

---

Exhibit 4–8 Critical Elements of Six Sigma

- Genuine focus on the customer.
- Data and fact driven management: the numbers speak.
- Processes are where the action is; processes are the key vehicle to success.
- Proactive management: acting in advance of a problem rather than reacting.
- Boundaryless collaboration: break down barriers between departments, organize work teams across the organization.
- Drive for perfection but tolerate failure.

Source: Data from Smith, B. (2003). Lean and six sigma—a one-two punch. *Quality Progress,* 37–41.

---

that determined a change in practice is the implementation of a service guarantee in various emergency departments across the country. CentraState, Oakwood Healthcare System, and St. Joseph Health Center examined practices in their emergency departments to determine what was effective and what resulted in patient dissatisfaction. A major complaint was wait time in the department before being seen by a physician or a provider. These facilities instituted processes enabling them to offer a service guarantee stating that a provider would see the patient, and/or treatment would be started, within 30 minutes. This has not only been an excellent success for the department, but it has also improved patient satisfaction, staff morale, and resulted in increased volume/revenue for each facility in the organization. (And we need to find additional ways to decrease wait time!)

Input and participation by staff are essential to the success of the project. Front-line staff are more familiar with the problems and opportunities in the department than anyone else and can be instrumental in identifying and implementing change or in orchestrating sabotage when not consulted. Involvement in performance improvement programs is often mandated in annual evaluations and reflected in bonuses for incentive plans.

Former patients are particularly valuable members on performance improvement committees. After all, the improvement effort is meant to improve the way we treat patients, and these committee members know what was important to them during their illness. It is also helpful if committee members have had a loved one experience all the difficulties inherent in a health care crisis within the health care system. Input from both patients and committee members who have had this experience is invaluable. They have the best ideas as to what needs to be done, or changed, to achieve value.

There is so much more to identify and eliminate or change for performance improvement. We have only identified the tip of the iceberg. It makes far more sense to be more proactive about patient safety by involving everyone in critically evaluating current practice patterns, current processes being used, potential environmental hazards, and anything else that might result in an unsafe situation *before* any incident occurs. The information can be included in the performance improvement goals, strategies can be implemented for prevention, and our patients will be safer. As an administrator we need to make sure that we are including these strategies in budget requests. We need to *be assertive and argue the importance of these expenditures.*

This means that we have to look around with new eyes to see potential issues that, if recognized, can be prevented. Consider the following list:

- Drug packaging looks the same for different drugs or drug names are similar. Barcoding is critical.
- According to The Joint Commission, 70% of errors involve breakdown in communication. Half of these occur during hand-offs such as shift change, patient transfer to another area, or transfer to another facility. Adopting a standard communication method is helpful.

Exhibit 4–9 provides an example of this method found to result in 96% to 100% retention of information.

- When staffing is inadequate, more safety issues occur. It may be better to find more staff, close beds, merge units, or some other strategy that is planned ahead of time so everyone knows what to do when this occurs.
- It is important for every RN to routinely do rounds and talk with the patients.
- Poor teamwork and ineffective leadership bring on a multitude of safety issues. Both Chapters 2 and 3 discuss ways to fix these issues.
- Sometimes an RN does not assume leadership of a team, for instance, perhaps this RN is a new graduate. This is where mentors or preceptors are so important.
- Woods and Doan-Johnson (2002) analyzed 21 disciplinary case files from nine boards of nursing to develop a taxonomy of nursing practice errors (**Exhibit 4–10**). Stress the importance of these with staff. All these errors can and should be addressed with education and process/performance improvement activities.
- Lack of critical thinking can cause errors. Here, staff members need to be educated to get beyond tasks to understanding the big picture and then determine actions.
- Miscommunication between professional groups can cause patient safety issues. Markey and Brown (2002) noted that a team of RNs, physical therapists, occupational therapists, patient care assistants, and physicians, when working together on teams, discovered that each discipline had a different vocabulary for the same items:

> Each department had its own activity and mobility vocabulary and because staff members' duties for mobilizing patients were not defined, creating a common language and clarifying responsibilities were essential to ensuring effective patient mobility plans. The group developed seven standard descriptions of mobility and activity levels ranging from "Total 100%/Be prepared to do everything" to "Independent/No assistance needed." With dressing, for instance, a patient who needs "total assistance" would meet the description, "Patient needs to be dressed," while a patient who needs "moderate" assistance would be noted as "Get dressing articles ready. Can put limbs in clothing but can't pull on completely" (p. 1).

They found that specific guidelines were most helpful in carrying out the activities specified by nurses, physicians, physical therapists, or occupational therapists. These guidelines were also shared with patients and families, accomplishing better consistency when working with patients, as, for example, the nurse aide understood specifically what to have the patient do and what the aide should do for the patient.

These guidelines provided a set of scripted behaviors that achieved a more consistent approach. This scripted format is becoming more popular in every health care setting, including the hospitals

---

Exhibit 4–9 SBAR Communication

S situation (the current issue)
B background (brief, related to the point)
A assessment (what you found/think)
R recommendation/request (what you want next)

Source: Data from Haig, K., Sutton, S., & Whittington, J. (2006). SBAR: A shared mental model for improving communication between clinicians. *Journal on Quality and Patient Safety, 32*(3), 167–175.

Exhibit 4–10 Categories of Nursing Errors

- Lack of attentiveness
  Attentiveness refers to the nurse's ability to find out and remember assessment data on each patient "paying attention to the patient's clinical condition and response to therapy, as well as potential hazards or errors in treatment" (p. 46).
- Lack of agency/fiduciary concern
  Lack of agency/fiduciary concern gets back to what the patient values. Here the nurse needs to be an advocate for the patient, by questioning physician orders, calling physicians, and paying attention to patient/family requests.
- Inappropriate judgment
  The nurse's judgment and clinical expertise is important if the nurse is to intervene on the patient's behalf.
- Medication errors
  A medication error is any preventable event that may cause or lead to inappropriate medication use or patient harm while the medication is in the control of the health care professional, patient, or consumer. Such events may be related to professional practice, health care products, procedures, and systems, includ- ing prescribing; order communication; product labeling, packaging, and nomenclature; compounding; dispensing; distribution; administration; education; monitoring; and use (p. 47). We know that many med- ication errors are never reported.
- Lack of intervention on the patient's behalf
  Often, symptoms that the nurse does not recognize or respond to in a timely manner result in a complica- tion or death that could possibly have prevented.
- Lack of prevention
  Teach all employees to identify any potential problems and rectify them as soon as the problems are noticed. Infection control, immobility hazards, and a safe environment are areas of concern.
- Missed or mistaken physician or health care provider orders
  Use of a provider order entry and a computerized documentation system could more effectively prevent this occurrence.
- Documentation errors (p. 46)
  Additional *documentation errors* are problematic in two areas:
  1. *Charting procedures or medications before they were completed.* Such a documentation error can cause a patient to miss a dose of medication or a treatment and can confuse, misrepresent, or mask a patient's true condition.
  2. *Lack of charting of observations of the patient* causes serious harm when a nurse fails to chart signs of patient deterioration, pain, or agitation or particular signs of complications related to the illness or therapies (p. 48).

Source: Data from Woods, A., & Doan-Johnson, S. (2002, October). Executive summary: Toward a taxonomy of nursing practice errors. *Nursing Management,* 45–48.

---

receiving the Malcolm Baldrige National Quality Award. In fact, part of their success is because the scripted format provides more consistent care regardless of the provider.

Being proactive, and preventing many mishaps, is very important. However, if mistakes occur, it is important to react from the Information Age perspective rather than from the patriarchal Industrial Age. In the past, the traditional approach to patient safety was to identify what an indi- vidual practitioner had done wrong. When very serious, this resulted in occurrences being "reported to the board for disciplinary investigation because of an error or breach in the standards of safe practice" (Woods & Doan-Johnson, 2002, p. 45). It was easy to get into blame and punishment with errors.

There are two issues here. First, blame does not accomplish anything except to encourage people to hide errors. Second, even when one person seemingly made the error, when the situation is examined, more than one person was involved in setting up the problem. Nor is it one factor that caused the error. It is really a combination of factors, or a lack of systems, that have caused the error. The IOM pointed out that often we do not look at the most important issue about those errors—what could we have done to prevent the error from occurring?

A more effective solution is to report the error and undertake a *root cause analysis* to determine what process changes—or patterns or trends—occurred that provide clues for immediate changes. Medical errors usually involve more than one person and require a systems approach in finding solutions. Usually, there is an organizational systems process that went wrong or a better process needs to be implemented. Then it is important to set up and implement systems to prevent this from happening again. Using a systems approach is best, as discussed in Chapter 3.

Establishing a "just" or blame-free culture is critical if organizations are to focus on process/system improvement instead of laying blame. Jim Conway with the Dana Faber Cancer Institute sums it up this way: "You have to set the tone," he explains, "provide a supportive, non-punitive environment for your staff. The goal is transparency—an atmosphere of open communication about safety concerns and incidents" (IHI, n.d., a). Without the opportunity for open discussion, too many opportunities for improvement are hidden or go unreported because team members are fearful of losing their jobs or getting into trouble. Then the problem will just reoccur.

Creating a just culture starts at the top and must be reinforced each time an incident occurs. But how do we accomplish this? First, we must be informed, and that starts with personal education. The American Hospital Association published a tool, *Strategies for Leadership: Hospital Executives and Their Role in Patient Safety* (Conway, 2000), that provides a checklist of actions that executives and leaders should use to help establish a just culture. Once informed, it is important to role model expected behaviors, speak publicly about safety, set expectations, establish policy, personally participate in significant event root cause analysis, and lead by example.

There are additional resources for nurse managers. The IHI offers some great resources to help managers implement programs to promote safety, and The Joint Commission has added an online resource for sharing patient safety practices. It provides valuable examples and tools that have been successfully used.

Another excellent source for patient safety is the *incident report*. These reports have been around for years but often have not been used as effectively as they could be. It is most often the incident report that alerts risk management personnel about significant problems. The risk management role has historically been to identify, manage, and reduce risk required to support the delivery of safe health care while reducing organizational legal risks. Because risk management more often occurs *after* the incident, it may not be the best or only approach to achieve safe care, but it is important to pay attention to this resource because this alerts everyone about additional organizational issues that need to be resolved to achieve patient safety.

A new emerging role in health care is the patient safety officer. This position promotes safety through education; examination of issues to determine better, safer organizational processes discovering the root cause; creating system changes to prevent future incidents of the same kind; and then be involved in implementing programs designed to foster safety. The IHI recommends this role be part of the executive team in the organization and solely be dedicated to patient safety with no overlapping duties. The patient safety officer works closely with risk management personnel in discovering the root cause and creating system changes to create a safer climate.

What Does It Mean to Be in the Information Age?

Performance improvement in the Information Age means that we need to make better use of technology. In the past, so many of our computer programs could not talk to one another. Moving to a fully integrated, computerized system moves the organization to a more viable status that allows for better flow of information and improved access to information. This integration allows for use of clinical decision support at the point of care that is crucial if we are to transform practice to evidence-based practice. This presents a major financial undertaking because these computer systems are expensive. Costs extend beyond the walls of the organization, making it more challenging. Physicians and other providers need access from multiple locations, not just in the facility. For true point of care access, computers must be mobile or at every patient bedside.

ONLINE CLINICAL DOCUMENTATION SYSTEMS

The Leapfrog Group identified the importance of a computerized physician order entry (CPOE) system. Actually, there are entire online clinical documentation systems that are even better with physician order entry as a part of the larger system. Online documentation provides integration of documentation from all disciplines. Because all disciplines chart together, there is immediate access to relevant information, as well as better continuity of care. In addition, preformatted charting presents an easier, time-saving format for the clinician to follow, and helps to achieve patient safety by indicating all possibilities associated with symptoms. Built-in clinical alerts identify abnormal results, allergies, stop dates on medicines, incompatible medicines, alerts that it is time to give medications, and a variety of other safeguards that promote patient safety and optimize quality.

Online systems also provide immediate and virtual access to laboratory and radiology results in both the health care facility and the physician's office. In addition, physicians can initiate the CPOE system from their office location. Prescriptions and discharge instructions can be generated. From a safety standpoint, the liability from legibility problems is decreased.

Using these systems, documentation is thorough and better reflects patient status, resulting in enhanced safety and increased reimbursement from accurate coding. The systems can even link cost and quality data.

An alert to clinicians using computers when in the patient's presence: A study found that patients often thought that clinicians were doing some computer activity not related to that patient, because clinicians gave no explanation of what they were doing. So it is important to explain to the patient that we are documenting care.

BAR-CODING

A closed-loop system comprised of a scanner to bar-code the medication, the clinician administering the medication, and the patient's armband has proven very successful in reducing medication errors related to the five rights of medication administration: right patient, right route, right dose, right time, and right medication. Medication dispensing systems such as Pyxis and Omnicell are available in many facilities to assist with medication administration. The medicine is categorized in drawers, and the appropriate drawer opens when the patient name and medication name are entered. Some facilities have implemented robotics to assist with medication identification in the pharmacy as well as with delivery from the pharmacy. This has greatly decreased the possibility of error. Although cost is significant, the savings realized from diverted errors, increased patient satisfaction, and promotion of quality more than substantiates the expense. In this era of health care shortages at crisis proportions, robotic help is needed.

Laptop computers and personal palm devices are being used more frequently to promote efficiency and decrease transcription errors. Access is available from remote locations and to decrease redundancy of information regarding demographics and insurance status asked during registration processes. In addition, clinicians can look up information about medications, diagnoses, and other health information immediately as needed (see Chapter 5 for more information).

Recognition of Value and Quality

There are a number of programs in health care. Some that pay attention to both the value and quality issues from the patient perspective have gained national awareness.

The Planetree Model

Planetree Inc. (2008) acknowledges the importance of environment, providing a more humanistic, personalized, patient-centered experience. The delivery is holistic, encompassing mental, social, and emotional dimensions as well as physical symptoms. The goal is to maximize health care by combining medical therapy with complementary alternatives using architectural and environmental designs in the process. Planetree embraces a novel concept in that the provision of compassionate, nurturing, personalized care is designed not only for patients and patient families, but also for staff. Thus, using the Planetree approach, the organization must embrace a culture that nurtures staff as well as patients (Planetree Inc., 2008).

The Planetree philosophy has two primary settings, acute care and continued care. Each setting has components that define their approach to care. Planetree facilities are challenged to incorporate these components to provide appropriate humanistic health care delivered in a caring environment (**Exhibit 4–11**). Planetree also provides measurement tools for continuous evaluation of quality of care, including patient satisfaction surveys and community image assessment.

The Eden Alternative

A philosophy similar to the Planetree model, instituted in long-term care, is the Eden Alternative. Developed by Dr. William Thomas, geriatrician, it is based on his belief that the focus of long-term care should be care and not treatment. Thomas further elaborates that the major problems in nursing homes are loneliness, boredom, and helplessness; the residents are overmedicated, deprived of the enjoyment of a pleasant meal by unnecessary dietary restrictions, and subject to endless activity programs developed to meet regulatory compliance rather than provide entertainment for the residents. His solution was the creation of an environment that allowed people to flourish by inundating them with life in the form of plants, animals, and children. The Eden Alternative offers a more humanistic, home-like environment; it offers residents opportunities to maintain and control the environment, and encourages interaction and compassion (Eden Alternative, 2008).

Magnet Hospital Status

Earning the esteemed designation of magnet hospital has become a renowned indicator of quality. This is an expensive process in terms of both money and resources for the facility. A magnet hospital voluntarily endures a strenuous evaluation of nursing services and successfully meets all criteria determined by nursing services and patient care in a hospital setting. Program objectives are to

---

Exhibit 4–11 Planetree Acute Care Components

- **Human interaction:** Human beings caring for other human beings, creating a healing environment for patients, families, and staff members.
- **Family, friends, and social support:** Contributes to the quality of the hospital experience by promoting caring connections between the patients and their support systems.
- **Information and education:** Patients, families, and community members are provided with increased access to meaningful information.
- **Nutritional and nurturing aspects of food:** Choice and personalized service, in combination with sound nutrition practices, add pleasure, comfort, and familiarity.
- **Architectural and interior design:** The Planetree design considers the patients' well-being. The hospital is welcoming and accessible, providing clearly marked signs for direction, comfortable and familiar rooms, and designs that engage the senses and break down barriers.
- **Arts and entertainment:** Music, artwork, theater, crafts, and clowns offer engagement and enjoyment to enhance the clinical environment.
- **Spirituality:** Planetree recognizes the vital role of spirituality in healing the whole person. From chaplains to meditation programs, hospitals can provide opportunities for reflection and support of spiritual needs.
- **Human touch:** Touch reduces anxiety, pain, and stress, benefiting patients, families, and staff members.
- **Complementary therapies:** Expand the choices offered to patients. Aroma and pet therapy, acupuncture, and Reiki are offered in addition to clinical modalities of care.
- **Healthy communities:** Expand the boundaries of health care. Working with schools, senior centers, churches, and other community partners, organizations are redefining health care to include the health and wellness of the larger community.

Source: Adapted from Planetree, Inc. (2008). *About Planetree*. Retrieved May 18, 2008 from http://www.planetree.org/ABOUT/ABOUT.html

---

- Recognize nursing services that use the scope and standards for nurse administrators to build programs of nursing excellence in the delivery of nursing care to patients.
- Promote quality in a milieu that supports professional nursing practice.
- Provide a vehicle for the dissemination of successful nursing practices and strategies among institutions using the services of registered professional nurses.

Performance Measurement

In an effort to contain costs, performance measurement became popular in the early 1990s when companies purchasing health plans could examine cost and quality data to determine which plan was best for the dollars spent. At first these plans were called report cards and published only summaries of various performance data. Report cards then started to be used internally by health care organizations to improve services. (For an example, see http://www.healthgrades.com.)

The idea behind performance measurement was that the patient outcomes could determine the effectiveness of organizational performance. Although this measurement was an improvement from past practices, there were several problems with this measurement: (1) future performance cannot be determined from the historical data; (2) no one asked the patient what the patient wanted or valued; (3) at times organizations were swimming in data that were collected, but no one figured out how to analyze the data or use then effectively; and (4) sometimes these data were used punitively when outcomes were not met, which only impeded future improvement occurring.

The following gives examples of how report card data are used:

1. The National Database of Nursing Quality Indicators uses a report card to compare voluntarily reported nursing sensitive outcomes such as fall rates related to nurse staffing and other organization characteristics.
2. Hospital Compare uses a report card format to compare outcomes for specific CMS measures. This is available for patients and families and can be used for selecting the facility of choice based on outcomes. Visit http://www.hospitalcompare.hhs.gov to learn more.

As report card data became available, the Joint Commission expanded performance measurement to include two sets of measures, core or standardized measures and noncore measures. Joining forces with CMS to align efforts, the Joint Commission requires organizations to report on a certain number of measures, depending on the populations served. The organization selects which measures to report, but the number varies depending on which measures are selected. For example, if an organization selects four of the core measures for reporting, then none of the noncore measures is required. If the organization selects only two of the core measures, then they must also report on six noncore measures. Measures are identified for hospitals, long-term care, and home care. The results are available to the public at www.qualitycheck.org.

Sentara Healthcare (Grayson, 2002) established performance improvement goals, and then went one step further. They tied it with the incentive plan. (We would take it one step further and tie it in with an incentive plan for all staff.)

> Our chief medical officer, who has worked in four institutions, said that this is the only place he's worked where he actually gets calls from the non-medical managers asking if we are making progress in the clinical quality indicators because their compensation is tied to these improvements. So it's a system to foster innovation with built-in accountability aimed at increasing the quality of care.... A good example is our remotely monitored electronic ICU. Intensive care specialists monitor ICU patients 19 hours a day for timely intervention. [From 7 a.m. to noon, physicians make rounds in the actual units.] The physician has computer access to the patient's records, including lab or radiographic tests, and can view the patient and talk with staff via in-room, high-resolution video cameras. The system enhances traditional rounds and on-site monitoring. Patient mortality rates have dropped 25 to 35 percent and it's achieved a 155 percent payback (Grayson, 2002, p. 36).

Benchmarking

Many health care organizations are benchmarking quality measures with other similar organizations. Often, when benchmarking, the organization sets a goal, such as to be in the top 25th quartile. However, be aware that benchmarking can be fraught with problems. Rudy, Lucke, Whitman, and Davidson (2001) report the following:

> Benchmarking is a common approach to establishing quality. However, the conclusions drawn from benchmarking depend heavily on whether the benchmark is obtained from the literature, from hospital-specific sources, or from an integrated hospital system. Benchmarking using the literature may appear the simplest, but often a literature-based benchmark is not available, is not sufficiently relevant, or differs in definitions, populations, or clinical practice.... An important but rarely addressed issue in literature-based benchmarking is assessing uncertainty, such as the standard error, in the benchmark itself.

> Internal benchmarking is available to hospitals with the relevant databases and statistical
> expertise, but it can provide an invalid assessment of performance when compared to other
> institutions....
>
> System benchmarking appears to avoid the pitfalls of these other two methods, but it
> requires coordinated database resources and sophisticated statistical analyses. System-
> based benchmarks without adequate adjustments for acuity put hospitals with higher acu-
> ity at a disadvantage. Hospitals with smaller censuses may have larger differences between
> hospital-specific and system-based estimates than do those with larger censuses (p. 189).

There is an additional problem with benchmarking. It compares current practices, not what has
value from the patient perspective. For instance, we benchmark the wait time for emergency rooms.
An hour wait time is considered normal. Think about this statement from the patient perspective. Does
the patient enjoy experiencing an hour or more waiting to be seen in the emergency room? From a
value perspective, wouldn't it be better to measure by eliminating the wait time and seeing the patient
immediately? After all, some are already using 30 minutes as the benchmark, and even 30 minutes is
not as valuable to the patient as no wait time. Remember, if we don't achieve it, someone else will!

Patient Satisfaction

Patient satisfaction has been one early performance measurement that pays attention to what the
patient values. Patient satisfaction instruments are a beginning measurement of value, although they
take place *after* the health care experience. Hospitals, particularly, have used patient satisfaction
measurement for some time because measuring patient satisfaction has been an important core outcome measure for Joint Commission accreditation.

Companies that provide patient satisfaction instruments, or services, to health care organizations
include both Gallop and Press Ganey. Generally, hospitals pay these companies to actually collect
and tabulate the data because patients are more likely to be honest with an outside group asking the
questions. This has some advantages in that the organization results are ranked in relation to other
similar organizations providing benchmarking opportunities. The 2007 Press Ganey report examined the experiences of more than 2.3 million patients treated at more than 1,700 acute care hospitals in 2006. The report provided data trending for the year and identified key priorities that would
help improve patient satisfaction. Using this information to identify opportunities for improvement
would help the organization focus on value for our patients.

To adequately assess patient satisfaction, both the patient's and the provider's expectations must
be clearly identified. Typically, in the past patients were seen as customers in need of health care;
now they are informed consumers looking for quality of care and noticing the method of delivery.
Health care has become a competitive business. Many facilities are using contract agencies to market their services and measure their success; they have implemented service excellence initiatives
to improve patient satisfaction. Some even have scripted behaviors and protocols to handle dialogue in difficult situations. (This is an example of the standardization issue discussed previously.)

The problem is that we are dealing with people. What has value to one person may not have value
with another. For example, one person may welcome talking about his or her emotions with a health
caregiver, whereas another person may find this invasive. One person may respond to pain by grin-
ning and bearing it, whereas another who experiences even mild pain loudly expresses this to all.

Staff, or department, evaluations may be directly linked to satisfaction results. Results from
patient satisfaction surveys can be very useful and can be used to

- Improve and measure the quality of care
- Manage complaints

- Implement strategic planning and marketing decisions
- Evaluate and/or provide bonuses to departments or individual (physician and nonphysician) staff
- Enhance public relations
- Meet accreditation standards
- Monitor for risk management
- Link survey results to clinical data
- Use survey results for contract payer negotiations
- Compare the results for benchmarking
- Link the results to financial data

Performance Measurement and Patient Value

We might question whether all the things we are measuring are really things that patients value. Certainly, CMS indicators and the Joint Commission National Patient Safety Goals are patient centered, but do they fully evaluate the patient's perception of how these standard measures add value? Press Ganey or Gallop measures satisfaction, but, again, they are not necessarily inclusive of the value perception. The Picker Institute, dedicated to the advancement of patient-centered care, created survey tools that focus on eight dimensions of patient-centered care. **Exhibit 4–12** lists these dimensions.

We need to keep coming back to what the patient values. If we lose sight of this, all our statistics are useless. We may be making a profit and have wonderful patient outcome statistics, such as preventing complications, but if the patients are not getting what they want or need, it is their choice whether or not to come back next time. This comes back to the patient and family advisory focus groups that we discussed earlier in this chapter. The data received from this

---

Exhibit 4–12   Picker Institute's Eight Dimensions of Patient-Centered Care for Inpatient Surveys

- **Access** (including time spent waiting for admission or time between admission and allocation to a bed in a ward)
- **Respect for patient's values, preferences, and expressed needs** (including impact of illness and treatment on quality of life, involvement in decision making, dignity, needs and autonomy)
- **Coordination and integration of care** (including clinical care, ancillary and support services, and "front-line" care)
- **Information, communication, and education** (including clinical status, progress and prognosis, facilitation of autonomy, self-care, and health promotion)
- **Physical comfort** (including pain management, help with activities of daily living, surroundings, and hospital environment)
- **Emotional support and alleviation of fear and anxiety** (including treatment and prognosis, impact of illness on self and family, financial impact of illness)
- **Involvement of family and friends** (including social and emotional support, involvement in decision making, impact on family dynamics and functioning)
- **Transition and continuity** (including information about medication and danger signs to look out for after leaving the hospital, coordination and discharge planning, clinical, social, physical and financial support)

Source: Adapted from Picker Institute. (n.d.). *Welcome to the Picker Institute.* Retrieved May 12, 2008 from http://www.pickerinstitute.org/index.html

group provide rich resources of data for both performance improvement and performance measurement.

As one collects data from focus groups, or even as one organizes the groups, it is important to think about the data in terms of populations served or the amount of data may easily get out of hand. This means that our focus moves from thinking about individuals to considering similar needs of larger groups of patients. If we examine populations of patients, it probably needs to go beyond groups with a certain disease or problem to some kind of subgroup population with similar concerns. For instance, parents of young children have different concerns from older adults experiencing chronic diseases on a fixed income or from certain populations who are more concerned with maintaining health. The focus group participants may need to be organized in a different way to better identify these populations.

Balanced Scorecard: Best Approach to Performance Measurement

Balanced scorecards are discussed in detail in Chapter 16. We advocate that this is the best way to conduct performance measurement. Metrics captured within the organization's balanced scorecard are tied directly to the strategic plan. A primary utility of the balanced scorecard is the tie between strategic management and performance management. Measurement of key financial, quality, market, and operational indicators provide management with an understanding of performance in relation to established strategic goals and graphically displays a snapshot of the institution's overall health (Health Care Advisory Board, 1999).

Utilization Review

Another measurement that occurs related to the care given is with *utilization review*. The Utilization Review Accreditation Commission (URAC) reviews health care operations to ensure business is conducted in a manner consistent with national standards. Similar to the Joint Commission, URAC evaluates organizations to see if they meet defined standards in one or more programs such as disease management, case management, credentialing, and so on.

The URAC defines utilization management in its 2008 Industry Report as "the evaluation of the medical necessity, appropriateness, and efficiency of the use of health care services, procedures, and facilities under the provisions of the applicable health benefits plan."

Utilization management is a quality dimension in that the primary purpose is to ensure appropriate use of available services and resources. Many organizations are integrating utilization management into the case management role, creating a more complete system of quality management. Historically, health care organizations established a person(s), or department, assigned to do utilization review—relaying clinical information to payers so the payers could determine whether they would pay for additional care for patients. In the managed care climate (managed care is further explained in Chapter 10), one cannot give the care and then submit the bill but instead must get preapproval for the care. The payers determine whether the care is allowable. Once the payers determine that the care meets their criteria, the patient is certified for payment.

Employee Issues

When discussing value and quality, we cannot ignore employees. When administrators value employees, employees will value patients. Thus this section includes issues in the value and quality arena that pertain to employees.

OSHA Standards for Employee Safety

The first employee issue is employee safety. There are so many possible hazards in the health care industry. The Occupational Safety and Health Administration (OSHA; www.osha-sic.gov) provides nationally mandated ongoing standards for the workplace. Thus health care staff must regularly orient to current OSHA standards. In addition, OSHA has record-keeping forms that someone in the organization must keep updated to document that OSHA standards have been followed. In larger health care systems, both quality and infection control personnel are often concerned with workplace compliance with OSHA standards. In smaller systems, this becomes another responsibility of staff who assume many roles. Either way, the nurse manager needs to be aware of the current standards, must make sure that staff have been oriented to these standards, and must be sure that the unit is in compliance with the standards.

Promoting a Healthy Workplace

Achieving a healthy workplace includes examining how the environment affects all present. It can be quite complicated. For instance, a nurse experiencing a needlestick when the patient has acquired immuno deficiency syndrome (AIDS) or hepatitis is a major hazard.

> Of the nearly 14 injury cases per 100 long-term-care employees, a significant number are related to patient lifting or repositioning tasks. OSHA recommends "that manual lifting of residents be minimized in all cases and eliminated when feasible."…Possible solutions…include using mechanical lifts and ceiling-mounted lift systems.…For patients with the ability to assist, or who are able to bear weight completely, equipment such as sit-to-stand devices, ambulation-assist devices, transfer boards, and lift cushions or chairs can minimize assistance needed in transferring. [This includes height-adjustable beds with electric controls rather than cranks and showering and bathing assistive devices.] (Weber, 2008, p. 30).

We also have members from the general public visiting or being admitted into health care facilities. These people may have a number of issues that could endanger others (i.e., have a gun, bring infections, threaten staff, and so forth). We have a responsibility to protect staff as well as patients in this environment.

Bioterrorism

A new issue that must be addressed in relation to patient and staff safety is bioterrorism. The intentional introduction of anthrax, smallpox, or other disease entities as a biological weapon would certainly play havoc on already short-staffed, financially burdened health care facilities. Procedures to address the identified emergency are dictated by the Federal Emergency Management Administration (FEMA), but facility-related issues such as lack of available nurses and methods to contain or quarantine are facility specific and should be addressed in policy before the need. Thus disaster planning and preparedness has assumed new significance. Sadly enough, this needs to also be considered at budget time to designate appropriate funds for protective apparel, vaccinations, preparation and training for staff, and public education.

Consider the Following

Change is occurring very fast these days. It is important to stay open to new information and to new ways of doing things to stay relevant. Our perspective is very important as we forge ahead. Thus we need to consider some other information.

Quantum Physics

> Quantum is defined as a "discrete quantity of electromagnetic radiation."…The science of quantum physics has demonstrated that our world actually occurs in very short, rapid bursts of light. What we believe we see as the swing of a baseball batter on home plate, for example, in quantum terms is actually a series of individual events that happen very fast and very close together. Similar to the many still images that make up a moving film, these events are actually tiny pulses of light called quanta. The quanta of our world occur so rapidly that although our eyes are capable of doing so, our minds do not discern individual bursts. Instead, the pulses are averaged together into what we see as one continuous event…Quantum physics is the study of these minute units of radiating waves, nonphysical forces whose movements create our physical world (Braden, 2000, p. 96).

If it seems like this is getting way out there, this is really fairly old information that goes back to Albert Einstein's research leading the way into our present reality. And the research continues to identify more about our world.

So if our world is actually a series of energy fields, let's look at the world around us. It is, "A vast porridge of being where nothing is fixed or measurable.…[There are] dynamic patterns continually changing into one another—the continuous dance of energy.…The universe begins to look more like a great thought than like a great machine" (Wheatley, 1992, pp. 31–32).

This means that the energy fields can be affected by our thoughts. Our thoughts create our reality. This quantum physics research aligns with another source:

> That which is, already has been;
> That which is to be, already is.
>
> *Ecclesiastics 3:15*

Both sources present us with a different way of viewing our world. Going on with the idea that our thoughts create our reality, "that which is" was caused by the thought we previously had. "That which is to be," our present thought, "already is" because we are thinking it, and it will be what happens next.

So, using this concept, what thoughts preceded our present reality? Do we actually have choices in our reality? How does this work? Let's go on with some additional research results:

> Under the right conditions, two atoms were occupying exactly the same place at precisely the same time! Until these studies were verified, such a phenomenon has been believed to be impossible. Now we know that it is not. The outcomes of our world at any given moment in time is made of people, machines, earth, and nature. At their most fundamental level, our outcomes are made of atoms. If two of the basic building blocks of our world may coexist at the same instant, then the doorway has been opened for many atoms, resulting in many outcomes, to do the same.…Through our refined language of quantum science, we now have the vocabulary to describe precisely how we participate in determining the outcome of our future.…Quantum physics suggests that by redirecting our focus—where we place our attention—we bring a new course of events into focus while at the same time releasing an existing course of events that may no longer serve us (Braden, 2000, p. 26).

This means that our thoughts create our reality, and at each moment there are several possibilities all present that we can choose from.

If this is the case, we need to really be careful what we think about. For example, many of us worry, worry, worry. Worry—giving thought to bad or awful events—gives energy to the awful event, which then could become our reality. Conversely, when we think about some positive event, we give energy to the positive event becoming reality. Let's take this a step further.

What thoughts resulted in the monetary cutbacks we are experiencing in health care today? Are we so caught up in scarcity of resources (our thought) that we have created that reality? How often are we saying, "There is not enough money for health care?" Should we change this thought?

> Accounting and finance are applied areas of microeconomics. The theory of economics forms the foundations upon which all financial management is ultimately built. The essence of economics is that society has a *limited amount of resources*, [our emphasis] with competing demands for them. The economic system attempts to allocate those resources in an optimal fashion (Finkler & Kovner, 2000, p. 4).

Microeconomic theory encourages us to believe our resources are limited. If we choose to believe this, our present reality is formed. So the question is whether this is the reality we want to create. Do we want to continue, like the ostrich with its head in the sand, with our present view of reality? It is something to ponder. A wonderful movie about this is called *The Secret* (available from www.thesecret.tv).

Let's consider another possible scenario for our present picture of health care. What if we substituted the word "abundance" for "scarcity"? Then our thoughts would create a different reality. We would have an abundance of resources and would not have to compete for those resources. We would have an abundance of nurses or other health caregivers. We can shun this idea...but what if it is true? We might be able to create a different, better reality. This might really result in better services for our patients/residents/clients, as well as a more satisfied workforce.

So, going on with our scenario, recently we have been involved with making budget cuts. What if we instead pictured that there *is* enough money and enough staff to give the services needed. Isn't that the reality that we would rather create?

Or take the argument that we cannot achieve quality when we have to make budget cuts. This thought means that we will get lower quality (our patients will suffer) along with budget cuts. Is this what we really want? Are we stuck in that box too?

We can change this thought to thinking about how much fun it is to work toward achieving quality and how rewarding it is when we feel we have achieved quality work. The choice is ours, and, according to quantum physics research, the outcome we think about happens.

Continuing this idea, we can choose to see our reality as a difficult challenge or as an opportunity to create our future. The choice is ours.

It is interesting that positive affirmations have become a common occurrence in our present reality. Things such as "I am in perfect health" or "I accomplish _____ easily and effortlessly". There are entire books (Hay, 1988) written on this subject, and they even link the negative thoughts to various diseases that occur from the thought. If one believes in affirmations, it is important to remember the "do no harm" clause in our nursing and medical professions because we live in a world of duality (i.e., good and evil, male and female, yin and yang). After all, we need to be ethical about this.

Perhaps this further explains the mind–body connection discussed previously in this chapter.

Chaos Theory

> Chaos is an essential constituent of all change. It works to unbundle attachment to whatever is impeding movement. Chaos challenges us to simultaneously let go and to take on. It reminds us that life is a journey of constant creation (Porter-O'Grady & Malloch, 2003, p. 2).

Another scientific field of thought presently is chaos theory. Chaos theory offers hope for our future. In this theory the world seems chaotic all around us. However, when all this seeming chaos "is plotted over millions of iterations," it plots out a perfectly proportioned picture (**Exhibit 4–13**). This offers great hope for us. Even when it seems like total chaos surrounds us, if we could rise above our present chaos and look down at it, there is order and perfection.

Sometimes when unexpected things happen or when we have setbacks or experience difficult situations, it can be comforting to know that these experiences accomplish good things for us as well. We can learn from such situations and become better persons. In addition, these experiences can lead us to something different or new that we probably would never have tried if the difficulties had not occurred.

When we think about planning change, chaos theory tells us that we cannot possibly plan, or map out, all the details of the plan because of chaotic occurrences. As these occurrences happen, they will necessitate a change in the plan. This is why all staff need to be involved in understanding the plan and need to be empowered to accomplish it—because the final product, or components of the

Exhibit 4–13   Three-Winged Bird: A Chaotic Strange Attractor

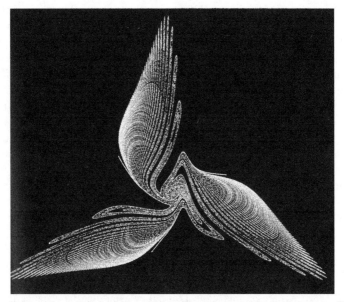

This is a self-portrait drawn by a chaotic system. The system's behavior is plotted over millions of iterations. The system appears to be wandering chaotically, always displaying new and different behavior. But over time, a deeper order—a shape—is revealed. This order is inherent to the system. It was always there, but not revealed until its chaotic movements were plotted in multiple dimensions over time.

From the work of Mario Markus and Bruno Hess, Max-Planck Institute, Dortmund, Germany. Used with permission.

Source: Wheatley, M. (1999). *Leadership and the new science: Discovering order in a chaotic world*, 2nd ed. San Francisco: Berrett-Koehler.

final product, will ultimately be different in the end. And really, there is no final product. Chaos will continue to change what was implemented. So we cannot rest on our laurels but need to continually move on into uncharted territory.

Many of us (administrative leaders) do not understand this concept of constant change. Instead, we still buy into the Industrial Age idea that everything is rational and can be planned out in minute detail and that we can just order others to follow through on our plan—and then get frustrated when people don't follow this to the letter. This is not reality. If we continue to believe this, we open ourselves up for a lot of unnecessary frustration, and the people that we supervise will be frustrated as well.

Instead, all of us need to be open to the reality around us, see the changes that are occurring, and help to interpret this for one another. For although we all have our own views of reality, if we do not pay attention to the chaotic reality that actually happens, the changes will occur and leave us behind. We will become obsolete and unfulfilled.

> Leaders now must incorporate the vagaries of complexity and chaos into the process of anticipating and planning for the future. Detailing the specifics of some future state is no longer a viable means of planning. Discernment and signpost reading are better skills to have than are those related to defining and direction setting. Leaders must realize that no real-time insight is sustainable, nor is it entirely accurate. It is simply a reflection of the particular point a person or organization is at in their continuous and relentless unfolding and becoming.
>
> A good leader is one who can read the signposts suggesting that a change is imminent and can discern the direction of the change and the elements indicating its fabric. The good leader synthesizes rather than analyzes and views the change thematically and/or relationally, drawing out of it what kind of action or strategy should be applied—the response, that is, that best positions for the organization to thrive in the coming circumstances.
>
> For a leader to act as a strategist today means not detailing the organization's future actions, but translating the signposts of change into language that has meaning for those who must do the work of the organization. Translating the signposts into understandable and inspiring language is more critical than almost any other strategic task. It is vital that a change have implications for those who are doing the work. Another way of saying this is that it must have meaning to them within the framework of their work activities so that they can commit to it, which they must do if they and the organization are to adapt to the change successfully. The leader's job is to describe the change in a way that allows the workers to understand its value and how it will affect their own efforts.
>
> In this new era, leaders need insights about contextual themes rather than step-by-step guidance on how to implement a minutely defined vision. They must understand that their organization is on a journey and that they need to continuously peruse the landscape for guidance rather than create a list of steps through which the organization will move on its way to a preset future. Becoming aware of the themes and undercurrents and reading the contextual signposts regularly is a wiser and more effective strategy for the new age leader than laying out a itemized plan that may or may not correspond with future conditions (Porter-O'Grady & Malloch, 2007, pp. 23–24). [See **Exhibit 4–14**.]

Exhibit 4–14 Interdependence

In nature everything is interdependent. There is an ebb and flow between all the elements of life. Leaders must see their role from this perspective. Most of the work of leadership will be managing the interactions and connections between people and processes. Leaders must keep aware of these truths:

- Action in one place has an effect in other places.
- Fluctuation of mutuality means authority moves between people.
- Interacting properties in systems make outcomes mobile and fluid.
- Relationship building is the primary work of leadership.
- Trusting feeling is as important as valuing thinking.
- Acknowledging in others what is unique in their contribution is vital.
- Supporting, stretching, challenging, pushing, and helping are part of being present to the process, to the players, and to the outcome.

Source: Porter-O'Grady, T., and Malloch, K. (2003). *Quantum Leadership: A Textbook of New Leadership*. Sudbury, MA: Jones and Bartlett, p. 22.

Discussion Questions

1. What can the nurse administrator do to improve the patient–provider relationship?
2. What are some things nurse administrators must do to create a culture of safety?
3. Why is it important to provide evidence-based care? Discuss some of the challenges nurse administrators face in creating an environment in which bedside nurses use evidence-based care.
4. Discuss some ways to identify what adds value for the patient and family in health care.

References

Academic Center for Evidence-Based Practice. (2007). Evidence based competencies. Retrieved June 3, 2008 from http://www.acestar.uthscsa.edu

Agency for Healthcare Research and Quality. (2008). *National Healthcare Disparities Report: 2007*. AHRQ Pub. No. 08-0041. Rockville, MD: U.S. Department of Health and Human Services.

Aiken, L., Clarke, S., Sloane, D., Sochalski, J., & Silber, J. (2002). Hospital nurse staffing and patient mortality, nurse burnout, and job dissatisfaction. *Journal of the American Medical Association, 288*(16), 1987–1993.

Alexander, R. (2002, October). A mind for multicultural management: Foster an environment that celebrates patient diversity. *Nursing Management, 33*(10), 30–34.

American Nurses Association. (2008). Nurse staffing impacts quality of patient care. Retrieved May 28, 2008 from http://www.nursingworld.org/FunctionalMenuCategories/MediaResources/PressReleases/2008PR/NurseStaffingImpactsQualityofPatientCare.aspx

Bargmann, J. (2002). The top hospital in america. *AARP. 77*(8), 44–53.

Braden, G. (2000). *The Isaiah effect: Decoding the lost science of prayer and prophecy*. Carson, CA: Hay House.

Cantor, J., Schoen, C., Belloff, D., How, S., & McCarthy, D. (2007). *Aiming higher: Results from a state scorecard on health system performance*. The Common Wealth Fund. Retrieved June 12, 2008 from http://www.commonwealthfund.org/usr_doc/StateScorecard.pdf?section=4039

Centers for Disease Control and Prevention. (2007). Estimates of healthcare associated infections. Retrieved June 8, 2008 from http://www.cdc.gov/ncidod/dhqp/hai.html

Centers for Disease Control and Prevention. (2008). Falls among older adults: An overview. Retrieved June 18, 2008 from http://www.cdc.gov/ncipc/factsheets/adultfalls.htm

Centers for Medicare and Medicaid Services [CMS]. (2008a). Hospital-acquired conditions (present on admission indicator). Retrieved June 1, 2008 from http://www.cms.hhs.gov/HospitalAcqCond/01_Overview.asp#TopOfPage

Centers for Medicare and Medicaid Services [CMS]. (2008b). Quality initiatives—general information. Retrieved June 1, 2008 from http://www.cms.hhs.gov/QualityInitiativesGenInfo/

Chapman, E. (2004). *Radical loving care: Building the healing hospital in America*. Nashville, TN: Baptist Healing Hospital Trust.

Committee on the Consequences of Uninsurance. (2001). Coverage matters: Insurance and health care. Institute of Medicine report brief. Retrieved May 28, 2008 from http://books.nap.edu/html/coverage_matters/reportbrief.pdf

Consumer Driven Health Care Institute. (n.d.). Home page. Retrieved May 28, 2008 from http://www.cdhci.org/index.php

Conway, J. (2000). Strategies for leadership: Hospital executives and their role in patient safety. American Hospital Association. Retrieved June 3, 2008 from http://www.ihi.org/NR/rdonlyres/B45B10FC-C371-4CAF-B5F2-5CBBE0C1B4E7/136/StrategiesforLeadershipTool2.pdf

Culhane-Pera, K., Vawter, D., Xiong, P., Babbitt, B., & Solberg, M. (2003). *Healing by Heart: Clinical and Ethical Case Stories of Hmong Families and Western Providers*. Nashville, TN: Vanderbilt University Press.

Dunton, N., Gajewski, B., Klaus, S., & Pierson, B. (2007). The relationship of nursing workforce characteristics to patient outcomes. *Online Journal of Issues in Nursing*. Retrieved May 28, 2008 from http://www.nursingworld.org/MainMenuCategories/ANAMarketplace/ANAPeriodicals/OJIN/TableofContents/Volume122007/No3Sept07/NursingWorkforceCharacteristics.aspx

Eden Alternative. (2008). About us: The Eden Alternative. Retrieved May 18, 2008 from http://www.edenalt.org/about/index.html

Finkler, S., & Kovner, C. (2000). *Financial management for nurse managers and executives* (2nd ed.). Philadelphia: W. B. Saunders.

Garcia, R. (2006). Five ways you can reduce inappropriate prescribing in the elderly: a systematic review. *Journal of Family Practice, 55*, 305–312.

Gerteis, M., Edgman-Levitan, S., Daley, J., & Delbanco, T. (1993). *Through the patients' eyes: Understanding and promoting patient-centered care*. San Francisco: Jossey-Bass.

Giger, J., & Davidhizar, E. (2004). *Transcultural Nursing: Assessment and Intervention*, 4th Ed. NY: Mosby.

Grayson, M. (2002, October). Forward motion. *Hospital and Health Services Networks*, 34–38.

Haig, K., Sutton, S., & Whittington, J. (2006). SBAR: A shared mental model for improving communication between clinicians. *Journal on Quality and Patient Safety, 32*(3), 167–175.

Hay, L. (1988). *Heal your body*. Carson, CA: Hay House, Inc.

Health Care Advisory Board. (1999). Balanced scorecards. Retrieved July 8, 2008 from http://www.advisory.com

Institute for Healthcare Improvement. (n.d., a). Health care leaders leading: A Dana-Farber Cancer Institute executive describes the crucial role of leadership in driving patient safety. Retrieved June 3, 2008 from http://www.ihi.org/IHI/Topics/PatientSafety/MedicationSystems/ImprovementStories/HealthCareLeadersLeadingADanaFarberCancerInstituteexecutivedescribesthecrucialroleofleadershipindriv.htm

Institute for Healthcare Improvement. (n.d., b). How to improve. Retrieved June 3, 2008 from http://www.ihi.org/IHI/Topics/ChronicConditions/AllConditions/HowToImprove/

Institute for Healthcare Improvement. (2006). Leadership guide to patient safety. Retrieved from http://www.ihi.org/IHI/Results/WhitePapers/LeadershipGuidetoPatientSafetyWhitePaper.htm

Institute of Medicine. (2000). *America's health care safety net, intact but endangered*. Washington, DC: National Academies Press.

Institute of Medicine. (2001). *Crossing the quality chasm: A new health system for the 21st century.* Washington, DC: National Academies Press.

Institute of Medicine. (2004a). *Health literacy: A prescription to end confusion.* Washington, DC: National Academies Press.

Institute of Medicine. (2004b). *Keeping patients safe: Transforming the work environment of nurses.* Washington, DC: National Academies Press.

Institute of Medicine. (2006). *Preventing medication errors.* Washington, DC: National Academies Press.

Institute of Medicine. (2007). *Creating a business case for quality improvement research: Expert views, workshop summary.* Washington, DC: National Academies Press.

Jackevicius, C., Li, P., & Tu, J. (2008). Prevalence, predictors, and outcomes of primary nonadherence after acute myocardial infarction. *Circulation, 117*, 1028–1036.

Joint Commission on Accreditation of Healthcare Organizations. (2008). Patient safety. Retrieved June 1, 2008 from http://www.jointcommission.org/PatientSafety/

Kaiser Commission. (2006). The uninsured and their access to health care. Retrieved May 28, 2008 from http://www.kff.org/uninsured/upload/The-Uninsured-and-Their-Access-to-Health-Care-Oct-2004.pdf

Kane, R., Shamliyan, T., Mueller, C., Duval, S., & Witt, T. (2007). *Nursing staffing and quality of patient care. Evidence Report/Technology Assessment No. 151.* AHRQ Publication No. 07- 005. Rockville, MD: Agency for Healthcare Research and Quality.

Kripalani, S., Henderson, L., Jacobson, T., & Vaccarino, V. (2008). Medication use among inner-city patients after hospital discharge: Patient-reported barriers and solutions. *Mayo Clinic Proceedings, 83*(5), 529–535.

Leapfrog Group. (n.d.). Fact sheet. Retrieved May 13, 2008 from http://www.leapfroggroup.org/about_us/leapfrog-factsheet.

Leonhardt, K., Bonin, D., & Pagel, P. (2007). How to develop a community-based patient advisory council. Aurora Health Care and CAPS Toolkit. Retrieved June 3, 2008 from http://patientsafety.org/page/109387/;jsessionid=7vhlrvtobuim2

Lindrooth, R., Bazzoli, G., Needleman, J., & Hasnain-Wynia, R. (2006). The effect of changes in hospital reimbursement on nurse staffing decisions at safety net and nonsafety net hospitals. Retrieved June 3, 2008 from http://www.pubmedcentral.nih.gov/articlerender.fcgi?tool=pubmed&pubmedid=16704508

Maniaci, M., Heckman, M., & Dawson, N. (2008). Functional health literacy and understanding of medications at discharge. *Mayo Clinic Proceedings, 83*(5), 554–558.

Markey, D., & Brown, R. (2002). An interdisciplinary approach to addressing patient activity and mobility in medical-surgical patient. *Journal of Nursing Care Quality, 16*(4), 1–12.

Melberg, S. (1997). Effects of changing skill mix. *Nursing Management, 28*(11), 47–48.

Miller, W., Vigdor, E., & Manning, G. (2004). Covering the uninsured: What is it worth? *Health Affairs*, W4157–W4167.

National Center for Patient Safety. (2006). *Falls toolkit.* Retrieved June 8, 2008 from www.va.gov/ncps/SafetyTopics/fallstoolkit/notebook/completebooklet.pdf

National Center for Policy Analysis. (2008). *Patient safety in American hospitals.* Retrieved June 8, 2008 from http://www.ncpa.org/sub/dpd/index.php?Article_ID=16556

Picker Institute. (n.d.). *Welcome to the Picker Institute.* Retrieved May 12, 2008 from http://www.pickerinstitute.org/index.html

Planetree, Inc. (2008). *About Planetree.* Retrieved May 18, 2008 from http://www.planetree.org/ABOUT/ABOUT.html

Pointe, P., Conlin, G., Conway, J., Grant, S., Medeiros, C., Nies, J., Shulman, L., Branowicki, P., & Conley, K. (2003). Making patient-centered care come alive: Achieving full integration of the patient's perspective. *Journal of Nursing Administration, 33*(2), 82–90.

Porter-O'Grady, T. (2003). Of hubris and hope: Transforming nursing for a new age. *Nursing Economic$, 21*(2), 59–64.

Porter-O'Grady, T., & Malloch, K. (2003). *Quantum leadership: A textbook of new leadership*. Sudbury, MA: Jones and Bartlett.

Porter-O'Grady, T., & Malloch, K. (2007). *Quantum leadership: A resource for health innovation* (2nd ed.). Sudbury, MA: Jones and Bartlett.

Press Ganey. (2007). *Patient perspectives on American health care*. Retrieved May 12, 2008 from http://www.pressganey.com/galleries/default-file/hospital-report.pdf

Purnell, L., & Paulanka, B. (2003). *Transcultural Health Care: A Culturally Competent Approach*, 2nd ed. Philadelphia: F. A. Davis.

Rhoades, J. (2005). The uninsured in America, 1996–2004: Estimates for the U.S. civilian noninstitutionalized population under age 65. AHRQ Statistical Brief #84. Retrieved May 28, 2008 from http://meps.ahrq.gov/mepsweb/data_files/publications/st84/stat84.pdf

Rudy, E., Lucke, J., Whitman, G., & Davidson, L. (2001). Benchmarking patient outcomes. *Journal of Nursing Scholarship, 33*(2), 185–189.

Shirey, M. (2006). Evidence-based practice: Impact on nursing administration. *Nursing Administration Quarterly, 30*(3), 252–265.

Simonson, W., & Feinberg, J. (2005). Medication-related problems in the elderly: Defining the issues and identifying solutions. *Drugs and Aging, 22*(7), 559–569.

Smith, B. (2003). Lean and six sigma—a one-two punch. *Quality Progress*, 37–41.

Stevens, J., Corso, P., Finkelstein, E., & Miller, T. (2006). The costs of fatal and non-fatal falls among older adults. Retrieved May 15, 2008 from http://injuryprevention.bmj.com/cig/content/full/12/5/290

St. Hill, P., Lipson, J., and Meleis, A. (2003). *Caring for Women Cross-Culturally*. Philadelphia: F. A. Davis.

Tennessee Hospitals & Health Systems. (2008). *THA develops nonpayment policy on serious adverse events.* Nashville, TN: Tennessee Hospital Association.

U.S. Department of Health and Human Services. (n.d.). Quick guide to health literacy: Fact sheet. Retrieved June 3, 2008 from http://www.health.gov/communication/literacy/quickguide/factsbasic.htm

Utilization Review Accreditation Commission [URAC]. (2008). What is care management? Retrieved June 3, 2008 from http://www.urac.org/resources/careManagement.aspx

U.S. Census Bureau. (2007). More diversity. Slower growth. Retrieved May 18, 2008 from http://www.census.gov/Press-Release/www/releases/archives/population/001720.html

Vanhey, D., Aiken, L., Sloane, D., Clarke, S., & Vargas, D. (2004). Nurse burnout and patient satisfaction. *Medical Care, 42*(2 Suppl), II57–II66.

Watson, J. (2004). *Postmodern nursing and beyond*. New York: Elsevier.

Weber, S. (2008, July). Ergonomics standards: An overview. *Nursing Management*, 28–31.

Wheatley, M. (1992). *Leadership and the new science*, San Francisco: Berrett-Koehler.

Whitman, G., Kim, Y., Davidson, L., Wolf, G., & Wang, S. (2002). The impact of staffing on patient outcomes across specialty units. *Journal of Nursing Administration, 32*(12), 633–639.

Woods, A., & Doan-Johnson, S. (2002, October). Executive summary: Toward a taxonomy of nursing practice errors. *Nursing Management*, 45–48.

CHAPTER 5

Pinpointing Evidence-Based Information: How to Find the Needle in the Information Haystack

Rick Wallace, MA, MDiv, MAOM, MSLS, EdD, AHIP

Martha Whaley, MSLS

Nakia Joye Carter, MSIS, AHIP

Janne Dunham-Taylor, PhD, RN

Hospital administrators are encouraged to use **higher ratios of RNs to non-licensed personnel** *to achieve their objective of quality patient outcomes and cost containment.*

- Significant *reductions in cost and length of stay* may be possible with higher ratios of nursing personnel in hospital settings.
- Sufficient numbers of RNs may *prevent patient adverse events* that cause patients to stay longer than necessary.
- *Patient costs were reduced* with greater RN staffing as RNs have higher knowledge and skill levels to provide more effective nursing care as well as reduce patient resource consumption (Thungjaroenkul, Cummings, & Embleton, 2007, p. 255).

Key Terms

- Bibliographic Database
- Case Control Study
- Case Study
- Cohort Study
- Evidence-Based Information (EBI)
- Informatics
- Levels of Evidence (LOE)
- Nursing Informatics
- PDA

- PICO (Population, Intervention, Comparison, Outcome)
- Proprietary Database
- Randomized Controlled Trial (RCT)
- Secondary Literature
- Strength of Recommendation (SOR) Ratings
- Systematic Review
- Translational Literature

This excerpt from a systematic review examining the impact of staffing changes illustrates just how important best evidence can be to the nurse administrator. What is the real value of evidence-based information? In some cases it may be worth only pennies, but in others it could be as invaluable as patients' lives. Those who have information (or access to information) have a powerful tool, one that can give them the confidence to make wiser, more cost-effective decisions. In this case the evidence can also be used to more effectively argue that better staffing is necessary to achieve better patient outcomes and higher cost savings for organizations.

Consider the following issues that nurse administrators frequently face:

- "Children's Memorial Hospital in Chicago reduced the turnover among new grads from 29.5% to 12.3% through the implementation of a multi-faceted orientation program" (Halfer, 2007, p. 7).
- "Researchers explored the relationship between nurse managers' leadership styles and organizational culture of nursing units within an acute care hospital that had achieved excellent organizational performance as demonstrated by a consistent increase in patient satisfaction ratings" (Casida & Pinto-Zipp, 2008, p. 7).
- "The short tenure of nurse managers is an urgent aspect of the leadership vacuum within the nursing shortage. [This article] describes the organizational factors that contribute to engagement for nurse managers and the applications for building cultures of engagement" (Mackoff & Triolo, 2008, p. 166).
- "Nurses are more satisfied with understanding, open, and accurate communication, especially with attending-level physicians" (Manojlovich & Antonakos, 2008, p. 237).
- "With demands to improve patients' clinical outcomes and decrease the escalating costs of inpatient care, nurse executives are focusing on how nurses spend their time rather than just raising staffing levels to positively impact patient outcomes.... More than one-third of nurses' time was considered non-value-added, averaging $757,000 per nursing unit in wage costs annually. Nurses spent more time on support activities (56%) than in providing patient care (44%) with the least amount of time being spent on patient teaching and psychosocial support" (Storfjell, Omoike, & Ohlson, 2008, p. 244).
- "12-hour shifts have become a common scheduling option for nurses.... Recent research suggests that 12-hour shifts are a potential hazard to patients" (Lorenz, 2008, p. 297).
- "Nursing highly values and exhorts its practitioners to function autonomously.... Magnet hospital staff nurses score significantly higher [in autonomy] than their counterparts in comparison hospitals" (Kramer, Maguire, & Schmalenberg, 2006, pp. 479, 487).
- Nurse administrators are often involved in designing new (or remodeling) facilities. "In this article, the author provides nurse leaders with examples of where to find data to guide decisions about the efficacy of specific design features in achieving desired outcomes" (Stichler, 2008, 153).

All these examples are current issues nurse administrators face while often not realizing that *evidence-based information might capture more solutions for their administrative practice.*

In addition, nurse administrators must *encourage staff nurses to consistently use evidence-based clinical information* as they care for patients. This is illustrated in Rauen, Vollman, Arbour, and Chulay's (2008) article, provocatively titled "Challenging Nursing's Sacred Cows." The authors discuss three examples of commonly performed practices that are not based on evidence:

1. Instilling normal saline solution into the patient's endotracheal tube before suctioning.
2. Turning critically ill patients manually every 2 hours.
3. Relying on the Glasgow coma scale alone for routine neurologic assessment.

According to Rauen et al. (2008), "When these practices were introduced, no research supported them. Yet many practitioners keep performing them despite recent research that suggests they should be changed" (p. 23).

Current evidence tells us that different approaches are necessary:

- "Instilling NSS [normal saline solution] before suctioning decreases oxygen saturation and forced expiratory volume (a sign of bronchospasm). This practice may increase the risk of hospital-acquired pneumonia" (Rauen et al., 2008, p. 23). So it is best not to do this.
- One longitudinal study "of a critical care unit found that over an 8 hour period only 2.7% of observed patients experienced position changes every 2 hours and more than half were supine for 4–8 hours" (p. 23). It was found that "turning every 2 hours isn't frequent enough to preserve the lung's oxygenating ability or prevent ventilator-acquired pneumonia" (p. 24). [Additional valuable information on positioning is also contained in this article.]
- "Although the GCS [Glasgow coma scale] has distinct benefits, scoring hinges on the patient's ability to respond to stimulation and interact with the clinician. The GCS doesn't assess brainstem reflexes, and has limited value for patients with deep sedation, neuromuscular block-ade, intubation and controlled ventilation, and some psychiatric or metabolic disorders" (p. 25).

Best-evidence information gives caregivers, managers, and administrators confidence in decision making. In fact, from a clinical perspective Klein, Ross, Adams, and Gilbert (1994) observed the following:

> Not only does information serve to trigger new or different diagnostic tests or therapeutic maneuvers, but as studies have suggested, its usefulness also exists in halting procedures or therapies that have been shown to be ineffective in similar situations (p. 492).

Klein et al. even suggested that database searching could be billed to third-party payers. We have discovered in the hospital setting that nurses often consult the professional literature for informa-tion. Some caregivers searched the literature and attached the resulting information to a patient's chart or medical record.

In this chapter we consider the information needs of nurse managers from an organizational and patient-centric perspective, and we review various resources for locating accurate, relevant information.

Nursing science is "information intense" from the first day of nursing school to the end of a career. We are now well into the 21st century, and print information is being converted continuously to digital formats. The study of how electronic information systems are used to improve nursing systems and ultimately patient care is referred to as *nursing informatics*. In a class we teach on nurs-ing informatics, we use the text *Essentials of Nursing Informatics* by Virginia Saba and Kathleen McCormick (2006)—an excellent reference. This text defines informatics as "a science that com-bines a domain science, computer science, information science and cognitive science" (p. 266).

Computer science and its application in information technology (IT) play a significant role in health care as a means to quickly access large volumes of information. This plethora of information presents a great challenge to nurse managers. How does one pinpoint the most relevant articles, books, and websites? The nurse manager's role involves being aware of and keeping updated on the following:

- How to find information needed to better manage the unit/department.
- How to encourage/require staff nurses to stay informed on current trends so they can follow best practices.
- How to provide consumer information for patients.

- How to choose, implement, and purchase new IT, and resources.
- How to ensure that staff nurses are adequately trained and involved in using all available resources.

Both the nurse manager and nursing staff need to use information resources so that ultimately the patient is served in the best possible manner. This means that the nurse manager fights several battles to make sure that all this is occurring and that adequate resources are available so this can happen. What an important responsibility!

Librarians are here to help you and your staff achieve all this. In this chapter we, as librarians, share our knowledge of information resources. Williams and Zipperer (2003) said, "Nurse administrators can establish partnerships with a medical librarian to help staff contribute to the safety of patients through improved access to the evidence" (p. 200). More on that later.

Evidence-Based Information

When we say that our decisions are evidence-based, what do we mean? The Joanna Briggs Institute, an international collaboration of organizations and institutions that promote evidence-based practice, defines evidence-based practice as "the melding of individual clinical judgment and expertise with the best available external evidence to generate the kind of practice that is most likely to lead to a positive outcome for a client or patient" (joannabriggs.edu.au). Nurse managers need to be sure that staff nurses are using best practices in their work.

The broader definition, however, goes beyond patient care to evidence that will help us better perform our work. As we look at the available information, it is important to glean the best evidence that applies to our work. For instance, a nurse manager needs to be aware of administrative and educational information that might influence or change administrative practices.

One more comment about evidence-based practice before we move on to another topic. It has a direct bearing on patient safety, a primary goal of nurse managers. This was articulated in a recent article by Williams and Zipperer (2003):

> Efficient and timely access to evidence-based medical literature is an important element in providing safe patient care. This knowledge base exists in primary sources such as the medication administration records and patients' medical records, from colleagues, and ideally, in the science reported in the biomedical literature. Given the complexity and time constraints involved in care delivery, seeking out the right information at the right time is an increasingly difficult goal for many health practitioners to reach. Frontline nurses are no exception to this dilemma. A key role for management therefore is to help improve access to evidence-based literature for nurses to enable them to interact more proactively for safety. Key to improving access to evidence from biomedical literature is the medical reference librarian or clinical librarian (p. 199).

Finding Information to Better Manage the Unit/Department

You need to find information on staffing ratios. You want help from the professional literature in making a decision, so you will not be relying solely on your own experience. Where do you turn? Outstanding databases are available for situations such as this.

Exhibit 5–1 lists selected resources that are gateways to the literature of nursing, informatics, and nurse management. The first is the online version (cinahl.com) of the Cumulated Index to Nursing and Allied Health Literature (CINAHL®). CINAHL has over 2,500,000 citations from more than 2,500

Exhibit 5–1 Selected Nurse Manager Resources

Focus	Website	Resource
Nursing and Allied Health	cinahl.com	Cumulative Index to Nursing and Allied Health Literature® (proprietary)
PubMed	ncbi.nlm.nih.gov/entrez	U.S. National Library of Medicine (free)
Business	il.proquest.com/products_pq/descriptions/abi_inform.shtml	ABI/Inform (proprietary)
Business	galegroup.com	Gale Group (proprietary)
Education	eric.ed.gov	ERIC (free)
Law	lexis-nexis.com	Lexis/Nexis (proprietary)
Statistics	cdc.gov/nchs/	National Center for Health Statistics (free)
Statistics	lib.umich.edu/govdocs/stats.html	Statistical Resources on the Web (free)
Medicare/Medicaid	cms.hhs.gov	Centers for Medicare & Medicaid Services (free)
Nursing Homes	medicare.gov/NHCompare	Nursing Home Compare (free)
General	scholar.google.com	Google Scholar (free)

journal titles. Its focus is nursing and allied health. It is a *proprietary* database, which means that it is privately owned and controlled. CINAHL may be purchased from several vendors, including CINAHL Information System, Data-Star, EBSCO Publishing, OVID Technologies, and ProQuest.

Another favorite resource of librarians is PubMed®, the National Library of Medicine's free database of more than 17 million citations to biomedical articles published from the 1950s to the present (pubmed.gov) **(Exhibit 5–2)**.

To start a search in any database, clearly define what you want to find. Write it down. Think of synonyms for your concept. Your search will only be as successful as your terms. Because we all use different terms for the same thing, here are some searching tips. First, use the *PICO format* **(Exhibit 5–3)** to help you better define your question. Let's say you wondered if there is a difference in patient outcomes when nurses work an 8-hour versus a 12-hour shift. Using the PICO format, you fill in each part as follows:

- Here the *Population* would actually be nurses who work the shifts, although as we thought about it we decided to further specify only registered nurses.

- We identify the *Interventions* as the 8- and 12-hour shifts. So in "I" we will put 8-hour shift, whereas in "C", *the Comparative intervention*, we will put 12-hour shift.

- We decided to start this search with the *Outcome* being patient satisfaction. (The Outcome in the original question was not precisely delineated. We could also do a different search using other *specific* patient outcomes, such as decubiti.)

After filtering this information through the PICO format, revise the question using the PICO terms you have determined to more specifically define the search. Our new question is, *For registered nurses, does working an 8-hour shift versus a 12-hour shift provide better patient satisfaction as measured by patient surveys?* You can see that the original question is quite "fuzzy" compared with the one that has been refined with the PICO format.

Exhibit 5–2 The National Library of Medicine's PubMed® Database

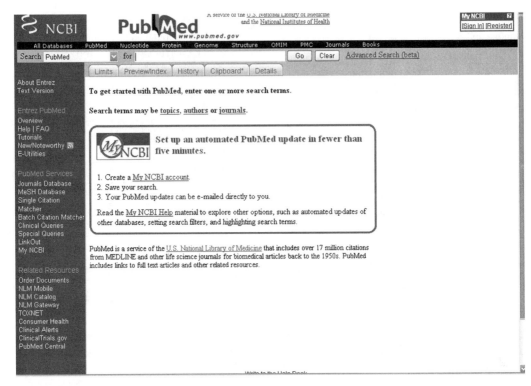

Source: http://www.ncbi.nw.nih.gov

Exhibit 5–3 PICO Format

Initial Question: Is there a difference in patient outcomes when nurses work an 8-hour versus a 12-hour shift?

P	*Identify the population or patient*	Registered nurses
I	*Intervention being considered*	8-hour shifts
C	*Comparative intervention being considered*	12-hour shifts
O	*Outcome desired for the population or patient*	Patient satisfaction measured by patient surveys

Revised Question: For registered nurses, does working an 8-hour shift versus a 12-hour shift provide better patient satisfaction as measured by patient surveys?

Second, be sure to use *limits* (**Exhibit 5–4**). For example, *date limits* can be very important. In health care, as you know, information has increased exponentially. Articles that are only 2 or 3 years old may be outdated and therefore may be of little value or even harmful. In our example we may want to limit the date of the retrieved articles to the last 5 years. *Language limits* are also

Exhibit 5–4 Summary of Limiting Techniques for Successful Database Search

Limiting Search Technique	Function
Subject headings	Allows a sharper focus in your search. Increases recall (getting all the articles on your topic) and precision (not getting articles that are irrelevant).
Date limit	Allows you to limit the time period in which you are searching.
Publication type limit	Very valuable for the advanced searcher. May want to restrict to clinical trials for therapy searches.
Language limit	Particularly valuable for PubMed, which indexes articles in journals written in over 40 languages.
Subheadings	A further refinement of subject headings that allows a tighter focus. For example, instead of retrieving every article on hypertension, you can limit to only therapy articles on hypertension.

useful, particularly in PubMed, which indexes articles from more than 40 languages. Unless you read Azerbaijani, this is an important tip. So, we want to limit our search to English. *Publication type* is another valuable limiter. In our example, we may want to limit the publication type to guidelines or systematic reviews. You may want to eliminate publication types such as letters to the editor or news and comments from your retrieval. (Note: Limits in PubMed are a function of indexing.) Using limits will *not* retrieve articles that are not indexed. In CINAHL you can use date published, language, publication type, peer-reviewed journal, and evidence-based practice to limit or refine your search.

A third tip is that *subheadings* bring a tighter focus to your search. A frequent problem in searching is finding too much information. Subheadings help you focus on one aspect of a topic. For example, in PubMed you may type the term "staffing" into the subject-heading index and click on it. Several choices are offered, and you select "personnel staffing and scheduling". You click on this term and notice that the subheadings are "classification, economics, ethics, history, legislation and jurisprudence, methods, organization and administration, standards, statistics and numerical data, trends and utilization". You choose the subheading "organization and administration" and "trends and utilization" because this is the type of information you need. Your retrieval of citations is more focused because you have chosen to eliminate articles with the other subheadings.

CINAHL and PubMed are not the only useful resources for nurse managers. (Refer again to Exhibit 5–1.) An excellent source for business information is ABI/INFORM, a proprietary database. According to the vendor website,

> Featuring over 4,055 journals, ABI/INFORM Complete™ is the most comprehensive business database on the market today. The combination of products forms a business database package that offers more than 2,965 full-text titles covering business and economic conditions, corporate strategies, management techniques, as well as competitive and product information.

The Gale Group of databases is proprietary and has several business databases such as Business & Company ProFile ASAP, Business & Company Resource Center, Business & Industry, Business & Management Practices, and Business Reference Suite. Gale also has the health databases Health Reference Center Academic and Health & Wellness Resource Center.

The Lexis/Nexis database is another proprietary database. It is an outstanding source of legal information and news.

State web pages are a superb source of information. In many instances they have the state code, health professional licensure verification, and rules and regulations from various state agencies.

A good source of statistical information is the National Center for Health Statistics®, produced by the Centers for Disease Control and Prevention (cdc.gov/nchs). Another exceptional site for statistical information is "Statistical Resources on the Web", produced by the University of Michigan (lib.umich.edu/govdocs/stats.html).

Specific information on Medicare and Medicaid can be found at cms.hhs.gov/ at the Centers for Medicare and Medicaid Services. Another useful database is medicare.gov, which has a link to a site that compares nursing homes.

ERIC (eric.ed.gov) is a premier education database. According to the ERIC website: ERIC provides free access to more than 1.2 million bibliographic records of journal articles and other education-related materials and, if available, includes links to full text.

If you are not searching for information on a specific topic but are looking for professional reading material for nurse managers, the *Journal of Nursing Administration* is an excellent publication. It is published monthly (July/August combined) by Lippincott Williams & Wilkins. Other first-rate journals are *Nursing Economic$, Nursing Management, Nursing Administration Quarterly, The Nurse Leader*, and *Seminars for Nurse Managers*. General business journals such as the *Harvard Business Review* are also good sources, as are generic business and administration textbooks. In addition, specific professional organizations have wonderful websites, giving administrative and clinical information for their specialty (**Exhibit 5–5**).

Exhibit 5–5 Selected Nursing and Informatics Organizations

Organization	Website
American Academy of Ambulatory Care Nursing (AAACN)	aaacn.org
American Association of Colleges of Nursing (AACN)	www.aacn.nche.edu
American Nurses Association (ANA)	nursingworld.org
American Nursing Informatics Association (ANIA)	ania.org
American Organization of Nurse Executives (AONE)	aone.org
American Public Health Association, Public Health Nursing Section (APHAPHN)	apha.org/membergroups/sections/aphasections/phn
Home Healthcare Nurses Association (HHNA)	www.hhna.org
National Association Directors of Nursing Administration in Long Term Care (NADONA/LTC)	nadona.org
National League for Nursing (NLN)	www.nln.org
Nursing Informatics Special Interest Group of the International Medical Informatics Association	www.imiani.org
Nursing Informatics Working Group of the American Medical Informatics Association	amia.org
Sigma Theta Tau International Honor Society of Nursing (STT)	nursingsociety.org

Do not forget to use *books* in this electronic age. One trick is to search for books in the subject area of your interest at Amazon.com. Copy the information and submit it to your librarian, who may be able to obtain the book on interlibrary loan. Please take time to search the online public access catalogs of large libraries. Almost all large libraries have made their catalogs available to search freely on the web. LOCATORPlus, the catalog of the U.S. National Library of Medicine, the largest medical library in the world, is available at locatorplus.gov. If you find a good title, ask your librarian to obtain it on interlibrary loan. In addition, the major publishers have very helpful websites (i.e., Jones and Bartlett, jbpub.com).

Finally, you should learn to use *search engines* such as Google, still the search engine of choice even though other search engines do have some features not contained in Google. Take time to look around in Google. If you are feeling mischievous, you may want to go to your neighbor's computer and click preferences in Google and set the retrieval to display in Klingon or Pig Latin. The *Google Images* tab is a great service because it restricts your search to only images. If you wanted an image of a pressure ulcer, for example, this would be a good place to look. *Google Scholar* provides a way of searching scholarly material across many subject areas, from nursing to music, in many formats, such as books, papers, abstracts, and conference proceedings.

Encouraging/Expecting Staff Nurses to Use Best Practices

While conducting a study to understand how healthy lungs protect against asthma attacks, a medical researcher did not thoroughly check the published research and missed the literature pointing out the potentially lethal side effects of the drug hexamethonium. A study volunteer died from complications caused by the drug. The supervising physician searched online resources, including PubMed, that only went back to 1964. This lethal side effect had been reported in the 1950s, so it was missed. This incident led to the development of search protocols by the institution to ensure that the researchers found all pertinent literature (newsbreaks.infotoday.com/nbreader. asp ?ArticleID=17534).

At this point we would like to insert a bit of philosophy. (Please do not change the channel. We promise to continue with more practical suggestions.) The guiding philosophy that nurse administrators, as well as health care librarians, should follow is that we must always focus on what is best for the patient. Our top priority is ordering our activities so that the greatest good is being done for patients.

Many people think of libraries and information as nice to have but ultimately nonessential. This is not true! Information is critical in providing the best health care. At our university we host a camp for high school students who are considering careers as health professionals. These students are reminded that only one group of people can tell you to take your clothes off or stab you with needles and knives and get away with it—health professionals. The rest of us would be arrested if we did that. The difference between health care professionals and the remainder of the world is what is between their ears—their knowledge, as well as caring. This one group has mastered a body of knowledge that gives them special rights in society. Of course, that professional degree does not give the one who earned it permission to coast along the information highway. Graduation is only the first step on a path of lifelong learning.

Many studies detail the deterioration of health care professionals' knowledge over time. One study (Shin, Haynes, & Johnston, 1993) found that a significant number of providers continued to use the treatment for hypertension that was standard in the year the provider finished formal training. Other studies identified the gold standard of therapy for a disease. Then health providers were chosen randomly and asked how they treated the disease. The treatments varied greatly. Although the study focused on physicians, the same assumption can be made about all professionals: Without frequent updating and retraining, knowledge and skill decline over time. The bottom line is this: *It is imperative for health care professionals to have the best information so everyone gets the best treatment.*

The goal for any health care professional should be to become an information master. This means not having to rely on outside expertise but instead being able to skillfully retrieve the highest quality information, appraise it, and apply it.

Here are five steps, presented as the "five "A's," to best practice information:

1. *Assess.* As you assess a situation, most often you have questions. No one learned it all in school; even if we did, we soon forget what we learn. Furthermore, if we learned it all and we did not forget, so much new information is being discovered that we are already behind as soon as we graduate.

2. *Ask.* It may be helpful to go through the PICO process explained earlier to develop precise questions (see Exhibit 5–3).

3. *Acquire.* The secret is to map your term from your PICO question to one of the controlled vocabulary terms in the database. This will help you get a much more successful retrieval. For example, in the PubMed database, the term for "heart attack" is "myocardial infarction", so if you used adult heart attack patients when you searched PubMed, you would need to change your term to "myocardial infarction" and, as a limit, to "adults". (Remember to ask your librarian if you need help with this step.)

4. *Appraise.* We will discuss critical appraisal in the next section, including levels of evidence and strength of recommendations.

5. *Apply.* In applying new information to the patient or management situation, you should ask the following questions:

   - How closely does the situation described in the literature match your situation?
   - What are the unique values of your patient or corporate culture?
   - How does the new information mesh with your values and instincts and past experiences?

Evaluating the Quality of Information on the Web

Now let's get back to filtering information once again. The web has a tremendous potential for the delivery of health information. Never before has such an opportunity been available to deliver current information to such a wide audience. But, there is a downside. Fraudulent health information exists on the web. You should keep several principles in mind when using web information. First, ask if it is produced by a reputable organization. What is the domain of the site? Is it an .edu (educational institution) or a .com (corporation)? A business corporation exists to make money, so have your "bias detector" turned on if you use a .com site. Often in health care, an .edu, .gov, or .org (an organization such as the American Heart Association) will have more reliable information. When was the site last updated? Is it current or out of date? There are certifications indicating the quality of health websites such as the Health on the Net Foundation code. However, be aware that these approval seals are usually self-reported, and any web page designer can copy the quality logo and paste it on his or her web page.

You should ask where the information originated and how it is selected. A good site has a purpose statement and clearly identifies its funding and creators. Is the site updated regularly? Is the site free from grammatical and typographical errors? Another thing to consider is the manner in which the site handles human interactions. Avoid a site that requires a lot of personal information before you are allowed to use it. Finally, glitz and glamour do not equal a quality website. A good site is easy to navigate, pleasing to the eye, and has minimal typographical and spelling errors.

Exhibit 5–6 Example of Research Study Types

Research Study Type	Features
Randomized controlled Trial	Experimental; equal chance to be in either group; blinded; considered most accurate; two arms (experimental and control); best type of study to answer etiology and therapy questions
Cohort study	Observational; starts in the present and followed to the future; best type of study to answer prognosis questions
Case control study	Retrospective; collects data from charts, data sets, and patient interviews
Case study	Detailed analysis of a person or group usually focused on a unique case
Systematic reviews	Combine the results of many randomized controlled trials; high level of evidence

Now let's go back to the staffing example discussed in the previous section. As we (or our helpful librarians) retrieve some possible articles, some basic principles will be helpful to aid you in critically appraising these articles.

Levels of Evidence

First, we want you to know that different types of research studies are used in the literature. Not all studies are created equal. A new trend is to evaluate studies based on rankings of evidence. These rankings are called levels of evidence *(LOEs)* (**Exhibit 5–6**). It is always best to use the highest LOE.

The *randomized controlled trial (RCT)* is the most accurate or "truthful" type of health information related to therapeutic topics. RCTs are carefully designed. They are blinded or double-blinded so that neither the participants nor the administrators know who is getting the experimental treatment and who is in the control group. They are randomized in the sense that everyone who is in the population being studied has an equal chance of being chosen to be in the experimental group (arm) or control group.

When many of these RCTs on the same topic are compiled, the result is termed a *systematic review*. Actually, the systematic review is the highest level because it puts together several randomized controlled studies. Although not RCTs, the first quote of this chapter is a systematic review of staffing and length of stay research.

A *cohort study*, the second LOE, is an observational study in which a group of people is identified in the present and followed into the future (a "prospective cohort study") or is identified from past records and followed from that time up to the present (a "retrospective cohort study"). An example of a cohort study is the famous Framingham study of heart disease, which has followed participant citizens of Framingham, Massachusetts, since 1948.

Case control studies are retrospective in nature and are the third LOE. They collect data from charts, data sets, and patient interviews. A good use of the case control study is for studies of harm. For example, we may choose patients with and without lung cancer and then examine the patients' records for a past exposure to a toxic substance.

A *case study*, the fourth LOE, is a detailed analysis of a person or group from a social, psychological, or medical point of view. It involves one case, usually one that is unique. The last LOE occurs

Exhibit 5–7 Example of a Levels of Evidence (LOE) Rating Scale

Level of Evidence	Explanation
Level I	Evidence obtained from at least one properly designed randomized controlled trial
Level II-1	Evidence obtained from well-designed controlled trials without randomization
Level II-2	Evidence obtained from well-designed cohort or case control analytic studies, preferably from more than one center or research group
Level II-3	Evidence obtained from multiple time series with or without the intervention. Dramatic results in uncontrolled trials might also be regarded as this type of evidence.
Level III	Opinions of respected authorities, based on clinical experience, descriptive studies, or reports of expert committees

Source: U.S. Preventive Services Task Force.

when individuals publish their expert opinions based on observation or research. **Exhibit 5–7** is another example of a LOE rating scale.

Strength of Recommendation Ratings

Just as there are ratings of studies based on study type, so also are there ratings to guide the reader as to the trustworthiness of the information. These are called *strength of recommendation* ratings (**Exhibit 5–8**) and may be found at guidelines.gov. Be warned that not all guidelines are evidence-based; some guidelines are *expert-based*. Cassey (2007) suggested the following:

> Once you find an important guideline related to your practice needs, consider working to incorporate the new guideline materials into your organization's practice manuals. Take a leadership role in bringing these relevant resources and new nursing knowledge to policy and procedures committees for active consideration (p. 303).

If critical appraisal concepts are overwhelming to you, welcome to the club. However, until you better understand the process, critical appraisal tools will guide you through the process. They can be found at the following urls from the Centre for Evidence Based Medicine, Duke University Medical Library, and Dartmouth Biomedical Library:

- cebm.net/index.aspx?o=1157
- mclibrary.duke.edu/subject/ebm?tab=appraising&extra=worksheets
- dartmouth.edu/~biomed/resources.htmld/guides/ebm_teach.shtml#worksheets

Well, now we have ruined your day. You probably thought you could just read the first journal article you found that was on your topic and that was sufficient. After all, are you not reading this book to make your hectic life easier? Do you need a new layer of guilt about something else you are not doing well?

Exhibit 5–8   Example of a Strength of Recommendation Table

Strength of Recommendation	Explanation
A	A strong recommendation, based on evidence or general agreement, that a given procedure or treatment is useful/effective, always acceptable, and usually indicated
B	A recommendation, based on evidence or general agreement, that a given procedure or treatment may be considered useful/effective
C	A recommendation that is not well established or for which there is conflicting evidence regarding usefulness or efficacy but which may be made on other grounds
D	A recommendation, based on evidence or general agreement, that a given procedure or treatment may be considered not useful/effective
E	A strong recommendation, based on evidence or general agreement, that a given procedure or treatment is not useful/effective, always acceptable, and usually indicated

Source: VA/DoD clinical practice guideline for management of ischemic heart disease.

Secondary Filters That Sort Out Best Evidence

Don't worry if you believe you do not have the skills to make critical appraisal judgments at this point. Critical appraisal skills take time to develop. An option is to turn to "secondary" or "translation" literature. These secondary databases really help us because only the highest LOE in summarized form goes into these databases. Therefore your search will produce only high quality results.

Secondary literature is based on dividing the literature into DOEs and POEMs. Most articles are DOEs, or **D**isease **O**riented **E**vidence, but these are *not* as helpful for the health professional. The most helpful secondary source, although they are not as plentiful, is the POEM, or **P**atient **O**riented **I**nformation that **M**atters. ("*Patient Oriented Information*" is used in the broad sense and includes many administrative as well as clinical studies.)

As we have mentioned before, health care professionals' poor utilization of the literature is not surprising considering the tendency of the health care system to put more and more work on fewer and fewer nurses. The health care literature is replete with articles that are discussions of DOEs. These articles do not help the caregiver, because the results described have not been proven in populations of people. They are often just the tedious manuscripts of academics and researchers yacking it up with each other.

In contrast, a POEM is important to the patient or administrator. POEMs are underutilized because clinicians are so overwhelmed with DOEs they miss POEMs. The secondary literature is a real advance because it attempts to create databases that are exclusively POEMs.

In a classic article, Slawson and Shaughnessy (1994) cited a good study on the diagnostic reliability of prostate-specific antigen for prostate cancer. This considers *only* one treatment for prostate cancer. Even though this might at first seem like an important article, this is a DOE because the *real issue* is if prostate cancer *should even be treated* if detected. A POEM would be a study that has compared two groups of men who were either *treated or untreated* and then compared for mortality and morbidity. The "sacred cows" mentioned in the introduction are good examples of quality POEMS that have changed practices.

Now, turning to information the nurse manager needs, the principles about POEMs also apply to management questions. For example, you might find an excellent article between two computerized systems that assist some management function. This would be a DOE. You still have to **assume** from the results that money will be saved, morale will be improved, patients will do better, or that other outcomes will occur that matter. A POEM is a study that showed that any computerized system *accomplished* these end results.

Some secondary databases (**Exhibit 5–9**) are Essential Evidence Plus, DynaMed, and Cochrane, among others. As you become a more experienced searcher, you will not always need to start with the primary literature databases such as CINAHL and PubMed. Along with an understanding of secondary or translational literature, knowing the concepts of evidence-based information can make information searching easier and more accurate.

The *Cochrane Database of Systematic Reviews* (CDSR) is part of a group of databases produced by the Cochrane Collaboration based in Oxford, England. We highly recommend that you become familiar with Cochrane. It consists of 5,320 systematic reviews of RCTs on therapy topics.

The Cochrane collection also includes the Database of Abstracts of Reviews of Effectiveness (*DARE*), that, unlike the systematic reviews database, covers topics other than therapy (such as economics, etiology, prognosis, and diagnosis). In addition, the Cochrane group of databases includes the Cochrane Central Register of Controlled Trials, which contains over one-half million reviewed RCTs. The summaries of CDSR and subscription information can be searched at no charge at cochrane.org. DARE can be searched at no charge at www.crd.york.ac.uk/crdweb.

Comprehensive evidence-based practice databases that include the CDSR are available. These can be purchased as an individual subscription or as a license for a group. One such product is *Evidence Essentials Plus* (essentialevidenceplus.com), which can be loaded onto a desktop computer or a handheld computer). A subscription to Evidence Essentials Plus allows access to the following:

- Cochrane systematic reviews
- A collection of practice guidelines
- A collection of summaries of POEMS
- Drug information
- An ICD-9 look-up
- Predictive calculators

Products similar to Evidence Essentials Plus are *Clinical Evidence* (clinicalevidence.com), *DynaMed* (dynamicmedical.com), *ACP Journal Club* (acpjc.org/), *Nursing Consult* (nursingconsult.com), and *UpToDate* (uptodate.com).

PubMed has a clinical queries filter on the sidebar. When this filter is used, a special search strategy is implemented in addition to the terms you enter. These filters have been designed to find the best evidence in the literature—whether it is a question on therapy, diagnosis, prognosis, or etiology. For example, when you do a "therapy" search, the filter adds additional terms such as "randomized," "placebo-controlled," and "blinded." Techniques exist in CINAHL, as well, to filter out the best evidence.

Many evidence-based nursing (EBN) sources are available. For example, the *British Medical Journal* publishing group produces an online journal called *Evidence-Based Nursing* (ebn.bmj.com). The product website states the following:

> Evidence-Based Nursing surveys a wide range of international medical journals applying strict criteria for the quality and validity of research. Practicing clinicians assess the

Exhibit 5–9 Sources for Finding Evidence-Based Information (Secondary Literature)

Name	Address	Comments
Cochrane Databases	cochrane.org	Database of systematic reviews of randomized controlled trials of therapy topics. Additional databases are DARE, has information other than therapy topics, and Controlled Trials Database, over 1/2 million validated randomized controlled trials. (Proprietary).
EssentialEvidencePlus	essentialevidenceplus.com	Cochrane's systematic reviews and POEMS plus guidelines, drug information, and clinical calculators. (Proprietary)
Evidence-based Nursing	ebn.bmj.com	Selects and examines every aspect of the very best international nursing research for your practice. (Proprietary)
PubMed, clinical queries	ncbi.nlm.nih.gov/entrez/ query/static/clinical.shtml	Filters added to PubMed searches queries filter designed to find the "best-evidence" information for therapy, prognosis, diagnosis, and etiology queries. (Free)
Centre for Evidence Based Nursing	www.york.ac.uk/healthsciences/ centres/evidence/cebn.htm	The Centre for Evidence Based Nursing is concerned with furthering evidence-based nursing through education, research, and development. (Free)
Online Journal of Clinical Innovations	cinahl.com/cexpress/ojcionline3/ index.html	Developed to provide up-to-date access to research reports and innovation implementation from conferences and communication with investigators and clinicians. (Proprietary)
Clinical Evidence	clinicalevidence.com	BMJ Clinical Evidence systematic reviews summarize the current state of knowledge and uncertainty about the prevention and treatment of clinical conditions, based on thorough searches and appraisal of the literature. (Proprietary)
DynaMed	dynamicmedical.com	DynaMed is a medical information database with nearly 3,000 clinical topic summaries. Designed for use at the point-of-care, providing best available evidence and updated daily. (Proprietary)
ACP Journal Club	acpjc.org	ACP Journal Club's general purpose is to select from the biomedical literature articles that report original studies and systematic reviews that warrant immediate attention by physicians attempting to keep pace with important advances in internal medicine. (Proprietary)

continued

Exhibit 5–9 Sources for Finding Evidence-Based Information (Secondary Literature) (continued)

Name	Address	Comments
Nursing Consult	nursingconsult.com	Mosby's Nursing Consult offers a single destination for the busy nurse. Easily search to seamlessly find information very quickly. It includes latest drug information, patient education, professional journals, reference books, current news, clinical practice, evidence-based content, and care planning tools. (Proprietary)
UpToDate	uptodate.com	UpToDate is an electronic information resource for getting specific, detailed answers to clinical questions. UpToDate covers more than 7,300 topics in 13 medical specialties and includes more than 75,000 pages of text, graphics, links to Medline abstracts, more than 250,000 references, and a drug database. (Proprietary)
UNC-Chapel Hill EBN	www.hsl.unc.edu/Services/Tutorials/EBN/index.htm	The goal of the site is the investigation of the field of evidence-based nursing (Free)

clinical relevance of the best studies. The key details of these essential studies are presented in a succinct, informative abstract with an expert commentary on its clinical application.

A good EBN site is the Centre for Evidence-based Nursing (www.york.ac.uk/healthsciences/centres/evidence/cebn.htm). The site lists its purpose as follows:

> The Centre for Evidence Based Nursing (CEBN) is concerned with furthering EBN through education, research and development. Evidence based nursing is the process by which nurses make clinical decisions using the best available research evidence, their clinical expertise and patient preferences, in the context of available resources (DiCenso, Cullum, Ciliska. Implementing evidence based nursing: some misconceptions [Editorial]. *Evidence Based Nursing* 1998; 1:38-40).

The *Online Journal of Clinical Innovations* (cinahl.com/cexpress/ojcionline3/index.html) is a peer-reviewed electronic journal published by CINAHL. It is "dedicated to harvesting new knowledge to be transformed into practice, and making sources of clinical innovation—new solutions or practices that solve problems—accessible to clinicians in varied roles and diverse settings." It is accessible by subscription, or you can purchase individual articles.

A final web resource that is a good source of information for evidence-based practice is the *Evidence-Based Nursing site at the University of North Carolina*, Chapel Hill. It may be found at (www.hsl.unc.edu/Services/Tutorials/EBN/index.htm). The goal of the site is as follows:

> … the investigation of the field of Evidence Based Nursing. Literature searching and web searching was conducted to discover useful articles and web resources about

evidence based practice targeted for nursing professionals and students. While it is not intended to serve strictly as a teaching module on EBN, the resources mentioned and the site layout may be helpful for those desiring to learn more about the topic and may be a useful starting point in the creation of a more expansive and in-depth teaching tutorial.

Providing Consumer/Patient Health Information

First, we must apologize for the last section. That was a lot to swallow. So let's take another break. Get up. Walk around the room three or four times. Get out your cell phone (unless you are in an area where it would interfere with equipment) and call a friend. Be sure to get another snack (watch the carbs) and maybe a cup of coffee or hot herbal tea. This section provides some practical tips to help you become a better information seeker. These are our very best secrets and if broadly distributed could result in widespread unemployment of librarians. Therefore you must promise to rip this chapter out and destroy it before we allow you to proceed. Our whole professional future depends on the ignorance of others.

Here is a scenario to get us going: You work for a fertility specialist. A patient's husband says to you, "My wife has been coming to this office for one year now and she is not yet pregnant. I have heard that acupuncture can help with infertility. Do you know anything about this?" What do you do?

We would like to climb on our soapbox. Consumer/patient information is important, and many people are appallingly illiterate when it comes to health knowledge. This is well documented and sad. The current literacy studies by government and research organizations estimate 75 to 90 million adults in the United States have low health literacy (Jones, 2007). Conditions like diabetes and obesity could be greatly reduced if consumers were better educated about their health and if they would practice what they learn. We believe that this lack of availability and use of health information is a national health crisis. (End of sermon.)

Back to you, your staff, and their patients. Where do you begin to find unbiased, practical information? Billions of consumer health information resources exist. Well, maybe not billions, but we could give you list after list of websites, books, and organizations that provide consumer/patient health information. We have found this flood of information to be confusing to information seekers. What we prefer is to offer a limited, but manageable, number of excellent resources.

By using gateways that have already been evaluated by librarians, you can save time, energy, and money. A good starting point for finding consumer/patient information is the database *MedlinePlus*® (medlineplus.gov). MedlinePlus is maintained by the National Library of Medicine, one of the National Institutes of Health of the federal government. MedlinePlus is an aggregator of the best consumer health information on the web. Because of its comprehensive nature, it usually makes possible "one stop shopping" for consumer health information.

When you search by topic in MedlinePlus, you retrieve a list of links from other websites that have been quality filtered. The information in MedlinePlus is grouped by topic and is easy to search. Some topics even have tutorials for those with poor reading skills as well as links to resources labeled "easy-to-read." The tutorials can be heard through computer speakers or through headphones while you watch a slide show that explains a procedure or condition.

MedlinePlus is a good source of drug information and includes directories and dictionaries as well. A Spanish version of the site is also available and includes an excellent encyclopedia and Spanish-language tutorials. One of MedlinePlus' newest enhancements is the audio feature for people with low health literacy or disabilities; the website is designed to read aloud the contents of a page in either English or Spanish.

Exhibit 5–10 MedlinePlus Health Topic Screenprint

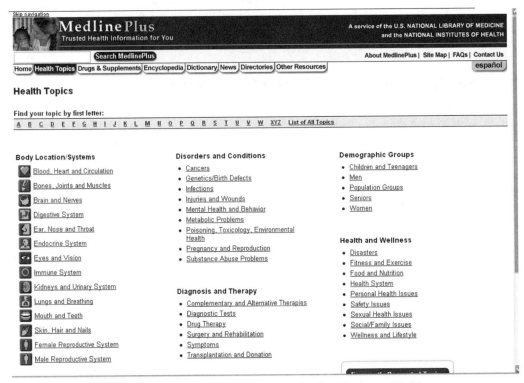

MedlinePlus is a service of the U.S. National Library of Medicine and National Institutes of Health.

MedlinePlus is now linked to consumer health information in over 40 languages. The National Library of Medicine continually updates, expands, and improves the site. A typical screen looks like that shown in **Exhibit 5–10**.

If you cannot find an answer from MedLinePlus.gov, we recommend that you use the *Medical Library Association's Consumer and Patient Health Information Section* (CAPHIS) site at http://caphis.mlanet.org. The people who maintain this site are the best of the best. They are professional librarians who spend a lot of their time providing consumer/patient health information on a daily basis. The group maintains a list of the top 100 consumer/patient health information web sites. According to CAPHIS:

> The purpose of the CAPHIS Top 100 List is to provide CAPHIS members and other librarians with a resource to use in their daily practice and teaching. Secondly, it is our contribution to the Medical Library Association so that the headquarters staff can refer individuals to a list of quality health web sites. Our goal is to have a limited number of resources that meet the quality criteria for currency, credibility, content, audience, etc., as described on our website.

Much fraudulent consumer/patient health information exists on the web. A site that exposes false and misleading health information on the web is *Quackwatch* (quackwatch.org). According to information found at the site, the mission of Quackwatch is as follows:

> Quackwatch, Inc., which was a member of Consumer Federation of America from 1973 through 2003, is a nonprofit corporation whose purpose is to combat health-related frauds,

myths, fads, fallacies, and misconduct. Its primary focus is on quackery-related information that is difficult or impossible to get elsewhere.

Choosing, Selecting, Implementing, and Purchasing New Information Technology

It is important for the nurse manager to keep up to date on IT trends. This is another example of the importance of having everyone in the organization stay connected, as discussed in detail in Chapter 3. Information can come from many sources: staff, patients/visitors, other administrators, physicians, suppliers, and your neighbor. Remind your colleagues to stay on the alert for better information options when they attend conferences, continuing education classes, and professional meetings. Books, newspapers, and journal articles on the emerging technologies abound. Professional organizations have websites that offer suggestions on what is available.

Share cutting-edge information with staff and encourage them to share their discoveries. A good website for finding new health care technologies is http://tie.telemed.org/europe/links/nursing.asp.

Perhaps your facility is considering whether to replace Pyxis systems. Do a web search to find similar systems that might be available. Look to see how long they have existed and who has used them. Get evaluations from users. Then contact the vendors to see if they are willing to arrange a demo of the product. It is helpful to establish pros and cons for each system before making a purchase. Interdisciplinary project teams are essential with such large purchases.

Any IT should be implemented only after the information system it is replacing is clearly understood and it can be shown to be an improvement (including the costs) over the previous system. (It would be scary to estimate the amount of money wasted by health care systems on IT that did not improve what it replaced.)

Chapter 19 in Saba and McCormick's *Essentials of Nursing Informatics* outlines how to implement and upgrade clinical information systems. Implementation is most successful if the nurse manager is very involved in the selection and execution of new IT. Users tend to adapt more quickly to the new technology when the supervisor is actively involved and interested in the new venture.

A nurse manager also needs to have a systems approach when purchasing new software. Let's assume that you have carefully evaluated all the available databases, have made your decision, and have negotiated a reasonable price with a vendor. When your purchase order reaches the Office of Information Technology (or its equivalent), the IT staff refuses to sign off on the order. (Gracious! You just got the money authorized to buy it, and now you cannot use it. Welcome to the wonderful world of online information.)

The IT office maintains that the hospital's firewall will not permit the access you need. The database vendors require that port 210 be open. You also want to give access through a proxy server so the nursing staff can access the information at home. Furthermore, you need a static IP address on the network for the computer at the nursing station. The IT folks will not allow any of this to happen, although the vendor promises you that the hospital's information system security will not be compromised. Furthermore, the vendor says that large hospital systems across the country use this product safely. What is your next move?

Beg? Cry? Resign? Purchase a billboard on the main highway in town that says, "IT stands for ignorant toad?" No, just take a deep breath and remember: IT folks are busy people, with great responsibilities, who must please a diverse group of users. Above all, they are concerned with the security of the information system. Therefore the cardinal rule when using IT products is to learn to *communicate with* IT. If you are considering purchasing a technology product, let them know about it in advance. They can tell you if it will work with the existing system. Meet with them frequently. Let them know what your needs are. Perhaps they have a solution for you that you never considered. Take them out to lunch. Thank them for their efforts.

Making Sure Information Resources Are Available

Part of the nurse manager role is making sure there are adequate information resources available. This is a big responsibility and one that the entire administration shares in an organization. In larger information systems, such as computerized documentation, or expensive technology, the expenditure needs to be an entire systems decision. It is important for staff nurses to have e-mail addresses and the ability to communicate quickly and efficiently (such as with a cell phone, personal digital assistant [PDA], computer, and/or some combination of all of them). They should also have up-to-date IT appropriate for the patient population served, and they should receive training so they will be able to use this equipment effectively. This is a tall order.

PDAs

Now let's do another scenario. You get a PDA for Christmas. What is a PDA? What do you do with it? A PDA is a handheld computer. There are two major platforms or operating systems for PDAs—the Windows mobile operating system and the Palm operating system. More products are made for the Palm system (**Exhibit 5–11**), which has been available for a longer time. (Some companies that make Palm-based PDAs are Palm, Sony, and Toshiba.) Windows Mobile is a Microsoft operating

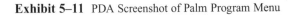

Exhibit 5–11 PDA Screenshot of Palm Program Menu

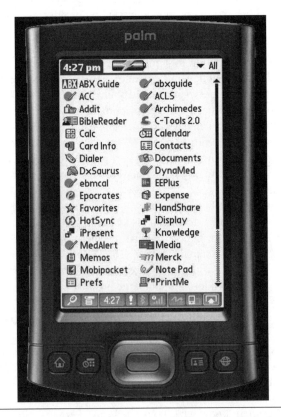

system and therefore works well with Microsoft products. (Some companies that sell Windows Mobile–based PDAs are Hewlett-Packard and Motorola.) A recent development is the combination of PDAs with cell phones. The resulting devices are called *smart phones*.

Are PDAs just fancy calendar devices for geeks? No! The calendar applications are, however, very useful. They can be made to synchronize with the calendar on your desktop computer and store all the names, phone numbers, e-mails, and addresses of your contacts. Your PDA can surf the Internet and send and receive e-mail wirelessly. If you are bored, you can play a game or listen to your favorite song on your PDA, or you can use it to make a video. In addition, PDAs have some wonderful applications in health care (**Exhibit 5–12**). They can be used for viewing health knowledge databases such as Essentials Evidence Plus, textbooks, drug databases, and just about every type of information resource that exists in print. Two sources for PDA health resources are skyscape.com and handheldmed.com.

Just a quick perusal of Skyscape shows featured nursing texts for PDAs such as RNotes (Nurse's Clinical Pocket Guide), Davis's Drug Guide for Nurses, Nursing Constellation: All-In-One Nursing Solution, and Nurse's Manual of Laboratory and Diagnostic Tests. This gives you a taste of the type of information that can be used on a PDA in a clinical setting

Like desktop computers, PDAs can be improved with accessories. You can buy keyboards and extra memory storage devices. The most common types of memory expansion cards are the secure digital cards. These are equivalent to compact disks on your desktop computers. PDAs work with

Exhibit 5–12 PDA Resources and Tools

PDA Resources	Comments
Skyscape.com	Good source for buying electronic textbooks
ePocrates.com	Free drug database for PDA
Dynamicmedical.com	Purchase Dynamed for PDA here
Essentialevidenceplus.com	Essential Evidence Plus for PDA
Immunizationed.org	Shots (immunization schedule) for PDA
Merckmedicus.com	Merck Manual and Pocket Guide for Diagnostic Tests
Handheldmed.com	Like Skyscape, a good source for PDA texts and databases
Administrative Tools	
Calendar function	Allows Outlook mail to be downloaded to the device
Note function	Useful for jotting down short notes instead of using paper
MS Word	Word documents can be saved, created, and read on PDAs. Staff regulations or guidelines could be carried around by each nurse with a PDA.
Excel spreadsheets	Useful for reviewing management data or for collecting data "on the spot"
Media	PDA devices will play audio and video files like IPods. Handwashing protocol videos could be maintained on each PDA
Internet access	Many PDAs have wireless capabilities. Some hospitals use this so clinicians can view patient data and order labs and tests using PDAs.

your desktop computer. A synching cradle or cable is used to pass information between the two devices. Information is entered into the PDA with a stylus. This skill is easy to acquire. We encourage you to invest in a PDA. They bring information wherever you go.

Suddenly you realize that PDAs would be helpful for each of the staff nurses to have. As they give care, they can look up information and get the call from the physician, family members, and pharmacy. They can give better care to patients. David Slawson, MD, a well-known proponent of EBN, equates a PDA to a stethoscope as a clinical tool. A quick Google search of "nursing PDA" retrieves a confusing number of sites that list PDA software for nurses.

We recommend that you definitely get Epocrates (epocrates.com). Epocrates is the free drug database that ignited the use of PDAs by clinicians (**Exhibit 5–13**). Any other programs you may choose to install on your PDA are a matter of personal preference.

In our institution the library allows PDA users to drop off their PDAs, and we load all the software for them. We install Dynamed (dynamicmedical.com) and Essentials Evidence Plus (essentialevidenceplus.com). These resources are outstanding best-evidence databases. They require an annual subscription. We also install the Merck Medical PDA resources, including the Merck Manual and the Pocket Guide to Diagnostic Tests (merckmedicus.com); Shots, which is a childhood and adult immunization schedule (immunizationed.org); the Johns Hopkins Antibiotic Guideline (hopkinsabxguide.org); and the American College of Cardiology Guidelines (acc.org/qualityandscience/clinical/statements.htm)

Exhibit 5–13   Epocrates

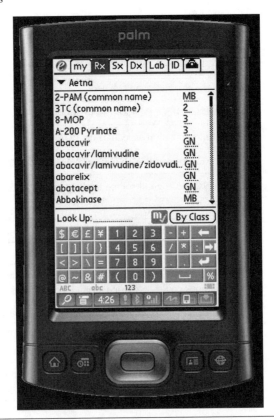

Many individual calculators can be purchased. Instead of downloading these individually, we recommend that you subscribe to the Evidence Essentials Plus program, which has hundreds of calculators. Also, remember that a selection of free calculators is included with Epocrates.

Information and Libraries/Librarians

Three nurses are out sick. Your census is up dramatically. You have more meetings than you have hours. You also need to find some information. What do you do? Often, the information need goes unfilled. We have a better idea—*use your librarian*. Do not hesitate to "bother" your librarian if there is one in your facility. Librarians are one of the world's best kept secrets. Librarians will do literature searches for you when you do not have time. They can order articles—including administrative articles—for you and your staff that the library does not have.

Some librarians are willing to come out to the clinical areas of the facility on a regular basis and interact with the staff. A current trend is for the electronic delivery of information through which librarians find information and e-mail it to you. One way, according to Reichel (1989), that librarians can meet the needs and obligations of the parent institution is by bibliographic instruction or teaching. Bibliographic instruction teaches library patrons how to locate and use library resources efficiently. Librarians love to teach. Schedule classes for them to work with you and/or your nursing staff. They can explain the information resources available at your facility and teach your staff how to properly use them.

OUTREACH LIBRARIANS

You work in a rural long-term care facility. You want better information resources for your staff, but cannot afford a library in the facility. What do you do?

Jensen and Maddalena (1985) note that, "The results of our work show that small rural hospitals (100 beds or fewer) have extreme difficulty in maintaining adequate on-site library resources and services over a period of time" (p. 60). Pifalo's (1994) research discovered that "In the United States, only 43.1% of hospitals have libraries, and in hospitals with less than 200 beds, the figure is 28%" (p. 30). Given the financial crunch on small hospitals, it is safe to bet that the number is even less. Often, unfortunately, when a hospital makes spending cuts, the library is a victim. A solution for these hospitals may be to contract the services of an outreach librarian who would spend varying amounts of time there, depending on the size of the hospital and its information needs. The outreach librarian visits several key areas throughout the hospital including nurses' stations, the physicians' lounge, the emergency room, the pharmacy, or outlying clinics. In Gordner's (1982) experience with outreach librarianship, nurses were the largest users of the information service.

Many regions of the country have Area Health Education Centers (AHECs). AHECs provide library services, continuing education programs, and many other services to health care professionals. AHECs are started with federal grant money and supported by user fees and state governments. You may have an AHEC librarian in your area who would be glad to provide library services to your facility. He or she may provide free service or in some cases may charge a reasonable fee to cover expenses. Fowkes, Campeau, and Wilson (1991) reported, "AHECs have demonstrated an ability to respond to current and emerging needs that distinguishes them from other institutions that have educational missions" (p. 219). AHECs responded better because they were more flexible than traditional academic bureaucracies and were more in touch with the communities they serve. Fowkes et al. continued: "Having both academic and community roots, AHECs know the needs and resources of each and how to use them in a manner that benefits both, thus strengthening and balancing the partnership between school and community" (p. 219).

Note: The National Network of Libraries of Medicine (NN/LM) is a division of the National Library of Medicine. NN/LM has centers throughout the country. Each center has trainers who will come out to your town and teach classes on PDAs, consumer health, public health information resources, and National Library of Medicine databases, just to name a few topics that are in their repertoire. The web address for NN/LM is nnlm.gov. To utilize the training, your organization must be an NN/LM member. Membership is free.

It is imperative that nursing leadership in rural areas provide organizational support for the enhancement of evidence-based practices. Munroe, Duffy, and Fisher (2006) reported that the overall knowledge of nurses in a rural community hospital increased significantly when evidence-based practice was promoted through personnel, education, and process interventions. An added bonus was a renewed "sense of professionalism and pride" among nursing personnel.

LIBRARIANSHIP IN THE CLINIC

Florance, Giuse, and Ketchell (2002) describe how Vanderbilt Medical Center librarians were trained in pharmacology, physiology, and biostatistics and actively participate in medical rounds. They not only gathered information for clinicians but also summarized it, appraised it, and offered commentary. This same practice could work with nurses. Williams and Zipperer (2003) said, "The occasional participation by the librarian in patient rounds with nurses and other clinical staff can engender trust in the relationship between the librarian and the clinical team" (p. 204). Your librarian could come on the floor once or twice every week. She could gather topics to be researched, meet new staff, update the staff about new developments in the library, and give one-on-one training. As a result, the nursing staff would save time and the librarian would become an important part of the clinical team.

We like to use the following illustration to explain why we believe librarians are an essential part of the health care team (Holtum, 1999):

> When health professionals request lab work, they turn to medical technologists. If an X-ray is needed, they direct the patient to a radiographic technician. The reason is simple: Even though the clinician is certainly capable of learning and performing these tasks (though at considerable time and expense), higher quality and greater cost-effectiveness are obtained by using the skills of specialists instead. Can the same not be said of the expertise and experience that librarians bring to the health care enterprise (p. 406)?

Although you may have learned some laboratory skills in school, you still send samples to a lab for analysis. It just makes sense to give a task to those who are trained and experienced at doing it. Libraries are similar. We hope you are good at finding information, but if a skilled professional is available to do it for you, then you can dedicate your time to what you do best—managing the unit and working with staff who are taking care of sick people.

Oh, and one more thing. Please be an advocate for libraries in your institution. Librarians need your support when budgets are cut, because administrators often consider eliminating the library first as a simple cost-cutting measure. Most small hospitals and health care institutions do not have a library because of the cost. If this is your situation, you may want to consider contracting for the services of an outreach librarian. Of course, you can also contact a librarian by e-mail or by telephone. Another option would be to contact your local academic health sciences library for assistance.

Summary

We have given you a lot of information. You are an official graduate of our crash course in access to knowledge-based health information. Congratulations! We hope we gave you enough exposure to different aspects of health information to know its value. We hope you can do a credible consumer search, a credible professional search, and a credible web search. We hope you understand the basics of best evidence information, the clinical value of PDAs, and the value of health sciences librarians. We hope you now can deal more fruitfully with information and technology, how to get it, and how to use it. We conclude by taking this opportunity to tell you that it is a great privilege to serve you. The exemplary care and comfort you give the sick makes taking care of your information needs a joy. Our goal is for you to master the theoretical concepts and practical uses of health care information for your own personal growth as a skilled health care professional and for the benefit of the patients you serve.

Discussion Questions

1. Use the following scenario to answer questions A through G:
    Your hospital is looking into implementing dedicated nurses to oversee the medication administration system to improve patient safety. You are not so sure this will help.
    A. PICO the question.
    B. Write out a well-formed clinical question that contains each part of the PICO.
    C. Map the PICO to either MesH in PubMed or subject-headings in CINAHL.
    D. Find an article that seems to answer the question.
    E. What type of study is the article (randomized controlled trial, cohort, etc.)?
    F. What level of evidence is it?
    G. Do dedicated medication nurses improve patient safety?
Answers:
A. *P* Staff nurse utilization
    I Dedicated medication error nurses
    C No dedicated medication error nurses
    O Improved patient safety
B. In hospital nursing staffs, does the use of a dedicated medication error nurse(s) reduce medication errors compared with hospital nursing staff who do not use a dedicated medication error nurse(s)?
C. *P* Nursing staff, hospital
    I Nurse's role
    C None
    O Medication errors/prevention and control
D. *Archives of Internal Medicine* 2003 Oct 27;163(19):2359–2367.

The impact of dedicated medication nurses on the medication administration error rate: a randomized controlled trial.

Greengold N, Shane R, Schneider P, Flynn E, Elashoff J, Hoying C, Barker K, Bolton L.

Department of Health Services Research, Cedars-Sinai Health System, Los Angeles, CA 90048, USA. NGreengold@WKHealth.com

BACKGROUND: Concerns about hospital medication safety mount as the pace of new drug releases accelerates.

METHODS: We performed a randomized study at two hospitals (A and B) to examine whether the medication administration error rate could be decreased by having "dedicated" nurses focus exclusively on administering drugs. "Medication nurses," after receiving a brief review course on safe medication use, were responsible solely for drug delivery for up to 18 patients each.

"General nurses," who did not attend the course, provided comprehensive care, including drug delivery, for six patients each. A direct observation technique was used to record drug errors, process-variation errors, and total errors.

RESULTS: At both hospitals combined, the total error rate was 15.7% for medication nurses and 14.9% for general nurses (P < .84). Comparing hospitals, the total error rate for medication nurses at hospital B was significantly higher than it was at hospital A (19.7% vs 11.2%; P < .04). At hospital A, there was a significantly lower error rate for medication nurses than for general nurses in the surgical units (P < .01) but no significant differences in total errors comparing nurse types in the medical units (P < .77).

CONCLUSIONS: This trial suggests that use of dedicated medication nurses does not reduce medication error rates. However, subgroup analysis indicates that medication nurses might be useful in some settings. The differences in findings at the two hospitals and their differences in medication-use processes reinforce the concept that medication errors are usually related to systems design issues.

   E. Randomized controlled trial
   F. Level 1
   G. No

2. You've been asked to serve on a committee that will plan a new neonatal intensive care unit for your hospital. Where can you find reliable information about state-of-the-art neonatal intensive care units?
    Answer: Go to the Health on the Net Foundation at www.hon.ch, click on "HONcode sites" and in the search box enter "neonatal intensive care unit 2008" (without the quotation marks).

3. You been assigned as manager of the orthopedic nursing unit at your hospital. Where can you find best practice guidelines to help you in your new role?
    Answer: Go to guidelines.gov and in the search box enter "orthopaedic nursing."

4. A nursing staff member says, "The patient in room 2001 can't sleep because she thinks her daughter is growing a poisonous plant called castor beans in her flower bed. She is worried that her grandchildren might eat the beans." Where can you find trustworthy information about the plant including pictures so the patient can confirm the identification of the plant?
    Answer: Go to medlineplus.com and in the search box enter "castor bean." For more photos of the plant go to Google Images.

5. In your administrative role, what specific evidence-based information sites would be most helpful?

6. Specify the information technology that would enable you to better accomplish your administrative responsibilities.

Glossary of Terms

Bibliographic Database—a searchable collection of citations to publications. The publications may include books, journals, audiovisual materials, websites, etc. Most bibliographic databases include information *about* the publication, such as author, title, copyright date, etc. Often an abstract of the publication is included, but the full-text of the article must usually be located elsewhere.

Case Control Study—a retrospective study that collects data from charts, data sets, and patient interviews.

Case Study—a detailed analysis of a person or group from a social, psychological, or medical point of view.

Cohort Study—an observational study in which a group of people is identified in the present and followed into the future or identified from past records, and followed from that time up to the present.

Evidence-Based Information (EBI)—the melding of individual judgment and expertise with the best available external evidence to generate the kind of information that is most likely to lead to a positive outcome.

Informatics—a science that combines a domain science, computer science, information science, and cognitive science.

Levels of Evidence (LOE)—a method of ranking evidence for better decision making.

Nursing Informatics—the study of how electronic information systems are used to improve nursing systems and patient care.

PDA—personal digital assistant or handheld computer.

PICO (Population, Intervention, Comparison, Outcome)—a method of formatting a focused question resulting in a more productive search and a more relevant answer.

Proprietary Database—a privately controlled and distributed database. Access is through subscription or on a pay-per-view basis.

Randomized Controlled Trial (RCT)—a carefully designed blinded or double-blinded experiment. Randomized controlled trials are randomized in the sense that everyone who is in the population being studied has an equal chance of being chosen to be in the experimental group (arm) or control group.

Secondary Literature—articles that filter the best information from the primary literature.

Strength of Recommendation (SOR) Ratings—guides to the trustworthiness of information.

Systematic Review—a compilation of randomized controlled trials on a single subject.

Translational Literature—see Secondary Literature.

References

Casida, J., & Pinto-Zipp. (2008). Leadership-organizational culture relationship in nursing units of acute care hospitals. *Nursing Economic$, 26,* 7–16.

Cassey, M. (2007). Incorporating the national guideline clearinghouse into evidence-based nursing practice. *Nursing Economic$, 25*(5), 302–303.

DiCenso, C. Implementing evidence-based nursing: some misconceptions. *Evidence Based Nursing. 1,* 38–40.

Florance, V., Giuse, N., & Ketchell, D. (2002). Information in context: Integrating information specialists into practice settings. *Journal of the Medical Library Association, 90*(1), 49–58.

Fowkes, V., Campeau, M., & Wilson, S. (1991). The evolution and impact of the national AHEC program over two decades. *Academic Medicine, 66*(4), 211–220.

Gordner, R. (1982). Riding the rural library circuit. *Medical Reference Services Quarterly, 1*(1), 59–74.

Halfer, D. (2007). A magnetic strategy for new graduate nurses. *Nursing Economic$, 25,* 6–12.

Holtum, E. (1999). Librarians, clinicians, evidence-based medicine and the division of labor. *Bulletin of the Medical Library Association, 87*(4), 404–407.

Jensen, M., & Maddalena, B. (1985). Implications of an AHEC library program evaluation: Considerations for small rural hospitals. *Bulletin of the Medical Library Association, 73*(1), 59–61.

Jones, J. (2007). Patient illiteracy. *AORN Journal, 85*(5), 951–955.

Klein, M., Ross, V., Adams, D., & Gilbert, C. (1994). Effect of online literature searching on length of stay and patient care costs. *Academic Medicine, 69*(6), 489–495.

Kramer, M., Maguire, P., & Schmalenberg, C. (2006). Excellence through evidence: The what, when, and where of clinical autonomy. *Journal of Nursing Administration, 36,* 479–491.

Lorenz, S. (2008). 12-hour shifts: An ethical dilemma for the nurse executive. *Journal of Nursing Administration, 38,* 297–301.

Mackoff, B., & Triolo, P. (2008). Why do nurse managers stay? Building a model of engagement. *Journal of Nursing Administration, 38,* 166–171.

Manojlovich, M., & Antonakos, C. (2008). Satisfaction of intensive care unit nurses with nurse-physician communication. *Journal of Nursing Administration, 38*(5), 237–243.

Munroe, D., Duffy, P., & Fisher, C. (2006). Fostering evidence-based practice in a rural community hospital. *Journal of Nursing Administration, 36,* 510–512.

Pifalo, V. (1994). Circuit librarianship: A twentieth anniversary appraisal. *Medical Reference Services Quarterly, 13*(1), 19–31.

Rauen, C., Vollman, K., Arbour, R., & Chulay, M. (2008). Challenging nursing's sacred cows. *American Nurse Today, 3*(4), 23–26.

Reichel, M. (1989). Ethics and library instruction: Is there a connection? *RQ, 28*(4), 477–480.

Saba, V., & McCormick, K. (2006). *Essentials of nursing informatics* (4th ed.). New York: McGraw-Hill.

Shin, J., Haynes, R., & Johnston, M. E. (1993). Effect of problem-based, self-directed undergraduate education on life-long learning. *CMAJ, 148,* 969–976.

Slawson, D., & Shaughnessy, A. (1994). Becoming a medical information master: Feeling good about not knowing everything. *Journal of Family Practice, 38*(5), 505–513.

Stichler, J. (2008). Finding evidence to support facility design decisions. *Journal of Nursing Administration, 38,* 153–156.

Storfjell, J., Omoike, O., & Ohlson, S. (2008). The balancing act: Patient care time versus cost. *Journal of Nursing Administration, 38,* 244–249.

Thungjaroenkul, P., Cummings, G., & Embleton, A. (2007). The impact of nurse staffing on hospital costs and patient length of stay: A systematic review. *Nursing Economic$, 25*(5), 255–265.

Williams, L., & Zipperer, L. (2003). Improving access to information: Librarians and nurses team up for patient safety. *Nursing Economic$, 21*(4), 199–201.

PART III

Workload Management

Workload management is an integral component of hospital operations. Relying on experience, intuition, and historical usage to manage workloads is not viable in an age of plentiful information and customer expectations for value-based services. The focus has necessarily shifted to managing the data to guide effective decision making, specifically *evidence-based staffing*.

Chapter 6 examines the workload management cycle: patient care needs (patient classification systems/benchmark data), core scheduling (staffing plan), daily staffing (nurse–patient assignments, skill mix, and variance management), evaluation (patient outcomes, quality), and budget management (budget and productivity monitoring). Nurse administrators are guided through this process and given key information on how to effectively manage our most valuable resource, the staff.

As a nurse administrator manages workload, there are certain ethical and legal considerations that are important to consider or that might aid in guiding decision making. Chapter 7 discusses *organizational ethics*. This chapter provides an historical perspective of ethics development in the health care system, presents ethical concerns of nurse administrators, and suggests insights into the development of ethical leadership.

Chapter 8 outlines some common *legal issues* facing nurse administrators. This chapter discusses the nurse practice act, the law that regulates nursing practice; standards of nursing practice, how these standards are applied, and how they are used as evidence during malpractice litigation; the legal significance of your nursing license; and your legal responsibility with delegation rules.

CHAPTER 6

Workload Management

Kathy Malloch, PhD, MBA, RN, FAAN
Janne Dunham-Taylor, PhD, RN
Janelle Krueger, MBA, BS, RN

Key Terms

- Acuity
- Case Mix Method
- Comprehensive Unit of Service
- Content Validity
- Construct Validity
- Core Schedules
- External Validity
- Face Validity
- Factor Evaluation Method
- Internal Validity
- Job Analysis
- Patient Classification
- Position Control
- Productivity
- Prototype Approach
- Relative Value Unit
- Reliability
- Sensitivity
- Skill Mix
- Staffing Plan
- Validity

Introduction

Workload management is an essential concept for health care leaders. Because nursing constitutes the majority of the workforce in health care facilities, nurse leaders in particular are faced with the ever-increasing demand to ensure efficient and effective service delivery. For years nurse leaders have relied on their experience, intuition, judgment, and traditions to create and justify optimal workload management systems, workload management systems that include an effective method to assess and predict patient care needs, a staffing plan core schedule, daily staffing processes, productivity monitoring tools, budget parameters, and quality evaluation criteria (Figure 6–1). However, with the explosion of clinical information system applications, clinical and financial data are now readily available. The focus has necessarily shifted to managing the data to guide effective decision making, specifically *evidence-based staffing*. Further, the challenge for nursing continues to escalate as the health care industry struggles with patient safety, pay for performance initiatives, demands for staffing ratio legislation, and increased collective bargaining units.

Centers for Medicare and Medicaid Services (CMS) have embarked on a *pay for performance system*. The purpose of this initiative is to link reimbursement programs to patient care improvements and not pay for our mistakes. In addition, there have been recommendations to CMS to

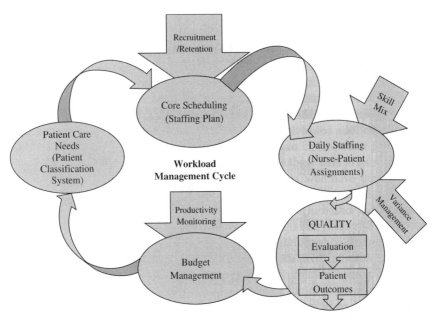

Figure 6–1 Workload Management Cycle

separate out nursing costs and hours of care and identify nursing personnel by license class to allow construction of a cost-to-charge ratio independent of the existing room and board cost center.

The need for leaders to develop and sustain valid and reliable workload management tools has never been greater. Understanding the role of each of the elements in the workload system is an important step in this process. Relying on experience, intuition, and historical usage to manage workloads is not viable in an age of plentiful information and customer expectations for value-based services. Systematic, replicable systems to track and monitor caregiver skill mix and hours of care are an expectation for effective leadership. In this chapter, the essential components of an effective workload management system include

- A way to determine and validate patient care needs
- A staffing plan for core scheduling
- A daily staffing plan and process
- Outcome evaluation that includes productivity monitoring
- A supporting budget

Open Systems Model

The systems model is helpful to understand the complexities of health care workload management. The fundamental elements and principles specific to the environment in which work occurs along with the inputs, throughputs, outputs, and feedback loops provide clarity to this process (Figure 6–2). To be sure, each of these elements has an impact on quantity, quality, and productivity of the health care system.

The environment or setting in which health care occurs is complex and ever changing. Inputs, throughputs, outputs, and feedback loops exist in an environment that includes economic, political,

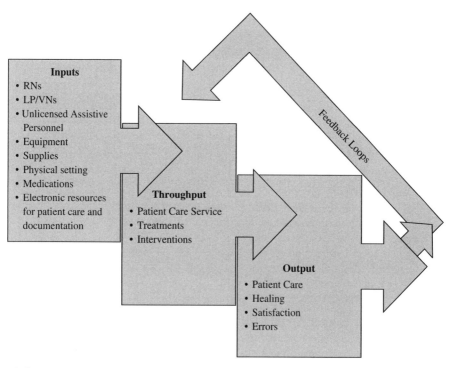

Figure 6–2 Open Systems Model

social, and cultural influences. The *inputs* include the resources, human and nonhuman (materials, equipment, buildings), that come together to provide the desired service. In health care, inputs might be staff labor hours, number and skill mix of nursing staff, other staff needed for various services, technology, equipment, supplies used, and remodeling or building expense. *Throughputs* are the processes or work that people do to achieve the output, the final product, or service. In the health care system, throughputs are the patient care services provided to the patient and family. Throughput processes use the available inputs to create work processes. *Output* results from the interaction of inputs in the throughput process. The output is the material, goods and/or services, produced. Outputs can be both qualitative and quantitative in health care. Reimbursement in health care is driven by the quantitative outputs or documented services produced by the system, regardless of the quality of the output or errors that might have occurred.

Measuring Patient Care Workload

Measuring human work is a complex process. *Workload measurement systems* consist of several distinct techniques that quantify the time associated with tasks performed by workers. There are at least 25 techniques that assist in the study and measurement of work (Myers & Stewart, 2002). These techniques are used to understand the nature and true cost of work processes and to address the ongoing challenge to reduce costs, reduce effort, and improve the work environment. Often times, there is confusion between motion and time techniques in measuring work. An overview of the differing types of techniques and those with specific application in health care are presented in **Exhibit 6–1**.

Exhibit 6–1 Time and Motion Study Technique / Definitions

Time Study Techniques		Motion Study Techniques
	Health Care Applications	
Predetermined Time Standards System (PTSS) *All work is reduced to basic motions (bend, reach, walk, etc.) and each motion is reduced to a specific time value.*		Process charts
Stopwatch Time Study *Use of stopwatch to determine time required by a skilled, well trained operator working at a normal pace doing a specific task.*	Army Workload Management System for Nursing (WMSN)	Flow diagrams
Work Sampling *Randomly observing people working to determine how they spend their time and then drawing broad conclusions based on laws of probability.*	Logging Factor	Multi-activity charts
Standard Data Formula Time Standards *Catalog of standards developed from a database collected over years of study.*	DRG ICD-9 HPPD RVU RUG Prototype	Operation charts
Expert Opinion *A person with a great experience base estimates time to perform a specific job within his/her area of expertise.*	CUS (Comprehensive Unit of Service)	

The five workload measurement techniques often used in health care—motion and time study, work sampling, self-reporting, standard data setting, and expert opinion—are discussed briefly.

The first technique, *motion and time studies,* involves continuous timed observations of a single person during a typical time period or shift of work (Burke et al., 2000). An observer for occurrences and duration of the specific activity measures primary tasks performed. Motion study is for cost reduction; time study is for cost control. Motion studies focus on design, whereas time studies focus on measurement. Both studies create a cost consciousness that is desired by the industry. Many of the common measures, such as the National Aeronautics and Space Administration Task Load Index, were developed for use in aviation, particularly studies of aircrew workload, although they have also been applied elsewhere, such as the nuclear and other safety-critical industries.

A *motion study* is designed to determine the best way to complete a repetitive job. Examples of techniques to study motion include process charts, flow diagrams, multi-activity charts, operation charts, workstation design, motion economy, and predetermined time standards system. Workload measurement via motion and time studies has been applied to a number of military and industrial problems. Interestingly, these are not often used in health care to help identify time standards. Rather, these techniques are more often used in the process improvement area. A *time study* measures how long it takes an average worker to complete a task at a normal pace. Examples of time study techniques include predetermined time standards system, stopwatch time study, standard data formula time standards, work sampling time standards, expert opinion, and historical data time standards. In health care, using worked hours per patient day (HPPD) or procedures per year to budget or staff for the next year would be consistent with the standard data set approach.

Second, *work sampling* is a time study technique that samples work activities at systematic or random intervals. It is the process of randomly observing people working to determine how they spend their time. The type and percentage of observations is assumed to represent the typical workload at any given point in time. It does not, however, determine the duration of a particular activity.

In health care, work sampling forms the foundation for some computerized patient classification systems. In work sampling, the caregiver's work is examined for the entire shift or event of care for a selected number of times to achieve a representative range of services. Once representative data are collected, the percentage of time spent on specific activities, such as taking and recording vital signs, performing assessments, administering medications, or managing intravenous fluid therapy and discharge planning, is determined. These amounts then form the time standards for determining patient acuity on a daily basis (**Exhibit 6–2**).

Third, *self-reporting* is another technique used to determine time associated with employee activities. Generally, the employee is asked to log the work performed using a data collection tool where start and stop times of each activity are recorded along with a brief description of the activity. Self-reporting may be subjective, but it has been shown to have high face validity (Burke et al., 2000).

A fourth technique, *standard data setting,* uses time standards developed from past experiences. It is a common term given to any collection of time values and is defined as a catalog of elemental time standards developed from a database collected over years of motion and time study. From the factory perspective, machine names or numbers and job descriptions organize the catalog of time standards. When a new part is designed and the fabrication steps have been identified, the time study person looks up the machine in the catalogue and identifies the source of variance and area in which new measurements are needed. These time standards are specific to the environment and

Exhibit 6–2 Example Patient Care Activity Groups: 8-Hour Shift

Activity / Time	Level 1	Level 2 Minutes / Shift	Level 3	Average Total Spent / Shift	Time (%)
Vital signs	5.0	9.5	5.0	19.5	5%
Assessments	10.0	19.0	10.0	39.0	10%
Treatments	20.0	38.0	20.0	78.0	20%
ADLs	20.0	38.0	20.0	78.0	20%
Documentation	20.0	38.0	20.0	78.0	20%
Medication administration	15.0	28.5	15.0	58.5	15%
Teaching	5.0	9.5	5.0	19.5	5%
Other	5.0	9.5	5.0	19.5	5%
Total	100	190	100	390	100%

ADLs, activities of daily living.

not readily transferable to another environment. Standard data time standards are typically the most accurate and least costly to determine.

Finally, *expert opinion* or *expert panel* is another technique used to determine time standards. A panel of experts, individuals with a great deal of experience and ability to estimate time in their area of expertise, identifies the time requirements for certain work. This consensus approach uses professional judgment to assess staff required and provides a flexible approach that focuses on a critical review of nursing practice, staffing, and the use of both supply and demand information (Dunn et al., 1995). Service work and one-of-a-kind jobs make setting time standards with the more traditional techniques cost prohibitive. Some workers never do the same thing twice, but goals are needed. An expert is needed to estimate every job and to maintain a log of estimates. The *best estimation technique* is a low cost, fast, and initially acceptable way of quantifying information using estimation and self-reporting techniques. The expert opinion technique attempts to remedy the criticism of the inability of the work sampling technique to capture professional judgment required in health care (Dunn et al., 1995). Because it can easily become biased and not always reflect current conditions, the expert opinion is reliable only if the results obtained approximate those results generated by experts, and the estimates are valid and reliable.

In health care the expert panel approach has been used to create a *comprehensive unit of service* as the foundational workload unit of measure (Malloch & Conovaloff, 1999). Experienced nurses create workload standards from a comprehensive perspective of the work performed; expert nurses compile the nurse interventions, provided to a patient for an entire shift or event, and identify the time required to provide this care as a unit rather than as summation of tasks. This approach integrates the multitasking processes of nurses and avoids the risk of double counting tasks. Typically, the expert panel consists of nurses who practice in clinical, educational, research, and administrative roles such as experienced staff nurses, clinical nurse specialists, nurse managers, and associate nurse executives. The panel of nurses collaborates to estimate the amount of time and level of caregiver (skill mix) required to provide the total care in the comprehensive unit of service.

Many of these techniques are difficult to use in health care where both the worker and the work to be done are highly variable. Health care is very different from the factory model in which the work is assembly-line mechanical and most variation lies within the activities of the worker. Accurate and credible motion and time standards specific to the health care worker provide an average time standard specific to a procedure. The *flaw of this averaging* process for health care is that the average situation may never occur. According to Savage (2002), the averaging process distorts accounts, undermines forecasts, and dooms apparently well thought-out projects to disappointing results. In health care staffing, average caregiver needs are often used to create monthly schedules. Although this process is efficient, it may create more challenges in the long run. Consider the situation in which the average number of staff per shift is five and the range for each day of the week is three to nine on the basis of patient activity. No shift requires five staff persons, yet every day is staffed with five persons. **Exhibit 6–3** illustrates the flaw of averages.

Using the specific number within the range of relevant numbers, in this case a number between 3 and 7, rather than the average of 5, for each shift results in more accurate staffing. The wide range of time required for similar—but different—patient situations is often significant. The time

---

Exhibit 6–3 The Flaw of Averages: Daily and Weekly Caregiver Staffing Requirements

S	M	T	W	T	F	S	Weekly Average
3	6	6	7	7	4	3	5.1 Caregivers

required to determine specific time standards for the range of patient care profiles and combinations of needs in health care would be overwhelming and cost prohibitive to determine using motion, time, and standard data techniques. Given the range of capabilities of the workload measurement techniques, a comparison of the advantages and disadvantages is presented in **Exhibit 6–4**.

Exhibit 6–4 A Comparison of the Advantages and Disadvantages of Workload Measurement Techniques

Workload Measurement	Advantages	Disadvantages
Time and Motion	• Considered the gold standard in time estimation in the industrial environment • Accuracy of time standards for selected tasks	• High cost of one-on-one observations over extended periods • Potential for observer-induced bias (changing participants' behavior when observed) • Variable task difficulty/complexity of clinical testing and procedures not considered • Multitasking events not considered • Complex interactions of physical, social, ethical, emotional, and financial dimensions of patient care not incorporated
Self-Reporting/Logging	• Simple and inexpensive • High face validity • Low cost • Minimal training required	• Inherent bias • Participants have significant burden of reporting every activity performed in a time period
Factor Evaluation/Subjective	• High face validity and hence acceptance by operators • Most operators find it fairly easy to assign ratings	• Operators can rate changing demands of a given task but find it difficult to compare workload on qualitatively different types of tasks • No unanimous agreement on the nature of the components of workload, and hence the set of scales that should be used • Ability to capture the nursing process is questioned
Work Sampling	• Experts are hired to validate time standards making validity level high • Useful when new procedures and techniques are introduced	• Large numbers of observations are required to obtain reasonable precision in time estimates • Does not determine the duration of a work activity

continued

Exhibit 6–4 A Comparison of the Advantages and Disadvantages of Workload Measurement Techniques (continued)

Workload Measurement	Advantages	Disadvantages
Standard Data	• Quick, easy to use • Consistent and fair • Economical	• Data are unique to a specific company, and companies cannot normally use another's standard data
Expert Panel	• Easy, efficient • Can be reliable if results approximate those obtained by experts • Low cost • Considers uniqueness of situations	• Easily biased • Doesn't always reflect current conditions
Comprehensive Unit of Service	• Incorporates impact of multi-tasking • Relies on standardized nursing taxonomy for high validity • Includes the dynamic complexity of human phenomenon including physical, psychological, and contextual realities	• Requires use of expert or experienced nurses to develop comprehensive units of service of specific patient population • Data are unique to the setting and cannot quickly be generalized to other settings • Nurses are sometimes reluctant to give up task model for fear of not identifying work that is done

Health Care Classification Systems

Determining labor needs depends on a system for assessing requirements of patients and fitting these requirements to the appropriate level of staff expertise. Nurse leaders are required to provide quantitative reports on workload allocations and justify the staffing levels required. The expectation is that resources expended did indeed produce value to the patient, that there is a relationship between the nursing care provided and the functionality or improvement in the patient's clinical condition. Using a patient classification system has become a standard management practice for nurse leaders. A patient classification system measures workload, providing one component of a comprehensive workload management plan.

Simply stated, *classification is the ordering of entities into groups or classes on the basis of their similarity, minimizing within-group variance and maximizing between-group variance* (Gordon, 1998). *Patient classification* is a process of grouping patients into homogeneous, mutually exclusive groups to determine their dependency on caregivers or to determine patient acuity (Dunn et al., 1995; Finkler, 2001). *Acuity* is defined as the level of need or dependency of an individual patient. The process of classifying patients is an element of workload management, the comprehensive system that includes patient classification, scheduling, staffing, and budgeting systems.

Workload management system principles have their origins in scientific management and were first identified over 100 years ago. Much credit is given to Frederick W. Taylor, who in 1881 at the Midvale Steel Company was determined to change the management system so that the interests of the workmen and management should become the same, instead of antagonistic (Barnes, 1980). Taylor argued, "the greatest obstacle to harmonious cooperation between the workman and the management lay in the ignorance of management as to what really constitutes a proper day's work for a workman" (Barnes, 1980, p. 59).

Professionals were concerned about effective workload management and focused on questions such as, "Which is the best way to do this job?" and "What should constitute a day's work?" Taylor set out to define the proper method of doing a piece of work, teaching the worker just how to perform the work that way, while maintaining stability in all conditions surrounding the work so that the worker was supported in accomplishing the tasks expected.

Not surprising, this issue exists today in most work environments. Decades later, the health care industry still struggles to determine the best way to identify and measure effective staffing resource utilization. Health care costs continue to be a persistent and growing problem for both the public and private health care funding sources, as discussed in Part IV.

These challenges have been slowly addressed beginning with the creation of classification systems to better understand patient care needs in multiple settings from inpatient hospital care to skilled nursing home care to office care. The ICD-9 (International Classification of Diseases), diagnosis-related group (DRG), and case mix systems are examples of classification systems, each with advantages and disadvantages. Several other classification systems, such as the ambulatory payment classification (APC), resource utilization groups (RUGs), and Outcome and Assessment Information Set (OASIS) and home health resource groups (HHRGs), have emerged in recent years to address the need for classification of patient care needs (Shi & Singh, 2004). (For more detail in using DRGs, RUGs, and OASIS [HHRG] see Dunham-Taylor & Pinczuk [2006]; also see Chapter 10 for additional information.[1])

The ICD system is used to code and classify mortality data from death certificates. The International Classification of Diseases, Clinical Modification (ICD-9-CM) is used to code and classify morbidity data from the inpatient and outpatient records, physician offices, and most National Center for Health Statistics (NCHS) surveys. The NCHS serves as the World Health Organization Collaborating Center for the Family of International Classifications for North America and in this capacity is responsible for coordination of all official disease classification activities in the United States relating to the ICD and its use, interpretation, and periodic revision (see www.cdc.gov).

The DRG system categorizes the types of patients a hospital treats based on diagnoses, procedures, age, sex, and the presence of complications or comorbidities. This system was developed by a group of researchers at Yale University in the late 1960s as a tool to help clinicians and hospitals monitor quality of care and utilization of services and has been used by Medicare in the United States to pay hospitals. Briefly, DRGs work by taking more than 10,000 ICD-9-CM codes and grouping them into a more manageable number of meaningful patient categories. Patients within each category are similar clinically in terms of resource usage.

Case Mix Methods

As the industrial workload model emerged, people began to realize that there were issues with productivity measurement that involved efficiency. For example, a patient day for a normal obstetrics/gynecology delivery versus a patient day for an intensive care unit patient requires different staffing. The same is true for home care or ambulatory visits; an initial visit usually takes longer because staff members need to get to know and assess a new patient, whereas a follow-up visit often takes less time. Somehow, this needed to be added to the productivity measurement equation.

This prompted the movement to use *case mix methods*. "Case mix is a method of clustering patients into groups that are homogeneous with respect to the use of resources. Factors used to cluster patients have included diagnosis, prognosis, resource utilization, organ system, hospital department,

---

[1] "For more detail using DRGs, RUGs, and OASIS (HHRG) see Dunham-Taylor and Pinczuk (2006) *Health Care Financial Management for Nurse Managers: Applications from Hospitals, Long-Term Care, Home Care, and Ambulatory Care*, Sudbury, MA: Jones & Bartlett.

and patient demographic characteristics" (Sullivan & Decker, 2001, p. 120). Thus Medicare began to use case mix methods, such as DRGs for hospital reimbursement, RUGs for long-term care reimbursement, and a case mix method for the ambulatory area using an ambulatory payment classification system that has relative value units that reflect the complexity of each procedure.

The case mix cluster reflects patient acuity based on ordering procedures and can be integrated with budgeting information and used within the ratios. The predominant problem with this is that most often the finance department does not understand the significance of the patient classification system. Patient classification systems are not traditionally covered in finance and accounting programs.

Patient care providers in areas other than the acute inpatient setting have also identified the need for systems that identify and measure the variations in staffing needs. Clinic visits, surgical procedures, deliveries, skilled nursing facilities, home health, and other procedures have been identified as service units. The Medicare program has adopted a case mix method to reimburse skilled nursing facilities. This method provides a per diem prospective rate based on the acuity level of patients. The case mix index uses the relative value unit technique and refers to the overall intensity of conditions that require medical and nursing interventions. The patient's condition is assessed and an estimate of the actual amount of resources that the patient will need is determined.

The case mix for skilled nursing facilities is driven by the minimum data set, which consists of a core set of screening elements used to assess the clinical, functional, and psychosocial needs of each resident. Using the data gained from the minimum data set assessment, the classification system RUGs was created to differentiate residents by their use of resources. Variables include diagnosis, functional limitations, negative health conditions, skin problems, and special treatments and procedures needed. RUG-III classifies patients into 44 categories according to their health care needs.

HHRGs use 80 distinct groups to indicate the severity of the patient's condition. Reimbursement for episodes of home health services are bundled under one payment and adjusted based on the patient's HHRG. Each of these models attempts to identify the qualitative aspects of clinical care and translate the care into mathematical formulations.

Neither the DRG, the ICD classification, nor the case mix systems have included the fundamental work of nursing—namely the coordination of care, patient assessment, education, development of the plan of care, provision of a safe environment, and delegation and supervision of selected personnel. The challenge remains to identify the real and specific work of nursing, quantify it into health care's economic equation, and create workload management systems that assure buyers they are getting value for their commitment of resources. Buyers want to be assured that there is some common frame of reference for clinical decisions made throughout the health system. They want to know whether there are some normative standards of clinical practice, including price, to which all providers comply, standards that can continually be validated and replicated. Further, every provider is now under the same obligation to ensure that there is a connection between what one does and what is achieved; there is now a requirement that a clinical decision also be the most cost-effective choice that can be made. It is from these mandates that the continuing need for valid and reliable patient classification systems remains relevant.

Patient Classification Systems in Nursing

In 1984 the North American Nursing Diagnosis Association established the conceptual framework for a nursing diagnostic classification system (Figure 6–3). This definition and taxonomy helped to establish consistent terminology, making oral and written communication easier and more efficient. In addition, definitive nursing functions were identified and increased the nurse's accountability in assessing the patient, determining the diagnosis, and providing the treatment called for by the diagnosis.

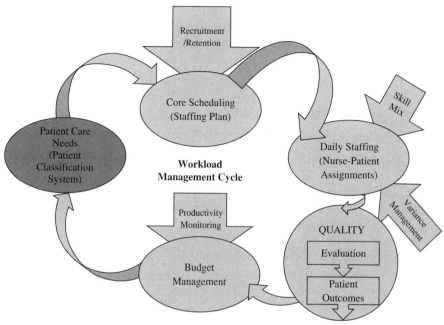

Figure 6–3 Patient Care Needs

Bulechek and McCloskey believed that the nursing process was a form of logical clinical inquiry and that the nurse made decisions about particular clinical phenomena (American Nurses Association [ANA], 1989). The nursing interventions identified and developed by the research team from the University of Iowa have become a highly regarded taxonomy for the work of nursing. Nursing intervention classifications (NICs) now represent an accepted and systemic approach to naming classes of nursing interventions, facilitating understanding, and communicating patient treatment plans. NIC is a comprehensive, standardized language that describes treatments that nurses perform in all settings and in all specialties. NICs include eight foundational domains: physiological (e.g., acid-base management), psychosocial (e.g., anxiety reduction), illness treatment (e.g., hyperglycemia management), illness prevention (e.g., fall prevention), health promotion (e.g., exercise promotion), interventions for individuals or for families (e.g., family integrity promotion), indirect care interventions (e.g., emergency cart checking), and interventions for communities (e.g., environmental management).

A standardized language for nursing provides the industry with tools to recognize the contributions and accomplishments of nursing. Using a standardized language is important in demonstrating contributions, influencing practice, and facilitating critical thinking. Nurses now have the necessary knowledge and instruments to clearly articulate the effects of their interventions on patient outcomes.

The increasing use of the electronic medical record has further impacted the classification process. Systematized NOmenclature of MEDicine (SNOMED) has gained increasing support as the acceptable language that can be used by all applications. Using the standardized language provides an excellent resource for data indexing, collection, analysis, interpretation, storing, retrieving, and aggregating clinical data.

Most recently, nurse leaders and informatics leaders created the Technology Informatics Guiding Educational Reform (TIGER) initiative as a mechanism to raise awareness of both the complexities and possibilities of informatics tools, principles, theories, and practices. It is believed that these efforts will support safer health care and more effective, efficient, patient-centered, timely, and equitable processes by interweaving enabling technologies transparently into nursing practice and education, making information technology the stethoscope for the 21st century (retrieved July 30, 2008 at https://www.tigersummit.com/Home_Page.html). Currently, over 500 nurses are working to bridge clinical practice quality with information technology.

Patient Classification System Characteristics

When selecting a patient classification system, several criteria are important:

- Interventions or indicator lists that provide an adequate representation of the current work of nursing
- Use of industry standardized language
- Consideration of the characteristics of facility geography (length of halls, available workspace, location of nurse workstations, etc.)
- Ability to determine skill mix and staff hours required for each patient
- A level of computerization and interface capability with the patient care record, patient registration systems, and scheduling systems
- A history of validity and reliability
- Flexibility so can be used with all patient care delivery models
- Identification of unique patient populations of the organization
- Consistent with the organization's mission and vision

When first introduced in the 1930s, patient classification systems were based on the industrial engineering model of nurses' time and nursing tasks. Engineers believed that patient activities could be quantified by identifying the time it took nurses to complete a task related to patient care. The identified timed tasks could then be summed to identify the number of staff needed.

Over the past 60 years, system users have identified that significant variables were omitted from these historic design structures, ones necessary to accurately determine either the patient acuity or the staffing requirements (Van Slyck, 2000). To address these shortcomings, health care leaders have also integrated factor, prototype, relative values, and comprehensive unit of service concepts into traditional systems to increase validity:

- The *factor evaluation method* identifies selected elements of care, critical indicators, or tasks with associated times that are most likely predictors of nursing care needs. Individual patients are then assessed for the presence or absence of these critical indicators and, based on this assessment, assigned to a category. Nursing is viewed as a series of tasks performed in a sequence. This method attempts to elicit a measure of overall workload. The factor evaluation system rates a number of indicators of care separately and then sums the ratings to designate the patient's acuity (Hasman, Wiersma, Halfens, & Algera, 1993). Examples of patient conditions or nursing interventions identified as critical indicators are activities of daily living, medications, monitoring, safety needs, and complex equipment. Some factor evaluation systems include as many as 400 items for the nurse to review before selecting the category that most accurately matches the patient. **Exhibit 6–5** is an example of the indicators in a factor patient classification system.
- The *prototype approach* identifies the characteristics of patients in each category. Individual patients are then assigned to the category that most closely reflects their nursing care requirements. This method generally offers profiles or descriptions of patients typical of those requiring a particular type and amount of nursing care. The system, developed by Walts and Kapadia (1996) to support their staffing algorithm, is a prototype system—it classifies patients into eight categories based on required nursing time. Examples of prototype

profiles or descriptions include simple or average, above average, and high or complex patient care needs. Each profile is assigned a designated number of hours for care. Typically, no skill mix differentiation is determined in the prototype method. **Exhibit 6–6** is an example of a prototype patient classification system. Unfortunately, because patients seldom fall into all of the categories in one level, this approach does not allow for partial selection, which often leads to inconsistent and inaccurate classification of patients.

- Another concept is the *relative value unit*. In addition to grouping patients into similar categories based on nursing care needs, a patient classification system can also quantify the workload within the categories by assigning a relative value to each category. A relative weight is assigned to each patient category; one category is assigned arbitrarily the value of 1.0 and all

Exhibit 6–5 Example of Factor Patient Classification System

Circle all that apply:

Self care	Restraints	4-6 IV Medications	Neuro check q shift
Partial care	Isolation	> 6 IV Medications	Neuro check q 2 hrs
Complete bath	Wound care—simple	Telemetry monitor	Medicate for pain x3
Ambulate with assistance x2	Wound care— complex	Suction q 2 hrs.	Medicate for pain >3 times
Ambulate with two person assist x1	1 peripheral IV line	Suction > q 2 hrs	Insert foley catheter
Assistance with meals	2 peripheral IV lines	I & O q 8 hrs	Enema
Total Feed	> 2 IV lines	I & O q 1 hr	Accucheck q 4 hrs
Skin care	Oral medications	Educate patient re: diabetes	Give 1 unit of blood
Heel care	1-3 IV medications	Educate patient re: surgery	Give > 1 unit of blood

Exhibit 6–6 Example of Prototype Patient Classification System: Levels 1–3

	Level 1–Average Needs	**Level 2–Above Average Needs**	**Level 3–High Needs**
ADL's	Minimal Assistance	Partial Bath; Assistance with feeding	Total Care
Medications	3–8 Oral Medications	9 or more oral medications 1–3 IV medications	More than 4 IV medications
Monitoring	Routine vital signs	Telemetry monitoring	Multiple monitors; telemetry, swan and / or ICP
IV Lines / Tubes	Less than 2 lines or tubes	3–6 lines and / or tubes	More than 6 lines and tubes

other categories are assigned values in relation to it. The relative value scale is then used to describe the workload for a given unit or organization.

- The *comprehensive unit of service*, developed by Malloch and Conovaloff (1999), is based on the standard data and the expert panel method. The comprehensive unit of service, an aggregate of eight categories of care, represents the total care provided by nursing during a shift or event of care and integrates a multitasking factor to account for the overlap of care in identified patient situations. This model is designed to address the lack of sensitivity to the unique holistic nature of patients and fluctuations in economies of scale or the impact of nurses doing more than one task or process at a time. **Exhibit 6–7** is an example of a comprehensive unit of service. The clinical profile based on care provided to the patient determines caregiver time and skill mix required for that the patient.

Once the standards are established using iterative summaries of expert nurse time estimations, nurses rate patients in eight categories, which represent the essence of patient care during or at the end of each shift. The hours and skill mix are generated for each patient and then summarized to identify the total unit staffing needs. Staffing hours and skill mix needed are then compared with available staff to determine adequacy of staffing or if adjustments are needed.

Benefits of Patient Classification Systems (Workload Measurement)

The benefits and rationale for valid and reliable patient classification include the following:

- *Understanding the relationship between patient care needs, nursing intervention, desired outcomes, and the skill level of nurses.* Determining the appropriate type and number of caregivers and support staff needed to provide safe and effective patient care is the foundation of

---

Exhibit 6–7 Comprehensive Unit of Service Example

Category	Caregiver Intervention	Rating
1. Cognitive needs	1-step commands; reorient every 2 hours	2
2. Self-Care needs	Transfer with 2 staff members; 1:1 feed; Complete bath	1
3. Emotional/Social/ Spiritual needs	Set limits 1:1; therapeutic communication > 45 minutes; reassure every hour	2
4. Comfort/Pain management needs	Assess /Monitor q shift; medicate x1 / shift	4
5. Family support needs	Update family x1/shift	5
6. Treatments	Wound care dressing change x2 / shift; 8 oral medications; 2 IV medications	3
7. Interdisciplinary coordination needs	Coordinate 4 providers; Delegate and supervise 2 caregivers	4
8. Transition needs	Assess x1 / shift	5
Time required: 3.0 hours	RN: 1.0; LPN: 1.0; NA: 1.0	

the workload management system (Behner, Fogg, Fournier, Frankenbach, & Robertson, 1990; Mark and Burleson, 1995).

- *Information to correlate the work of nursing and the outcomes of care.* Providing services that do not impact the outcome of patient functionality is no longer appropriate or affordable. When registered nurse (RN) levels are low, nurses may not have time to provide essential education or prevention oversight of patients or to supervise nonlicensed staff. Further, there are documented relationships between RN staffing and levels of medication errors, patient falls, new pressure ulcers, nosocomial pneumonia, urinary tract infections, length of stay, and unplanned readmissions (Aiken, Clarke, Cheung, Sloane, & Silber, 2003; Cho, Ketefian, Barkauska, & Smith, 2003; Harper & McCully, 2007; Needleman, Buerhaus, Mattke, Stewart, & Zelevinsky, 2002; Potter, Barr, McSweeney, & Sledge, 2003; Sasichay-Akkadechanunt, Scalzi, & Jawad, 2003; Seago, 2001; Unruh, 2003). (See Chapter 4 for additional information on quality.)
- Fixed staffing numbers (ratios) cannot be considered sufficient to manage variations in patient care and sustain quality patient care (Bolton et al., 2001). *Patient-to-nurse ratios identify the minimum staffing levels, whereas patient classification systems define the amount of staff needed for a particular situation.* Ratio-staffing levels are data derived from a valid and reliable patient classification system and from knowing the range of patient care needs. Ratio data are best used in the aggregate for budgeting and scheduling, not for day-to-day staffing.
- *Valid and reliable systems define and defend the work of professional nursing, increase visibility of professional nursing practice, protect patients from complications, and decrease the vulnerability of nurse staffing to budget cuts.* The integration of nursing science taxonomy into practice also explicates professionalism and the ethical obligations of nursing to use resources wisely while providing skilled services. The ANA Staffing Principles, developed in 1999 and updated in 2008, clearly identify and support the need for empirical data to guide decision making to identify and maintain the appropriate number and skill mix of nursing staff using valid and reliable systems. The nine principles identified by an expert panel for nurse staffing are as follows:

1. Appropriate staffing levels for a patient care unit reflect analysis of individual and aggregate patient needs.
2. Either retire or seriously question the usefulness of the concept of nursing hours per patient day (NHPPD).
3. Unit functions necessary to support delivery of quality patient care must also be considered in determining staffing levels.
4. The specific needs of various patient populations should determine the appropriate clinical competencies required of the nurse practicing in that area.
5. RNs must have nursing management support and representation at both the operational level and the executive level.
6. Clinical support from experienced RNs should be readily available to those RNs with less proficiency.
7. Organizational policy should reflect an organizational climate that values RNs and other employers as strategic assets and exhibits a true commitment to filling budgeted positions in a timely manner.
8. All institutions should have documented competencies for nursing staff, including agency or supplemental traveling RNs, for those activities that they have been authorized to perform.
9. Organizational policies should recognize the myriad needs of both patients and nursing staff (ANA, 2008).

In essence, the ANA has identified four critical factors essential in the creation of nurse staffing systems: patient characteristics, intensity of unit activity, context of care, and the expertise of caregivers.

Validity, Reliability, and Sensitivity of Patient Classification Systems

As previously noted, a patient classification system must be credible both to nursing staff and to those outside nursing, including administrators, financial officers, and directors of health care plans. The validity, reliability, and sensitivity of the system must therefore be clearly established and sustained. A valid, reliable, and sensitive patient classification system that defines patient care needs is the foundation of an effective workload management system.

VALIDITY

A system to determine staffing needs, typically a patient classification system, is said to have a high degree of validity when it accurately represents the work of the caregivers, correctly distributes patients among distinct classes, and defines the category of caregiver required for the care (Hernandez & O'Brien, 1996a, b). Nursing workload data must be accurate to make appropriate staffing and scheduling decisions and to make wise budget allocations. Accurate data cannot be obtained unless the patient classification system, the foundation of the workload management system, is both valid and reliable.

Validity of the patient classification can be described as the degree to which it actually measures what it intends to measure. The patient classification system is intended to measure the work of nursing. The work of nursing includes at a minimum the general categories of physiological care, behavioral support, safety measures, family education and support, coordination of care, documentation, and community integration (McCloskey & Bulechek, 2000). Validity is a matter of degree, not an all-or-none property, and the process of validation is unending (Hernandez & O'Brien, 1996a). Validity should be monitored annually, and the method of assessing validity will vary with the type of classification system (Hernandez & O'Brien, 1996b). Several types of validity are considered in a patient classification system, including face, content, construct, internal, and external validity. Each is briefly described.

Face validity is high when nurses believe that the system accurately reflects and represents the work they do or the dependency of the patients for whom they provide care. Face validity is lost when the nurses do not fully understand the system or the assumptions that underlie it. If the nurse does not understand the philosophy of the system (i.e., task or process) and does not believe that the system captures all of the workload, face validity is lost and the instrument is no longer credible or usable.

Content validity is the extent to which the tool includes all the major elements relative to the construct being measured. The evidence is typically obtained from three sources: literature, representatives from relative populations, and content experts (Burns & Grove, 2001). Most existing tools capture the procedural work of nursing but only minimally include the coordination, monitoring, and evaluation role of the professional nurse, thus resulting in a tool with less than acceptable validity.

Construct validity is the fit between the conceptual definitions and operational definitions of variables. Conceptual definitions provide the basis for the definition of operational definition of variables. The measure should provide a valid inference of the construct. Does the tool measure what it claims to measure? Does the category system explain the complexity of responsibility areas and total care required (Verran, 1986)? An example is a patient assessment. The construct is the assessment and the operational definition would include those elements that comprise a nursing assessment such as body systems, psychosocial status, safety needs, family support needs, and discharge planning. Thus the tool would necessarily include items or indicators specific to the operational definition of a nursing assessment to create construct validity.

Internal validity, or the extent to which the measures used in the tool are a true reflection of reality (and not the result of extraneous variables), is another key characteristic of the patient classification tool. Internal validity of a patient classification system considers the credibility of the tool or system within the organization. Inclusion of scheduling and staffing requirements into a patient classification system diminishes the internal validity because the variables of staff competence levels, indirect support time, and/or regulatory requirements cloud the specific patient care requirement. Incorporating system requirements into the patient classification system decreases the internal validity.

External validity, or the extent to which the findings can be generalized beyond the sample used, is a critical issue for patient classification systems. Although the industry is desperately seeking a measurement tool that can be used in all organizations with all patient populations and with high external validity, the achievement of this goal remains a challenge. There are some commonalities in the categories of nursing care interventions from organization to organization; there can also be significant variations in the operational definitions and processes of care for the same interventions. Whereas the comparisons appear appropriate, validity is uncertain until the definitions and associated time requirements are examined. This is not to imply that some degree of external validity cannot be obtained but rather to note that when external comparisons of data from setting to setting are made, the limitations to generalizations of comparability must be noted.

RELIABILITY

The *reliability* of the patient classification system tool addresses the consistency of rating. Different observers assessing the same patient at the same time should generate the same rating. According to Finkler (2001), prototype tools are more subjective, making this degree of reliability more difficult to achieve. Factor evaluation tools are more objective, but their reliability depends on clear definition and consistent interpretation of the critical indicators. Ongoing measurement of reliability is necessary and generally involves two or more raters independently (interrater reliability) assessing a defined percentage of classified patients at a specified interval. Reliability scores of 100% (no discrepancies in ratings) are always the target. There is disagreement about the necessary frequency for interrater reliability and the number of patients to classify when doing reliability checks. Recommended frequencies span from annually to monthly. To obtain the highest degree of system reliability, annual review of 100% of system users is recommended. However, authors agree that more frequent reliability monitoring is required if a high degree of interrater reliability is not maintained (Hernandez & O'Brien, 1996a).

With prototype tools, reliability addresses only agreement of type. With the factor evaluation tools, reliability ideally is demonstrated by agreement on both patient type and individual critical indicators. Interrater reliability scores of less than 85% seriously compromise the credibility of the system.

SENSITIVITY

Sensitivity typically refers to physiological measures and is related to the amount of change of a parameter that can be measured precisely (Gift & Soeken, 1988). If changes are expected to be very small, the tool must be able to detect the changes. For example, infant scales that differentiate ounces are appropriate in the nursery. Truck scales that measure hundreds of pounds would not be sensitive enough for the nursery. Patient classification sensitivity is about detecting those changes that determine time and type of caregiver and is a balance between estimation of time and precise time amounts. At best, the time for patient care can only be an estimation of requirements within certain ranges because patient events are unpredictable and patient responses to care vary. Estimates within 15 minutes of actual time required for patient care are adequate for the complex phenomena of patient care.

Patient Classification Systems: Limitations and Challenges

Skepticism about patient classification systems has existed since their introduction. With the variety of patient classification systems available and the years of testing new and innovative ways of capturing time estimation, the nursing profession still struggles with the creation of credible workload management systems. To be sure, the optimal solution for measuring caregiver workload is the attachment of time and skill mix standards to clinical interventions in an electronic documentation system. With documentation driving the calculations for patient needs, the issues of reliability are decreased significantly. Several sources of the patient classification system mistrust exist: low validity, misuse, failure to use the data generated, and lack of tool simplicity.

LOW VALIDITY

Task-based acuity systems do not always account for professional nursing care practices, such as patient education, interdisciplinary collaboration, family support, and delegation and supervision of other caregivers. As a result, although the system appropriately captures increasing patient severity, the assumptions used to structure staffing models are flawed (Shaha, 1995). Because much of nursing is mind-work rather than hand-work, it is not surprising that the task-based methods of some systems capture only a part of nursing work. Additionally, the effects of multitasking are not captured.

At present, there is no single agreed-on patient classification system that describes the commonly accepted nursing practice components of assessment, diagnosis, intervention, and outcomes. Because there is no agreed-on system, there are few, if any, empirical data sets to describe nursing practice across clinical settings, client populations, DRGs, medical diagnoses, geographical areas, or time. The lack of standardized nursing language makes it extremely difficult to know with any degree of accuracy which type of patient classification system provides the most valid and reliable data for workload management decisions.

MISUSE OF THE TOOL

The most common problems with classification systems relate to a phenomenon called *acuity creep*. Acuity creep occurs when the reported acuity of patients increases slowly over time but the actual care does not appear to change. In other words, acuity levels creep to higher and higher levels often to justify higher resource use by managers in affected areas. Creep becomes a problem because it assumes there is an ever-increasing need for patient care resources and labor in an industry where financial resources for such care are ever decreasing (Shaha, 1995).

The use of a system with low validity makes it difficult to distinguish inappropriate acuity creep from those changes in patient care that are real. Reimbursement changes and growth in alternative areas beyond the inpatient arena have not only changed the actual acuity of inpatients but also changed the typical model of patient care delivery. Nurse aides, for example, were not factored into original acuity systems but provide a significant portion of care in current inpatient and outpatient settings.

The lack of trust between administration and caregivers stems in part from the belief that patient classification systems are a vehicle to decrease staffing levels. Caregivers believe that initiatives in redesigning nursing work have emphasized efficiency over patient safety. Poor communication practices between staff providing patient care and health care leaders have also led to mistrust. This loss of trust has serious implications for the ability of hospitals and other health care organizations to make the fundamental changes essential to providing safer patient care (Page, 2004).

PROSPECTIVE VERSUS RETROSPECTIVE CHALLENGES

Patient classification data are best used in planning for the next shift. Planning for the next shift requires not only information about the patient needs, but also information about the oncoming staff competencies, the previous similar shift staffing (yesterday's afternoon shift to compare with the upcoming afternoon shift), facility support for housekeeping, pharmacy, transportation, teaching staff available, and anticipated admissions, discharges, and transfers.

The general consensus of nurse leaders and staff nurses is that they want a patient classification system that prospectively determines the amount of staff and skill mix that will be sufficient for meeting the patient needs on the following shift. Yet the greatest frustration with staff nurses is that there is no system that can accurately predict the staffing needs for the next shift, and when attempts to formulate estimations for the next shift are implemented, caregivers are quick to challenge the results.

Although there is a core of expected care for the next shift, *a minimum of 20% of the workload in most units is highly variable.* New admissions, unplanned clinical condition changes, family crises, and provider rounding times make the prediction process difficult—if not impossible—without a crystal ball! The most that a patient classification system can tell you is on average what the staffing should be based on history (Seago, 2002). The severity of patient illness, need for specialized equipment and technology, intensity of nursing interventions required, and the complexity of clinical nursing judgment needed to design, implement, and evaluate the patient's nursing plan are often not predictable.

UNITS OF MEASURE: TOTAL HOURS VERSUS SKILL MIX REQUIRED

The required skill mix for each patient is often an overlooked component of a patient classification system. The patient classification system must identify not only the needs of the patient and the hours required for this care but also what level of caregiver is required to perform the work. Despite the name implying a measurement of severity of illness, *patient acuity or patient classification is in truth more concerned with determining the time required for care*; the patient acuity level is *secondary* information. There is indeed some correlation between acuity and amount of care required, but the correlation is not absolute. A chronic ventilator-dependent paraplegic may score high in severity of illness but not require a large number of care hours due to condition stability and established plans of care. Many systems do not differentiate between the two measurements and make the leap from quality to quantity of nursing care a significant challenge.

FAILURE TO USE THE DATA GENERATED

The patient classification system is typically overseen by the nursing department and requires the input of staff supervisors, unit directors, and unit staff that will be affected by the data. Financial officers and leaders of other clinical services are typically not involved in the initial design and management of nursing systems. Oftentimes, the credibility of the data and the possibility of manipulating the data to the advantage of nursing are challenged, particularly if the data demonstrate increased workload and increased need for resources (Finkler, 2001). As a result, the fundamental trustworthiness of the system is questioned by non-nursing hospital leaders and the system is merely tolerated or ignored.

LACK OF TOOL SIMPLICITY

To address the credibility gap, clinicians have worked to develop all-inclusive, objective lists of interventions to create a valid system. Unfortunately, these systems become lengthy and risk losing reliability very quickly. Some systems require the user to review and select from 100 or more items for each patient event, a process that seldom results in good data. Classification systems that try to list every possible intervention become overwhelming, time consuming, and not worth the effort needed to ensure accuracy. When the system is not easily integrated into the workflow, it is seen as one more thing to do, and becomes a lower priority—often completed only after the shift is over. Systems that are easily misused, mismanaged, or generate inaccurate data cannot be used by managers to defend their staffing decisions. The time it takes to complete the tool can also be a significant barrier in the collection of accurate data.

This conundrum of attempting to identify every intervention but doing so in an efficient manner sets the stage for mistrust and inaccuracy in any patient classification system. The low validity achieved when nurses attempt to identify every intervention ultimately makes the product mistrusted by nursing staff, nurse leaders, financial managers, and administration. Many of the current models of patient classification systems continue to struggle with this challenge. Resolving conflicts that arise from the use of a patient classification system for staffing have often ended up at the bargaining table and in the regulatory arena (DeGroot, 1994).

Staffing Plan Core Schedule

The second component of a workload management system is the *staffing plan*. The staffing plan describes adherence to the ANA's Code of Ethics, Social Policy Statement, and Standards of Practice. The intended benefits of such a plan are (1) improved quality of patient care; (2) positive impact on patient outcomes; (3) improved work environment; (4) increased staff satisfaction, retention, professional growth, and development; and (5) improved organizational outcomes.

The staffing plan describes the structure and process by which responsibilities for patient care are assigned and how the work is coordinated among caregivers. In addition, it describes the mechanism for documenting and reporting staffing concerns. This integrated set of processes, or the patient care delivery model, integrates data from a valid and reliable patient classification system. For example, the patient classification system will identify the required skill mix necessary to best manage the typical patients on any given unit. Trended data may identify a need for a change in the skill mix and staffing plan that incorporates the use of greater numbers of RNs, or greater numbers of licensed practical/vocational nurses (LPNs/VNs) and nursing assistants providing adjunctive care.

Core schedules represent an aggregated average number and skill mix required for patient care and focus on having sufficient staff to care for the population served. Components include direct, indirect, and activity time. The *core scheduling* (Figure 6–4) is the long-range plan that becomes the organization's template for the required number of staff. The schedule incorporates the organization's goals; available staff; state and national legislation; scope of practice defined by licensure, regulations, and accreditation requirements; and planned patient demand (Gardner & Gemme, 2003).

Whenever possible, *direct care*, or interventions specific to patient care that can be directly attributed to the patient, as well as *daily planning* and *documentation* should be identified in the patient classification system. According to O'Brien-Pallas, Irvine, Peereboom, and Murray (1997), health care leaders are challenged to examine the traditional concept of direct and indirect care and to define the main constructs that may influence nursing work. Patient care work should include work that is directly attributed to the patient, whether it is at the bedside or in the conference room supporting the planning process. Support hours such as shift report and counting supplies and

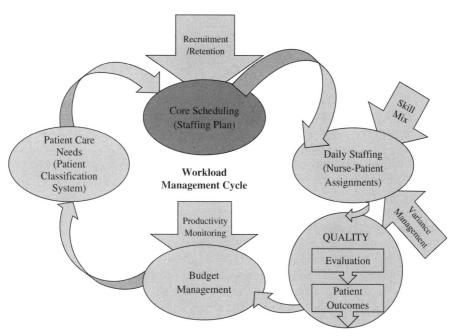

Figure 6–4 Core Scheduling

medications are typically a percentage of time and are calculated for inclusion in the core schedule. Once patient needs are determined and validated, the department director can then determine the core staffing hours and skill levels needed to run the department efficiently and effectively.

The staffing plan includes the person who is in charge during a shift. This person provides leadership, makes assignments, and deals with unusual incidents or difficult situations. This person supports the leadership on issues as they occur during a shift or for a specified length of time.

Staffing plans may need to temporarily change when new employees are hired. As the new employee is oriented or if the staff member is just out of school, this person will not be able to take care of as many patients. If a preceptor is used, the preceptor will need to work the same schedule as the new employee.

The staffing plan also considers *indirect caregiver role requirements* such as the health unit secretary. Those roles that support the operations of the unit should be categorized in the schedule portion of the workload management plan. This time, traditionally labeled as indirect time, is defined and measured in a variety of ways in organizations. Regardless of how it is defined, indirect time must be measured consistently.

Once basic staffing levels are determined, one can set up several scenarios within the staffing plan to determine when the staffing would change as patient volume increases or decreases. For instance, Hollabaugh and Kendrick (1998) at Good Samaritan Regional Medical Center in Arizona developed a five-level pyramid to staff for peak times (winter) as well as low census/acuity times (summer), a hiring plan for the varying census times, and a more equitable cancellation policy. This plan achieved cost savings, more continuity and job satisfaction, fewer patient and physician complaints, and established a more effective way to adequately staff despite large variations in census. The amount of patient care staff, skill mix, and necessary support staff needed to assist in providing the care is adjusted based on patient needs (the daily staffing process).

When the patient volume goes *below* the minimum staffing level (as explained in Chapter 13), staffing cannot be cut further, and other options, such as combining services with another cost center, must be considered. Ideally, if a reliable and valid patient classification system is available, the staffing plan is based on patient acuity. Typically, the nurse executive, in collaboration with key stakeholders, is responsible for establishing an overall staffing plan for the division or departments of nursing and should include levels of patient care needs identified in the patient classification system. The plan describes the professional practice model used in the hospital and indicates how that model supports the delivery of patient care and the environment in which care is delivered.

If patient classification data are not available, comparative data such as benchmarking with other units serving a similar patient population can be used. Benchmarking data are available from other health care organizations, the literature, patient classification system companies, professional organizations, or group purchasing organizations such as VHA and Premier. When benchmarking secondary data it is very important to ensure data consistency (Garry, 2000; Hall, Pink, Johnson, & Schraa, 2000). Dunham-Taylor and Pinczuk (2006) *Health Care Financial Management for Nurse Managers: Applications in Hospitals, Long-Term Care, Home Care, and Ambulatory Care* devoted a chapter on developing staffing plans for a hospital using benchmark data.

Evidence for optimal, or at least adequate, staff is emerging. Research is now available to substantiate *staffing plan effectiveness*. Pinkerton and Rivers (2001) identified an extensive list of contextual factors impacting staffing effectiveness (**Exhibit 6–8**). Staffing is not simply providing a schedule for staff so they know when to show up for work. Effective staffing is the result of careful consideration of multiple variables and an examination of their relationship to outcomes. *Effective staffing* practices integrate historical evidence about performance from patient, family, staff, and operational perspectives. *Efficient staffing* uses the least costly level of caregiver to achieve the desired patient outcomes.

As a nurse administrator establishes a staffing plan, it is important to have this plan reflect productive hours actually worked (as defined in Chapter 13). It is best if the budget can reflect productive hours separately from nonproductive hours.

Exhibit 6–8 Understanding Contextual Variables/Factors Impacting Staffing Needs

I. Support

  A. Interdepartmental
    1. Number of support staff from other disciplines.
    2. Adequacy of support services, for example, patient transport team, volunteers.
    3. Ineffective discharge planning.
    4. Quality and/or evidence of pre-hospital patient teaching.
    5. Presence or absence of services in the hospital that support nursing care 24 hours.
    6. Increased ancillary service utilization.
    7. Quality of relationship with physician.
    8. Changes in other departments impacting nursing.
    9. Effectiveness of interdisciplinary teams.
    10. Effectiveness of communications.
    11. Accuracy and thoroughness of patient education by other disciplines.

B. Intradepartmental
  1. Number of unit-based support staff.
  2. Number of orientees scheduled (training time).
  3. Teamwork or no teamwork/unit cohesiveness.
  4. Communication from patient to nurse (is there a person answering call light who can adequately communicate problems to nurses)?
  5. Ineffective discharge planning.
  6. Full or part-time, shift worked.
  7. Number of tasks per staff type.
  8. Health of nurse, pregnancy, work restrictions.
  9. Skill mix.
  10. Patient care modality.
  11. Consistency of patient care assignment.
  12. Staff turnover.
  13. No working preferred shift/rotating shifts.
  14. Paperwork expectation—nursing documentation.

II. Care Environment

  1. Bed turnover (combined number of admits and discharges).
  2. Environmental layout impacting efficiency.
  3. Presence of extender system (for example, tube systems, fax machines, PCs).
  4. Availability of patient safety devices (fall prevention, restraint reductions measures) or is the nurse required to have direct sight?
  5. Shift of patients from one level of care to another.
  6. Midnight census may be an outdated way of tracking workload because so many patients have early evening discharge and midnight census does not reflect work between 7 am-7 pm when most patients come and go.
  7. Medication delivery system.
  8. Having weighted factors for outpatients housed on impatient units. Most care provided in first 6 to 10 hours. If they go home at 2300, only partial credit given for intensive care.
  9. Impact of academic presence/students.
  10. Technology development: automatic blood pressure machines at bedsides, auto charting, medication dispensing, etc.
  11. User-friendly technology.
  12. Information systems: data retrieval.
  13. Information systems: order entry.
  14. Chaos factors impacting the delivery of nursing care.

III. Professional Competency.

  1. Experience level of staff, new graduates especially with diverse patient population.
  2. Organizational skills of the nurse.
  3. Delegation skills of the nurse.
  4. Level of education (degree): continuing education certifications.
  5. Charge capable (charge nurse).

continued

Exhibit 6–8 Understanding Contextual Variables/Factors Impacting Staffing Needs (continued)

   6. Philosophy and leadership style of the nursing leadership team.

   7. Participation on hospital/unit/community related activities: gets overall richer understanding of nursing.

   8. Frequency of new procedures produced (learning curve).

   9. Impact of generalist vs. specialist practice.

  10. Number of float/temporary staff.

  11. Professional attribute/professional practice model.

  12. Autonomy level of the nurse.

  13. Cultural competence/diverse composition of teams (correlate with diversity of patient population).

IV. Physician Driven

   1. Number of consultants on case (writing excessive orders and/or conflicting orders requiring confirmation re-work).

   2. Number of different physician groups, with greater impact when patients are off service.

   3. Variation in physician practice/medical staff rules and regulations.

V. External

   1. Changes in nursing workforce.

   2. Declining nurse productivity with an aging workforce.

   3. Decreased commitment to suffering.

   4. Aging workforce.

   5. Generational differences.

   6. Regulatory requirements.

   7. Legal/liability for RNs.

   8. Fatigue

   9. Frequency and complexity of changes.

Source: Pinkerton, S., and Rivers, R. (September–October, 2001). Factors influencing staffing needs. *Nursing Economic$,* 19(5), 237.

Dunham-Taylor and Pinczuk (2006) provide samples of staffing plans included in *Health Care Financial Management for Nurse Managers: Financial Applications in Hospitals, Long-Term Care, Home Care, and Ambulatory Care* (Dunham-Taylor & Pinczuk, 2006). There are several staffing plans available in other literature as well (Douglas & Mayewski, 1996; Fralic, 2000; Schmidt, 1999; Strickland & Neely, 1995).

Considerations in Creating the Core Schedule

NURSING STAFF SKILL MIX

An important factor in determining appropriate staffing is the *nursing staff skill mix,* the various types of nursing staff by job classification necessary to care for the patient population. To determine the skill mix one should ask several questions: What are the interventions needed by the patients and which skill level has the authorization and ability to provide the care? How do we deliver the care? Who is best to deliver the care? How is the care divided among the various caregivers? What skill mix provides the safest care? Which is cost effective? Unfortunately, there are no ideal answers. What works best in one setting (i.e., in a stepdown unit) may not be best in another (i.e., a skilled unit). And the answer to any one of these questions may depend on current circumstances such as patient acuity, turnover of patients, discharges pushed to Fridays, admissions arriving on the evening shift, staff competencies or availability, or budget deficits. Both this and the next section present further information to answer these skill mix questions.

Caregiver Roles—Advanced Practice Nurses

This group includes many different kinds of nurses with advanced degrees (most often master's degrees). Acute nurse practitioners, clinical specialists, and clinical leaders can plan, educate, coordinate, and provide care for the more complicated hospitalized patients, whereas primary care nurse practitioners and clinical specialists can see patients in various settings, prevent health care complications, teach patients, and encourage prevention of disease. Nurse anesthetists provide anesthesia under the guidance of an anesthesiologist. In some states nurse midwives can actually deliver babies; in other states they function more like a clinical specialist.

Clinical specialists are presently underused in health care organizations and in community settings. They provide clinical leadership for complex patients in a cost-effective way, as well as educate staff on ways to better care for patients. It is important to note that the Institute of Medicine recommends more extensive use of advanced practice nurses.

The clinical nurse leader is a new role developed by the American Association of Colleges of Nursing (AACN). This advanced practice role functions within the health care delivery system and assumes accountability for health care outcomes for a specific group of clients within a unit or setting through the assimilation and application of research-based information to design, implement, and evaluate client plans of care (AACN Working Paper on the Role of the Clinical Nurse Leader, 2004).

Caregiver Roles—RNs

"The role of the Professional Nurse is to establish a therapeutic relationship with the patient that includes responsibility for managing the patients' care over an episode of care" (Manthey, 2001). The RN areas of expertise—assessment of the patient, discharge planning, and patient teaching—are those that other nursing caregivers do not have. It is important to "articulate the unique contributions of the RN in meeting patient outcomes so that these aspects of the work of RNs are preserved if addressing nursing shortages involves fulfilling non-RN tasks with other licensed or certified personnel" (American Organization of Nurse Executives [AONE], 2000, p. 16).

One advantage noted with high RN mix was that less time was needed to communicate with less skilled workers. RNs save patient care costs in other ways. RNs possess an extensive knowledge base and assessment capability that places them in a position of significance to the patient. Outcomes research so far is showing that a higher RN skill mix results in lower length of stay and fewer complications, safety, and legal issues (Aiken et al., 2003; Aiken, Clarke, Sloane, Sochalski, & Silber, 2002; ANA, 1997, 2000; Blegen & Goode, 1997; Blegen, Goode, & Reed, 1998; Blegen & Vaughn, 1998; Blegen, Vaughn, & Goode, 2001; Bliesmer, Smayling, Kane, & Shannon, 1998; Bolton et al., 2001; Hendrix & Foreman, 2001; Kerr, 2000; Melberg, 1997; Needleman, Buerhaus, Mattke, Stewart, & Zelevinsky, 2001; Shullanberger, 2000).

Research linking RN skill mix with patient outcomes, a quality dimension necessary to consider in workload management (see Figure 6–5) has been an exciting ongoing process with more information becoming available each month. To date, with one exception, these studies generally found that higher RN ratios make a big difference in the quality of patient care. This started with ANA's *Implementing Nursing's Report Card* (1997), followed by ANA's *Nurse Staffing and Patient Outcomes* (2000). This last study used data from nine states—using all-payer data sets (9.1 million patients in almost 1,000 hospitals) for six states (Arizona, California, Florida, Massachusetts, New York, and Virginia) and just using a Medicare sample (3.8 million patients in more than 1,500 hospitals) for an additional three states (Minnesota, North Dakota, and Texas). As nurse staffing increased, the outcomes—length of stay, pneumonia, postoperative infections, pressure ulcers, and urinary tract infections—decreased. There was close congruence between data from each hospital regardless of payer mix. The exception is reported by Bolton et al. (2001), who found that fall rates and occurrence of pressure ulcers were not significantly lowered in California after mandated nurse ratios went into effect.

It is important to remember that additional variables impact the quality of care delivered. Number of traveler nurses, facility leadership, nurse–physician relationships, and available technology, or lack of it, impact care as well.

The RN scope of practice is specifically defined in each state. Although there are individual differences in this definition, there is a consistent core definition that includes the nursing process (assessment, diagnosis, planning, intervention, and evaluation), expert knowledge or professional judgment, and specialized skills needed for this independent, professional role. "The RN has the responsibility and accountability to delegate or not delegate direct patient care activities based on such factors as the complexity of the task, potential for harm, abilities of the [LPN or] UAP, and the necessary problem solving skills" (Kido, 2001, p. 28).

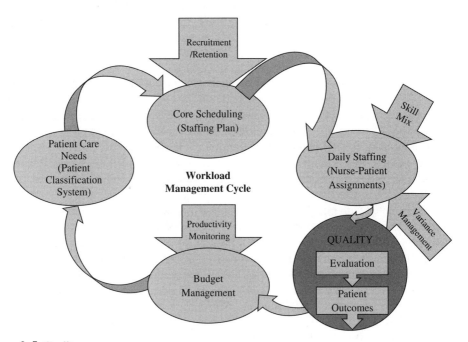

Figure 6–5 Quality

Perhaps this difference in perception comes partially from the educational preparation of the nurse; only 31% of RNs in the United States have Bachelor of Science degrees in nursing (BSNs). Goode and colleagues (2001) reported a survey of 43 hospital chief nursing officers who defined a difference between associate degree/diploma RNs and BSN RNs. They rank ordered the differences by describing the BSN RN as having greater critical thinking skills, less task orientation, more professionalism, stronger leadership skills, more focus on continuity of care and outcomes, greater focus on psychosocial components, better communication skills, and greater focus on patient teaching (Goode et al., 2001, p. 58). In this study, only 43% of hospital employers paid a salary differential for educational credentials.

Caregiver Roles—LPN/VNs

The LPN/VN provides an intermediate level of care as delegated by the RN and in accordance with state nurse practice acts. The role of the LPN is most appropriate in highly functioning teams, skilled nursing facilities, and office settings.

Caregiver Roles—Unlicensed Assistive Personnel (UAP)

Unlicensed assistive personnel assist the RN to carry out professional activities. Health care organizations use these workers in a variety of roles, some that are more focused on supporting the patient care environment rather than the patients themselves. The use of lower cost workers in delivering nursing care is a concept that has taken on a greater importance to hospitals and other health care institutions grappling with real and threatened declines in reimbursement, coupled with an aging nursing force. UAPs have been used in a variety of roles, in addition to the traditional primary support functions at the bedside; some perform simple housekeeping or secretarial tasks, and others perform higher level clinical or technical tasks such as electrocardiograms and phlebotomy. Because there is no one accrediting body common to all types of UAPs and because state laws vary regarding their use, hospitals have been relatively free to experiment with different care models under the guidance of their internal nursing leadership (McClung, 2000, p. 531).

The Omnibus Budget Reconciliation Act of 1987 (OBRA 87) required states to certify nursing assistants in long-term care facilities and to define the knowledge base and competencies required for nurse assistant certification. State requirements vary (training may be less than 1 week to 4 or more weeks) but must include those requirements federally mandated. Some boards of nursing require certified nursing assistants to submit proof of additional education to the state board to be recertified. (So in long-term care a nursing assistant must be certified, whereas hospitals can hire noncertified nursing assistants.)

Caregiver Roles—Volunteers

Another important role to support safe and effective staffing is the volunteer. Volunteers are used most often by hospitals but can be used in any setting or by individual units. This is a fairly untapped resource. Specific guidelines need to be developed as to their qualifications, training, and specific services they would provide.

COMPETENCY

Nurses and health care leaders are challenged to ensure individual nurse competency and to develop systems to address the reality of variability in caregivers and patients. There is a wide range of the levels and achievements of skill acquisition for caregivers. Incorporating the evolutionary roles of novice, advanced beginner, competent, proficient, and expert practitioners is essential to further increase the effectiveness of a workload management system. Examples of caregiver competency indicators are listed in **Exhibit 6–9**.

Exhibit 6–9 Caregiver Competency Indicators

1. **Years of experience**
   a. In the organization
   b. In the profession
   c. In the specialty
   d. In related disciplines (LPN/VN, certified nurse assistant)

2. **Certifications**
   a. ACLS/ BLS/PALS
   b. Specialty—Critical Care (CCRN), Rehabilitation (CRRN), Monitor Tech, Wound/Ostomy (Wound, Ostomy, and Continence Nursing (WOCN) and Enterostomal Therapy (ET) Nurse)

3. **Continuing education**
   a. Skills lab
   b. Course work (dialysis, chemotherapy)
   c. Inservices (internal)
   d. Workshops (external)

4. **Other**
   a. Critical thinking skills
   b. Ability to delegate effectively
   c. Manual dexterity
   d. Attitude
   e. Relationship building skills
   f. Organizational skills

To determine how to define *competency* within an organization, the ANA suggests, "The specific needs of various patient populations should determine the appropriate clinical competencies required of the nurse practicing in that area.… All institutions should have documented competencies for nursing staff, including agency or supplemental and traveling RNs, for those activities that they have been authorized to perform" (2003a, p. 5).

Other sources for establishing clinical competency are the nurses who have a great deal of experience caring for a patient population, professional nursing organizations, the literature (LaDuke, 2000; McConnell, 2001; Taylor, 2000), benchmarking, and regulatory agencies. Meretoja and Leino-Kilpi (2001) reviewed the available competency instruments and found that most measured "nurses' self-perception of competence.… It is important to have more comparative studies of nurse competence from managerial, patients,' and other health e-team members' points of view" (p. 351). Within each organization, nurse administrators need to determine how to measure staff competency, to document that this competency has been met, and to make appropriate educational opportunities available for staff.

Additional references for staffing adequacy, skill mix/outcome research follows:

- ANA Safe Staffing Saves Lives (retrieved July 18, 2008 from www.safestaffingsaveslives.org) summarized legislated staffing plans, staffing ratios, and requirements for public reporting as well as other activities related to proposed legislation.
- Kane, Shamliyan, Mueller, Duvan, and Wilt (2007) summarized research studies specific to RN staffing levels and patient outcomes.

- Blegen and Goode (1997) found that when there were more RNs proportionately, medication errors decreased as did respiratory and urinary tract infections, skin breakdowns, and patient complaints. A year later, two other studies (Blegen et al., 1998; Blegen & Vaughn, 1998) found that there "were the fewest number of patient and family complaints, patient falls, medication administration errors, and observable decubiti" when the RN to non-RN ratio was 85% to 87% (Shullanberger, 2000, p. 147). Blegen, Vaughn, and Goode (2001) further reported that "controlling for patient acuity, hours of nursing care, and staff mix, units with more experienced nurses had lower medication errors and lower patient fall rates" (p. 33).
- Needleman and colleagues (2001) sampled 799 hospitals from 11 states and found consistent relationships between nurse staffing levels and "patient outcomes, urinary track infections, pneumonia, length of stay, upper gastrointestinal bleeding, and shock in medical patients" and death in major surgery patients (p. ii). A weaker relationship was found for urinary track infections and pneumonia in surgery patients.
- Similarly, "Sochalski, Aiken, and Fagin (1997) found that 'magnet hospitals,' those known for first-rate nursing care, had significantly lower mortality rates than matched (similar size and type) hospitals. They had slightly higher RN-to-patient ratios and a considerably richer skill mix than equivalent hospitals. They also enjoyed higher rates of patient satisfaction, lower nurse burnout, and a safer work environment" (Shullanberger, 2000, p. 132).
- Another variable that has an influence on patient outcomes is the organizational context in which nurses practice. Aiken and Patrician (2000) developed and established reliability and validity for a revised nursing work index instrument to measure the organizational context. Subscales within this instrument measure autonomy, control over the practice setting, the nurse–physician relationship, and organizational support. Other research using these variables found that magnet hospitals—known for good nursing care—have a lower patient mortality rate of 9 fewer deaths per 1,000 Medicare discharges (Aiken, Smith, & Lake, 1994).
- Brewer and Frazier (1998) conducted a multivariate analysis of RN staffing in western New York and found that the type of unit, nursing model, rural location, and use of aides and unit secretaries affected RN staffing. Intensive care, pediatric, and maternity units had higher levels of RN staffing than medical/surgical/gynecological units. Rural hospitals used more RNs than other hospital settings. Adding nurse aides increased the RN ratio, whereas use of LPNs did not significantly change the RN ratio. A unit secretary decreased the RN ratio.
- Mark, Salyer, and Wan (2000) examined the skill mix in 67 hospitals in 11 southeastern states. They found that "high-tech services and a larger percentage of admissions in which managed care organizations were the primary payer were associated with a higher proportion of RNs on the unit. Lower RN skill mix was associated with more regular stay admissions. One nursing unit characteristic, complexity of patients' needs for nursing care, was predictive of nursing unit skill mix, with increasing complexity associated with a higher proportion of RNs" (pp. 557–558).
- In the long-term care setting, Bliesmer and coworkers (1998) found that greater use of licensed nurses in the first year of admission resulted in improved functional ability, increased probability of discharge home, and decreased probability of death. There was no difference found with chronic patients who had been in long-term care over a year.
- Hendrix and Foreman (2001) found that nurse aides have substantially more impact than RNs on minimizing long-term care decubitus costs, but both were significant. This study shows that the average nursing home operator would need to spend approximately $380 per resident for RNs and $569.98 to $1,820.32 per resident for nurse aides to achieve this staffing ratio. Increased LPNs did not achieve fewer decubiti, so this study advocated reducing or eliminating

LPNs. When staffing was not at the minimum suggested by this study, the researchers found that the nursing homes spent $84,085,167 within the industry on decubiti—*a cost that could have been eliminated with adequate staffing.*

- After 8 years of research on nursing home patient care levels, federal health officials (Pear, 2000) found that 54% of all nursing homes fall below minimum nurse staffing standards and further said that patients were endangered with low staffing levels. They found that staffing levels were much higher in nonprofit nursing homes compared with for-profit nursing homes. In their study results, federal officials advocated that minimum staffing standards for all care facilities should be 2 hours per day per patient of nurse aide time and 12 minutes per day per patient of RN time. Outcome measures in this study included decubiti, malnutrition, weight loss, dehydration, need for hospital admissions, and possible death. When there were low staffing ratios, the staff turnover rate increased.
- Aiken and colleagues (2003) found that patients had a greater chance of survival when more highly educated nurses were providing the direct patient care.
- Aiken et al. (2002) linked survey data from 10,184 staff nurses with 232,342 general, orthopedic, and vascular surgery patients from 168 Pennsylvania hospitals and found that 50% of the hospitals had patient-to-nurse ratios that were 5:1 or lower. "Each additional patient per nurse was associated with a 7% … increase in the likelihood of dying within 30 days of admission and a 7% … increase in the odds of failure-to-rescue (deaths within 30 days of admission among patients who experienced complications—examples included aspiration pneumonia and hypotension/shock). After adjusting for nurse and hospital characteristics, each additional patient per nurse was associated with a 23% … increase in the odds of burnout and a 15% … increase in the odds of job satisfaction" (p. 1987).
- Correspond this with a telephone survey of 601 RNs reported by Peter D. Hart Research Associates, Inc. in 2003: "Three in five hospital nurses (59 percent) say that the staffing level at their hospital is having a negative impact on the quality of care patients receive. More than half (54 percent) say that when it comes to the quality of care, understaffing at their hospitals is a very or fairly serious problem, and Med-Surg nurses with higher patient-to-nurse ratios (more than 6:1) are especially likely to agree. When it comes to nurse burnout, fully three in five (62%) nurses have considered leaving the patient-care field during the past two years, and Med-Surg nurses with higher patient-to-nurse ratios are more likely than average to have considered leaving the patient-care field…. Med-Surg nurses report that on average they are caring for 8.0 patients per shift, with 50 percent caring for more than six patients and 82 percent caring for more than four. [When asked] how many patients they should be caring for, [they indicated] an average of 5.2 patients" (pp. 1–2).

These data would generally indicate that part of the problem causing the nursing shortage is that hospitals are not adequately staffing units, so nurses decide to leave and work in other settings. Note that the March 2004 issue of *Research in Action* from the Agency for Healthcare Research and Quality reviews the literature on hospital staffing and quality of care (www.ahrq.gov).

FULL-TIME AND PART-TIME STAFF

To schedule most effectively, it is generally best to have both full-time and part-time staff. If there are too many full-time staff, there are not enough staff available to cover weekends, vacations, and sick time. If there are too many part-time staff, continuity of care suffers. For an inpatient unit it is preferable to have *approximately 60% to 70% full-time and 30% to 40% part-time* staff to allow for some flexibility yet still have continuity (for more details see Chapter 13). Part-time staff can be helpful and, in addition to working a regular schedule, may be willing to work extra shifts as long as it fits with their other life circumstances.

ADMISSION, DISCHARGE, AND TRANSFER PATIENT ACTIVITY

As a rule of thumb, areas where there are a lot of admissions, discharges, and transfers generally need a higher RN ratio to do the necessary assessment. Rural hospital staffing also has a greater number of RNs because patient needs vary widely. One fallacy that can occur is that RNs are more expensive than unlicensed nursing staff. On the surface one might believe RNs are expensive because their salaries are higher than LPNs and aides. Research is beginning to refute this notion (McClung, 2000). Melberg (1997) showed that a hospital budget with a 96% RN staff mix is less expensive than another hospital budget with a 64% RN mix. In fact, the hospital with the highest costs had the lowest RN skill mix (64%):

> A high RN mix [96 percent] does not correlate with higher nursing costs per patient day in acute or critical care. Diluting the RN mix does not always reduce staffing costs. Although hospital A has a 96 percent RN-skill mix, the highest in the system, total nursing salary per patient day falls exactly in the middle. The highest costs occurred at hospital C where, in fact, the 64 percent RN mix is the lowest in the system. This finding is consistent in acute care, in critical care and on the orthopedic units, specialty nursing areas found in all five hospitals and therefore used for comparison. This difference is not explained by regional variations in RN salary, since RN salary at hospital A during the period of study was higher than at any hospital in the system except hospital E (p. 48).

The turnover of patients on one shift has increased dramatically. Patient acuity also continues to increase, whereas length of stay has decreased. "Norrish found that nurses reported patient turnover rates of 40 percent to 50 percent in a single shift. Lawrenz found similar unpredictability with the number of admissions, discharges, and transfers averaging from 25 percent to 70 percent of midnight census" (Mark, 2002, p. 240). Thus staffing might be adequate at the beginning of the shift, but insufficient later in the workday, causing poorer, more expensive patient outcomes or patient safety issues.

Although the transfer activity factor is generated from patient activity, these data are a component of the scheduling plan. Failure to understand and manage unit activity or unit turbulence results in chaos and frustration of even the most organized and experienced nursing staff. Specific trend data include the results of historical data from admission, discharge, and transfer activity by day of the week and time of the day. A factor for each admission is incorporated into the core schedule to minimize unit chaos and to adequately provide needed patient care services.

It is interesting to note that some health care leaders still believe that the transfer activity is a nonissue. They believe that because staffing has been allocated for the patient being discharged, time for the admitted patient is available from the unused time of the discharged patient; it is essentially a wash as admissions replace discharged patients. The reality is that the *admission process is significantly more intense than the discharge process and requires an additional 45 minutes of RN time and 15 minutes of unlicensed time* (Cavouras & McKinley, 1998). As the environment becomes less stable with frequent admissions and discharges, the patient classification system becomes less accurate at predicting workload. The notion of taking data from a population (annual data) and applying it to a single point in time (shift) means that you will be correct (or nearly so) on average (Seago & Ash, 2002). Given the current health care turnaround time and inpatient length of stay at 3.5 to 4.0 days, the need to trend and integrate these data into the core schedule is essential.

OVERTIME

Overtime is often used when there are not enough staff present. Standard policies regarding the use of overtime should exist because it can become abused and really burn up staff and budget dollars. However, overtime is useful for occasional use and is less expensive than other options such as hiring an additional person for peak times or paying for agency staff. As the nursing shortage has exacerbated, *mandatory overtime* has become an issue. It is best *not* to resort to this measure—it is a "quick fix" that will backfire because patient safety issues and turnover may result as staff become tired, overworked, and burdened. ANA, and some states, advocate restrictions on mandatory overtime, further specifying that "no staff member in a health care organization should be required or forced to accept work in excess of a predetermined schedule. Any employer who violates the provisions would be subject to sanctions. Nurses do not want to be forced to work overtime when they are tired or when they have other commitments" (ANA, 2001, p. 2).

Another issue with overtime is that the federal government recently passed a law that salaried "white collar" workers are entitled to overtime pay. This new law ("FairPay") was passed to cover workers making $23,660 a year or less. This could apply to LPNs or other health care workers who are salaried, rather than being paid on an hourly basis.

POSITION CONTROL

Organizationally, *position control* is the process used by human resources and specifies actual full-time equivalents (FTEs) assigned to a unit. Generally, there is a position control format, computerized or paper trail, that tracks each person filling every FTE in the organization. **Exhibit 6–10** shows a typical position control document that specifies the total number of FTEs and lists all staff members, their positions, and their correct FTE designation. The authors recommend that the nurse manager be sure that records are updated, noting such things as leaves of absence, vacancies, new employees, changes in FTE designations for positions, and any other issues that would impact the FTEs. If a question arises regarding actual number of FTEs, the nurse manager has the documentation to show the accurate amount. Usually, a nurse manager can decide to split the FTEs differently, but the main issue would be that the total FTEs still remain the same.

JOB ANALYSIS

Job analysis is an assessment of the job responsibilities included in a specific role and includes tasks, knowledge, and skills and competencies required for a particular job. Job analysis is helpful in situations in which work is expanding or decreasing to determine the most appropriate combination of duties in a single role. For example, a person may have *so many* job responsibilities that he or she cannot do the job well. One example of this is a nurse manager responsible for 150 FTEs. In this case, it becomes necessary to create another nurse manager position. In fact, the industry standard is approximately *50 FTEs or less* as the cut-off point for nurse managers. In this case, two additional nurse managers are needed. In fact, the industry standard is below 50 FTEs depending on unit

Exhibit 6–10 Position Control

Position Title	FTE	Hours/Year	Hours/Week	Name
Nurse Manager	1.0	2,080	40	S. Rutherford (8/19/82)
RN	1.0	2,080	40	J. Smith (2/14/95)
RN	0.6	1,248	24	C. Jones (0.3) (4/25/01), K. Wilson (0.3) (10/7/01)
LPN	1.0	2,080	40	T. Blair (11/17/98)
Nurse Aide	1.0	2,080	40	D. Dixon (6/3/04)
Nurse Aide	0.8	1,664	32	R. Thomas (6/18/97)
Unit Secretary	1.0	2,080	40	E. Simmons (7/15/03)

complexity, size, patient acuity, case mix, and scope of responsibilities. One study found that the best average was 36.8 FTEs per nurse manager (Altaffer, 1998, p. 37).

Evaluating the Core Schedule Staffing Plan

Staffing plans need to be evaluated at least annually or when significant patient or staffing issues have occurred. Examination of the numbers of staff and outcomes achieved guide this examination.

This evaluation includes availability of support staff as well as the effectiveness of adjustments to changes in patient census or needs. However, if this is not occurring, the staffing plan needs to change to more accurately schedule staff when needed. For instance, perhaps the patient population has changed and the acuity and/or patient census has increased, which results in a recurrent under-staffing problem. Perhaps there are not enough staff or not enough of the right kind of staff present at the right times to adequately staff the unit.

Professional organizations provide further guidelines for evaluation. The AONE *Perspectives on the Nursing Shortage* (2000) recommends that regular evaluation reflect the value of nursing services. "Patients, providers, payers and policymakers will demand to know that changes in health care delivery in response to the diminishing size of the nursing workforce have not adversely affected patient care" (p. 15). They stress the importance of actual quantitative data and evidence-based policies that can be used to demonstrate the quality of the care given to patients:

> [These data] must provide a solid foundation for decisions on staffing and financing. Voluntary initiatives should incorporate:
>
> - Collecting of nurse-sensitive indicators, especially those seeking to associate patient outcomes with care delivery models and staffing patterns.
> - Collecting data on workforce supply, employment patterns and vacancy rates on an ongoing basis.
> - Evaluating state practice acts to recommend policy changes that facilitate innovation in patient care.
> - Working with regulatory bodies to facilitate communication between patients and health care providers within systems that cross state lines (p. 15).

The ANA, in *Principles for Nurse Staffing* (2008), drawn up by an expert panel of nurses, provides more specifics about evaluation data to be collected:

> Changes in staffing levels, including changes in the overall number and/or mix of nurs-ing staff, should be based on analysis of standardized, nursing-sensitive indicators. The effect of these changes should be evaluated using the same criteria. Caution must be exercised in the interpretation of data related to staffing levels and patterns and patient outcomes in the absence of consistent and meaningful definitions of the variables for which data are being gathered. [Thus the following data should be used to determine staffing levels.]
>
> - Number of patients,
> - Level of intensity of the patients for whom care is being provided,
> - Contextual issues including architecture and geography of the environment and avail-able technology, and
> - Level of preparation and experience of those providing care (2008, pp. 5–6).

Measuring staff satisfaction provides additional data about existing issues that need to be addressed that can affect the core schedule. If staff satisfaction ratings are low, further discussion is needed with the staff group to both identify problems and potential solutions. Sometimes the actual staffing numbers may not be the issue (i.e., staff do not help each other). Or the problem may be at a higher level where there is ineffective leadership or where there are organizational process issues that need to be resolved.

After evaluating and determining the solution(s), it might be necessary to develop a new budget and different staffing requirements using the average NHPPD needed for adequate staffing. (Chapter 12 shows how to create a budget from acuity data.) A change in budget, staff mix, or better use of staff resources might result.

Staffing Legislation

There has been increasing reliance on legislation to ensure adequate staffing. Regulatory issues vary depending on the regulatory body, as discussed in Chapters 4 and 8. Regulatory issues related to national accreditation and licensure emphasize the importance of (1) adequate staff credentialing to do the assigned work, (2) policies and procedures describing how nursing assignments are completed on a shift-by-shift basis, and (3) adequacy of nurse staffing. As a required part of the regulatory process, the nurse administrator needs to demonstrate each of the above with a comprehensive workload management system that includes accurate records of actual staffing.

The Patient Safety Act of 1999 (H.R. 1288/S. 966) requires Medicare providers (health care organizations) to make public information on the following:

- Number of RNs providing direct care
- Numbers of UAP
- Average number of patients per RN
- Patient mortality
- Incidence of adverse patient care incidents
- Methods used for determining staffing levels and patient care needs (American Organization of Nurse Executives, 2000)

Several states have mandated all or parts of this Act to be required for all health care organizations, even if they are not certified for Medicare.

At the state level, some states have legislated staffing numbers and policies. California has implemented minimum nurse-to-patient ratios for each unit of every hospital. The impact of this legislation is emerging (Upeniks, Akhavan, Kotlerman, Esser, & Ngo, 2007).

There is a growing trend toward legislating nurse staffing to address patient safety issues. Legislators have responded by both studying the issues and enacting laws to prevent harm to patients and support safe staffing. The first legislation related to safe staffing, developed in California in 1995, is the most comprehensive approach, calling for institutions to develop valid staffing systems. The California Assembly Bill 394 was enacted in 1999. This legislation requires specific standards for UAP, patient classification systems, and minimum nurse staffing ratios. UAP cannot be assigned to perform nursing functions in lieu of RNs in acute care facilities (see www.applications.dhs.ca.gov/regulations).

According to Curtin (2003), there is some merit to legislatively mandated nurse-to-patient staffing ratios. More and more research indicates that nurse staffing has a definite and measurable impact on patient outcomes, medical errors, length of stay, nurse turnover, and patient mortality

(Aiken et al., 2003; Cho et al., 2003; McCue, 2003; Needleman et al., 2002; Seago, 2001). Yet, the evidence for what the specific numerical ratio should be continues to vary widely.

However, modification of the ratios is needed based on the nurses' level of experience, the organization's characteristics, leadership issues, and the quality of clinical interactions between and among physicians, nurses, and administrators (Curtin, 2003). Many believe that legislating staffing ratios is good for nursing (Mason, 2003). Leaders of the ANA have noted that if hospitals could be trusted to staff properly, they would have done so.

Proponents for staffing ratios do not believe that minimum legislated ratios will become the maximum but rather that the best hospitals will exceed those standards and the worst will be forced to stop assigning eight or more patients to the medical-surgical nurse. Further, failing to set minimum standards will not be impossible due to the shortage; rather, *poor staffing is a cause of the shortage* and will continue until staffing is fixed.

Opponents to staffing ratios have been equally strident about the ineffectiveness of this approach. Their belief is that nurse-to-patient ratios are counterproductive to evidence-based decision making and inappropriate as a staffing methodology for the complex phenomenon of patient care. Ratios assume that care is constant within each level of care, regardless of length of stay, skill mix, care delivery model, cost, competence, and unit geography. This assumption is clearly counterintuitive and contrary to what nurses tell us about patients—that they can all be very different, require very different interventions, and have a variety of holistic needs while residing within the same unit. When nursing units adopt standards that are not appropriate, a continuous cycle of unfulfilled expectations can result (DeGroot, 1994). Further, some leaders may actually lower current effective RN staffing to the required minimum. Using the legislated minimum ratios is particularly ineffective in rural settings and trauma settings with wide ranges of patient care needs. The potential for failure to rescue patients in possible danger increases dramatically in these situations and results in unplanned negative patient consequences—consequences for which the nurse is often blamed but which are really unavoidable because of the minimum staffing.

Even the proponents of staffing ratio mandates recognize that ratios do not resolve all the issues; hence the requirement to institute a patient classification system along with the minimum ratios. *If hospitals had ensured the use of a valid and reliable patient classification system and relied on that system as a tool for determining nursing workload management, the lack of trust that historically has misaligned the credibility of staff, managers, and administration would not exist.* Staffing would thus be based on patient needs rather than the need to comply with mandated ratios that are arbitrary and without empirical support. Despite the best of intentions in which legislated nurse-to-patient ratios were created, the complexity of staffing is yet to be addressed adequately. Competence, experience, and education all affect productivity and patient outcomes. These variables have not been addressed in legislated staffing ratios. The debate continues regarding the staffing ratio laws enacted. **Exhibit 6–11** gives a synopsis of the advantages and disadvantages of staffing ratios.

The Joint Commission provides recommendations to organizations through standards. Current efforts to ensure that staffing effectiveness is achieved using an evidence-based approach reinforces the need to enhance current practices. The Joint Commission standards require organizations to assess the number, competency, and skill mix of their staff by linking staffing effectiveness to clinical outcomes. This approach relies on the use of multiple clinical and human resource indicators rather than a single data element. Organizations collect and analyze data on multiple screening indicators, which are believed sensitive to staffing effectiveness such as overtime, vacancy rates, and adverse drug events. The Joint Commission standards do not rely on arbitrary ratios but rather emphasize the need for an ongoing informed review of staffing based on credible screening indicators (The Joint Commission, 2002).

Exhibit 6–11 Staffing Ratios: Advantages and Disadvantages

Advantages	Disadvantages
Consider historical average patient acuity	Do not consider the range of patient care acuity and fluctuations in daily care
Incentives for nurses to return to the bedside	Assume nurses are available.
Simple to regulate specific numbers	Minimum ratios could become maximum ratios; facilities can manipulate ratios by moving patients to units that have higher ratios when staff are not available
Alleviate nurse stress (short term)	Do not reflect the differing skills of nurses
Decrease the need to justify nurse staffing	Will force closure of hospital beds in the annual budgeting process
Increase nurse satisfaction	Devalue the role of nurse critical thinking and judgment
Improves patient safety/outcomes	Assume a manufacturing model is appropriate for patient care
Marginally supported by evidence	Remove staffing accountability from the organization to the government
Nurses traditionally support equal numbers of patients assigned to each nurse, not taking activity into account	Patient care is widely varied in required hours and caregiver skill level

Consideration: Collective Bargaining Units

Another strategy to address safe staffing has been the use of collective bargaining. Ongoing changes in health care have subjected nurses to the effects of cost cutting, shuffled duties, reorganization, and the chronic nursing shortage. This has prompted nurses to turn to the collective bargaining process to ensure safe staffing conditions for nurses and to correct inconsistent staffing. Unions have taken on the challenge to mandate organizations to provide not only adequate staffing but also to provide valid and reliable patient classification systems within their contracts. Another reason nurses organize is to protect the patients under their care.

As long as nurses continue to feel disenfranchised, unprotected, and under siege by doctors and health care administrators, interest in unions will grow stronger. The protection of collective bargaining and the belief that greater benefits are extracted with an intermediary provide a powerful force for health care workers. Increasing numbers of nurses believe that their voice in decision making is best heard through a legally binding contract between the employer and a bargaining unit. The contract prevents arbitrary decisions by the employer and enforces the right to participate in determining wages, hours of work, standards of practice, pension and benefits, and all other terms of employment.

Given the complex nature of health care staffing and the strident nature of collective bargaining units, *new and visionary partnerships between health care organizations and collective bargaining units are desperately needed*. The mutuality of goals for safe staffing positions incite both groups to rise to the challenge to address this pressing need and make recommendations to modify the health care system processes and beliefs to achieve the desired goal in a way that is beneficial to both nurses and patients.

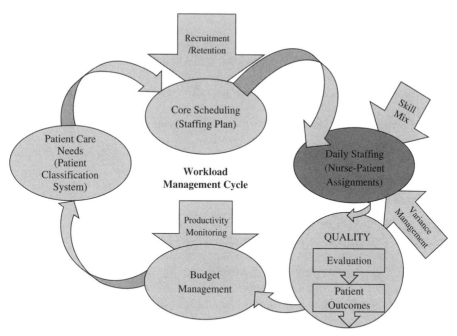

Figure 6–6 Daily Staffing

Daily Staffing Guidelines

Daily staffing (Figure 6–6) is the real-time adjustment of the schedule based on current census, acuity, and the mix of available resources (Gardner & Gemme, 2003). When patient census fluctuates, a common practice is to give staff excused absences without pay for that shift or to have staff float to another unit. Policies or guidelines that identify who floats under what conditions and how staff are cross-trained are important considerations.

The increasing availability of computerized applications for data collection and analysis greatly assists nurse leaders and managers in evaluating staffing adequacy. Data from multiple sources can be quickly integrated and analyzed to optimize decision making (Hyun, Bakkan, Douglas & Stone, 2008). It is important to maintain records showing that nursing staff are working within the scope of practice determined by the state licensing board, meet current health requirements such as appropriate immunizations, and that staff are safe, competent practitioners. The state licensing board sets minimum standards for nurse competency.

Staffing Office Center

The coordination and documentation of scheduling and staffing typically occurs in a central location. In a centralized model, there may be a daily staffing meeting attended by the chief nursing officer, directors of nurses, nurse managers, the shift supervisors, and other administrative personnel such as the nursing office staffing person and the chief executive, operating, and financial officers. These meetings are used to identify unusual situations, to work out solutions, to find out bed availability, to share staffing concerns, and to share what positions are open or filled, along with other administrative issues.

Staffing and Scheduling Policies

As a nurse manager decides what staffing and scheduling options to use, it is helpful to have some policies. Often, these are established organizational policies for such things as use of vacation time, how many staff can be on vacation at one time, how to make requests for time off, when and how to use overtime, and self-scheduling guidelines. It is important that policies enhance staffing and scheduling, because guidelines are helpful. However, too many policies can often impede creativity and discourage someone from working for us. Instead, *if we give staff more freedom to determine work time (this includes shift times) and time off, staff are more satisfied, retention greatly improves, and turnover lessens.*

Nurse-to-Patient Assignments

The assignment of patients to specific caregivers is currently the responsibility of the nurse manager or staff nurse because there are multiple variables to be considered. This process includes giving consideration to (1) the competency of caregivers; (2) yesterday's assignment (continuity of care); (3) preference of the caregiver; (4) previous shift staffing (RN follows LPN/VN); (5) pending admissions, discharges, and transfers; and (6) geography of the unit, or proximity of patients to the central station (or having all the resources needed at the bedside). The ultimate goal is to match patients with a nurse who has the experience, qualifications, competencies, and interest required to provide the care that is needed and will support the best possible outcomes.

Assignment planning should also include time allotment for those indirect and administrative unit activities that support the operations of the unit, such as shift report, narcotic counts, and crash cart checks. Time devoted to the routine tasks needed to keep the department operating can be as much as 30% of the human resource time, whether there is related patient volume or not (Brady, 2001). In the NIC taxonomy, indirect care interventions are described as treatments that direct care providers perform away from the patient but on behalf of a patient or group of patients. Administrative interventions, in comparison, are actions performed by a nurse administrator, nurse manager, or middle manager to enhance the performance of staff members to promote better patient outcomes (McCloskey & Bulechek, 2000). *Failure to include time in the core schedule of the workload management system for indirect and administrative interventions can result in feelings of inadequate staffing due to an undocumented but very real variance.*

In many organizations, a staffing or ratio grid is used for daily staffing. It is important to remember that staffing solely on ratios is incomplete. Ratios do not consider or recognize caregiver delegation ability, critical-thinking skills, experience, motivation, organizational skills, technical skills, or attitude. Even if the total number of care hours might be sufficient with a certain ratio, differentiation among the type of caregivers required to meet the patient needs is not identified. The fallacy of mandating licensed nurse-to-patient ratios rather than RN-to-patient ratios assumes that all licensed nurses are equal—specifically, the RN is the same as the LPN. As the literature continues to recognize the improved outcomes with the use of RNs, staffing ratios may be of lesser value than intended. Assuming all patients are alike and all nurses are alike is an inappropriate and faulty assumption.

Nurse retention is positively impacted when staff believe their assignments are doable and equitable. Experiencing a sense of accomplishment at the end of a shift and believing that appropriate care was given enhance staff satisfaction and ultimately retention. *Recruitment* becomes the result of satisfied employees who share these perceptions with other potential employees. The environment is noted for its sensitivity to quality patient care and safe staffing.

Variance Management

This essential step is often overlooked or minimized in importance. When this analysis is not done, the entire work of patient classification is, in fact, negated or at best ignored. The reality of the routine mismatch between patient care needs and available staff is an issue for the organization as a collective rather than the individual caregiver. Expecting the caregiver to do one's best in an impossible situation continues to fuel the flames of caregiver dissatisfaction, and he or she will ultimately exit from the workforce.

Variance data for each day should be examined to determine significance and appropriate interventions. Typically, a *variance* is significant when the difference between required staff and available staff is greater than one-half of the length of a shift: 4 hours for an 8-hour shift and 6 hours for a 12-hour shift. A variance is also significant if the classified hours and available staff are adequate but the skill mix available is not consistent with the classified skill mix. Existing staff can usually manage variances below one-half of a shift. When the variance exceeds one-half of a shift, the team should identify actions to manage the variance, then document and address them. Examples of variance actions include postponing or rerouting admissions, calling in additional staff, floating existing staff, reevaluating the patient acuity ratings, postponing nonemergent care, and overtime. **Exhibit 6–12** is an example of a variance management form.

Trend data for variances identify patterns and frequency of occurrences for each patient care area and define acceptable levels of variance from suggested staffing. These data are important in knowing where and when staffing problems occur and thus allowing managers to focus on fixing only problem areas rather than developing whole system changes. *Analysis of aggregate variance data should be done at least quarterly and more often if significant variances are occurring.* Variances specific to day of week (e.g., Mondays and Fridays may require additional labor hours due to increased admission, discharge, and transfers, or Tuesdays and Thursdays may be higher procedure days), by season (e.g., winter vs. summer), by skill mix (e.g., additional unlicensed hours needed rather than licensed hours), and by shift (e.g., additional nurse aides needed on day shift vs. night shift) become readily apparent in this analysis.

Managing the daily variances between patient care needs and available staff is but one strategy to address the shortage of nursing and will not rectify all challenges of staffing **(Figure 6–7)**.

Exhibit 6–12   Calculating the Variance: Comparison of Patient Classification and Actual Staff Hours

	Patient Classification Hours	**Actual Staffing Hours**	**Variance**
RN Hours	28.0	36.0	+8.0
LPN/VN Hours	30.0	24.0	−6.0
NA Hours	35.0	24.0	−11.0
Total	93.0	84.0	−9.0

Variance Management Actions:

_____ Control of work flow by re-routing admissions	_____ Reassess patient classifications for possible overestimation of staff needs
_____ Call in additional help	_____ Re-define the workload and eliminate or postpone nonessential tasks
_____ Staff overtime	_____ Other
_____ Utilize Resource Nurse	

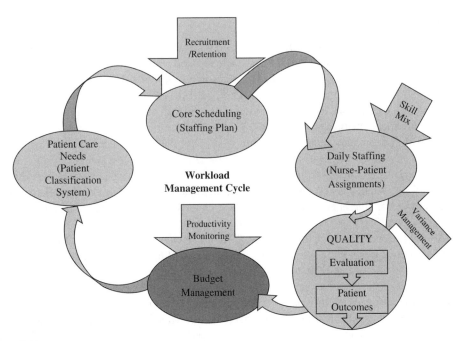

Figure 6–7 Budget Management

Indeed, other essential long-term strategies are needed, including building better communication systems between leaders and staff, new staffing patterns, flexible scheduling, flexible benefits, technology, new partnerships with nursing schools, and involvement in policy issues that impact patient safety and nurse staffing. These strategies are essential to address this long-standing challenge.

In **Exhibit 6–13**, seven steps are presented to describe both the flow of data and the analysis of data as patient care needs change:

- Step 1 provides summative data from a valid and reliable patient classification system and shows the associated labor costs for direct care for RNs, LPNs, and nursing assistants. Indirect costs are factored in once direct care needs have been determined. The range of patient care needs is noteworthy because these ranges serve to guide the core scheduling process for allocation of resources on a daily basis.
- Step 2 displays data using the projected volume and associated patient care need categories. Total salary dollars, average cost of care per patient day, total projected hours, total projected FTEs, and the average HPPD are identified in this step.
- In Step 3, changing patient care needs are identified and the budget is modified to reflect the changes.
- Step 4 includes recalculated salary dollars, average cost of care per patient day, total projected hours, total projected FTEs, and the average HPPD.
- Steps 5 to 7 present analyses of the changes in costs of care, FTEs, skill mix, and average HPPD.

Before finalizing changes based on these data, the impact on patient care outcomes must be examined to ensure optimal patient safety and desired clinical outcomes.

Exhibit 6–13 Putting It All Together: Translating Patient Classification System Data to the Annual Budget

Step 1. Patient Classification System Summary Data: Unit A 2003

	Hours			Total Hours	Cost / Job Role			Total Cost
	RN	LPN	NA		RN ($25.00/hr)	LPN ($15.00)	NA ($8.00)	
Patient Type A	1.00	0.50	1.00	2.50	$25.00	$7.50	$8.00	$40.50
Patient Type B	1.50	1.00	1.50	4.00	$37.50	$15.00	$12.00	$64.50
Patient Type C	2.00	2.00	1.50	5.50	$50.00	$30.00	$12.00	$92.00
Patient Type D	4.00	2.50	1.50	8.00	$100.00	$37.50	$12.00	$149.50
Patient Type E	6.00	3.00	2.00	11.00	$150.00	$45.00	$16.00	$211.00
Range of Hours / Job Role	1.0 - 6.0	0.5 - 3.0	1.0 - 2.0	2.5 - 11.0				

Notes

Individual patient care staffing needs form the foundation for the unit budget. The patient types A–E are used to reflect common patient care needs for calculation purposes only and do not reflect the myriad patient care needs profiles that exist on patient care units. Knowing the skill mix for each patient, the range of needs as defined by hours and skill mix are essential elements for a realistic budget. In this example, hours of care range from 2.5 to 11.0 hours per patient. The average cost per patient ranges from $40.50 to $211.00 per patient.

Step 2. Calculating the 2004 Budget: Unit A: Dollars and FTE's

	Unit Volume	Cost/Patient	Total Cost / Patient Type	Total Hours	Hours	FTE's
Patient Type A	3,300	40.50	$133,650.00	8,250	2.50	3.97
Patient Type B	3,500	64.50	$225,750.00	14,000	4.00	6.73
Patient Type C	1,500	92.00	$138,000.00	8,250	5.50	3.97
Patient Type D	1,200	149.50	$179,400.00	9,600	8.00	4.62
Patient Type E	500	211.00	$105,500.00	5,500	11.00	2.64
Projected Patient Days	10,000					
Total Projected Labor Cost			$782,300.00			
Average Cost / Patient Day					$78.23	
Total Projected Hours				45,600		
Total Projected FTEs						21.92

Average HPPD   4.56

Notes

The budget for 2004 is created based on actual patient care needs and skill mix experienced in the prior year. Calculations for total hours and dollars estimates for the 2004 budget year are based on the estimated volume of patient days (10,000) and percentages of patient care types expected by categories A through E. The range of hours (2.5 to 11.0 hours) used by skill category provides information from which to create the daily staffing plan. The total budget for RN/LPN/NA salaries for direct patient care for this unit are $782,300. The average cost of care for each patient day is $78.23. Total annual hours of care are 45,600 hours. Total FTE's are 21.92. Average HPPD are 4.56 hours. Indirect hours (e.g. unit support, employee education) are added to the core patient care needs labor budget. Typically, indirect hours range from 8–15% of the total dollars budgeted.

Step 3. Patient Classification System Summary Data (Actual): Unit A 2004

	Hours			Total Hours	Cost / Job Role			Total Cost
	RN	LPN	NA		RN ($25.00/hr)	LPN ($15.00)	NA ($8.00)	
Patient Type A	1.50	0.50	1.00	3.00	$37.50	$7.50	$8.00	$53.00
Patient Type B	2.00	1.00	2.00	5.00	$50.00	$15.00	$16.00	$81.00
Patient Type C	2.50	1.00	1.50	5.00	$62.50	$15.00	$12.00	$89.50
Patient Type D	4.50	2.00	2.00	8.50	$112.50	$30.00	$16.00	$158.50
Patient Type E	7.00	3.50	2.50	13.00	$175.00	$52.50	$20.00	$247.50
Range of Hours / Job Role	1.5 - 7.0	0.5 - 3.5	1.0 - 2.5	3.0 - 13.0				
Range of Cost / Job Role					$37.50 - $175.00	$7.50 - $52.50	$8.00 - $20.00	

Notes

The actual hours and skill mix used during the current year 2004 are then compared to the 2004 budgeted hours and skill mix.

From 2003 to 2004 the range of hours of care increased from 2.50 to 11.0 to a range of 3.0 to 13.00.

The range of direct salary cost per patient day increased from $40.50-$211.00 (as shown in Step 1) to $53.00-$247.50.

continued

Exhibit 6–13 Putting It All Together: Translating Patient Classification System Data to the Annual Budget (continued)

Step 4. Revising the Budget for 2005: Unit A: Dollars and FTE's

	Unit Volume	Cost/Patient	Total Cost / Patient Type	Hours	Total Hours	FTE's
Patient Type A	3,300	37.50	$123,750.00	3.00	9,900	4.76
Patient Type B	3,500	81.00	$283,500.00	5.00	17,500	8.41
Patient Type C	1,500	104.50	$156,750.00	5.00	7,500	3.61
Patient Type D	1,200	173.50	$208,200.00	8.50	10,200	4.90
Patient Type E	500	247.50	$123,750.00	13.00	6,500	3.13
Projected Patient Days	10,000					
Total Projected Labor Cost			$895,950.00			
Average Cost / Patient Day				$89.60		
Total Projected Hours					51,600	
Total Projected FTEs						24.81
Average HPPD						5.16

Notes
The 2005 hours, skill mix and dollars budget is revised to reflect the increase in patient care needs and skill mix changes.
The number of patient days remains the same at 10,000.
The budget increased 17% from $768,300.00 to $895,950.
The average cost per patient day increased 17% from $76.83 to $89.60.
The projected hours increased 26% from 45,600 to 51,600 hours.
The total FTE's increased 24% from 21.92 to 24.81.
The average HPPD increased 13% from 4.56 to 5.16.

Step 5: Analysis of Annual Hours, Dollars and Skill Mix Changes

	2003	2004	Percentage Change
Labor Cost	$768,300	$895,950	17%
Average Cost / Patient Day	$76.83	$89.60	17%
Total Projected Hours	45,600	51,600	13%
Total Projected FTEs	21.92	24.81	13%
Average HPPD	4.56	5.16	13%
RN hours	19,350	24,600	27%
LPN hours	12,650	10,800	-15%
NA hours	13,600	16,200	19%

Notes
From this analysis, it is concluded that both the cost and hours increased during 2004 but at differing rates. Labor cost increased 17% while total hours increased 13%. The RN % increased 27%, the LPN % decreased 15% and the NA % increased 19%.

Budget Planning

Once the patient needs and staffing plan are created, the budget can be developed. The data collected from the workload management system provide the baseline for preparing the labor component of the nursing budget. The primary responsibility for this process belongs to the nurse executive, but nursing supervisors and unit managers are accountable for direct and worked productive hours. Resource allocation decisions begin with the assumption that the budget will be met and not exceeded.

Budgeting for staffing needs requires historical patient classification trend data, core scheduling staffing plans, and information from staffing variance analysis specific to the following:

- Census for each unit including average and ranges for each shift
- Admissions, discharges, and transfer activity for each shift
- Actual direct hours and indirect hours per patient day
- RN hours as a percent of the total hours worked
- Education hours, orientation, and training hours by unit
- Overtime hours both scheduled and incidental
- Anticipated sick time
- New staff orientation hours

The initial patient care hours estimate is adjusted for any changes in assumptions for the upcoming budget year, such as increases in expected patient volumes, new patient care programs, or equipment purchases that would impact staffing requirements, as well as decisions made based on the above analysis. It is evident that this phase cannot be achieved as planned without success at the previous levels. Failure to respect the order of the process often results in inaccurate forecasting and financial overruns.

Productivity Monitoring

An important component in the workload management system is the evaluation of productivity of the workforce. In this section, the use of comparison data to assess the effective use of resources is presented. The American Productivity and Quality Center defines *productivity* as "a process of getting more out of what you put in. It's doing better with what you have" (Health Care Education Associates, 1987). From the health care perspective, we want "to achieve positive health outcomes at the lowest possible cost" (Chang, Price, & Pfoutz, 2001, p. 433). Using these definitions is helpful in examining both the quality and quantity of the outcome, as well as the resources and processes necessary to achieve that outcome. Enhancing productivity involves achieving more *efficiencies*—time or resources saved to deliver a service—and must be linked with *effectiveness*—the degree to which the final result achieves the desired outcome. Productivity is one of those elusive things that is hard to measure and where, no matter how well we accomplish it, there is still room for improvement.

Productivity is calculated from several perspectives: nationally, organizationally, and individually. *Nationally*, when there is high productivity, higher standards of living result. When productivity increases and costs remain the same, the country benefits. However, often when productivity increases, costs can increase. Then, purchasing power can decrease and inflation can occur. When productivity decreases, labor costs often go up, and a less competitive position results.

Organizational productivity is necessary to stay competitive. It is an aggregate calculation of both the individual product and the ability of those involved to work effectively as a team. Productivity is a reflection of the dynamic complexity of multiple smaller systems that form the greater system. Historically, our first attempts were to only quantify productivity. Many organizations still do this. Although this measurement provides useful data, it is only a partial measurement. As we have already said, both efficiency and effectiveness are part of productivity, so quality must be added to the measurement. Presently, quality measurements include patient outcomes and patient satisfaction.

Individual productivity reflects a person's performance. This is influenced by the person's ability to do the work, support that is available, and the amount of effort the person is willing to put into accomplishing the work.

Productivity measurement can include such things as staff/RN HPPD, per test, per visit, per treatment or per procedure; FTE-to-bed ratios, sometimes written as FTE per adjusted occupied bed; or cost per unit of service (i.e., the cost per home visit, the cost per DRG, or the number of patients per overall facility budget amount), within a specific time period. When measured at regular intervals over time, these data can provide an idea as to whether the productivity level has improved. If productivity has improved, more outputs (patient days, visits, etc.) were able to be produced using fewer resources (inputs—staff hours or FTEs). If productivity worsened, more resources were used without significantly increasing the outputs.

Measuring and managing productivity in health care presents considerable challenges. First, *our service product is not well defined*. Are we providing disease care, or are we providing health care? More often, we treat disease, and, as we do this, our client experiences more discomfort. Our client may achieve better health as a final outcome, although better health may never be discussed. In fact, the best outcome may be to lessen pain or to achieve a peaceful death. Most often it is the insurer(s), by defining what will be reimbursed, that determines what services will be provided.

Second, it continues to be a challenge to *quantify* our service output. We can measure patient days or visits, but it is more difficult to say that we cured *x* number of people with pneumonia or *x* number of clients with heart disease. If there is a cure, chances are it happens after the patient no longer needs our services.

Third, *did the patient achieve what he or she wanted and valued*? Or was something else provided and measured that the patient did not even want? Patient satisfaction is one component of what is valued. It implies client expectancy. But the actual value piece, what the client actually wanted as an expected outcome, may remain unknown. The other problem with value is that *we presently do not have enough research to know whether present practices actually affect the client outcome*. For example, what specific actions enhance or detract from healing? Why do some patients respond positively to treatment whereas others do not? How can we anticipate whether a particular patient will experience side effects of a medication, whereas another patient will not? Why do some patients who believe they will die actually do, whereas other patients who are expected to die live? So the significant question, "Were desired patient outcome(s) achieved?", is difficult to answer at best.

Fourth, Letvak and Buck (2008) identified how factors influencing work productivity, such as the chemistry or adequacy of relationships between coworkers, affect quality. Administratively, this becomes very complicated because staff, administrators, and physicians differ in the way they respond to situations, to each other, and to patients and their families. In fact, the same person can respond differently when part of a different work group, when the person has a different boss, or with different patients. In fact, organizationally

> Improving only one component of an agency will not affect overall productivity. Productivity improvement involves a systematic assessment of the entire organization rather than just a staffing review. For example, a physical therapist's job tasks may be tied to secretaries who answer the phones and screen calls, to data processing (records may not

be transcribed and given back to the therapist for use during the scheduled visit), and to other disciplines. The therapist may have to wait for the home health aide to arrive to supervise the visit or to meet with an RN regarding the client. One provider group cannot improve or change productivity unless other components of the system are evaluated. *Therefore, do not expect the RN staff to increase productivity unless productivity improvements occur in other components of the system in which RNs work* (Harris, 1997, p. 471).

There are many factors that can enhance or decrease productivity. As previously noted, every chapter in this book not only has financial implications but affects productivity. Poor leadership, poor management, and poor performance all result in productivity ineffectiveness, and vice versa. For example, productivity is affected by such things as staff issues: their level of experience, amount of staff scheduled, not being oriented properly, not having been taught how to do something, or not having enough information about something they are expected to do. Tardiness and absenteeism, sick and vacation time, conference time, overtime, and use of agency staff can all affect productivity. Staff mix could be inappropriate for the work that needs to be done—either overqualified personnel are doing a task or staff are underqualified to do the required work. Sometimes lower productivity has environmental causes, such as not having enough supplies, equipment, or technology to properly do the work; there are problems with the physical layout; or there are long distances for staff to travel in home care.

At times low productivity may be apparent overall, even when productivity seems high. For example, if not enough staff are available to work, staff may be doing as much as possible for patients yet know that more needs to be done. As staff frustration mounts, it is easy to start missing important things that should happen. In this case efficiency looks wonderful but effectiveness suffers. Putting all productivity measurements together, the result is actually low productivity.

Low productivity may occur due to interorganizational issues. For instance, perhaps an insurer has not paid for the care a patient received in a timely manner. Perhaps the physician did not put the diagnosis on the insurance claim, or a coder put the wrong CPT code on the claim, or the patient did not give the correct address as to where the payment should be sent. In such instances, this problem will take more of the patient's time, more of the insurer's time, and more of the provider's time, and even after all this, the outcome—payment—may not occur, even after several people, and organizations, were involved in trying to resolve the issue.

Another question is to ask, what is necessary?

> Look for the best outcomes and the best practices in all areas—clinical and administrative—and seek to replicate those practices throughout the organization.... And stop doing and stop paying for things that do not contribute to quality.... Basically, what the cost of quality boils down to is the cost that is involved that would be eliminated in your organization if there were absolutely no quality problems. Studies of administrative and service industries dealing specifically with healthcare show that 20% to 50% of the activities are nonreal work. What is nonreal work? It does not mean that you and your staff are not busy; you are busier than ever. But the tasks that many are doing do not necessarily contribute to quality care. A few examples:
>
> * System delays such as laboratory tests that come back late and delay discharges, which can increase patient days and staffing;
> * Variations in physician practices, which generate medically unnecessary patient days and test procedures;
> * Drug doses that are discarded because they are mislabeled or put on the wrong cart;

- Skill mix problems—not just in the context of nurse versus unlicensed staff; nurses have taken over a lot of the tasks that a few years ago were done only by physicians; and

- Excess inventory, such as hoarding supplies on the floor because you cannot quite count on your ordering delivery system to get you the product you need when you need it.

All these things cost. Every time you have staff turnover, patient falls, infections, litigation, in short, any time that you are doing any reprocessing or rework activities, that is a cost of quality....

Look for ways to cross departmental boundaries to achieve your strategic goals. When you get your staff working together, they can be a gold mine of information. They know exactly where the rework and reprocessing occurs because they do it everyday, day in and day out (Van Slyck, 1999, p. 53).

Productivity Misconceptions

There are some misconceptions about productivity that can lead to viability issues if they get too far out of hand. As with all concepts, at times, even though we all use the same words, we are actually operating using different definitions. These differences should be identified and clarified early. When allowed to continue over years, the effects of the misconceptions can be considerable. We identify some common misconceptions about productivity here. Porter-O'Grady and Malloch (2007) identify three misconceptions that involve staff productivity (see **Exhibit 6–14**):

> Business still operates under questionable assumptions regarding productivity—that the more hours employees work, the more productive they are; that the faster employees work, the more they accomplish; and that the more employees are paid, the more motivated they are to be productive—leaders are challenged to better understand the reality of employee productivity. Health professionals in this country are working more hours than ever before and getting less done. In fact, Americans have the dubious distinction of being first in the number of hours worked each year. The U.S. Department of Labor, Bureau of Labor Statistics, noted only a slight increase in productivity from 1960 to 1990, and the productivity increase in the last 10 years is attributed to technological advances, particularly the development of the Internet.
>
> Health care employees are burning out faster than the replacements are coming in, yet they are still being pushed to become more productive. They are working 12-hour days, are commuting up to 2 hours a day, and are held by an electronic leash to the office. Their opportunity to relax is almost nonexistent.
>
> Contrary to popular beliefs, we need to learn how to slow down our thinking at times, not speed up. Time for reflection and contemplation of ideas and issues is sorely missing in health care. The never-ending checklist is always present and demanding attention. Further, experts report that pay is not the chief motivator for productivity. In general, employees desire to do meaningful work most of all, next they desire opportunities for collaboration through group decision making, and then they want equitable pay (pp. 317–318).

This provides us with three important ways (questions to ask) to enhance productivity. First, is our work meaningful? Do staff feel that way about their work? If not, what is the problem? Are they

---

Exhibit 6–14 Myths and Truths About Employee Productivity

Accepted Notions

- If employees work more hours, they will be more productive.
- If employees work faster, they will be more productive.
- If employees are paid more, they will be motivated to work harder and produce more.

The Reality

- Employees perform optimally for six to seven hours and may be able to work longer in a burst of energy or inspiration, but then they must rest.
- Employees need balance; they need a life outside of work.
- Slower, intuitive thinking is often more effective in solving problems than mental agility.
- Studies show that, in Germany, where individual performance is not rewarded with pay increases, productivity is often higher than in the United States.
- Employees are most productive when their employers pay them *equitably* and then do everything possible to help the employees put money out of their minds.

Source: Johnson, C. B. (2000). When working harder is not smarter. *Inner Edge, 3*(2), 18–21.

---

doing work that does not match their gifts? Do others treat them like they are unimportant? Second, do staff have opportunities for collaboration? Does group decision making occur? Third, is the pay equitable? How can we, as administrators, improve these issues in our workplace?

A fourth misconception is that quantitative measurements are "the be all and end all" to measure productivity. In other words, quantitative measurement is assumed to be the most effective measurement. In reality, quantitative productivity measurements provide a barometer about productivity but need to be considered with other qualitative and efficiency data. More importantly, the quantitative measurement may not include other important productivity or quality factors. Using quantitative measures only provides an incomplete picture of productivity.

A fifth issue with productivity measurement is that in some cases productivity has gotten a bad reputation with some nursing staff, as the word "productivity"—as defined by the finance department—has been used synonymous with budget cuts or with unrealistic increases in workload. The short-term result can be not having enough staff to safely deliver care; dissatisfied nurses, physicians, and patients; and more patient safety and legal issues.

> Slash-and-burn cost cutting brings only a series of onetime efficiencies. In the end, there's only one encore—another round of cost cutting. And that's the catch. This approach leads to increasingly hollow companies that ultimately are unable to maintain market share in an ever-expanding global economy (Roach, 1998, p. 154).

This view of productivity by nursing staff is unfortunate because the true meaning of productivity is that, chances are, all could be more efficient and effective. But the slash-and-burn tactics are not the way to accomplish this goal. These tactics devalue staff and do not follow what employees most want—to have meaningful work, to collaborate in decision making, and to have adequate pay. Following these three precepts, if budget cuts are needed, all need to be involved in the identification of where the cuts will occur. And maybe staff will have other ideas as to different ways to make money and offer better services that will negate the need to cut the budget.

A sixth misconception is that budget cuts always result in negative outcomes. This is not necessarily the case. This is related to a seventh misconception: that as productivity increases, quality suffers. For example, when at 7 a.m. there are too many staff but by 10 a.m. there are not enough staff, productivity could be improved by having staff start work at 10 a.m., and, if necessary, add another staff person to provide care during the peak load time only.

Another organizational issue is that support services are a problem. Why are the beds not being cleaned promptly? Depending on worker function, this may involve the housekeeping department or nurse aides. But it also might come right back to the nurses and unit secretary who have not communicated ahead with those workers that a discharge is about to occur. If everyone involved can get together and discuss both their frustrations and suggestions for improvement, chances are better efficiencies can be achieved.

An eighth misconception with productivity is that when a department experiences productivity problems, the department head is directed to fix the problem. Here the department in question tries to either increase their productivity number (i.e., number of visits or patient days; or spends time attacking the quality of the data), while a larger, more important problem is not being dealt with at all. It is a silo mentality to believe that poor productivity lies within that department alone. Chances are that although the department needs to improve, there are other organizational systems problems that need to be fixed as well.

There is another misconception that the productivity issue is an individual employee issue, not a management issue. The administrative role goes beyond personal examination. Part of our responsibility involves our looking at the system, identifying issues that need improvement, involving staff to be doing the same, and then getting everyone involved to bring about the changes necessary to fix the problems.

The staff, or the administrators, or the finance department may hold a tenth misconception, that productivity improvement is the only way of improving income generation in the organization. If this were true, why is it so important to change and add new services? Using this scenario, we would just continue doing the same thing until we eventually went out of business from our antiquated business practices.

Eleven, just paying attention to internal issues can be another misconception. It is possible, for instance, that the supply chain has malfunctioned and the organization cannot get needed supplies and equipment in a timely way, thus causing serious productivity problems. Here the problem lies with the supplier, although, chances are, staff in the organization are helping to cause the problem as well. For instance, as something becomes scarce, staff squirrel it. They hide whatever they cannot get easily, and this may actually cause the shortage to get worse. Additionally, the paperwork is so ponderous that it is impossible to get needed supplies quickly. Perhaps someone is forgetting to order promptly. We are all in this together! Each of our actions can affect the outcome.

Evaluate Factors Affecting Productivity

Thus, when measuring productivity, it is important to always examine the factors that have affected current productivity levels. For instance, if one month our productivity level was not as good, what factors might have accounted for this change? Perhaps since the budgeted hours were established, a significant event(s) occurred that might increase or decrease the number of staff needed to accomplish the work. Factors might include such things as a new procedure for patient safety was implemented; staff are caring for different, more acute patients; a new staff member is orienting; a new computerized documentation system has been implemented; a change has been made in a work process; a new physician is using different treatments; or more staff are needed temporarily while implementing a new change. Any of these factors could explain why the productivity level was not as high.

Another factor that can significantly change productivity measurement is nonproductive time. When determining productivity measurements, it is important to know whether nonproductive time is included. (Nonproductive time, nonworked time such as sick and vacation time or annual leave time, is further explained in Chapter 13.) If nonproductive time is figured into the productivity level, then any time someone uses sick or vacation time, the productivity level drops. If this is the case, staff productivity may actually be the same from day to day, yet the productivity measurement may look like productivity has decreased whenever staff take nonproductive time. If one can actually have two separate staff budgets, one reflecting worked time and the other reflecting nonproductive time, productivity measurement is more accurate. If it is not possible to separate out the two, the nurse manager may have to manually refigure productivity just using productive time.

Benchmark data, such as staff per patient ratios, NHPPD, and budget information, used by facilities can also be affected if one facility counts nonproductive time and another does not. If you are benchmarking with other organizations, be sure to clarify that all benchmark facilities are reporting nonproductive time in the same way, or you may be comparing apples and oranges. Benchmarking on productivity data can also be affected by other factors (i.e., staff getting more vacation time at one facility, or staff getting education days at one location and not at another).

One other issue with productivity is that occasionally nonproductive time is not included anywhere in the budget. In this case, appropriate staffing will be impossible on most days because there will not be enough FTEs to cover staff that take annual leave time. Then the nurse manager must figure actual nonproductive time needed, immediately discuss this with the nurse executive and the finance department, and by the next budget year get the base budget recalculated to add a line for nonproductive time to the budget. In the meantime it could be dealt with as a variance.

Linking Quantitative Productivity Measures with Performance Evaluation Data

Productivity measurement in health care is most effective if it does not stand alone. It needs to be linked with patient outcomes. Otherwise, how do we know that the productivity levels have been effective? For instance, if productivity figures are wonderful but patients are having a lot of complications, something is wrong with the *effectiveness* component of productivity. This comparison is complicated by the fact that sometimes poor patient outcomes occur after a patient is discharged and we may never be aware that they occurred. Furthermore, we do not know, and have not measured, what the patient wants or values.

One way we have tried to add the effectiveness dimension is by using patient satisfaction instruments, discussed in Chapter 4. Patient satisfaction measurements provide additional data on how patients have viewed their health care experience. Unfortunately, most instruments are designed to find out historical data, so it is difficult to rectify problems as they occur. Ideally, more direct feedback is needed during the actual patient experience. Patients may be afraid to give negative information for fear that this will adversely affect their care. So we need more accurate data.

Although not ideal, today the most effective productivity evaluation measurements combine financial, organizational, and patient outcome data and are called *performance evaluation*. This includes patient-related outcome data such as length of stay, readmission rates, patient falls, adverse reactions, complications, infections, deaths, number of medications per patient, client condition on discharge, and consumer satisfaction/complaints. (Performance data are described in more detail in Chapters 4 and 16.) Performance data do not yet measure whether the patient received what was wanted and valued. It also may only measure complications that we are aware of while the patient is with us—not what occurs after we have seen the client. Then in performance evaluation, the outcome data (effectiveness) is compared with the processes influencing those outcomes (efficiencies). Process data measuring efficiency can include numbers and skill mix of staff; staff turnover; cost of the staffing; overhead costs; quality/safety measures implemented, including adding technology; and/or equipment and supplies consumed.

Hall and colleagues (2000) suggested a nursing productivity tool that measures nursing knowledge indicators (educational preparation, experience, career planning and development, autonomy, organizational trust, organizational commitment, and satisfaction), nursing productivity system indicators (nursing costs, turnover, absenteeism, orientation costs, and education costs), and patient indicators (nursing errors related to patient safety, and patient satisfaction). Unfortunately this still does not find out or measure whether the patient received what was wanted and valued.

As more performance data have become available on a national level through the CMS, these published summaries of various performance measures have provided performance data to regulators, payers, and consumers via the Internet. Consumers can choose their providers based on these data, if the consumer is aware the data exist. Payers use these data in two ways: (1) to compare providers, choosing to have contracts only with providers who have the best performance data, and (2) to pay only for positive performance, not paying for problems that health care facilities caused for patients (*pay for performance*). This is called *performance-based reimbursement evaluation*.

When health care systems share this valuable historical performance data with employees for evaluation and improvement, everyone benefits. Enhanced productivity effectiveness results. So far, however, a lot of this is historical and does not capture the information soon enough to rectify the situation immediately. Additionally, these data do not indicate future performance.

Although there are currently no absolute standards or guidelines as to actual criteria to use or how well a provider needs to perform, undoubtedly there will be considerable development in this arena. It will be exciting to see where this leads us because the research results have started to provide us with more effective assessment data, all essential for productivity measurement.

Obtaining performance data is just the first step and, aside from the value question, brings up more questions: Do the processes currently used and measured have an actual effect on the outcome? Does patient preoperative teaching actually result in fewer complications, quicker recovery, and higher patient satisfaction following surgery? Are there fewer medication errors when patients give themselves their own medication(s) when possible? There are hundreds of these questions that we need to ask. We may believe intuitively that we know the answer. However, our research does not prove it. Research results can surprise us. It would be nice to know what processes specifically make a difference in our patient outcomes. Effectiveness and efficiency need to be measured in tandem and considered together for the greatest effectiveness.

Coming back to the patient perspective, consider the following questions: What does the patient want, need, and value? What does the patient need to achieve safety and good patient outcomes? What can the patient afford? Was the patient satisfied with what he or she received? Do patients value what staff currently do? Can staff reasonably give the patient what the patient wants?

Course Correction: After the Initial Evaluation, What Comes Next?

While evaluating current practice and determining productivity standards, the need for some changes or improvements may become obvious. In addition, once the productivity standards are set, it is important to measure against that standard to make sure the standard is met or exceeded. If it not met, other productivity improvement measures may be needed. But productivity improvement does not stop there. It must permeate everything we do.

Then implementation begins. For example, new care paths may need to be developed for certain patients, educational programs may need to be implemented so staff are using the most efficient or effective approach with clients, paperwork may be eliminated or streamlined by purchasing new technology, new programs may be started with present programs being eliminated or revamped, or new incentives may be implemented to encourage staff to improve productivity.

Productivity Improvement

Productivity improvement is everyone's responsibility. In this book we stress the importance of involving staff at all levels in the decision-making process. This continues to be true with productivity:

> Remember the basic assumptions when [improving] productivity. First, productivity improvement is not completed in a vacuum. Improving only one component of an agency will not increase overall productivity, so consider an agencywide program. Second, involve all staff, particularly direct caregivers, in planning and evaluating the productivity of an agency. Third, management holds the key to effective productivity through effective supervision and the ability to create environments that challenge and motivate staff (Benefield in Harris, 1997, p. 479).

As all staff are involved, it is important that they understand that productivity is linked with organizational viability (see **Exhibit 6–15**).

Productivity improvement is more easily accomplished when we feel that we do meaningful work:

> What drives people to work at their best? How can health care leaders revitalize the lost passion of employees? What are the retention strategies that will support the rebuilding of a hopeful culture? Interestingly, the answer is simple. When employees believe their work is meaningful—productive in the sense of producing beneficial results—then they will be motivated to work harder and will experience a renewal of passion and hopefulness. Productivity is not only about quantity; it is also about quality.
>
> Optimizing employee performance takes on a whole new meaning in this context. All human beings have a need to express their uniqueness and their talents in the work they do and be recognized for their contributions. Therefore, employees are typically motivated

---

Exhibit 6–15 Optimizing Performance: Productivity or Fruitfulness?

Productivity

- Productivity is mechanistic.
- In a productivity-driven organization, employees are treated like machines and judged on the quantity of their output.
- The predominant concern is getting more "bang for the buck."
- Efforts to increase employee motivation are dependent on external sources, pay, benefits, etc.

Fruitfulness

- Fruitfulness is humanistic.
- Fruitfulness involves a respectful, holistic view of each person that recognizes values, beliefs, and expectations.
- Fruitfulness honors the inner need of each person to express his or her uniqueness and talents and to develop and expand.
- Fruitfulness engages the inner selves of employees and causes them to grow and be sustained naturally and enduringly.

Source: Johnson, C. B. (2000). When working harder is not smarter. *Inner Edge, 3*(2), 18–21.

employees are typically motivated by jobs that develop their skills and expand their minds, demand individual initiative, involve working on teams, benefit others, and spark a desire to make a difference in the world. Jobs that have these characteristics possess what Cedric Johnson (2000) called fruitfulness—work flows from one person to another in a way that is both respectful and valued. To ensure that health care workers possess fruitfulness, leaders need to do the following:

- Continually examine services, measures, and systems to assess their impact on patient outcomes. Retain those that improve patient outcomes, and eliminate those that have no effect or a negative effect.
- Believe that hope can be restored to care providers through restoring value to the work they do.
- Believe intensely that individuals will give their best when treated like adults.
- Be alive and be committed to doing what is best for patients.
- Consistently expect only value-adding services to be delivered to patients. Publicly recognize individuals who are able to focus on value, and guide those who require assistance in eliminating unnecessary and non-valued-adding work.
- Believe that all health care providers intuitively know that restoring value to work is the right path but have not been able to translate their perceptions into practice. Believe that most, but not all, will eventually make the transition. Believe that the health care system will not only support but will require increases in the value of health care services. Know that colleagues support caring, healing work that makes a difference (Porter-O'Grady & Malloch, 2003, pp. 317–318).

Information Systems

When patients always receive exactly the care they need at the appropriate time, health care achieves its ultimate altruistic goal—the holistic, humanistic, and seamless integrated health care delivery system (Malloch & Porter-O'Grady, 1999). This lofty goal is often overwhelming and considered impossible by many in health care because of lack of predictability and uncertainty of future patient care needs. Yet, as information technology continues to advance, progress in meeting this goal is becoming more apparent.

Information systems now play a central role in providing efficient clinical services. Bedside computers and clinical information systems promise to revolutionize hospital nursing (Shi & Singh, 2004). The use of bar coding for supply charging and medication dispensing/administration, instant test result retrieval and analysis via computer systems, hand-held charting devices, transcription options, and telemedicine technology have all impacted care outcomes and the structure and processes of health care delivery. Using technology for real-time matching of patient care needs with caregiver skill profiles from staffing and scheduling systems will be the focus of the next generation of patient classification systems.

The challenge is to integrate nursing informatics with engineering principles using a scientific inquiry aspect to create a better future (Huber, 1996). The engineering aspect applies technology to perform a function or uses computers for very specific functional purposes. The scientific inquiry aspect determines the necessary data and information and how this information should be captured, represented, processed, and stored so that it provides a realistic reflection of practice, adequate support of decision making, effective management of resources and knowledge, and sound hypothesis testing.

Computerized systems can record the actual times of all direct and indirect nursing care activities. The next challenge is to interface documented caregiver interventions and their associated time standards with scheduling systems. Time computations and acuity ratings can be automatically calculated and updated in real time. Once all activities of caregivers can be labeled and documented, the computer can capture actual activity performed for the patient. It can rapidly and automatically calculate data and determine patient needs, interventions required to meet those needs, and the time associated with those processes. Staffing can then be calculated while avoiding subjectivity and information delay (Huber, 1996). Indeed, such technology would render the calculation of staff hours and skill mix transparent in the process and eliminate the need for caregivers to rate, score, or select interventions in a separate process. It would be the end of patient classification systems as we know them today!

Summary

Patient care executives need reliable management measurement tools for nursing practice. Although tools such as patient classification systems were initially developed decades ago, much work is still needed to make these tools useful and trusted. The updates to current tools reflect some of the changes in technology, care delivery, and patient populations being served and unfortunately still result in varying degrees of success.

With the development of new approaches to patient care, new parameters with corresponding methodology to measure the resources required for that care would be essential to progress in the technological age. The measurement of patient care services has moved away from the specific cost accounting approaches popular 10 years ago to the analysis of data from relational databases. Collaboration with management engineers and financial experts is necessary to advance current systems. At the patient care and caregiver level, variance from predicted, expected, or best practices provides data needed by not only nurse executives but also by financial officers, managed care plan administrators, and state and federal governments administering health benefits. At the service and system level, data that provide insight into cause, effect, and system interactions are more useful for improving care. At the organized delivery system level, data specific to the extent to which processes and management methods influence the quality of practice can provide new insights into resource utilization, prioritization of services, and patient safety.

Discussion Questions

1. Evaluate a staffing plan for a unit.
2. If you had to choose a patient classification system for a nursing unit, which type would you choose? Give your rationale.
3. Explain how you would establish validity and reliability of a patient classification system.
4. How would you determine the skill mix for an inpatient unit? Give your rationale.
5. Do you believe there should be state legislation concerning RN staffing ratios? If so, describe what it should contain. Give a rationale for this answer.
6. How does pay for performance effect staffing?
7. How can you determine whether there is staffing adequacy?
8. Describe the components to establish competency for a staff nurse in your work area.
9. Describe staffing variances that occur. How would you deal with them effectively?
10. Give an example of productivity measurement in your facility? Evaluate it.
11. How could you improve productivity in your work unit?

12. Are any of the productivity misconceptions occurring in your workplace? If so, what are they and how could a nurse administrator more effectively influence productivity measurement in that setting?

Glossary of Terms

Acuity—the level of need or dependency of an individual patient.

Case Mix Method—a method of clustering patients into groups that are homogeneous with respect to the use of resources.

Comprehensive Unit of Service—an aggregate of eight categories of care, represents the total care provided by nursing during a shift or event of care and integrates a multitasking factor to account for the overlap of care in identified patient situations.

Content Validity—the extent to which the patient classification tool includes all the major elements relative to the construct being measured.

Construct Validity—the fit between the conceptual definitions and operational definitions of the variables.

Core Schedules—an aggregated average number and skill mix required for patient care focusing on having sufficient staff to care for the population served; the long-range plan that becomes the template for the required number of staff.

External Validity—the extent to which the findings can be generalized beyond the sample used.

Face Validity—is high when nurses believe that the system accurately reflects and represents the work that they do or the dependency of the patients for whom they provide care.

Factor Evaluation Method—identifies selected elements of care, critical indicators, or tasks with associated times that are most likely predictors of nursing care needs.

Internal Validity—the extent to which the measures used in the patient classification tool are a true reflection of reality.

Job Analysis—assessment of the job responsibilities included in a specific role, including tasks, knowledge, and skills/competencies required for a particular job.

Patient Classification—a process of grouping patients into homogeneous, mutually exclusive groups to determine their dependency on caregivers or to determine patient acuity.

Position Control—the process used by human resources to specify actual FTEs assigned to a unit or department.

Productivity—a process of getting more out of what you put in. It's doing better with what you have; achieving more efficiencies linked with effectiveness.

Prototype Approach—identifies the characteristics of patients into categories. Individual patients are then assigned to the category that most closely reflects their nursing care requirements.

Relative Value Unit—in addition to grouping patients into similar categories based on nursing care needs, a patient classification system can also quantify the workload within the categories by assigning a relative value to each category.

Reliability—addresses the consistency of rating in a patient classification system.

Sensitivity—refers to physiological measures and is related to the amount of change of a parameter that can be measured precisely.

Skill Mix—the various types of nursing staff by job classification necessary to care for the patient population.

Staffing Plan—describes the structure and process by which responsibilities for patient care are assigned and how the work is coordinated among caregivers.

Validity—the degree to which a patient classification system actually measures what it intends to measure.

References

Aiken, L., Clarke, S., Cheung, R., Sloane, D., & Silber, J. (2003). Educational levels of hospital nurses and surgical patient mortality. *Journal of the American Medical Association, 290,* 1617–1623.

Aiken, L., Clarke, S., Sloane, D., Sochalski, J., & Silber, J. (2002). Hospital nurse staffing and patient mortality, nurse burnout, and job dissatisfaction. *Journal of the American Medical Association, 288*(16), 1987–1993.

Aiken, L., & Patrician, P. (2000). Measuring organizational traits of hospitals: The revised nursing work index. *Nursing Research, 49*(3), 146–153.

Aiken, L., Smith, H., & Lake, E. (1994). Lower Medicare mortality among a set of hospitals known for good nursing care. *Medical Care, 32*(8), 771–787.

Altaffer, A. (1998). First-line managers: Measuring their span of control. *Nursing Management, 29*(7): 36–39.

American Nurses Association. (1989). *Classification systems for describing nursing practice.* Kansas City, MO: Author.

American Nurses Association. (1997). *Implementing nursing's report card: A study of RN staffing, length of stay and patient outcomes.* Washington, DC: American Nurses Publishing.

American Nurses Association. (2000). *Nurse staffing and patient outcomes: In the inpatient hospital setting.* Washington, DC: American Nurses Publishing.

American Nurses Association. (2001). *2001 ANA staffing survey.* Washington, DC: American Nurses Publishing.

American Nurses Association. (2003a). *Nurse staffing plans and ratios.* Kansas City, MO: Author.

American Nurses Association. (2003b). *Workplace issues: ANA: The right choice for organized and collective bargaining.* Retrieved December 1, 2003 from http://www.nursingworld.org/dlwa/barg/

American Nurses Association. (2008). *Principles for nurse staffing with annotated bibliography.* Kansas City, MO: Author. Retrieved August 2, 2008 from http://www.nursingworld.org/MainMenuCategories/HealthcareandPolicyIssues/Reports/ANAPrinciples/NurseStaffing.aspx

American Organization of Nurse Executives. (2000). *Perspectives on the nursing shortage: A blueprint for action.* Monograph Series. Chicago: AONE.

Barnes, R. M. (1980). *Motion and time study design and measurement of work* (7th ed.). Hoboken, NJ: Wiley & Sons.

Behner, K., Fogg, L., Fournier, L., Frankenbach, J., & Robertson, S. (1990). Nursing resource management: Analyzing the relationship between costs and quality in staffing decisions. *Health Care Management Review, 15*(4), 63–71.

Blegen, M., & Goode, C. (1997, Spring). Nurse staffing effects on patient outcomes: Results of main/mnrs joint collaborative grant. *MAINlines, 7,* 22.

Blegen, M., Goode, C., & Reed, L. (1998). Nurse staffing and patient outcomes. *Nursing Research, 47*(1), 43–50.

Blegen, M., & Vaughn, T. (1998). A multisite study of nurse staffing and patient occurrences. *Nursing Economic$, 16*(4), 196–203.

Blegen, M., Vaughn, T., & Goode, C. (2001). Nurse experience and education: Effect on quality of care. *Journal of Nursing Administration, 31*(1), 33–39.

Bliesmer, M., Smayling, M., Kane, R., & Shannon, I. (1998). The relationship between nursing staffing levels and nursing home outcomes. *Journal of Aging & Health, 10*(3), 351–372.

Bolton, L., Jones, D., Aydin, C., Donaldson, N., Brown, D., Lowe, M., McFarland, P., & Harms, D. (2001). A response to California's mandated nursing ratios. *Journal of Nursing Scholarship, 33*(2), 179–184.

Brady. (2001). Sitting in the dark. *Organizational Effectiveness, 1*(7), 1–3.

Brewer, C., & Frazier, P. (1998, September). The influence of structure, staff type, and managed-care indicators on registered nurse staffing. *Journal of Nursing Administration, 28*(9), 28–36.

Burke, T., McKee, J., Wilson, H., Donahue, R. M., Batenhorst, A., & Pathak, D. (2000). A comparison of time-and-motion and self reporting methods of work measurement. *Journal of Nursing Administration, 30*(3), 118–125.

Burns, N., & Grove, S. (2001). *The practice of nursing research: Conduct, critique & utilization* (4th ed.). Philadelphia: Saunders.

Cavouras, C., & McKinley, J. (1998). Annual survey of hours. *Perspectives on Staffing and Scheduling, 17*(3), 3.

Chang, C., Price, S., & Pfoutz, S. (2001). *Economics and nursing: Critical professional issues*. Philadelphia: F.A. Davis.

Cho, S., Ketefian, S., Barkauska, V., & Smith, D. (2003). The effects of nurse staffing on adverse events, morbidity, mortality and medical costs. *Nursing Research, 52*(2), 71–79.

Curtin, L. (2003). An integrated analysis of nurse staffing and related variables: Effects on patient outcomes. *Online Journal of Issues in Nursing*. Retrieved November 30, 2003 from http:// www.nursingworld.org/ojin/topic22/tpc22_5.htm

DeGroot, H. (1994). Patient classification systems and staffing: Part 1. Problems and promise. *Journal of Nursing Administration, 24*(9), 43–51.

Douglas, D., & Mayewski, J. (1996). Census variation staffing. *Nursing Management, 27*(2), 32–36.

Dunham-Taylor, J., & Pinczuk, J. (2006). *Health care financial management for nurse managers: Applications from hospitals, long-term care, home care, and ambulatory care*. Sudbury, MA: Jones and Bartlett.

Dunn, M., Norby, R., Cournoyer, P., Hudec, S., O'Donnell, J., & Snider, M. (1995). Expert panel method for nurse staffing and resource management. *Journal of Nursing Administration, 25*(10), 61–67.

Finkler, S. (2001). *Budgeting concepts for nurse managers* (3rd ed.). Philadelphia: Saunders.

Fralic, M., (Ed.). (2000). *Staffing management and methods: Tools and techniques for nursing leaders*. Chicago: AHA Press.

Gardner, A., & Gemme, E. (2003). Virtual scheduling: A 21st century approach to staffing. *Nursing Administration Quarterly, 27*(1), 77–82.

Garry, R. (2000). Benchmarking: A prescription for healthcare. *Journal of Nursing Administration, 30*(9), 397–398.

Gift, A., & Soeken, K. (1988). Assessment of physiologic instruments. *Heart & Lung, 17*(2), 128–133.

Goode, C., Pinderton, S., McCausland, M., Southard, P., Graham, R., & Krsek, C. (2001). Documenting chief nursing officers' preference for BSN-prepared nurses. *Journal of Nursing Administration, 31*(2), 55–59.

Gordon, M. (1998). Nursing nomenclature and classification system development. *Online Journal of Issues in Nursing*. Retrieved November 19, 2003 from http://www.nursingworld.org/ ojin/tpc7/tpc7_1.htm

Hall, L., Pink, G., Johnson, L., & Schraa, E. (2000). Development of a nursing management practice atlas: Part 2, variation in use of nursing and financial resources. *Journal of Nursing Administration, 30*(9), 440–448.

Harper, K., & McCully, C. (2007). Acuity systems dialogue and patient classification systems essentials. *Nursing Administration Quarterly, 31*(4), 284–299.

Harris, M. (1997). *Handbook of home health care administration* (2nd ed.). Gaithersburg, MD: Aspen.

Hasman, A., Wiersma, D., Halfens, R., & Algera, J. (1993). Evaluation of a patient classification system for community health care. *International Journal of Bio-Medical Computing, 33,* 109–118.

Health Care Education Associates, (1987) *Basic budgeting for nurse managers*. St. Louis: Mosby.

Hendrix, T., & Foreman, S. (2001). Optimal long-term care nurse staffing levels. *Nursing Economic$, 19*(4), 164–175.

Hernandez, C., & O'Brien, P. (1996a). Validity and reliability of nursing workload measurement systems: Review of validity and reliability theory. Part 1. *Canadian Journal of Nursing Administration, 9*(3), 16–25.

Hernandez, C., & O'Brien, P. (1996b). Validity and reliability of nursing workload measurement systems: Review of validity and reliability theory. Part 2. *Canadian Journal of Nursing Administration, 10*(3), 16–23.

Hollabaugh, S., & Kendrick, S. (1998). Staffing: The five-level pyramid. *Nursing Management, 29*(2), 34–36.

Huber, D. (1996). *Leadership and nursing care management*. Philadelphia: Saunders.

Hyun, S., Bakken, S., Douglas, K., & Stone, P. (2008). Evidence-based staffing: Potential roles for informatics. *Nursing Economic$, 26*(3), 151–173.

Johnson, C. (2000). When working harder is not smarter. *The Inner Edge, 3*(2), 18–21.

The Joint Commission. (2002). Health care at the crossroads: Strategies for addressing the evolving nursing crisis. Retrieved December 2, 2003 from www.jcaho.org

Kane, R., Shamliyan, T., Mueller, C., Duval, S., & Wilt, T. (2007). The association of registered nurse staffing levels and patients outcomes: Systematic review and meta-analysis. *Medical Care, 45*(12), 1195–1204.

Kerr, P. (2000). Comparing two nursing outcomes reporting initiatives. *Outcomes Management for Nursing Practice, 4*(3), 144–149.

Kido, V. (2001). The UAP dilemma. *Nursing Management, 32*(11), 27–29.

LaDuke, S. (2000, April). Nurses' perceptions: Is your nurse uncomfortable or incompetent? *Journal of Nursing Administration, 30*(4), 163–165.

Letvak, S., & Buck, R. (2008). Factors influencing work productivity and intent to stay in nursing. *Nursing Economic$, 26*(3), 159–165.

Malloch, K., & Conovaloff, A. (1999). Patient classification systems, Part 1: The third generation. *Journal of Nursing Administration, 29*(7), 49–56.

Malloch, K., & Porter-O'Grady, T. (1999). Partnership economics: Nursing's challenge in a quantum age. *Nursing Economic$, 17*(6), 299–307.

Manthey, M. (2001). A core incremental staffing plan. *Journal of Nursing Administration, 31*(9), 424–425.

Mark, B. (2002). What explains nurses' perceptions of staffing adequacy? *Journal of Nursing Administration, 32*(5), 234–242.

Mark, B., & Burleson, D. (1995). Measurement of patient outcomes: Data availability and consistency across hospitals. *Journal of Nursing Administration, 25*(4), 52–59.

Mark, B., Salyer, J., & Wan, T. (2000). Market, hospital, and nursing unit characteristics as predictors of nursing unit skill mix: A contextual analysis. *Journal of Nursing Administration, 30*(11), 552–560.

Mason, D. (2003). How many patients are too many? Legislating staffing ratios is good for nursing. *American Journal of Nursing, 103*(11), 7.

McCloskey, J., & Bulechek, G., (Eds.). (2000). *Nursing interventions classification (NIC)* (3rd ed.). St. Louis: Mosby.

McClung, T. (2000). Assessing the reported financial benefits of unlicensed assistive personnel in nursing. *Journal of Nursing Administration, 30*(11), 530–534.

McConnell, E. (2001). Competence vs. competency. *Nursing Management, 32*(5), 14.

McCue, M. (2003). Nurse staffing, quality and financial performance. *Journal of Health Care Finance, 29*(4), 54–76.

Melberg, S. (1997). Effects of changing skill mix. *Nursing Management, 28*(110), 47–48.

Meretoja, R., & Leino-Kilpi, H. (2001). Instruments for evaluating nurse competence. *Journal of Nursing Administration*, *31*(7/8), 346–352.

Myers, F., & Stewart, J. (2002). *Motion and time study for lean manufacturing* (3rd ed.). Upper Saddle River, NJ: Prentice Hall.

National Center for Health Statistics. (2003). Centers for Disease Control and Prevention. Retrieved November 20, 2003 from http://www.cdc.gov/nchs/about/otheract/icd9/abticd9.htm

Needleman, J., Buerhaus, P., Mattke, S., Stewart, M., & Zelevinsky, K. (2001). *Nursing staffing and patient outcomes in hospitals*. Final Report, US Department of Health and Human Services, Contract No. 230–99–0021.

Needleman, J., Buerhaus, P., Mattke, S., Stewart, M., & Zelevinsky, K. (2002). Nurse staffing levels and the quality of care in hospitals. *New England Journal of Medicine, 346*(22), 1715–1722.

O'Brien-Pallas, L., Irvine, D., Peereboom, E., & Murray, M. (1997). Measuring nursing workload: Understanding the variability. *Nursing Economic$, 15*(4), 171–182.

Page, A. (2004). *Keeping patients safe: Transforming the work environment of nurses*: Quality Chasm series. Institute of Medicine, The National Academy of Sciences. Washington, DC: National Academy Press.

Pear, R. (2000, July). U.S. recommends strict new rules at nursing homes: Concern over staffing: Officials say patients may be endangered by shortages of both nurses and aides. *New York Times*.

Pinkerton, S., & Rivers, R. (2001). Factors influencing staffing needs. *Nursing Economic$, 19*(5), 236–237.

Porter-O'Grady, T., & Malloch, K. (2003). *Quantum leadership: A textbook of new leadership*. Gaithersburg, MD: Aspen.

Porter-O'Grady, T., & Malloch, K. (2007). *Quantum leadership: A resource for health care innovation* (2nd ed.). Sudbury, MA: Jones and Bartlett.

Potter, P., Barr, N., McSweeney, M., & Sledge, J. (2003). Identifying nurse staffing and patient outcome relationships: A guide for change in care delivery. *Nursing Economic$, 21*(4), 158–166.

Roach, S. (1998). In search of productivity. *Harvard Business Review*, 153–160.

Sasichay-Akkadechanunt, T., Scalzi, C., & Jawad, A. (2003). The relationships between nurse staffing and patient outcomes. *Journal of Nursing Administration*, *33*(9), 478–485.

Savage, S. (2002). The flaw of averages. *Harvard Business Review, 79*(11), 20–21.

Schmidt, D. (1999). Financial and operational skills for nurse managers. *Nursing Administration Quarterly, 23*(4), 16.

Seago, J. (2001). Nurse staffing, models of care delivery, and interventions. In Shojania, K. Duncan, B., McDonald, K., & Wachter, R. (Eds.). *Making health care safer: A critical analysis of patient safety practices, evidence report*. Technology assessment No. 43. Rockville MD: AHRQ.

Seago, J. (2002). The California experiment: Alternatives for minimum nurse-to-patient ratios. *Journal of Nursing Administration, 32*(1), 48–58.

Seago, J., & Ash, M. (2002). Registered nurse unions and patient outcomes. *Journal of Nursing Administration*, *32*(3), 143–151.

Shaha, S. (1995). Acuity systems and control charting. *Quality Management in Health Care, 3*(3), 22–30.

Shi, L., & Singh, D. (2004). *Delivering health care in America: A systems approach* (3rd ed.). Sudbury, MA: Jones and Bartlett.

Shullanberger, G. (2000). Nurse staffing decisions: An integrative review of the literature. *Nursing Economic$, 18*(3), 124–148.

Sochalski, J., Aiken, L., & Fagin, C. (1997). Hospital restructuring in the United States, Canada, and Western Europe: An outcomes research agenda. *Medical Care, 35*(10), OS13–OS25.

Strickland, B., & Neely, S. (1995). Using a standard staffing index to allocate nursing staff. *Journal of Nursing Administration, 25*(3), 13–21.

Sullivan, E., & Decker, L. (2001). The effect of LPN reductions on RN patient load. *Journal of Nursing Administration, 33*(4), 120.

Taylor, K. (2000). Tackling the issue of nurse competency. *Nursing Management*, 35–37.

Unruh, L. (2003). The effect of LPN reductions on RN patient load. *Journal of Nursing Administration, 33*(4), 201–208.

Upeniks, V., Akhavan, J., Kotlerman, J., Esser, J., & Ngo, J. (2007). Value-added care: A new way of assessing nursing staffing ratios and workload variability. *Journal of Nursing Administration, 37*(5), 243–252.

Van Slyck, A. (1999). Improving productivity: A payer/provider debate. *Journal of Nursing Administration, 29*(1), 51–56.

Van Slyck, A. (2000). Patient classification systems: Not a proxy for nurse "busyness." *Nursing Administration Quarterly, 24*(4), 51–59.

Verran, J. (1986). Testing a classification instrument for the ambulatory care setting. *Research in Nursing and Health, 9*, 279–287.

Walts, L., & Kapadia, A. (1996). Patient classification system: An optimization approach. *Health Care Manager Review, 21*, 75–82.

CHAPTER 7

Ethics in Nursing Administration

Lois W. Lowry, DNSc, RN, ANEF
Jo-Ann Summitt Marrs, EdD, RN

A society cultivates whatever is honored there. It is important for us to know what we honor.

—*Plato*

Key Terms

☞ Autonomy
☞ Beneficence
☞ Business Ethics
☞ Clinical Ethics Committees
☞ Code of Ethics
☞ Deontology
☞ Distributive Justice

☞ Ethical Climate
☞ Ethical Principles
☞ Ethics
☞ Justice
☞ Morality
☞ Moral dilemma
☞ Moral distress
☞ Nonmalfeasance

☞ Organizational Ethics
☞ Organizational Ethics Committees
☞ Profession
☞ Teleology
☞ Utilitarianism

Introduction

Nurse executives today find themselves in rapidly changing and challenging health care systems in which personal ethics and organizational ethics often are in juxtaposition. Whatever happened to the health care culture of our youth when the institutions were primarily nonprofit and the medical profession comprised the governing body? In those *good old days*, professionals employed in organizations followed codes of ethics endorsed by their respective professions to guide their behavior. Individual ethics were framed by these codes—taught in the professional schools—and governed practice. These codes, then and now, affirm the professional ideals of conduct and commit members to honor them. They have two primary functions: first, to provide an enforceable standard of minimally decent care and, second, to maintain one's own professional competence to safeguard patients from incompetent or unethical practice.

If these codes were sufficient to frame the care we gave in the past, why are they seemingly inadequate in the health care organizations of today? This chapter provides an historical perspective of ethics development in the health care system, presents ethical concerns of nurse administrators, and suggests insights into the development of ethical leadership.

Setting the Stage: An Historical Overview

> We may not know what our destiny will be, but one thing we do know: the only ones among us who will be really happy are those who've sought and found how to serve.
>
> —*Albert Schweitzer*

Were there ever good old days? Probably not, except in our reverie; the days were just different and perhaps simpler than today. Nightingale exhorted her nurses to "be sober and honest... devoted... to have a respect for her own calling, because God's precious gift of life is placed in her hands" (Nightingale, 1859, p. 71). These wise words were based on the need for personal morality so that a high quality of life could be maintained for oneself, society, and the individuals for whom one was caring.

Concern with moral values and expectations led to the development of the discipline of *ethics*, whose focus is the systematic study of and reflection on morality. All health professions, by virtue of their fiduciary relationships with patients, have developed codes of ethics to set forth moral principles as standards for behavior.

Ethical codes have been present in societies since ancient times, originating from religious principles like service to others without exploitation. The Hippocratic oath is one of the earliest codes (4 B.C.) accepted as a covenant between physicians and patients in the ancient world. This code became the dominant ethical document for all professional medicine in the Western world and is still acknowledged by medical students.

The first code of medical ethics was drafted by the American Medical Association in 1847 and for the next 150 years committed the American Medical Association physician to "render service to humanity" within a paternalistic framework. The patients' rights movement in the 1960s influenced the American Medical Association to update its code of ethics from a *paternalistic* to a *patient-centered* focus (Veatch, 2002). The most recent American Medical Association code of ethics, written in 1981, considers commitment to the rights of patients first (Veatch, 2002).

Nursing, on the other hand, established *dignity and respect for persons* as the most fundamental principle in its original code written in 1976, with *self-determination* as the second most important principle. The American Nurses Association House of Delegates revised the *Code of Ethics for Nurses With Interpretive Statements* in 2001, setting forth the profession's values and standards of conduct for nursing practice (**Exhibit 7–1**). Codes of ethics imply duties and rights and thus stem from the ethical theories of deontology.

Deontology implies that one is acting correctly when guided by rules and duties that come from universal moral principles that undergird religions, such as the Ten Commandments and the Golden Rule. The German philosopher, Immanuel Kant (1724–1804), introduced the concept of "categorical imperative," implying that there is a right and wrong. Persons have an obligation to act morally based on laws (e.g., do right for right's sake). *Obeying the rules is more important than the consequences of the act.* Every individual has inherent dignity and deserves respect; thus professionals have a duty to treat their patients as ends in themselves and never as a means to an end.

Thus it is clear how professional codes of ethics were influenced by this theoretical perspective. The strengths of deontological thinking are that the rules are clearly stated and thus enforceable. Living by rules and codes of behavior maintains a high moral quality of life within communities, because all humans will be respected and treated with dignity.

There are weaknesses within deontological thinking, however. Deontology is based on the assumption that we live in a homogeneous society and not only know what the rules and duties are but are rational and autonomous beings who can understand the rationale for them. Because there

---

Exhibit 7–1 Code of Ethics for Nurses

American Nurses Association Code of Ethics for Nurses

1. The nurse, in all professional relationships, practices with compassion and respect for the inherent dignity, worth, and uniqueness of every individual, unrestricted by considerations of social or economic status, personal attributes, or the nature of health problems.

2. The nurse's primary commitment is to the patient, whether an individual, family, group or community.

3. The nurse promotes, advocates for, and strives to protect the health, safety, and rights of the patient.

4. The nurse is responsible and accountable for individual nursing practice and determines the appropriate delegation of tasks consistent with the nurse's obligation to provide optimum patient care.

5. The nurse owes the same duties to self as to others, including the responsibility to preserve integrity and safety, to maintain competence, and to continue personal and professional growth.

6. The nurse participates in establishing, maintaining, and improving health care environments and conditions of employment conducive to the provision of quality health care and consistent with the values of the profession through individual and collective action.

7. The nurse participates in the advancement of the profession through contributions to practice, education, administration, and knowledge development.

8. The nurse collaborates with the other health professionals and the public in promoting community, national, and international efforts to meet health needs.

9. The profession of nursing, as represented by associations and their members, is responsible for articulating nursing values, for maintaining the integrity of the profession and its practice, and for shaping social policy.

Source: American Nurses Association. *Code of Ethics for Nurses with Interpretive Statements.* (2001). Washington DC: American Nurses Foundation/American Nurses Association.

---

are no exceptions to the rules or any guiding principles that give instruction what to do, we are faced with ethical dilemmas when there is a conflict between two principles (Aiken, 2004). For example, if one cannot tell a lie, should we tell the patient that he or she is getting a placebo?

Ethical problem solving at this individual level is relatively simple but does illustrate the conflicting principles of truth telling with patient autonomy. How does the deontological approach, however, enable professionals to act morally and ethically when serving in more complex systems, such as a hospital that employs many levels of workers and professionals, provides services to many types and cultures of patients, and must demonstrate fiscal responsibility in the delivery of services?

The hospital systems in the early 20th century were managed by physicians and staffed primarily by nurses, both professions being guided by their respective codes of ethics. These codes guided physician and nurse behaviors and moral duties to the patients so that competent care could be delivered. Further, most of the hospitals of the day were operated as nonprofit entities, and many were supported financially by religious systems; thus the professionals in charge of patient care did not have the burden of balancing the budget. Further, the age of technology had not dawned, so patient care was primarily comfort care.

Society accepted that there was a natural life span: a time to be born and a time to die. There were few dilemmas surrounding prolongation of life at either end of the age spectrum. Not only were decisions about life and death simpler but less costly. Conflicts were few between the principle of *justice* (being fair to all in the delivery of treatments) and *autonomy* (the individual's right to freely choose what he or she wants). Thus the deontological approach was generally sufficient for guiding ethical behaviors of the health care professionals.

As hospitals grew into more complex systems, however, management shifted from physician models to business models. The business model gave rise to business ethics, that is, the application of general ethical rules to business behavior such as the *Ethical Policy Statement* issued by the American college of Healthcare Executives. If society's ethical rules say that dishonesty is unethical and immoral, then anyone in the business who is dishonest with employees or customers is acting unethically. On the other hand, recalling a defective product to avoid public harm is an example of an ethical business behavior.

As the management of hospitals shifted from physicians to business administrators, the key to ethical decision making in the hospital system rested with the business administrator. These individuals had the opportunity to set the ethical tone for the organization, depending on their personal values and ethical standards, rather than from a code of ethics (Frederick, Davis, & Post, 1988).

As hospital systems became more complex, *teleological* theories were considered more appropriate to guide ethical decision making within hospitals. These frameworks focus on the ends and on the consequences of actions rather than the means to an end.

The most important teleological theory for health care ethics is *utilitarianism*. Its premise considers that an act or behavior is right if it promotes the best consequences overall. Ethical decisions are based on the principle of providing the greatest good for the greatest number. Actions are right to the degree that they promote overall happiness to the majority. No act is intrinsically good or evil; only the *consequences* of the act are considered (e.g., what consequence brings the most happiness to the greatest number of people). Individual good is considered less important than aggregate.

The theory was developed by two philosophers, Jeremy Bentham (1748–1832) and John Stuart Mill (1806–1873), who were contemporaries of Kant but did not agree with his premises. The strengths of utilitarianism for hospital managers are that ethical decisions are not based on the evaluation of right and wrong behaviors but on policies that promote the general welfare (Purtilo, 2005). For example, when budgeting for scarce resources, it is more likely that purchases of equipment that will serve the most persons will be selected over that which is used by a few (e.g., a computed tomography scanner over six neonatal intensive care unit beds). It is obvious that conflicts are inevitable for health care professionals who are functioning by their codes of ethics based on treating all patients as equals (*deontology*) and are employed within systems that are governed by utilitarianism (*teleology*).

Organizational Ethics

> The patient ideally has a right to a relationship that assures that he/she will be treated with respect and the medical knowledge will be used to further his/her own plans and values.
>
> —*Brody: The Healer's Power*

Business ethics proved to be a limiting system for health care organizations, because the goal of business is primarily an economic, not a service, orientation. Health care organizations have a dual purpose: the delivery of competent, safe care to all patients by committed professionals and faithfulness to the mission of the organization. Thus the philosophy of *organizational ethics* in health care that has emerged since the 1990s and become the best guiding framework for health care institutions has a unique focus on both moral analysis of the individuals in the organization and on the moral life of the institution.

A helpful analogy for thinking about organizational ethics is *ecology*, which considers interactions among cells, organisms, and ecosystems. Similarly, organizational ethics takes into account individuals, teams of health care workers, institutions, integrated delivery systems, and the entire health care environment. Health care organizations possess a distinctive organizational ecology characterized by "their mission of service to alleviate pain and restore patient health, a highly complex regulated environment, many professional cultures, and a rapidly changing healthcare market" (Boyle, DuBose, Ellingson, Guinn, & McCurdy, 2001, p. 10).

The terms *morality* and *ethics* are often used interchangeably but are differentiated in organizational ethics. Morality is defined as the lived experience of making choices and ethics as the systematic reflection on that lived experience. Within health care systems that ascribe to organizational ethics, a method of moral analysis is incorporated into the life of the organization. Moral norms of both the individuals and the organization are evaluated as they apply to the attitudes and goals of the organization. Thus the scope and character of *organizational ethics* includes consideration of the interactions between ethical theories: utilitarianism and deontology; usefulness of the principles of beneficence, nonmaleficence, justice, and autonomy in resolving ethical dilemmas; personal virtues; and formal structures to resolve ethical dilemmas (Boyle et al., 2001).

Ethical Principles

Ethical principles, like ethical theories, represent moral considerations of health care professionals to respect the wishes of competent patients. Some of these, such as veracity, fidelity, dignity, and respect, listed in the professional codes of ethics, refer to attributes of the professional nurse. The four major principles that focus on the patient and family—beneficence, nonmaleficence, autonomy, and justice—are accepted by all health care organizations as basic guides to creating the ethical caliber of the practice environment.

Two ethical principles that undergird prevention or curing of disease and assist patients to maintain their functional abilities are *beneficence* and *nonmaleficence*. Both of these have their origin in the Hippocratic Oath and are foundational to the duties of health care professionals to help persons in need and to refrain from causing harm. Beneficence occurs when the nurse administrator tries to determine what good care is. Generally, good care includes making allowances for the patient's beliefs, feelings, and wishes, as well as those of the family and significant others (Aiken, 2004). Nonmaleficence means that health care providers do no harm to their patients. In real practice this principle is violated as the patient often suffers short-term pain for long-term treatment. This principle also extends to the health care provider protecting those who are vulnerable such as children, the mentally incompetent, the unconscious, and the elderly (Aiken, 2004).

In Western culture the principle of *autonomy* is highly valued. We believe that persons are the best decision makers in matters that affect their life and health. Even advocates of evidence-based medicine conclude that the patient can assess benefits and risks to treatment more adequately than physicians. Under certain circumstances the right to autonomy may be taken away, especially if there is potential harm for someone else's health, well-being, or rights (Aiken, 2004).

The fourth principle, *justice*, refers to a social contract between persons in society as described by John Rawls. This principle supports the obligation to treat one another fairly and to expect to be treated equally regardless of sex, race, marital status, medical diagnosis, social standing, economic level, or religious belief. This principle brings into focus the arguments for a right to health care, a subject too large for the scope of this chapter.

All these principles are important to nurse administrators from the perspective of their relationship to nursing staff rather than to patients. Nurse administrators must do good for the personnel under their jurisdiction and do no harm. All nursing staff have the right to be autonomous in their decision making in matters that concern them.

The most important principle for administrators, however, is justice because they must make decisions about the delivery of services to collective groups of patients. Thus understanding the principle of *distributive justice* is essential for nurses in management. For example, staff nurses are primarily concerned about staffing on their unit, but the administrator must consider the needs on all units and allocate staff accordingly, recognizing that there are greater and lesser needs within the institution. Perhaps some beds must be closed when there is not sufficient staff.

It is helpful for administrators to be familiar with the six parameters of distributive justice. Each approach embodies different values and is used in different situations that lead to different actions as described:

1. *Justice renders to each the same thing.* All persons must be treated the same way, irrespective of age, sex, race, or religion. However, all services are not unlimited, so how does one differentiate need?
2. *Justice renders to each according to his or her work.* This implies that one must discern the best approach for proportional treatment, not equal treatment.
3. *Justice renders to each according to his or her merits.* This principle bases decisions on the basis of personal excellence, like merit raises or career ladder advancement. It is less applicable in instances of distribution of institutional resources.
4. *Justice renders to each according to rank.* This statement presupposes that "rank has its privileges" and could be applied to salary ranges based on educational preparation and experience.
5. *Justice renders to each according to his or her legal entitlement.* Although this approach requires that all persons be accorded their rights under the law and under legally binding contracts, there are many conflicts of legal rights that are difficult to solve.
6. *Justice renders to each according to his or her need.* Considering this principle, it is fair to allocate institutional resources based on patient need, but more questionable to allocate educational resources to promote a person based on personal need only (Curtin & Arnold, 2005).

Another example that illustrates how the parameters of distributive justice can be considered involves a current issue before the American Organization of Nurse Executives. Members of the American Organization of Nurse Executives are recommending that hospitals unbundle inpatient nursing care from daily room and board charges, as has been suggested by the Centers for Medicare and Medicaid Services, to hospital inpatient prospective payment systems (Kerry Weems, Acting Administrator, Centers for Medicare and Medicaid Services, personal communication, June 3, 2008). By following the American Organization of Nurse Executives' recommendation, actual nursing care hours and estimated costs for individual patients will be assigned; thus less complex cases will receive less compensation and more complex cases will receive greater compensation when factoring in the diagnosis-related group relative weights (Dalton, 2007).

If this proposed action is taken, there will be less tendency for hospitals to overvalue services for less complex cases, which can create unwanted incentives for hospitals to specialize in more profitable cases, and to eliminate admission of more complex cases. This is an obvious ethical dilemma, according to parameter 2, *Justice according to work*, and parameter 6, *Justice according to need*. First, it is ethical to give more compensation to a nurse who spends 8 intensive hours caring for a patient than to a nurse who may spend 2 hours caring for a less complex patient. Both nurses should not receive the same compensation. Further, the patient with more complex needs requires more intensive nursing care to promote healing, which may result in a shorter length of stay. This results in cost savings for the hospital in an ethical way.

When nurse administrators consider the six parameters of distributive justice, they are basing their ultimate decisions on meeting the greatest need, even though they may recognize the needs of all.

The four universal ethical principles give us direction and purpose to solve ethical dilemmas. None is absolute, but principles do help us to organize our thoughts, justify our actions, and formulate resolutions to competing claims. Sometimes there are conflicts between the principles. For example, a father feels a moral obligation to donate one of his kidneys to save the life of his daughter (*beneficence*). On the other hand, he desires the freedom to make his own decision because of the risk to his own health and survival (*autonomy*) (Veatch, 2002). When conflicts occur, it is essential to weigh risks and benefits in each situation, taking into account all parties involved and using a decision-making process accepted by the organization. There is not an *a priori* ranking of moral principles. Each situation must be considered individually with input into the resolution by all persons involved in the decision. Some of the considerations are the stakeholders, who wins, who loses, costs, risks, and benefits.

The question arises, "Which principle takes precedence over other principles when weighing issues in an ethical dilemma?" Social workers find *the ethical principles screen* helpful in listing all the principles that are common to patient-centered dilemmas (Dolgoff, Loewenberg, & Harrington, 2005). A multidisciplinary group of health care professional educators reprioritized the list as a teaching tool for nurses, physicians, and social workers (**Exhibit 7–2**).

Nurse administrators could benefit from using this hierarchy in their decision-making process. The first principle is to choose an option that causes the least permanent harm or one that promotes a better quality of life for all persons. The risk-to-benefit ratio will help one to resolve whether autonomy applies and when it is more ethical to ignore one party's decision. Be honest and provide truthful information. Maintain confidentiality because we owe privacy to each other.

Clinical ethics committees function to assist families, patients, and physicians in identifying, analyzing, and resolving ethical dilemmas. Persons on the committees represent physicians, nurses, other professional disciplines, and community members, whose purpose is to foster awareness of clinical ethical issues and to provide insight into solving ethical dilemmas. These dilemmas usually fall into the following areas of consideration: conflicting rights, end-of-life decisions, prioritizing values, family conflicts, decisional-making capacity, and substituted judgment.

Ethics committees vary in their structure from formal entities that meet regularly, providing a forum for discussions, to informal meetings of physicians and nurses when an ethical dilemma is identified. Usually, the ethics committees have developed a process for ethics consults and use a decision-making model to assist in resolving ethical dilemmas. These committees, however, have a relatively narrow focus directed toward dilemmas associated with patient conditions and decisions.

Considering the range of issues within organizations at a macro level, such as employee issues, conflicts of interest, resource management, and external pressures, there is a need for organizational ethics committees to address the challenges of the organization. The American College of Healthcare

---

Exhibit 7–2 Hierarchy of Ethical Principles

1. Do the most good and the least harm.
2. Promote quality of life.
3. Protect life.
4. Promote justice.
5. Consider autonomy and freedom.
6. Be truthful and fully disclose.
7. Respect privacy and confidentiality

Source: Dolgoff, R., Loewenberg, S., & Harrington, E. (2005). *Ethical decisions for social work practice* (p. 65). Belmont, CA: Brooks Cole.

Executives supports the development of mechanisms to deal with general ethical issues and decisions. As leaders in their respective organizations, the executives have a primary role in the development and operation of these ethical mechanisms (American College of Healthcare Executives, 1993).

Thus a code of ethics for health care executives was written in 1995 that contains standards of ethical behavior in their professional relationships. As executives, nurse administrators must embrace this broader code of ethics as well as the American Nurses Association Code for Nursing. The Joint Commission on Accreditation of Healthcare Organizations requires health care organizations to have a mechanism in place to address ethical issues present in health care settings. *Administrative ethics* is distinct from *clinical ethics*, yet the two are interrelated. Nurse administrators are held to a higher responsibility than their employees because they must have loyalty to aggregates of patients as well as to the nursing staff.

Charting the Direction

It is easy to catch the wave, but difficult to stay on top.

—Anonymous

Traditionally, chief nurse executives defined their ethical behaviors governing their practices based on universal values with a focus on the delivery of competent and effective nursing services to all patients. As hospitals become more complex, administrators must be concerned about both nursing ethics and business ethics. Management decisions are strongly influenced by economics, with social and legal ramifications. Administrators must size up the organizational culture or "personality" early in their tenure. Does the culture include an "ethical climate," defined as a pervasive moral atmosphere of a social system (Bell, 2003)?

The *ethical climate* is characterized as shared perceptions of right and wrong and collective assumptions about how moral concerns should be addressed. Organizations with an ethical climate interact responsibly, model integrity, share organizational purpose and direction, and value stakeholder perspectives (Bell, 2003). Nurse administrators in the 21st century hold positions that demand knowledge (the know *what*) and skills (the know *how*) of navigating organizational cultures. Foundational to successful navigation is the development of ethical integrity within the nurse administrator role.

Ethical Leadership of Nursing Administrators

Those who lead in health care must do so by their own example and through actions ensuring that core ethical principles—beneficence, nonmaleficence, honesty, and justice—are embedded into their daily work (Johnson, 2002).

Administrators are nurses first who are obligated to professional codes and outcomes that are duty driven by the standards of the profession to act in the patient's best interest as advocate, to maintain competence, and to keep confidences. *Profession* (from the Latin, *profitere*) literally means "public promises" and implies nurses' social contract. Impose business ethics onto the professional obligations and it is clear that there will be resulting tensions.

Business ethics are generally outcome oriented, stemming from utilitarian principles through the lens of results, aims, and purposes. Functioning within health care organizations, nurse administrators are obligated to act for the common good and to be accountable for the outcomes of their decisions. The dual role of professional and business manager sets up tensions and dilemmas in which both perspectives must be considered. How can administrators lead well in this environment? Six steps are suggested:

1. *Reflect.* Leaders must reflect on the internalized values of the profession and the values of the organization. "Taking time to reflect, taking time to be, allows for profound insights and for breakthrough ideas to arise from the stillness of the leader's being" (Cashman, 2000). Reflection accompanies goal setting, problem solving, and real action. After becoming clear on values and principles, the leader is more able to behave in ways that are more congruent with the priniciples.

2. *"Walk the talk."* The leader must be a role model for the organization in a visible way, living out the values and principles of the organization. Not walking the talk sends a negative message to employees that it is acceptable to stretch the limits of ethical behavior.

3. *Lead like Socrates.* Strong ethical leaders ask difficult questions and create forums in which the ethical dilemmas can be discussed openly. One who leads the way and promotes and participates in the dialogue sends an important message about the importance of ethics in the organization.

4. *Demonstrate courage.* Do the right thing for the right reasons. Foster integrity and fear will be driven from the organization.

5. *Create processes to ensure ethical integrity.* An example is to initiate a review of all operations from an ethical viewpoint.

6. *Search for simplicity.* Consciously move past the complexity to simpler analysis and reflection. Each decision can be broken down into parts, each of which can be analyzed. Maintain one set of values for your life and your work (Johnson, 2002, pp. 6–8).

Organizations with integrity have truly learned that there is no choice but to walk the talk of their values and to be accountable for them (Boyle et al., 2001; Wheatley, 1999). The leader's task is to embody the principles and then to help the organization to understand and become the standard that it has declared. If leaders do not practice what they preach, there is a breakdown of ethical integrity.

Several studies support the fact that top management establishes the ethical tone for the organization. If transgressions are ignored or rewarded in the organization, then others are more likely to take advantage in the future (Kronzon, 1999). If corporate ethics are more transparent, then employees are more perceptive of situations with ethical undertones (Marta, 1999). Leaders can develop moral virtues or character by managing their own motivations and developing integrity (Torres, 2001). An ethical leader must first "know thyself."

Ethical Principles of Nurse Administrators

Administrators frequently must deal with their own ethical dilemmas as a result of their concomitant duty to patients and to the employing institution. When patient and corporate goals are not congruent, administrators face difficult choices (Seifert, 2002). Leah Curtin (2000b) proposes 10 principles for ethical administration that can align the dual roles and duties as patient advocates and organizational managers. These principles reflect universal values and include both utilitarian and deontological points of view:

1. *Frugal and therapeutic elegance*—promotes the right degree of economy of means with the right amount of resources necessary to ensure competent care (respect for life, wisdom, stability, and fairness)

2. *Clinical credibility through organizational competence*—requires disciplining professional practice through the application of current practice guidelines, regular self and peer evaluations, mutual teaching and counseling, and promoting

a. *Organizational competence* through consistent policies that advance the welfare of employees and provide discriminating and flexible staffing and scheduling patterns designed to safeguard patient care (tolerance, responsibility, freedom, women's place, and equity)

3. *Presence*—promotes mutually trusting and beneficent relations with peers, collaborating professionals, patients, families, and members of the general public through communicating decisions in person and monitoring and altering decisions as necessary (love, responsibility, and unity)

4. *Responsible representation*—ensures that the clinical and ethical concerns of nurses are heard at the highest level of organizational decision making (courage, truthfulness, and justice)

5. *Loyal service*—forbids exploiting the organization or the staff to advance one's own career (justice, responsibility, love, and stability)

6. *Deliberate delegation*—demands that the delegation of tasks and duties includes enough authorization to accomplish them; requires an act of trust (fairness, unity, and courage)

7. *Responsible innovation*—requires that organizational change be examined before it is implemented for its impact on patient care and employee morale (respect for life, love, and tolerance)

8. *Fiduciary accountability*—provides value for the dollar in terms of the safety, quality, and relevance of services offered to the community (justice, truthfulness, freedom, responsibility, and hospitality)

9. *Self-discipline*—ensures that decisions made and actions taken are based on careful deliberation, never made in anger or fear, and never for retribution or vengeance (love, tolerance, and responsibility)

10. *Continuous learning*—recognizes that time and resources must be invested in self and staff to ensure continued competence of care and excellence in organizational performance (love, truthfulness, and fairness) (**Exhibit 7–3**).

These principles are not commands so much as they are guides to decision making. When times are difficult, they serve as the "voice of conscience" within each of us.

Typical Ethical Issues of Nurse Administrators

Nurse administrators incur ethical responsibilities for their organization, patients, nursing staff, and the profession. Their obligation is to make decisions within the limited resources available; thus

---

Exhibit 7–3 Curtin's Ten Ethical Principles for Nurse Administrators

1. Frugal and therapeutic elegance.
2. Clinical credibility through organizational competence.
3. Presence.
4. Responsible representation.
5. Loyal service.
6. Deliberate delegation.
7. Responsible innovation.
8. Fiduciary accountability.
9. Self-discipline.
10. Conscious learning.

Source: Curtin, L. (2000). The first ten principles for the ethical administration of nursing services. *Nursing Administration Quarterly, 25*(1), 7–13.

closing beds may be the right thing to do when staffing is unsafe, even though this action may adversely affect the organization's bottom line. Nurse administrators are faced with the same type of problems that other organizational executives have, namely, problems with human relations, potential injustices to minorities, resource management, conflicts between the right thing to do and organizational policy, failure to speak up when unethical practices occur, and supporting the corporate hierarchy as opposed to doing the job well (Boyle et al., 2001).

Studies of administrator dilemmas in the decade of the 1990s focused on the use or allocation of resources and concerns about the quality of care (Borawski, 1995; Cumunas, 1994; Harrison & Roth, 1992; Sietsema & Spradley, 1987; Silva & Lewis, 1991). Demands to decrease budgets "no matter what" led to nurse-to-patient ratios that were unsafe, the use of less skilled personnel for patient care rather than registered nurses, hiring traveling nurses, inadequate salaries, greater workloads, and other economic pressures. Management decisions are strongly influenced by economic, social, and political factors. Riley (2001) found that *nurse administrators experienced three types of ethical conflict—professional role conflict, organizational conflict, and interpersonal conflict.*

In a study by Redman and Fry (2003) the six most frequently experienced issues by New England nurse administrators (in order of frequency) were "protecting patient rights and human dignity (62.7 percent); respecting/not respecting informed consent to treatment (41.4 percent); use/nonuse of physical/chemical restraints (31.7 percent); providing care with possible risks to the registered nurses' health (TB, HIV, violence) (28.3 percent); following/not following advance directives (25.5 percent); and staffing patterns that limit patient access to nursing care (21.9 percent). Note that five of these are patient rights issues, and the sixth is a patient care issue, demonstrating that the influence of one's professional ethics are so imprinted that they often take precedence over organizational ethics" (p. 152).

The six least frequently encountered ethics issues reported by New England nurse administrators were "participating/not participating in euthanasia/assisted suicide; reporting unethical/illegal practices of health professionals or agencies; caring for patients/families who are uninformed or misinformed about treatment, prognosis, or medical alternatives; ignoring patient/family autonomy; discriminatory treatment of patients; and breaches of patient confidentiality or privacy. The first issue is an end-of-life issue; the remaining issues are patient care issues" (Redman & Fry, 2003, p. 152). In organizations where there are ethics committees, the patient care dilemmas are usually addressed within these structures, thus freeing administrators to focus on the broader issues that affect the organization.

A more extensive survey of 4,000 members of the American Organization of Nurse Executives, conducted about the same time, revealed that *quality of service* continued to be the most pressing issue. For example, more than 50% of the respondents agreed that the organization failed to provide quality service consistent with professional standards, failures were due to economic restraints, and that these failures in quality were acknowledged by the health care providers in the organization.

Despite its importance as a causative agent, *economic constraints were not the key cause of the widespread disappointment in quality; it was the conflict between the organizational philosophy and the professional philosophy and standards.* The lack of knowledge or skills to competently perform one's duties (reflecting resource limitations on continuing education and the hiring of less qualified nurses due to the nursing shortage) was ranked higher by nurse executives than by the health care organization. The authors of this study concluded that the quality issues were present because of the conflict between clinical and organizational ethics and the lack of ethics committees to provide input into these dilemmas (Cooper, Frank, Gouty, & Hansen, 2002). Nurse executives were cautioned, however, to manage costs effectively because if this was not done, their organization would not be in business and there would be no worry about quality and outcomes.

A qualitative research study by Gaudine and Beaton (2002) identified four themes of ethical conflict between nurse managers and their organizations. *Voicelessness* was a major concern. Nurse managers were invited to administrative meetings yet were treated as "invisible" members of the group. Comments of the managers included the following:

- Nursing is not valued.
- Nursing is not understood.
- No effort is made to understand nursing.
- Nurse managers are hired because they are perceived to "toe the party line."
- Nurse managers are not present during decision making on issues that affect nursing.
- Nurse manager positions are radically decreased, resulting in minimal nursing input.

Fiscal allocation for resources was the second area of conflict as demonstrated by the following comments:

- Money is spent on acute care instead of long-term care.
- There is a failure to invest in staff development; the focus is on short-term issues instead of the quality of nurses' work life.
- Quality is sacrificed (e.g., substandard patient care or patient/family rights are secondary to a balanced budget).
- Crisis management occurs rather than long-term budgetary planning.

Third, rights of individuals were less valued than operational needs. Nurse managers must be concerned with all nursing staff, not only their workloads but personal concerns such as salary, benefits, and opportunities for career advancement. The managers interviewed in this study stated the following:

- Policies support the hospital's legal needs as opposed to patients' and nurses' needs as perceived by the nurse manager.
- The nurse manager is forced to make decisions that serve the needs of the organization but have negative implications for nurses.

The fourth theme reflected *unjust practices* on the part of senior administration and/or the organization. Interestingly, more comments were made on this issue than on the other issues:

- There are unfair policies used for the promotion and termination of nurse managers.
- Workloads for direct-care nurses and nurse managers are unfair.
- Senior administration fails to act even when aware of a problem.
- Decision making is centralized rather than decentralized.
- Non-nurses are given priority over nurses for first-line supervisory positions.
- There is a punitive absenteeism policy.
- There is a punitive medication-error policy.
- Nurse managers are underpaid.
- The hospital's stated values (e.g., integrity, consultation) are not upheld by the administration and the board.
- There seems to be a lack of interest and lack of information on the part of the board of directors (Gaudine & Beaton, 2002, p. 22).

When nurse administrators did submit suggestions to resolve some of the above dilemmas, they claimed there was negative fallout with the organizational administrators. There was an inability to resolve issues surrounding poor and unsafe patient care, treatment of patient's friends and relatives, and issues of downsizing nursing management. The nurses claimed that their inability to resolve ethical dilemmas was due to personal factors, situational factors, and issues related to the nurse manager:

Personal factors
- Inability to speak out or to act
- Unwillingness of staff nurses to speak out, often due to fear
- Inability to make the needs of nursing understood
- Knowing that senior management is aware of a problem but will do nothing
- Knowing that documenting required changes has been a waste of time

Situational factors
- Fear that the situation will escalate if the nurse manager speaks out
- Poor communication with senior administration, either because of the organization's size or because the administration does not value nursing management
- Some people refuse to negotiate
- Opinions of physicians more valued than those of nurses
- Uninformed board of directors
- Salary inequities among nurse managers
- New nurses for whom nursing is just a job
- Difficulty in recruiting and retaining nurses
- Nurses complain instead of taking constructive action
- Unfair comparisons with other hospitals regarding staffing levels
- Staff aware that other hospitals have better resources or have eliminated their deficits
- Staff aware that other hospitals go beyond the contract
- Staff see money spent on physician retention
- Silence on the part of professional associations and other directors of nursing on an issue for which they are aware
- Staff aware that nurse manager's situation is not unique and that nursing in Canada is in trouble
- Smear campaign against a nurse manager

Factors relating to the nurse manager
- The nurse manager is unable to identify what is right and what is wrong.
- Staff remember when nursing used to be valued.
- Staff need to have a mentor.
- Nurse managers feel trapped because of their number of years in nursing management.
- Nurse managers do not know if they are doing the right thing.
- Nurse managers feel responsibility to improve a situation.
- Nurse managers fail to inform staff nurses of one's efforts to resolve issues of concern to nurses (Gaudine & Beaton, 2002, p. 26).

In this study, nurses provided some insight into factors that would mitigate the nurse managers' ethical conflicts with hospitals: support, problem solving, and refocusing. Actual comments included the following:

Support
- Support from other nurse managers, hospital administrators, physicians, hospital ethics committees, staff nurses, family, and public
- Internal strength gained from knowing that one is morally right
- Internal strength gained from knowing that one is following the Canadian Nurses Association's Code of Ethics

Problem solving and growth
- Problem solving with other nurse managers, hospital administrators, physicians, hospital ethics committee, staff nurses
- Learning to separate personal values from professional responsibilities
- Developing and presenting a proposal to senior administrators

Refocusing
- Hoping that the next generation (of better-educated nurses) will improve nursing
- Focusing on one's own goals and on what one can do
- Focusing on the high quality of care that nurses do provide
- Dwelling on the positive when senior administration begins to address a problem (Gaudine & Beaton, 2002, p. 27)

Negative feelings, such as frustration, anger, fear, resentment, stress, loneliness, demoralization, lack of fulfillment, and powerlessness, arise from being in conflict. Managers may develop a poor self-image because they are undervalued and unsupported. They are concerned about patient safety and the well-being of the staff. Many times they are torn between viewpoints of staff nurses and those of senior administration (Gaudine & Beaton, 2002). These study results are disturbing and have implications for nurse retention.

When conflict exists between managers and the organization, the initial reaction is disappointment from the *moral dilemma* (recognizing more than one right thing to do). If the conflicts are not resolved, nurses experience *moral distress* (knowing the right thing to do but being prevented from doing it). Some may choose the road of being silent, whereas others may leave the institution, contributing to nursing shortage and the lack of problem resolution. The helplessness, hopelessness, powerlessness circle continues. Some administrators are empowered to acknowledge the problems and address them through better work hours, increased salaries, implementing shared governance, and increased autonomy for their staff. Nurse administrators claim they are supported by their professional organizations and look to them for strategies for preventing or coping with ethical conflicts.

Fast forward to 2009 and a snapshot of the health care arena of today. In the classic publication, *To Err Is Human* (Kohn & Donaldson, 1999), issues of hospital errors, unsafe practices, and risks to patients were candidly presented. The result of this publication influenced hospitals to change practice standards that would ensure safety and ethical delivery of care. This publication had indirect effects on the nursing profession and the issues described by the studies quoted above. Two requirements for health care institutions developed and provided incentives to promote a nurturing, therapeutic, and ethical environment. First, to achieve accreditation, the Joint Commission on Accreditation of Healthcare Organizations required that institutions develop and operate under an organizational code of ethics and create ethics committees. Second, the American Nurses Credentialing Center (2003) conceived the magnet hospital program for recognizing excellence in nursing. The expectation is that "knowledgeable, strong, risk-taking nurse leaders follow a well-articulated, strategic and visionary philosophy in day-to-day operations of nursing services" (p. 1). The attributes of magnet hospitals reflect the establishment of a therapeutic work setting in which nurses are recognized as moral agents with rights and duties to provide quality patient care. Organizational chief executive officers must demonstrate evidence that the nurse administrators serve as influential members of the organization's highest decision-making body for strategic planning and operations. In other words, chief nursing officers may not be voiceless. They must give proof of their contributions to decisions that affect staffing, fiscal, and administrative decisions. Their role is vital in decentralization, shared governance, multidisciplinary, and collegial working relationships. Staffing policies must adapt and flex to internal and external factors. Evidence must be demonstrated that ethical codes, theories, and principles are followed by nursing staff in magnet-designated hospitals (see http://www.nursingworld.org/ancc/magnet.htm).

Outcomes, Opportunities, and Challenges

> The need is not only to call attention to the conflicts and problems facing us as a profession and confronting us personally, but also to offer a process for examining these confusing areas and a new way to view change and growth.
>
> *—Diann Ustal*

How Should We Interpret These Findings?

This issue arises again in a study done by Cooper and colleagues (2004) in which they affirm that quality of service continues to be an issue and that the perception of the concern extends beyond the nursing profession to include other providers as well. To overcome the problem in quality, nurse administrators need to examine their own personal contributions to the problem by asking the following questions:

1. Am I taking all appropriate steps necessary to help work through key ethical problems?
2. Am I seeking more information regarding problems that have been identified by staff?
3. Am I helping staff to see the need for the changes in nursing practice, and am I providing them with resources needed for the change?
4. Am I encouraging staff to take risks?
5. Am I motivating staff to focus on new opportunities created by change?
6. Am I participating in and encouraging others to participate in ethics committees?
7. Am I advocating changes to senior managers to improve productivity and job stability?
8. Am I advocating changes to senior managers that I believe are essential in order to provide the best quality patient care?

Shared governance (explained in Chapter 3) can serve as a starting point to change the work environment to one that more closely resembles both organizational ethics and professional ethics.

Nurses in administrative roles tended to report that *39% of the time they had experienced ethical issues*; this was more frequent than that for the staff nurses. The most distressing issue for the nurse administrators was lack of patient access to nursing care, followed by that of prolonging the dying process with inappropriate measures.

Guidelines for Ethical Decision Making

There is little doubt that addressing ethical issues consumes a large amount of the nurse administrator's time and energy and that making these decisions is very difficult. When an ethical leader must grapple with the "rightness" of a decision, he or she must look at possible solutions from all points of view. The best leaders realize that there are few "best" decisions. There will always be those who disagree with the course of action decided upon. For a decision to be good, it must be subjected to analysis and must consider all the stakeholders.

Most ethical leaders choose their battles wisely. There may be times that accepting a less than optimal decision saves political capital and power for issues of significance. This does not mean that a leader should accept actions that are unethical; however, it does mean that ethical decisions are often in the gray area, not black and white. Competent decision-making skill is needed to differentiate between when flexibility is acceptable and when "right is right" without compromise (Sanford, 2006).

Taft (2000) proposed the following guidelines for making decisions in ethical dilemmas:

- Consciously acknowledge the separate but related domains of philosophy, religion, economics, law and government regulation, culture, industry and disciplinary effects, and individual context as they contribute to ethical decision and action.
- Understand that conflicting obligations are the rule, not the exception. In any presenting situation, differentiate one's personal from societal values.
- Identify the ethical value hierarchy of authority that should prevail. Unless a compelling likelihood of immediate or future harm to others is present, the principles of law, government regulation, and explicit organizational policy should rule—in that order.
- When a compelling likelihood of harm to others does exist that is insufficiently addressed by law, regulation, or organizational policy, identify and discuss the ethical situation with trusted peers and managers. Consider both present and future scenarios, and acts both of commission and omission.
- Identify the process and people to engage in addressing the ethical challenge. Marshall peer support and initiate action.
- Understand the contingencies of the situation, including inherent risks for you, the nurse. Know what risks you can assume and what actions you personally are prepared to take as the situation moves toward a valid, or flawed, resolution (pp. 18–19).

These guidelines can be used by the nurse administrator as personal principles to consider on the job.

In addition to these considerations, Sanford (2006) suggests seven steps to ethical management decision making.

1. Identify the issue/question.
2. Identify the stakeholders who will be affected by solution/answer. Consider:
   a. Customers/patients
   b. Staff/employees
   c. The organization
   d. The community
   e. Medical staff
   f. Others
3. List possible solutions/answers.
4. Evaluate each solution from each stakeholder's viewpoint.
5. Identify the organization's decision-making rules.
   a. Do the values and mission of the organization specify or imply greater weight to the good of certain stakeholders? Example: Is individual patient welfare given greater weight than individual employee welfare?
   b. Which solution(s) best serve the common (rather than individual) good?
6. Make a decision.
   a. Are you able to explain why you chose this solution?
   b. Would you feel proud of the decision if it was reported on the front page of your local newspaper (along with your rationale)?

7. Act and reflect on the action.

   a. Evaluate the results of the decision.

   b. Learn from the evaluation to improve ethical decision making in the future.

Note that these steps take into account all stakeholders and the perspective of each. Choices made by the hospital have economic and social effects on the entire community. The moral imperative may not be clear in all cases. All solutions must be considered to ascertain which is most beneficial or least harmful to the organization, the community, the staff, and the individuals involved.

The best decision-making criteria for an organization are often determined before a final decision is made. The leadership teams who are serious about ethics in the management ranks thoroughly examine decisions for ethical content (Sanford, 2006). Institutions who manage themselves by the principles of *organizational ethics* add a "triple bottom line," in which the organization's effects on the environment and societal good are as important as finances (Boyle et al., 2001).

Conclusions

The 21st century demands that ethics should be part of every decision. Health care administrators who choose to lead their organizations from an organizational ethics frame of reference require innovation and departure from doing things as usual. They need to assess the culture and then promote ethical consciousness and conduct among the staff. The administrator must support an environment conducive to providing high-quality, cost-effective health care that also encourages individual ethical development. It is important to seek support from internal and external sources so that success occurs. The administrator has an obligation to accomplish the organization's mission in a way that respects the values of individuals and maximizes their contributions. Competency in ethical decision making is what will make health care a healthier place for everyone.

Discussion Questions

1. Nurse administrators must be attentive to personal codes of ethics and organizational ethics in the management of their job. How do the theories of deontology and utilitarianism inform ethical decision making?
2. Select two ethical conflicts identified in the qualitative study by Gaudine and Beaton. Describe the steps you would take to resolve each dilemma.
3. The chief nursing officer (CNO) of a large community hospital is interested in applying for magnet status, thinking that going through this process would raise the status of nurses in the hospital and the quality of nursing care. What strategies would the CNO use to move the organization in this direction?
4. The CNO of St. Elsewhere Hospital, located in a multiracial area, believes she could serve the community better if she took steps to be more sensitive to her constituents by providing translators for patients, putting up signs in Spanish, and hiring some bilingual staff. The chief executive officer (CEO) and Advisory Board of the hospital verbally agreed to the idea. Time passed and there was not evidence of any of the steps being taken. Then one evening a Spanish-speaking man came to the emergency department with gunshot wounds, was turned away, and almost bled to death. The CNO expressed her ethical concerns about the situation and demanded to know why the recommendations for better cultural care had not been implemented. The CEO replied, "I agree with your concern, but the recommendations are too costly for this hospital."

    a. What are the ethical challenges for all the stakeholders? Who wins? Who loses?
    b. Which priorities are in conflict?
    c. How could the ethical principles hierarchy assist the administrators in resolving the dilemma?
    d. In what circumstances should costs outweigh benefits?

Glossary of Terms

Autonomy—an individual's right to freely choose what she or he wants. In Western culture, the principle of autonomy is highly valued.

Beneficence—occurs when the nurse administrator tries to determine, *what is good care?* Generally, good care includes making allowances for the patient's beliefs, feelings, and wishes, as well as those of the family and significant others.

Business Ethics—the application of general ethical rules to business behavior. Business ethics is primarily outcome oriented. One issue is that the goal of business is primarily economic rather than service.

Clinical Ethics Committees—function to assist families, patients and physicians in identifying, analyzing, and resolving ethical dilemmas. Persons on the committees represent physicians, nurses, other professional disciplines, and community members whose purpose is to foster awareness of clinical ethical issues and to provide insight into solving ethical dilemmas. Usually, the ethics committees have developed a process for ethics consults and use a decision-making model to assist in resolving ethical dilemmas. These committees, however, have a relatively narrow focus directed toward dilemmas associated with patient conditions and decisions.

Code of Ethics—sets forth moral principles as standards for behavior; implies duties and rights.

Deontology—implies that one is acting correctly when guided by rules and duties that come from universal moral principles that undergird religions, such as the Ten Commandments and the Golden Rule.

Distributive Justice—an important principle for nurse administrators who must make judgments about the delivery of services to collective groups of patients. *Understanding the principle of distributive justice is essential for nurses in management.* For example, staff nurses are primarily concerned about staffing on their unit, but the administrator must consider the needs on all units and allocate staff accordingly, recognizing that there are greater and lesser needs within the institution.

Ethical Climate—a pervasive moral atmosphere of a social system; shared perceptions of right and wrong, and collective assumptions about how moral concerns should be addressed.

Ethical Principles—represent moral considerations of health care professionals to respect the wishes of competent patients. Some of these, such as veracity, fidelity, dignity, and respect, are listed in the professional codes of ethics. The four major principles are accepted by all health care organizations as basic guides to the ethical caliber of the practice environment, in which commitment to patients and families is primary.

Ethics—the systematic study of and reflection on morality.

Justice—being fair to all; a social contract between persons in society. This principle supports the obligation to treat one another fairly and to expect to be treated equally regardless of sex, race, marital status, medical diagnosis, social standing, economic level, or religious belief.

Moral dilemma—recognition that there is more than one choice that is right (moral).

Moral distress—recognition of the right thing to do and being prevented from doing it.

Morality—the lived experience of making choices

Nonmaleficence—means that health care providers do no harm to their patients. In real practice this principle is violated as the patient often suffers short-term pain for long-term treatment. This principle also extends to the health care provider protecting those who are vulnerable such as children, the mentally incompetent, the unconscious, and the elderly.

Organizational Ethics—focuses on both moral analysis of the individuals within the organization and on the moral life of the institution. The scope and character of organizational ethics includes consideration of the interactions between ethical theories: utilitarianism and deontology; usefulness of the principles of beneficence, nonmaleficence, justice, and autonomy; personal virtues; and formal structures to resolve ethical dilemmas.

Organizational Ethics Committees—considering the range of issues within organizations at a macro level, such as employee issues, conflicts of interest, resource management, and external pressures, there is a need for organizational ethics committees to address the challenges of the organization. The American College of Healthcare Executives supports the development of mechanisms to deal with general ethical issues and decisions. As leaders in their respective organizations, the executives have a primary role in the development and operation of these ethical mechanisms.

Profession—from the Latin, *profiteer*, literally means "public promises" and implies nurses' social contract.

Teleology—focus on the ends and on the consequences of actions, rather than the means to an end.

Utilitarianism—when an act or behavior is right if it promotes the best consequences overall. Ethical decisions are based on the principle of providing the greatest good for the greatest number.

References

Aiken, T. (2004). *Legal, ethical and political issues in nursing* (2nd ed.). Philadelphia: F. A. Davis.

American College of Healthcare Executives. (1993). *Ethical policy statement.* Chicago: American College of Healthcare Executives.

American College of Healthcare Executives. (1995). *Code of ethics.* Chicago: American College of Healthcare Executives.

American Nurses Association. (2001). *Code of ethics for nurses with interpretive statements.* Washington, DC: American Nurses Foundation/American Nurses Association.

American Nurses Credentialing Center. (2003). *Magnet recognition program standards.* Washington, DC: American Nurses Association.

Bell, S. (2003). Ethical climate in managed care organizations. *Nursing Administration Quarterly, 27*(2), 133–139.

Borawski, D. (1995). Ethical dilemmas for nurse administrators. *Journal of Nursing Administration, 25*, 60–62.

Boyle, P., DuBose, E., Ellingson, S., Guinn, D., & McCurdy, D. (2001). *Organizational ethics in health care.* San Francisco: Jossey-Bass.

Cashman, K. (2000). *Leadership from the inside out.* Provo, UT: Executive Excellence Pub.

Cooper, R., Frank, G., Gouty, C., & Hansen, M. (2002). Key ethical issues encountered in healthcare organizations. *Journal of Nursing Administration, 24*(6), 331–337.

Cooper, R., Frank, G., Hansen, M., & Gouty, C. (2004). Key ethical issues encountered in healthcare organizations. *Journal of Nursing Administration, 34*(3), 149–156.

Cumunas, C. (1994). Ethical dilemmas of nurse executives, Part I. *Journal of Nursing Administration, 24*(7/8), 45–51.

Curtin, L. (2000a). Ethics & nursing administration: Part I. *Curtin Calls, 3*(6), 4–5.

Curtin, L. (2000b). The first ten principles for the ethical administration of nursing services. *Nursing Administration Quarterly, 25*(1), 7–13.

Curtin, L., & Arnold, L. (2005). A framework for analysis, Part II. *Nursing Administration Quarterly, 29*(3), 288–291.

Dalton, K. (2007). A study of charge compression in calculating DRG relative weights. RTI Project Number 0207964.012.008, Prepared for Centers for Medicare and Medicaid Services, Office of Research, Development, and Information. Baltimore, MD: RTI International.

Dolgoff, R., Loewenberg, S., & Harrington, E. (2005). *Ethical decisions for social work practice.* Belmont, CA: Brooks Cole.

Frederick, W., Davis, K., & Post, J. (1988). *Business and society.* New York: McGraw Hill.

Gaudine, A., & Beaton, M. (2002). Employed to go against one's values: Nurse manager's accounts of ethical conflict with their organizations. *Canadian Journal Nursing Research, 34*(2), 17–34.

Harrison, J., & Roth, P. (1992). Ethical dilemmas faced by directors of nursing. *Journal of Long Term Care Administration, 20*(2), 13–16.

Johnson, J. (2002). Six steps to ethical leadership in health care. *Patient Care Management, 18*(2), 1, 5–9.

Kohn, L., & Donaldson, M., (Eds.). (1999). *To err is human.* Washington, DC: National Academies Press.

Kronzon, S. (1999). *The effect of formal policies and informal social learning on perceptions of corporate ethics: Actions speak louder than codes.* Doctoral dissertation, Princeton University, 1999. Dissertation Abstracts International, 60, 1897.

Marta, J. (1999). *An empirical investigation into significant factors of moral reasoning and their influences on ethical judgment and intentions (marketing ethics, Hunt-Vitell model, religiousness).* Doctoral dissertation, Old Dominion University, 1999. Dissertation Abstracts International, 60, 1229.

Nightingale, F. (1859). *Notes on nursing: What it is and what it is not.* Reprinted. Philadelphia: J.B. Lippincott.

Purtilo, R. (2005). *Ethical dimensions in the health professions* (4th ed.). Philadelphia: Elsevier.

Redman, B., & Fry, S. (2003). Ethics and human rights issues experienced by nurses in leadership roles. *Nursing Leadership Forum, 7*(4), 150–156.

Riley, J. (2001). Nurse executives' response to ethical conflict and choice in the workplace. *Nursing Ethics Network.* Retrieved August 8, 2001 from http://www.aone.org/practiceresearch/evolving nurse executive.htm

Sanford, K. (2006). The ethical leader. *Nursing Administration Quarterly, 30*(1), 5–10.

Seifert, P. (2002). Ethics in perioperative practice: Duty to foster an ethical environment. *Association of perioperative Registered Nurses, 76*(3), 490–497.

Sietsema, M., & Spradley, B. (1987). Ethics and administrative decision-making. *Journal of Nursing Administration, 17*(4), 28–32.

Silva, M., & Lewis, C. (1991). Ethics, policy, and allocation of scarce resources in nursing service administration: A pilot study. *Nursing Connections, 4*(2), 44–52.

Taft, S. H. (2000). An inclusive look at the domain of ethics and its application to administrative behavior. *Online Journal of Issues in Nursing.* Retrieved from June 13, 2008 from http://www.journaldatabase.org/articles/91294/An_Inclusive_Look_at_the_.html

Torres, M. (2001). *Character and decision-making.* Doctoral dissertation, University of Illinois at Chicago, 2001. Dissertation Abstracts International, 62, 2485.

Veatch, R. (2002). *The basics of bioethics* (2nd ed.). Upper Saddle River, NJ: Prentice Hall.

Wheatley, M. (1999). *Leadership and the new science.* San Francisco: Berrett-Kohler.

CHAPTER 8

Contemporary Legal Issues for the Nurse Administrator

Frances W. "Billie" Sills, MSN, RN, ARNP, LNC

Any law that takes hold of a man's daily life cannot prevail in a community unless the vast majority of the community are actively in favor of it. The laws that are the most operative are the laws which protect life.

—*Henry Ward Beecher*

Key Terms

- Abuse
- Administrative law
- Burden of Proof
- Case Law
- Civil Actions (Torts)
- Common Law
- Constitutional Law
- Criminal Actions
- Defendant
- Expert Witness
- Felonies
- Fraud
- Intentional Tort
- Malpractice
- Misdemeanor
- Nurse Practice Act
- Plaintiff
- Qui Tan Whistleblower Statute
- Reasonable Nurse
- *Res Ipsa Loquitur* (The Thing Speaks For Itself)
- Respondeat Superior
- *Stare Decisis* (Precedent)
- Statutory Law
- Unintentional Tort

As a nurse manager it is important to have fundamental knowledge of the laws that affect the practice of nursing. This chapter includes: 1) discussion of the Nurse Practice Act, the law that regulates nursing practice; 2) standards of nursing practice, how these standards are applied, and how they are used as evidence during malpractice litigation; 3) the legal significance of your nursing license; and your legal responsibility with delegation rules.

Knowledge regarding the law as it pertains to nursing practice is the best defense a nurse can have. The 21st century is proving to be a century of change. It seems that nurses are finding themselves in a constant state of chaos. The challenge of keeping up with the ongoing technological advances in equipment and procedures; acquiring knowledge on emerging diseases, medications, and diagnostic studies; and evidence-based practice becomes overwhelming. When you add to this the new push for cost containment that forces us to work faster and more efficiently, we often make immediate, crucial choices during high pressure patient care situations. This gives the nurse little time to reflect on the legal and ethical consequences of her or his actions before performing them. Nurse managers not only have to know the law as it pertains to nursing practice, but they need to know the level of under-standing each member of the nursing staff has of the law that governs their practice.

Becoming a registered nurse (RN) means that you have achieved a new status under the law. You now have a license to practice nursing. This license means that each of us is responsible and held accountable for our nursing practice. It is not only important but *essential* that the professional nurse know these standards and the scope of our practice. If we violate the standards and/or practice outside our scope of practice, the state has the authority to suspend or revoke our license to practice nursing.

As a professional you can also be sued for negligence and/or malpractice. When a professional's behavior is negligent and someone gets hurt as a result, the stage is set for a lawsuit. It is also impor-tant to understand that working as a professional, the expectations for your behavior are higher than those of being a "reasonable" person. You are expected to perform as a *reasonable nurse* (one that practices within the scope of practice and upholds the standards of nursing practice). If your actions are determined *not* to be what a right and reasonable nurse would do and your actions cause some-one to be injured in some way, you can be sued for malpractice.

There are three documents that each nurse should have and be familiar with:

1. The Nurse Practice Act for the state in which she or he works
2. American Nurse Association's Standards and Scope of Practice
3. Speciality organizations' standards for the appropriate areas in which she or he works

Each individual nurse (RN, licensed practical/vocational nurse, and advance practice RN) who holds a license to practice nursing is responsible and accountable for his or her own actions. In addi-tion, supervisors are responsible for what they delegate to staff members, ensuring that it is within the individual's scope of practice and that the individual is competent to perform the task delegated.

Legal Aspects of Licensure

Receiving a license to practice nursing is a privilege, not a right. Graduation from an accredited edu-cational program and passing the National Council Licensure Examination for Registered Nurses (NCLEX-RN) does not guarantee that a license will be granted. The state grants a license after the candidate has successfully met all the requirements in that particular state. The license is intended to guarantee public safety while the level of expertise necessary to pass the test is the minimum level needed to provide safe care. The state continues to monitor your practice and to investigate any complaints regarding your practice.

In most states the Nurse Practice Act does the following:

- Describes how to obtain licensure and enter practice in that state
- Describes how and when to renew your license
- Defines the educational requirements for entry into practice
- Provides definitions and the scope of practice for each level of nursing practice
- Describes the process by which individual members of the board of nursing are selected and the categories of membership
- Identifies situations that are grounds for discipline, or circumstances in which a nursing license can be revoked or suspended
- Identifies the process for disciplinary actions, including diversionary techniques
- Outlines the appeal steps if the nurse believes the disciplinary actions taken by the board are not fair or valid

The practice acts vary from state to state; some are very specific and detailed, and others simply grant the board of nursing authority to declare the rules and regulations (administrative law) and to establish the details. To understand the scope of practice within the state that you wish to practice in, you must obtain a copy of the state's nurse practice act that includes the law, rules, and regulations that the board or administrative agency has established in that state.

Remember that knowledge is the best defense against any lawsuits. Each nurse on your staff has the individual responsibility to know the parameters of practice and the rules and regulations that govern their practice that will pay off in the long run.

The power of the board to discipline is power that can have an adverse effect on your ability to practice. Boards of nursing have the authority to censure, to suspend, to revoke, or to deny licensure. You can avoid liability by using caution and common sense and by maintaining a heightened awareness of your legal responsibilities.

Change can be frightening, and there is a tendency to behave like an ostrich and bury one's head in the sand. Although this may seem like a good solution to some who believe *What I don't know cannot hurt me*, nothing could be further from the truth. Ignorance of the law is no excuse when you find yourself in the middle of a lawsuit. A much safer approach is to learn all you can about how the law can affect your ability to practice. The law can be a very helpful tool in ensuring safe nursing practice with positive outcomes. When you know about the law, you are in a better position to protect yourself if you find yourself in a position where you have to deal with some legal issues. It is also important to remember, like everything else in healthcare, the law is always changing, and it takes effort and continuous vigilance to keep up. The first step is to learn what the law is, where it comes from, and the implications of each type.

Definition of the Law

The most common type of law that affects nurses is *statutory law* or *statutes* or *laws*. These are documented rules that govern living in your state (state laws) or the United States (federal laws) that are passed by state legislatures and Congress. Statutes cover the rules for our relationships with each other and can be viewed as the ethics of our society written down. The most important part of a statute is the section on definitions. Here the authors of the statute explain what they meant when they use a certain word. This is very useful because we all use words differently, but in reading the law a more precise understanding is necessary. (For example, *reasonable care* is defined as "the level of care or skill that is customarily rendered by a competent healthcare worker of similar education and experience in providing services to an individual in the community or state in which the person is practicing.") The issue comes up frequently in lawsuits when the question is asked, "What is the difference between the RN and the licensed practical nurse?" The answer lies in the Nurse Practice Act of the state in the scope of practice definition.

The Nurse Practice Act of each state is an example of *state statutory laws* and can be found from the state board of nursing, the public library, or on-line on the state's government website. It is imperative to see how your state defines an RN, an advanced practice nurse, and a licensed practical nurse. In most cases the definition provides you with what the state says a nurse can or cannot do. It is important, however, to keep in mind that as a rule these laws are quite general and may or may not answer a specific question. When in doubt, the best rule of thumb is to contact the state board of nursing and get an answer to your specific question.

Constitutional law refers to the rights, privileges, and responsibilities that are stated in, or have been inferred from, the U.S. Constitution, including the Bill of Rights. States may not pass laws or institute rules that conflict with these constitutionally granted rights or rules because the Constitution is the highest law of our country. Examples of these rights are freedom of speech and religion. The right to privacy is a right that is inferred from the Constitution.

Administrative law is that in which the body of law is made by administrative agencies that have been granted the authority to pass rules and regulations and render opinions, which explain in more detail the state status on a particular subject. Rules and regulations passed by the state board of nursing to control the practice of nursing are an example of administrative law.

Common law is a type of law that includes decisions made by judges in court cases or established by rules of custom and tradition.

Case law is composed of the decisions rendered in court cases by appeals courts. When a decision is reached by an appeals court, a record of the court's opinion and reasoning is recorded. Cases that are appealed to a higher court are ones that involve an issue of statutory law. When a case is appealed and there is a recorded court opinion, the result is the legal principle of *stare decisis*. This means that if an issue has been decided, all other cases concerning the same issue should be decided the same way. This is also known as a *precedent*. Each state has its own body of case law and it differs from other states because it is based on decisions of individual judges who base their decisions on differing state statutes and may resolve issues in a different way.

Classifications of Legal Action

There are two major classifications of legal action that can occur as a result of either deliberate or unintentional violations of legal rules or statutes. The first category is *criminal actions*. A criminal action occurs when an individual has done something that is considered harmful to society as a whole. These cases involve a trial with a prosecuting attorney, who represents the interests of the state or the United States (the public), and a defense attorney, who represents the interests of the individual accused of the crime (defendant). These actions can usually be identified by the title, which will read "*State v. (name of the defendant)*". Examples of criminal action are murder, drug violations, and some violations of the Nurse Practice Act such as misuse of narcotics, abuse, and neglect. Felonies and misdemeanors are the two types of criminal action. *Felonies* are serious crimes that result in the perpetrator's imprisonment. A *misdemeanor* is a crime that results in a fine with no jail time.

The second category of legal claims is *civil actions*. These actions concern private interests and rights between the individuals involved in the case. Civil actions are also known as *torts*. A tort is a civil wrong or injury resulting from a breach of a legal duty that exists by virtue of society's expectations regarding interpersonal conduct or by the assumption of a duty inherent in a professional relationship (as opposed to a legal duty that exists by virtue of a contractual relationship). *Malpractice* refers to a tort committed by a professional acting in a professional capacity.

The law broadly divides torts into two categories: unintentional and intentional. An *unintentional tort* is a civil wrong resulting from the defendant's negligence. An *intentional tort* is a deliberate invasion of someone's legal right. In a malpractice suit involving an intentional tort, the plaintiff doesn't need to prove that you owed him or her a duty. The duty at issue (for example, not to touch an individual without his or her permission) is defined by law, and you are presumed to owe him or her this duty. The plaintiff still must prove that you breached this duty and this breach caused him or her harm. **Exhibit 8–1** shows the actions that can lead to claims in the two categories of tort claims.

The most common unintentional tort action brought against nurses is a malpractice claim. The National Practitioner Data Bank 2003 report stated that 16,339 nurse and nurse-related practitioners had a report made against them between the years 1990 and 2003 (National Practitioner Data Bank, 2004). This number represents claims where payment is made on behalf of a specifically named

---

Exhibit 8–1 Tort Claims and Actions That Lead to Tort Claims

Unintentional Tort

Negligence

- Leaving foreign objects inside a patient after surgery
- Failing to observe a patient as ordered by the physician
- Failing to obtain informed consent before a treatment or procedure
- Failing to report a change in a patient's vital signs or status
- Failing to report a staff member's negligence that you witnessed
- Failing to provide for a patient's safety
- Failing to provide the patient with appropriate teaching before discharge

---

Intentional Tort

Assault

- Threatening a patient

Battery

- Assisting in nonemergency surgery performed without the consent of the patient
- Forcing a patient to ambulate against his or her wishes
- Forcing a patient to submit to injections
- Striking a patient
- Inappropriately restraining a patient

False imprisonment

- Confining a patient to a psychiatric unit without a physician's order
- Refusing to let a patient return home

Invasion of privacy

- Releasing private information about a patient to third parties
- Allowing unauthorized person to read a patient's medical record
- Allowing unauthorized persons to observe a procedure
- Taking pictures of a patient without his or her consent

Slander

- Making false statements about a patient to a third party, which causes damage to the patient's reputation

---

nurse and so does not touch on the number of claims in which a specific facility or corporation was named yet involved nursing actions. Recent reports show an increasing trend in reports against nurses. As a nurse you may worry about being sued for something when, in the eyes of the law, no malpractice has occurred. Not every poor outcome is a case of malpractice. Healthcare professionals can make an error in judgment. For this reason it is important to know the basic elements that must be proven before malpractice can occur.

Our legal system's view of malpractice evolved from the premise that each person is responsible, or liable, for the consequences of his or her actions. *Malpractice law* deals with a professional's liability for negligent acts, omissions, and intentional harm.

An unintentional tort is a civil wrong resulting from the defendant's *negligence*. If you are sued for negligence, the plaintiff must prove four things:

1. You owed him or her a specific duty. In nursing malpractice suits this duty is equivalent to the standards of care.
2. You breached this duty.
3. The plaintiff was harmed (the harm can be physical, mental, emotional, or financial).
4. Your breach of duty caused harm.

Using a hypothetical case, let us look at the four elements to determine if there is a case of malpractice.

Case Study

You are working the 3- to 11-P.M. shift in an acute care hospital and it is time to give one of your patient's his 8 P.M. hydrocortisone IM injection. You make sure that the physician's order in the medical record has not been changed, and when you remove the drug from the medication cart, you check it against the physician's order and find it to be correct. You go to the patient's room, call the patient by name, and check his hospital ID bracelet to ensure that it is the right patient. You give the injection in the patient's left upper outer quadrant of the buttocks and document this on the medication administration record in the medical chart.

The patient leaves the hospital and a year later you are notified by Risk Management that a lawsuit has been filed against the hospital. The patient is claiming that the injection you gave him has caused sciatic nerve damage and his whole leg is numb. Who may have malpractice liability in this situation and why? Is it the nurse, the physician, the hospital? What defenses may be available to you? *Remember the four basic elements that must be present in each malpractice case.* The plaintiff's attorney needs to prove to a jury that each element has occurred. Your attorney defends you by proving that all, or even just one, element did not happen. It is important to understand that this is not always a black and white process, which can often be frustrating and confusing. It is important for the nurse to be able to evaluate the events using the four elements and know how they are proven in court.

1. *Do you have a professional duty?* To make a claim of malpractice against a nurse the plaintiff must establish a nurse–patient relationship or, stated in legal terms, that you had a professional duty to the patient. A *duty* implies that you are employed by and rendered services at a healthcare facility, such as a hospital, clinic, long-term care facility, home health, as a school nurse, or in a physician's office. The first element has been proven. In cases where a nurse has given aid at the scene of an accident or volunteers at sports events or other activities where professional services may be needed, it is important to know what your status would be under such circumstances in your state and/or if you have immunity and/or are covered by malpractice insurance. The contents of a Good Samaritan Act in the state in which you work are good to know.

2. *What was the professional duty owed?* Once it has been established that a professional duty was owed, the question then becomes what is that duty? A nurse's duty owed is different from that of a physician or a nursing assistant. The duty of the nurse is to act as a reasonable nurse under the same or similar circumstances. How does the attorney prove that the nurse acted as a reasonable nurse? Several things are considered when attempting to establish duty using evidence about what the standard of care for that nurse might be:

   a. The *Nurse Practice Act* is probably the most important guideline for what nurses do. Most acts outlines the activities, or scope of practice, that the nurse can legally perform within the jurisdiction. These tend to be described in fairly general terms. Things that are considered unprofessional conduct are generally more specific. A violation of any of these acts means that you have fallen below the standard of care set by the state for nurses. It can also mean that you risk action against your license. Not knowing the contents of the practice act of your state puts you in jeopardy. Therefore it is in your best interest that you keep up with the licensing standards of the state.

b. *Expert witnesses*: The most common method to establish the duty owed by a nurse is by the testimony of an RN, with training and background similar to yours. The expert nurse will testify regarding what a reasonable nurse in the same or similar circumstances would be expected to do and that you did not do it. Testimony by experts is an essential ingredient in malpractice cases for both the plaintiff and defendant, in lawsuits involving nursing care issues.

1. The court's position is that a nurse is the most appropriate expert witness when dealing with the action or decisions made by a nurse. Before 1980 it was common for physicians to testify about the standards for nursing care. In the case of *Young v. Board of Hospital Directors, Lee County* [#82-429 (FL 1984) p. 212], the court concluded that physicians may not determine nursing standards of care. The physician, being unfamiliar with the daily practices of nurses, is unable to set a standard or to testify as to deviation from common nursing practice. The nurse expert witness can explain technology or nursing care in the language jurors can understand. This type of testimony is important to dispel common misconceptions and/or to explain scientific facts as they pertain to nursing care and the care at hand.

2. There is a type of malpractice case in which an expert is not required. This type of claim is called *res ipsa loquitur*, or *the thing speaks for itself*. This claim is very difficult to prove because the patient must have enough evidence to show that (1) the injury would not have occurred unless someone was negligent, (2) the instrumentality causing the injury was within the exclusive control of the defendant, and (3) the incident was not owing to any voluntary action on the part of the plaintiff. If an individual can prove that all these exist, the burden then shifts to the defendant to prove that malpractice did not take place. Cases in which a sponge or instrument was left in a patient or a wrong body part was operated on fall into this category of claims.

c. *Established policies and procedures*: Next to the Nurse Practice Act, established policies and procedures of the institution in which you work are the most crucial pieces of evidence for establishing a *standard of care*. In looking at the case study the attorney would request the hospital's or facility's policies on documentation and administration of medications. If you did not follow the policy of the institution, then you fell below the standard of care set by the institution. It is important that you know and read the policies within your healthcare facility or corporation. These policies are an important resource when you have questions about how to do a certain procedure or what your rights are in certain situations. *Policies* are the laws under which you work. It is important for you as a professional to participate in making or changing policies so that they accurately reflect what nurses are doing in your facility. Because the policies set standards for providing quality and consistent patient care, it follows that it can be used to proactively prove that you followed the standard of care set by your institution.

d. *Accreditation and facility licensing standards*: Most healthcare facilities and other healthcare organizations such as health maintenance organizations (HMOs) must go through a process whereby they become licensed and/or accredited. The Joint Commission and the

National Committee of Quality Assurance (NCQA) are two such organizations that set standards for healthcare organizations. State licensing requirements such as those needed for facilities to admit and treat Medicare and Medicaid recipients also define standards of care. These standards are often used as evidence of a standard of care for nurses working in such facilities.

e. *Textbooks and journals*: If you are involved in a lawsuit, either as a defendant or deposed as a witness, you may be asked about textbooks that are used in the workplace, such as the *Physician's Desk Reference* (*PDR*). You can also be asked if you subscribe to any nursing journals. Articles or portions of such publications may be used as evidence of the standard of care for nurses to follow. The fact that a *PDR* is available to the nurses on the unit might be used to demonstrate that a source for the correct dose, side effects, and the correct administration of the medication was/is immediately available to you at your workplace.

f. *Professional standards for organizations*: Professional organizations, such as the American Nurses Association, (ANA) and the nursing specialty organizations, such as the American Association of Neuroscience Nurses, have published certain standards of care and/or practice guidelines. These may be used as evidence for what a reasonable nurse should do under certain circumstances.

In summary, there are many different types of evidence used by plaintiff attorneys to demonstrate an expected standard of care. The individual nurse and the nurse manager need to remember that these documents can be your *friend* or your *enemy* depending on your knowledge of them and the importance they play in the determination of whether or not the standard of care was met.

Looking again at our case study, the plaintiff will have to find a nurse who can testify to the correct method of giving intramuscular injections. If you did not give the injection the correct way, the jury can then infer that you did not act reasonably. However, if the correct method is to give the injection in the upper, outer quadrant of the buttocks and you have documented that you did this, the testimony of the expert will not prove anything. Also being able to demonstrate that you followed the facility's policies in the administration of medication, there will be no proof of falling below a standard of care.

3. *Was there a breach of professional duty?* The plaintiff must prove what the standard of care is in a given situation and that the nurse did not meet the standard of care. Other legal reasons that are sometimes used are "the nurse fell below the standard of care" or "the nurse breached the duty owed the patient." This means that the plaintiff must demonstrate through the evidence listed that you did not act as a reasonable and prudent nurse under the circumstances.

4. *Did the breach of duty cause the injury? Causation* is the element that is often overlooked by the nurse, and yet it is the issue most often hotly argued by attorneys. Was the injury caused by the nurse improperly administering an intramuscular injection, or did the patient subsequently injure him- or herself after medical care was administered? The causation requirement must be proven by the plaintiff's attorney, and this is not always easy. Certain well-documented observations will make it *impossible* for the plaintiff's attorney to show causation.

a. Clearly document the patient's physical and mental condition upon admission to discharge from your facility. These observations can be used to demonstrate that either the patient had the symptom when she or he came and/or did not have the symptom upon discharge.

b. After any incident, such as a patient fall, the patient's physical and mental condition must be documented. This demonstrates that any subsequent complaints cannot be attached or caused by the incident.

c. Document clearly any actions of a patient that demonstrate noncompliance with medical directives. When a patient is noncompliant with the prescribed treatment, it, rather than the treatment itself, can cause therapeutic failure. A documented "no show" at an outpatient clinic can dispel later claims that the complaints were ignored and therefore caused the injury.

d. It is important to document clearly when a patient complains and when they do not. Again, looking at the case study, if it is documented that the patient had no complaints after the injection, was resting comfortably, and was discharged home with no complaints, it would be difficult to prove that the injection caused the problem.

e. Use caution when documenting what a patient states as opposed to what you believe may have happened. If the patient states that an injection caused the problem, the correct documentation is, "patient states 'my leg has felt numb since I received the injection'" rather than "hospital injection caused patient's leg to become numb."

f. Document clearly the discharge instructions given to the patient and/or a member of the family and the level of understanding demonstrated by the patient and/or the member of the family.

g. Allergies, or lack of, is another important piece of information that needs to be documented. Neither the nurses nor the physicians cause an individual to have allergies. They have a duty to ask, and not give, any medications when the individual has experienced an allergic reaction to it in the past. The documentation of "No Known Allergies" can completely eliminate a claim involving an allergic reaction.

Applying Causation to the Case Study

Let us go back to the case study. The patient will have to prove that the injection given by the nurse caused the numbness in his leg. There are many factors that could have caused the numbness. As the defendant in the case, you do not have to prove anything because you do not have the *burden of proof*. The plaintiff may have a difficult time, especially if there are no documented complaints by the patient at the time of the injection or shortly thereafter. In the case study the nurse documented clearly where she administers the intramuscular injection. Her action was supported by policy and guidelines for the proper administration of an intramuscular injection. The opinion of a nurse expert would further validate this.

It is important to remember that a patient's claim that you or another healthcare provider caused a problem or injury should not automatically be assumed to be true. Untoward events, problems, and/or injuries have many causes and many stories behind them. There are four important things to remember regarding documentation that can protect you from litigation:

1. Document the facts.
2. Document what you see and do.
3. Your role is to provide nursing care and not to judge.
4. Leave the determination of fault to the courts.

Your actions and truthful documentation will be your best defense. In the case study the proper documentation was the evidence needed to demonstrate that the intramuscular injection was not the cause of the numbness in the patient's leg.

Did the Patient Suffer Damages or Injury?

The fourth element of negligence that must be proven is that the actual physical loss or damage was caused by the defendant's negligent conduct. In the case study, numbness of the leg may be difficult to prove. Nerve conduction studies could demonstrate that the injection could not have caused the neurological injury. Numbness does not mean lack of function and would not usually prevent any activity of daily living. The age and status of the plaintiff play an important role, as would your documentation of the lack of patient complaints and the daily ability to ambulate.

Who Is at Risk for Liability (Responsibility) in a Claim?

Personal Liability

Many nurses have asked the question, "Who is responsible for my actions as a nurse?" The simple answer is, "You are." However, how many times have we heard a supervisor, physician, or other healthcare provider say, "Don't worry, I'll take responsibility for this". It is essential that each individual nurse understand that in the eyes of the law, *each individual is accountable for his or her own actions.* There is no defense in the statement, "She made me do it." Even if you are not named in a lawsuit, you will be questioned as to your involvement in the case and you will have to be able to defend your actions under oath. "I was just following orders" does not explain why you as a professional nurse made a medication error. As a professional you are held to a professional standard of care to know about the medication you are administering, including the correct dose, side effects, and action of the drug. If you administer the wrong dose of the medication to a patient, you are going to be held accountable for the error and would most likely have liability.

Physician and Other Independent Practitioner Liability

In the past, the physicians were seen as the "captain of the ship" and thus ultimately responsible for everything that happened to the patient. This doctrine is no longer true. Each professional is responsible and accountable for his or her actions under their individual scope of practice. Many nurses are under the misconception that if they are following the "doctor's orders" they are not accountable if an error occurs. It is true that nurses do have a duty to carry out the physician's orders under most circumstances; however, if the nurse believes or has reason to believe that the order is unsafe for the patient or not within the nurse's scope of practice, it is her or his responsibility *to **refuse** to* carry out the order. For example, if the physician gives an order for the nurse to administer intravenous conscious sedation, it does not relieve the nurse of the duty to determine whether this is in her or his scope of practice.

In a situation where the nurse is hired directly by a physician to work in an office practice, the physician, as an employer, can be held liable on a theory of *respondeat superior*, meaning that the employer is responsible for acts of the employee. The physician then would be named in the lawsuit, but the nurse is still responsible for his or her actions.

Another issue in today's healthcare arena is what the nurse should accept as delegated or ordered by other independent healthcare practitioners, such as nurse practitioners and physician assistants. States have different rules as to who can give orders to the RN, so it is important that you know what the rule is in the state that you are working. The general rule is that the RN can accept orders from other licensed healthcare providers who are working within their scope of practice. It is important to remember that when you accept a delegated duty, you should only accept those that you are competent to carry out and that are within your scope of practice.

Supervisory Liability

The standard of care for a supervisor is to act as a reasonable supervisor under the same or similar circumstances. A supervisor is expected to ensure the following:

- The task was properly assigned to a worker competent to safely perform it.
- Adequate supervision was provided should the worker need it.
- The nurse provided appropriate follow-up and evaluation of the delegated task.

The *delegation of nursing duties* to unlicensed personnel presents supervisory nurses with some special risks. Changes in our healthcare delivery system and its financing are providing us with some unfamiliar categories of unlicensed caregivers with a variety of skills and expertise. Most boards of nursing hold the position that the individual nurse remains personally liable for any task delegated to an unlicensed worker on the theory that the delegated task is considered still to be the nurse's responsibility, rather than within the scope of practice of the unlicensed worker. Certain nursing responsibilities, such as assessment, nursing diagnosis, planning, evaluation, documentation, and teaching, should not be delegated to nonlicensed staff. It is important to contact the board of nursing in your state to better understand your responsibilities in the delegation of nursing duties.

Institutional Liability

Healthcare facilities, such as hospitals, are usually sued under the theory of respondeat superior for the actions of its employees. Almost all healthcare institutions carry insurance to cover the acts and omissions of their employees because the institution cannot do any act that would cause a lawsuit except through its employees. For the most part it is the institution, and not the individual nurse, that is named as the defendant in a lawsuit. This does not relieve the nurse from having to formally answer to the court for his or her actions or inaction. An institution's policies, or lack of them, are also common claims in a lawsuit.

Student/Instructor Liability

Nursing students have responsibility for their own actions and can be liable. The old adage that "students practice under their instructor's license" is no longer true. At the beginning of the nursing program the student will have an instructor supervising the individual closely, but as the student progresses the supervision lessens. Student nurses are held to the same standard of an RN for the tasks that they perform. It is important that students never accept assignments that are beyond their preparation and that they communicate frequently with their instructors for assistance and guidance. *Instructors, like supervisors, are responsible for reasonable and prudent supervision*, a standard that may be higher than that of a work supervisor because of the students' lack of experience.

Liability in Special Practice Settings

If you are a nurse manager in a specialty unit or setting, such as critical care units, emergency departments, or labor and delivery, it is important that you know that nurses are judged by additional standards. Although errors can happen in virtually any practice setting, nurses who work in certain settings are more vulnerable to malpractice charges because the errors are more costly for the patients. The courts may also expect a higher standard of care from nurses who practice in a specialty setting. The nurse manager in these settings must be familiar with the standards of practice set forth by the specialty's professional organization. It is important to remember that the newly graduated nurse has been prepared to be a generalist and not a specialist.

CRITICAL CARE NURSING

Compared with nurses that work on a general floor, nurses who work in the intensive care unit spend more time in direct care of a critical patient, whose condition can change at a moment's notice, increasing the opportunity for errors and the number of potential lawsuits. There are many invasive and potentially harmful procedures performed in this setting; critical care nurses are more vulnerable to charges of *negligence* and *battery*. If for some reason they perform duties or procedures that are outside their scope of practice, they can be accused of practicing without a license. The unilateral severance of a professional relationship with a patient without adequate notice, when the patient still needs attention, or the nurse fails to observe the patient closely for subtle changes in their condition can lead to charges of *abandonment*. Two additional tort claims that can be filed against critical care nurses are *invasion of privacy*, and *failure to obtain informed consent*.

EMERGENCY DEPARTMENT NURSING

The day-to-day practices of emergency department nurses fall into somewhat of a legal gray area because the law's definition of a true emergency is open to interpretation. For example, healthcare workers who treat a patient for what they regard as a true emergency may be liable for *battery* or *failure to obtain informed consent* if the court ultimately concludes that the situation wasn't a true emergency. One of the most common charges filed against emergency department nurses is *failure to assess and report a patient's condition*; however, inadequate triage may be considered *negligence*. Other tort claims that can be made against emergency department nurses include the following:

- *Failure to instruct a patient adequately before discharge*
- *Discounting complaints of pain from a patient who's mentally impaired by alcohol, medication, or injury*
- *Failure to obtain informed consent, giving rise to claims of battery, false imprisonment, and invasion of privacy*

PSYCHIATRIC NURSING

The most common tort claim against psychiatric nurses is *failure to obtain informed consent*. It is wrongly assumed that informed consent is not required, especially if the patient's condition interferes with his or her awareness or understanding of the proposed treatment or procedure. Violation of a patient's right to refuse treatment may stem from the mistaken belief that all mentally ill patients are incompetent. It is important to remember that *the right to refuse treatment is not absolute*: It can be abrogated if a drug or treatment is required to prevent serious harm to self or others. Generally, a physician, not a nurse, makes this decision, and in many cases the court makes the decision.

Malpractice claims may also stem from *failing to protect a patient from inflicting foreseeable harm to him- or herself or others*. Protecting a patient or his or her potential victims from harm may include a duty to *warn the patient's family* that he or she is a threat to him- or herself or a duty to *warn a potential victim*. This duty is a standard of care in mental health practice that has been incorporated as either case law, statutory law, or both in many states. If a nurse fails to report information given to her or him in confidence that could have prevented harm, she or he could be held liable for breaching her or his duty to appropriately assess the patient and for failing to comply with her or his duty to warn.

OBSTETRIC NURSING

Cases that involve labor and delivery *may have at least two plaintiffs: mother and child.* An obstetric nurse may be held liable for the following:

- *Negligence through participation in transfusion of incompatible blood, especially in relation to Rhesus factor incompatibility*
- *Failure to attend to or monitor the mother or the fetus during labor and delivery*
- *Failure to recognize labor symptoms and to provide adequate support and care*
- *Failure to monitor contractions and fetal heart rate, particularly in obstetric units which has internal monitoring capabilities*
- *Failure to recognize high-risk labor patients who demonstrate signs of preeclampsia or other labor complications*

Evidence That Assists in a Lawsuit

Medical Record

It is estimated that *one in four malpractice cases are decided on the basis of what is in the medical record* (Sullivan, 2004). You can become a nurse star or find yourself in deep trouble based on your timely and accurate documentation in the medical record. It is the first piece of evidence the plaintiff attorney asks to see. The nurses' notes are often the first part of the medical record to be examined. The integrity, accuracy, and completeness of the medical record go a long way in making the claim defensible or indefensible.

When the nurse records the care administered, the specific time it was given, the patient's response, and the overall condition of the patient, the nurse can demonstrate that the standard of care was met. We have all heard the adage, "If it is not documented, it wasn't done." In reality, simply, it is difficult to prove that it was done if there is no documentation and the plaintiff claims it was not done. The more accurate statement would be, "If it is documented, then it was done." Once the action has been documented at the time of the event, it is presumpted that the documentation is accurate and whatever a patient says to the contrary is simply not true. This is why it is so important to document extensively, accurately, and factually in the medical record, especially when there is an adverse event.

There are several documentation systems that are used by healthcare facilities:

1. *Source orientated system*: Documentation in this system has each professional's notes kept in a separate system.
2. *Problem-orientated system*: Documentation in this system focuses on the problems identified by all members of the treating team and all members of the treating team document to the problem if appropriate on the progress notes. The notes are formulated using the mnemonic "SOAP" (Subjective data, Objective data, Assessment, Plan).
3. *Traditional narrative format*: The healthcare professional documents the assessment data, interventions, and patient responses in chronological order.
4. *Focus charting*: The patient care problem(s) is the focus of concern and the documentation is specific to the focus.
5. *PIE charting*: In this system information is grouped into three categories: problem, intervention, and evaluation.
6. *Charting by exception*: This system requires the health professional to document only abnormal or significant findings. It relies on written standards of practice that identify nurses' basic responsibilities to patients and protocols for intervention. It includes a standardized care plan based on a nursing diagnosis, in addition to several flow sheets, which allows you to easily track trends.

Charting by exception is the one system that carries with it several legal risks. Because this system relies on written standards of practice that identify the nurse's basic patient responsibilities, there must be well-defined guidelines and standards, and the use of these must be clearly understood by all staff members and used consistently.

Lama v. Boras (P.R. 1994) (p. 75) illustrates what can happen when nurses do not follow accepted standards of care when using charting by exception:

> On May 15th, 1995, R. Romero Lama had surgery for a herniated disk. Two days later, a nurse wrote in his chart that the bandage covering the surgical wound was "very bloody". An entry for the next day indicated he had pain at the incision site. On May 19th, a nurse documented the bandage was "soiled again". The next day Mr. Romero Lama began to complain of severe back discomfort; he passed the night screaming in pain. On May 21st the physician diagnosed an infection in the space between the vertebral disks, and ordered antibiotics. The patient was hospitalized for several months to treat the infection. Mr. Romero Lama sued the hospital and the physicians treating him, alleging that they failed to prepare and monitor proper medical records. The hospital did not dispute the charge that the nurses did not supply the required notes, instead they pointed out that they followed the hospital's official CEB policy.

The court ruled against the hospital on the grounds that Puerto Rican law requires qualitative nurse's notes for each nursing skill, and the violation of this regulation caused Mr. Lama's injury. The court reasoned that a more complete picture of his evolving condition was unavailable because the hospital's charting by exception policy called for nurses to note qualitative observations only when needed to chronicle important clinical changes. Although objective aspects of the patient's care and condition (temperature, vital signs, and medications) were charted regularly, important details, such as the changing condition of the surgical wound and the patient's reports of increasing pain, were not (*Lama v. Boras* [P.R. 1994], p. 75).

The medical record is presumed to be accurate if there is no evidence of fraud or tampering. Evidence of tampering can cause the record to be ruled inadmissible as evidence in court. Medical records may be corrected if the portion in error remains legible; deleting or rendering the entry illegible can impose liability. Late entries are usually acceptable if they are clearly marked "late entry" when made. Loss of the medical record raises a presumption of negligence (which can be overcome by contrary evidence). Nursing documentation must be complete, accurate, and timely to foster continuity of care. It should always cover the following:

- The initial assessment using the nursing process and applicable nursing diagnoses
- Nursing actions, particularly reports to the physician
- Ongoing assessments, including their frequency
- Variations from the assessment and plan of action
- Accountability information, including forms signed by the patient, location of patient's valuables, and patient education including patient's understanding of material taught
- Notation of care by other disciplines, including physician visits, if appropriate
- Health teaching including content and response
- Procedures and diagnostic tests
- Patient's response to therapy, particularly to nursing interventions, drugs, and diagnostic tests
- Statements made by the patient
- Patient comfort and safety measures

There are many factors that influence nursing documentation standards that include

- Federal statutes and regulations
- State regulations and statutes, including licensing statutes and nurse practice acts
- Custom
- Accrediting bodies
- Standards of practice issued by professional organizations
- Institutional policies and procedures

As a facility develops policies and procedures regarding documentation, it has integrated the appropriate laws, regulations, and standards into its own policy and procedure manual. Your best assurance of following the law is to adhere to the facility's policy, which should describe who is to maintain each portion of a patient's record and by which system. A good way for the nurse manager to be aware of the quality and content of the documentation in each patient's record and the quality of the documentation done by the nursing staff is to have periodic chart audits done by the staff on randomly selected charts of the patients on the unit.

DEFENSIVE CHARTING: A GOOD DEFENSE

All healthcare professionals should know some *simple guidelines for good defensive charting*. It is one way to protect you from liability. Some tried and true guidelines are as follows:

1. All entries must be accurate and factual.
2. If a correction is needed, it should be done appropriately and according to the facility's policies.
3. Never obliterate or destroy any information that is, or has been, in the chart.
4. If you realize that you forgot to include something in your documentation, you should make a "late entry," noting the time the "late entry" charting actually occurred and the specific time the actual charting occurred. For example, (7/22/08) "2200 late entry, charting to reflect that on 7/22/08 at 1200."
5. Identify all patient problems, nursing actions taken, and patient responses. A patient problem should not be documented without a nursing action and the patient response also charted.
6. Document why you did not do something you would routinely do. For example, "Pt. refused to ambulate because of...."
7. Be as objective as possible in your charting. The note should read, "Patient ambulated to the end of the hall, tolerated well, no shortness of breath noted, R-22, P rate 98, no complaints of discomfort," rather than, "Patient ambulated, tolerated well."
8. In the case of a fall or some other untoward event, chart exactly what happened, what action was taken and the patient's response, the time the physician was notified, the time she or he responded, any orders given and the follow-up of those orders, and any other individuals notified, such as family members.
9. It is important that your notes are legible and clearly reflect the information you intend.
10. It is equally important to review notes from other providers as the medical record is used for communication and it should demonstrate that the team members are coordinating efforts and thought.

Situations That Put the Nurse at High Risk for a Lawsuit

Equipment Failure

In today's healthcare environment nurses can feel that more time is spent nursing the equipment than the patient. It is true that we now practice in a very "high-tech" world, and with all the advances in medical technology comes more responsibility for the nurse. There is a certain standard of care that is connected to the equipment that we use. *It must be used as directed by the manufacturer, and the nurse has a duty to know what that is and follow such directions.* There is also a duty to make sure that the equipment is free from defects.

As the nurse manager you are responsible to see that the equipment used on your unit is in correct working order and that your staff understand the importance of reporting (and taking out of service if possible) any piece of equipment that is not working properly. The hospital procedure for repairing equipment that is not working properly should be followed with the proper documentation. Nurses also need to exercise reasonable care in selecting equipment for specific procedures and patients. For example, if your patient is obese and a regular blood pressure cuff does not fit properly, you need to have available a large cuff for such patients. This is because if it does not fit properly, the reading could be inaccurate, thus placing the patient in jeopardy. This jeopardizes your practice as well because it does not meet the standard of patient care. The nurse can also be held liable for improper use of equipment that is functioning properly. This liability often occurs with equipment that cause burns.

Healthcare Facility's Responsibility for Patient Safety

Each healthcare facility shares responsibility for the patient's safety. This institutional responsibility for patient safety rests on the two most frequently used doctrines of malpractice liability.

The first doctrine, *corporate liability*, holds the healthcare facility liable for its own wrongful conduct—for breach of its duties as mandated by statutory laws, common law, and applicable rules and regulations. Over time, the courts have expanded the concept of an institution's liability for breaching its duties. In a landmark case, *Darling v. Charleston Community Hospital* (1965) the Illinois Supreme Court [33III, 2nd 326, 211 N.E. 2d 253 (1965), pp. 55–56] expanded the concept of hospital corporate liability to include the hospital's responsibility to supervise the quality of care given to its patients. In *Thompson v. The Nason Hospital* (1991) [527 PA. 330 A.2d 703 (1991)] the courts went further and discussed four general areas of corporate liability:

1. A duty to use reasonable care to maintain safe facilities and equipment
2. A duty to staff the hospital with only competent physicians
3. A duty to oversee all individuals practicing medicine within the hospital
4. A duty to develop and enforce policies and procedures designed to ensure quality patient care

The second doctrine of institutional malpractice liability is *respondeat superior*. Under this doctrine the facility is liable for an employee's wrongful conduct. Basically, this means that both the employee and the facility can be found liable for a breach of duty to the patient, including the duty of ensuring his or her safety.

Medication Errors

A study of 36 hospitals and nursing homes found that 20% of all medications administered involved some sort of mistake. All of them involved a violation of the classic five "rights" of medication administration—the failure to administer the right drug to the right patient, in the right amount, by the right route, and at the right time (Lafleur, 2004). Another study claimed that 770,000 hospital patients experienced an adverse drug event yearly and that almost half of these were preventable, such as those attributable to miscalculations, drug interactions, or drug allergies (Guido, 2001). The increased costs for these errors may be $2 billion for the nation as a whole (Kohn, Corrigan, & Donaldson, 2000). Claims involving medication errors are increased when the nurse fails to record the medication administration properly, fails to recognize side effects or contraindication, and/or fails to know the individual patient's allergies.

The Joint Commission's 2004 and 2005 national safety goals require that institutions develop bar code technology for matching patients with their medications and other treatments. Initiatives that improve patient safety also lower the chance of someone being sued. But, it also sets a new standard on which the standard of care may rest and therefore it is important for every nurse to know and follow. *The nurse's ability to listen to a patient or a family member who mentions that the medication is new or to recheck when anything about the patient seems unusual may prevent a serious error.* Although many nurses believe they just don't have the time to recheck something, making that check a priority will prove to be time well spent. Dealing with the error and the many consequences it can cause will take more time and can place the patient and the nurse in jeopardy.

Providing a Safe Environment for the Patient

Safety is being recognized more and more as a duty of healthcare institutions (The Joint Commission, 2004). The nurse manager plays multiple roles in this area. Staff must know how equipment should work and not use it if it is not functioning properly; removing obvious hazards such as chemicals, which could be mistaken for medications; and making the environment free of hazards such as inappropriately placed furniture or equipment and spills on the floor. *An important preventive measure is knowing how to document correctly if an incident occurs,* so that there can be no doubt regarding the facts of what happened and all you did to protect the patient.

Patient falls represent one of the primary risks in this category, second to medication errors, in numbers of untoward events. The following case study illustrates how inattention to the safety of your patient and the environment can not only endanger the patient but make you and the facility liable for injuries that the patient may incur:

> *Cooper v. Rehabilitation Facility at Austin* (1998) [d/b/a/ Appeal from 353rd District Court of Travis County], the plaintiff, Ms. Cooper, age 71 had a history of rheumatoid arthritis but was found to be a good candidate for a knee replacement. In preparation for her upcoming surgery, she was admitted to a rehabilitation hospital to increase her mobility. While nurses attempted to transfer her from a wheelchair to a bed, she complained of pain, nausea and fainted. Eventually, she was transferred to a bed, given pain medication and O_2 by mask, while her physician was notified of the incident. Later that day, it was determined that she had a fractured right tibia and fibula. The next day, after she continued to complain of pain in her left leg, her left tibia and fibula were found to also be fractured. The patient sued the hospital, nurses, and physician. She settled her case against the physician and agreed to a non-suit regarding her claim against the nurses, but went to trial against the hospital alone on a charge of negligence. The jury found the hospital vicariously liable for the nurses' negligence in transferring her to the bed as well as for the other healthcare professionals who failed to diagnose and treat her injuries in a timely manner. They found in favor of Ms Cooper for the amount of 1,200,000 dollars. The hospital appealed but the verdict was upheld. The considerable sum of damages was based on the pain and suffering that Ms Cooper experienced as well as the change in her circumstances. Prior to the fractures, she still had the ability to perform some activities herself and hoped by having the surgery she would be able to do even more. It was obvious from the medical records that she was making progress before the fractures occurred. The court found that she entered the hospital to gain mobility and independence, not to lose it.

This case is a good example of how nurses and the facility failed to protect the patient either by being involved in the patient's fall or by failing to assess a patient's risk for falling. Generally, a lawsuit is brought when the fall results in a serious injury such as a fracture and/or head injury.

Nurses are best able to defend themselves in these cases when the institution has a policy regarding the protection of patients against falls. In many facilities it is call a "fall protocol." These policies establish levels of risk for patients, taking into account factors such as age, confusion, sedation, and/or preexisting conditions that might cause the patient to be unstable. Assessment for fall risk at the time of admission and periodically depending on the level of risk is one of the most important activities the nurse can do. The next most important thing is the documentation completed when a patient falls. The nurse's first duty when a patient falls is to the patient. This involves the following:

- Assess the patient immediately for possible injuries.
- Notify the physician about the fall and your assessment findings.
- Make sure that the patient is protected from further injury.
- Notify the family as soon as possible.

Documentation is extremely important and the following should be considered:

- Factually document how the fall was discovered, where the patient was found, and any other fact surrounding the fall.
- Document what the patient says regarding the fall.
- Document who you notified and the time.
- Document what was done for the patient, such as your assessment, the exam by a physician, any x-rays taken and the time, monitoring after the incident, and any changes in the current plan of care.

Failure to Adequately Assess, Monitor, and Obtain Assistance

There continues to be an increase in the number of cases when there is an inadequate nursing assessment or a failure to monitor and/or reuse and obtain needed medical assistance for a patient whose condition is changing or has deteriorated. Delegation of the RN's responsibility of assessing and evaluating patient care is being seen more and more in the healthcare system today. If some portions of this duty are done by others (such as another RN, licensed practical nurse, or unlicensed personal), the nurse primarily responsible for the care of the patient must still be aware of the findings and confirm them when they indicate a change in the patient's condition or progress. Again, the documentation of the changes and events surrounding them is critical. When it is necessary to report these changes to a physician or other healthcare professional, sometimes this involves challenging the physician/other professional staff. This can cause discomfort for you as the nurse manager or your experienced staff, not just the new graduate. The nurse must have current and accurate information. These situations require the difficult balance between assertiveness and diplomacy. These are skills that can be taught but are perfected with practice and experience.

Failure to Communicate

Communication is perhaps the most important role of everyone on the healthcare team. The Joint Commission (2005) included improved communications in its *National Patient Safety Goals.* The patient's total care rests on whether the communication occurs in the medical record or through verbal communication. One of the most frequent claims against nurses in this area is the failure to communicate changes in the patient's condition to a professional with a need to know. This communication needs to be documented and should include the time, who you spoke to, what was reported, and the individual's response.

Failure to Report

Several states have statutes that require healthcare professionals to report certain incidences or occurrences. If the provider fails to report as required and an individual is injured, there can be negligence per se, and no expert testimony is needed to prove the case. In addition, both institutional and professional licensure can be affected. Nurses need to be aware of the reporting statutes in the state in which they practice. In some states it is not only a duty but the law to report certain incidents. Institutional policies and Nurse Practice Acts on these topics are invaluable and make excellent topics for review at an educational meeting or seminar.

Short Staffed or Understaffing

What is adequate staffing? Unfortunately, there are few legal guidelines to help you, the nurse administrator, to answer this question. There are a few guidelines that do exist; however, they vary from state to state and are limited mainly to specialty care units (such as the intensive care unit). Even the Joint Commission offers little help. Its staffing standard sets no specific nurse-to-patient ratio. It just generally states, "The organization provides an adequate number of staff whose qualifications are commensurate with defined job responsibilities and applicable licensure, law, regulation, and certification."

California lawmakers have taken note of this and in 1999 passed a bill that required hospitals to meet minimum nurse-to-patient ratios in all units based on patient acuity, prohibiting nurses from being assigned to areas for which they lack adequate orientation or clinical training. In 2002 the California Department of Health Services announced nurse-to-patient ratios, but other states have not followed suit. This gives the courts no reliable standard for ruling on cases of alleged understaffing. Each case has been decided on an individual basis.

There have been some important court rulings regarding understaffing. The decision in the landmark case *Darling v. Charleston Community Memorial Hospital* (1965) [33III.2nd 326, 211 N.E. 2d 253 (1965), pp. 55–56] was based partly on the issue of understaffing. The case dealt with a young man who broke his leg playing football and was taken to Charleston's emergency department where the on-call physician set and casted his leg. The patient began complaining of pain almost immediately. Later, his toes became swollen and dark, then cold and insensitive, and a stench pervaded his room. Nurses checked his leg only a few times a day, and they failed to report the worsening condition. When the cast was removed 3 days later, the necrotic condition of the leg was apparent. After several surgical attempts to save the leg, it was amputated below the knee. The court found the hospital liable for failing to have enough specially trained nurses available at all times to recognize the patient's serious condition and alert the medical staff.

Since this case there have been several similar cases cited: for example, *Cline v. Lun* (1973) [31, Cal App.3d 755, 107 Cal Rptr.629 (1973), pp. 98–99, 189], *Sanchez v. Bay General Hospital* (1981) [172 California Rptr. 342], and *Harrell v. Louis Smith Memorial Hospital* (1990) [(197 Ga App. 189) (397 SE2nd 746)]. Almost every case involved a nurse who failed to continuously monitor the patient's condition—especially vital signs—and report changes to the attending physician. In each of these cases, the courts have emphasized

- The need for sufficient numbers of nurses to continuously monitor a patient's condition
- The need for nurses who are specially trained to recognize signs and symptoms that require a physician's immediate intervention

Hospital Liability

Courts have held hospitals primarily liable in lawsuits in which nurse understaffing is the key issue. A hospital can be found liable for patient injuries if it accepts more patients than its facilities or nursing staff can accommodate. The hospital controls the budget and, in the court's view, is the only party that can resolve the problem. That being said, there are many different defenses that have been offered by the hospitals (for example, there were no extra nurses available or lack of funding for additional nursing staff). The courts have been hesitant to accept either of these defenses, particularly when the hospital has allowed the understaffing condition to exist for a long period of time.

Nurse Administrator, Nurse Manager, or Charge Nurse Liability

You as the nurse administrator/nurse manager/charge nurse, for a specific amount of time, may find yourself personally liable in understaffing situations:

1. You know that the unit is understaffed but you fail to notify administration.
2. You fail to assign your staff properly and then fail to supervise their actions continuously.
3. You (or your staff) try to perform a nursing task for which you (or she or he) lacks the necessary training and skills.

It is important to understand that *you are not automatically liable for mistakes made by a nurse on your staff* even though it may seem like it by now. Most courts won't hold you responsible unless you knew or should have known the nurse who made the mistake:

1. Had previously made similar mistakes
2. Was not competent to perform the task
3. Had acted on the manager's erroneous orders

Remember, the plaintiff-patient has to prove two things, that you failed to follow customary practices, thereby contributing to the mistake, and that the mistake caused the patient's injuries.

Other staffing situations that you, as the nurse manager, can find yourself facing include the following:

1. *Sudden overload of patients*: You begin the shift and suddenly find yourself with more patients than you have staff to safely care for. What do you do?
   a. First, make every effort to protest the overload and get it reduced. Begin by asking your supervisor or director of nursing services to supply relief. If they can't, or won't, your next step is to notify the hospital administration. Whether you receive help or not, it is important to write a memorandum detailing exactly what you did and the answers that you received. *Do not* walk off the job as you can be charged with patient abandonment. Instead, do the best you can. After the shift is over, prepare a written report of the facts and file it with the director of nursing.
2. *Floating*
   a. If your facility "floats" nurses to other units than they have been assigned to, then the facility should have established policies that clearly state the competencies required of nurses asked to float to a unit other than the one where they usually work.
   b. The facility should also have a contingency plan if no such nurses are available. The policy should also delineate the method of orientation for nurses who are floated to another unit.
3. *Mandatory overtime*
   a. Most nurses, and particularly nurse managers, would agree that mandatory overtime is a chronic, inappropriate response to poor staffing policies. It raises safety issues when the nurse has already worked a 12-hour shift and is too tired to continue to work safely. The practice of requiring nurses to work mandatory overtime spread throughout the country beginning in 2000 and is still continuing in some areas. In studies of

mandatory overtime in other industries, the U.S. Department of Labor found that increasing scheduled work time increased time lost to absenteeism and increased injuries, and it usually required 3 hours of work to produce an additional 2 hours of productivity (Thomas, 1990).

In the healthcare arena mandatory overtime by medical residents is implied to be linked to significant number of patients' deaths as a result of care being delivered by exhausted residents.

Realistic concerns about nurses' ability to provide safe care were amplified by the release of the three Institute of Medicine documents: *The Adequacy of Nurse Staffing in Hospitals and Nursing Homes* (Wunderlich, Sloan, & Davis, 1996), *To Err is Human: Building a Safer Health Care System* (Kohn, Corrigan, & Donaldson, 2000), and *Keeping Patients Safe: Transforming the Work Environment of Nurses* (Page, 2004). The number of nursing staff available to provide inpatient nursing care is linked to patient safety as shown by a substantial growing number of research studies. Aiken, Clarke, Sloane, Sochalski, & Siber (2002) showed that an increased patient load is directly related to more patient deaths, as well as higher levels of stress and burnout in nurses. These documents and studies provide you, the nurse manager, with sound evidence to advocate for appropriate staffing which improves both patient and financial outcomes.

4. *Temporary employees*
   a. The addition of agency or traveling nurses presents its own unique set of challenges for the nurse manager. Each time that you have a "temporary nurse" assigned to your unit, you must provide orientation and assess the competencies before making patient care assignments. Failure to appropriately assess the competencies of the nurse can open the door to breakdown in the standard of care, especially if the temporary nurse lacks the requisite competencies and thereby causes harm to a patient.

The mistaken belief that "a nurse is a nurse is a nurse" is constantly being disproven in this 21st century of high-tech patient care. The ongoing increase of potential lawsuits holds testimony to this. The above issues regarding staffing are certainly not inclusive of the multitude of problems and challenges you face on a daily basis as you struggle to provide safe, evidenced-based, high-quality clinical care to the patients on your unit.

Fraud and Abuse

Unfortunately, within our current healthcare system, there are many examples of fraud and abuse in healthcare that go way beyond the nurse administrator role. Sometimes nurses will become involved with these, so it is important to be aware of them and to avoid getting involved with them at all costs.

The Centers for Medicare and Medicaid Services (CMS) describes fraud as "the intentional deception or misrepresentation that an individual knows to be false or does not believe to be true and makes, knowing that the deception could result in some unauthorized benefit to himself/herself or some other person" or agency. *Fraud* typically involves the following:

- Overutilization—providing unnecessary services
- Upcoding—assigning a current procedure terminology code that reflects a higher level of service than actually was provided
- Billing for services not provided—the only issue to be resolved is whether the bill was submitted intentionally or through oversight
- Failing to provide necessary services—capitation penalizes the healthcare professional for overutilization; thus, providers may be monetarily encouraged to underserve patients

- Filing false cost reports—typically filed by providers who are paid under Medicare Part A, including hospitals, skilled nursing facilities and home health agencies (e.g., disguising an unallowable cost as an allowable cost)
- Enrolling fictitious participants in health maintenance organizations (Lovitky, 1997, pp. 42–44)
- Misrepresenting the patient's diagnosis to justify the services or equipment furnished
- Unbundling or exploding—altering claim forms or billing for separate parts of a single procedure to obtain a higher payment or using split-billing schemes
- Looping—using insurance benefits of one member for billing for services provided for another. This is known to be more frequent when services are provided for more than one family member at the same time
- Double billing—deliberately applying for duplicate payment, that is, billing Medicare and a private insurer for the same services
- Phantom billing—billing for services rendered by an agency that is not certified as a Medicare participant through one that is certified
- Kickbacks—soliciting, offering, or receiving rebates/remunerations and bribes from other healthcare agencies or durable medical equipment companies (Tahan, 1999, p. 19).

A Medicare statute, "otherwise known as the Anti-Kickback Act" (Lovitky, 1997, p. 44) now deals with this last issue. Examples of this are when a physician refers a patient for laboratory tests to a lab owned by the physician or a family member or "several physicians have been prosecuted for accepting payment from hospitals in exchange for referring Medicare patients to those hospitals. Similar types of prosecutions have occurred with respect to illegal payments made by durable medical equipment suppliers to nursing homes and home health agencies" (Lovitky, 1997, pp. 44–45). Furthermore:

> Distinguishing between fraud and mere negligence is imperative. Fraud generally occurs when individuals knowingly disregard the truth by submitting intentionally false claims. A mere oversight or an inadvertent error will not rise to the level of fraud; however, a pattern of oversights or errors may increase the likelihood of fraud liability. One cannot escape liability merely by intentionally not learning the truth about health claims being submitted. The government will prosecute "ostrich" behavior. Similarly, liability may not be avoided merely by outsourcing billing functions to a billing company. Typically, the government will assert its claims against both the principal and the agent in this type of circumstance (Lovitky, 1997, pp. 42–44).

Abuse, which is not easy to prove, is billing for excessive charges, services not provided or not medically necessary, or undocumented care. CMS defines abuse as "incidents or practices… that are inconsistent with accepted sound medical practices, directly or indirectly resulting in unnecessary costs… or improper payment… for services that fail to meet professionally recognized standards." Familiar examples are the unnecessary surgery issue with hysterectomies, tonsillectomies, caesarean sections, and coronary bypass surgeries and unnecessary hospitalizations, unnecessary tests, unnecessary medications, or unnecessary physician visits. Abuse can also occur when patients are denied their rights, experience verbal or physical abuse, or are restrained unnecessarily.

Fraudulent claims are probably costing billions of dollars—both for insurance companies and from our tax dollars. Medicare fraud was found to be 14% when the federal government did the first comprehensive audit of Medicare. This prompted the federal government to start The National Health Care Anti-Fraud Association in 1985, both to discover fraud and abuse and to teach about it. Several additional acts have aimed at increasing the federal government's effectiveness in this issue. Meanwhile, both the Attorney General's office and the Department of Health and Human Services have begun investigating and heavily fining persons or organizations involved in fraudulent claims.

In 1998 "as part of its Medicare fraud-busting campaign, [CMS] launched a program … that enlists the country's 39 million Medicare beneficiaries. As the program's 'eyes and ears in the field,' …seniors can report a suspected case of fraud to the agency and collect a bounty of up to $1,000. The money comes from funds recovered from providers.… [Seniors are doing just that, and] not all of them want money.… They see it as their personal responsibility" (Haugh, 1999, p. 16). This is called the "qui tan whistleblower statute." This law allows private individuals to sue on behalf of the U.S. government when they become aware of fraudulent activities. "The private citizen bringing the suit obtains a reward—usually 15 percent to 30 percent of any amounts collected by the government. Qui Tam suits have resulted in several large dollar awards in which millions have been paid to the whistleblower (Lovitky, 1997, pp. 42–44).

The False Claims Act remains the keystone of fraud and abuse prosecutions. Between the years 1987 and 2005 $15 billion were spent in False Claims Act settlements and judgments. Healthcare was responsible for 33% or $5 billion. In 2006 alone, it was $3.17 billion with healthcare in excess of $2.2 billion or over 70%. We wonder why healthcare costs continue to spiral out of control.

Where does the nurse come into all this?

> The ethos of the corporation and the urgency for profit maximization place pressures on healthcare corporations to act in a way that may be incompatible with ethical practice. Profit-driven incentives often result in corporate deviance and criminal behavior. Nurses may be pressured to go along with schemes that may be unethical or illegal and because of shaky job markets may be unable to adhere to professional ethical guidelines.… Dirty hands cases are those instances in which one agent is morally forced by someone else's immorality to do what is, or otherwise would be, wrong.… Problems of this kind have been labeled by some as "dirty hands" situations, because the circumstances are such that the agent is left with a "moral stain" after taking an action (Mohr & Mahon, 1996, pp. 28–29).

As a nurse manager in the 21st century you are challenged to manage units that are constantly admitting and discharging higher acuity patients, to motivate and coordinate a variety of diverse health professionals and nonprofessionals, to embrace change that will develop work environments that are safer and more conducive to professional nursing practice, and to manage limited resources and shrinking budgets. Basic knowledge of the law as it pertains to nursing practice is another tool to add to your management skills arsenal.

Your role as a nurse manager places you in the position to affect change not only in providing quality patient care but having a work environment that nurses want to be part of. As a role model, mentor, counselor, financial manager, and negotiator, you are one of the most important pieces of the puzzle that has to fit together to provide the safe, quality care. Remember,

> The law is good, if a man uses it lawfully.

> *—The First Epistle of Paul the Apostle to Timothy 1:8*

Useful Web sites and References

www.nursingworld.org (American Nurses Association)
www.ncsbn.org (National Council of State Boards of Nursing)
www.ashrm.org (American Society for Healthcare Risk Management)
www.fda.gov (Federal Food and Drug Administration)
www.jcaho.org (The Joint Commission)

www.cms.hhs.gov (Centers for Medicare and Medicaid Services)
www.ahrq.gov (Agency for Healthcare Quality and Research)

Brennan, J., Jr. (2007). *Update on fraud and abuse issues impacting hospitals and physicians.* Baltimore: AHLA Institute on Medicare and Medicaid Payment Issues.

Cherry, B., & Jacob, S. (2005). *Contemporary nursing: Issues, trends & management* (3rd ed.). St. Louis, MO: Elsevier Mosby.

Clark A. (May 2003). Malpractice prevention and technology expertise. *Clinical Nurse Specialist, 17*(3), 126–127.

Helm, A. (2003). *Nursing malpractice: Sidestepping legal minefields.* Philadelphia: Lippincott Williams & Wilkins.

Nurse's Legal Handbook (5th ed.). (2004). Philadelphia: Lippincott Williams & Wilkins.

Discussion Questions

A 9-year-old boy was admitted to the emergency room with an acute asthma attack. Solu-Medrol, magnesium sulfate, and breathing treatments with albuterol did not open his airway so that he could breathe on his own. The young man became combative from lack of oxygen. Lidocaine and ketamine were given in preparation for a rapid sequence intubation. Then, one of the nurses gave succinylcholine, which immediately paralyzed the respiratory muscles. It was clearly contrary to hospital policy for the nurse to administer succinylcholine, as opposed to the physician doing the intubation. No one started bagging the boy for 4 minutes; then it took almost 20 more minutes to intubate him, during which time he went into a full-blown cardiac arrest. He was successfully resuscitated but suffers from brain damage as a result of oxygen deprivation.

1. Identify what kind of constitutional law has been broken and why.
2. Using the basic elements of malpractice, discuss if the case meets the criteria for causation.
3. In the case study, who may have malpractice liability in this situation and why? The nurse, the physician, the hospital? Discuss the defenses that may be available to you.
4. The medical record provides legal proof of the nature and quality of care that the patient receives. Using the case study, discuss what documentation you should find in the chart regarding this incident. What finding do you believe would be key in the plaintiff's case?

Answers to the Discussion Questions

1. Identify what kind of constitutional law has been broken and why.
Administrative law. The Nurse Practice Act, which defines the scope of practice of the RN. The question that needs to be answered is did she function outside the scope of practice as defined in the state practice act. The fact that it is against hospital policy does not make it against the law but certainly puts the nurse in the position of disciplinary action by the hospital and she could also be reported to the board for "unsafe practice."
2. Using the basic elements of malpractice, discuss if the case meets the criteria for causation.
   a. Did the nurse have a professional duty? Yes, a nurse–patient relationship began when treatment was started.
   b. What is the professional duty owed? The duty of the nurse is different from the physician or EMT. The duty of the nurse is to act as a reasonable nurse under the same or similar circumstances.
   c. Was there a breach of professional duty? Yes, the nurse violated hospital policy and possibly the Nurse Practice Act.

d. Did the breach of duty cause the injury? Yes, the patient suffered brain damage as a result of the injection of the medication.

e. However, even though it may seem clear that malpractice occurred, the causation requirement must be proven by the plaintiff's attorney and this may not be easy.

3. In the case study, who may have malpractice liability in this situation and why? The nurse, the physician, the hospital? Discuss the defenses that may be available to you.

It could be all three depending on the situation. The plaintiff's attorney would have to prove that the nurse gave the injection, on her own, without directions from the physician to do so. The hospital's policy would have to be clear as to whether there were any circumstances in which the nurse would be allowed to administer the drug and what were the parameters. The physician would have to defend his actions, if he gave the order for the nurse to administer the drug. It is important to remember that not all poor outcomes are the result of malpractice.

4. The medical record provides legal proof of the nature and quality of care that the patient receives. Using the case study, discuss what documentation you should find in the chart regarding this incident. What finding do you think would be key in the plaintiff's case?

a. Admission time, immediate assessment findings, drugs given, time, dosage, and route

b. Actions of the members of the team as the patient continued to deteriorate

c. The key findings in this case are the time frames and the action of the nurse

Result: Besides the nurse's error the court faulted the whole treatment team for rapid sequence intubation not being started until 12 minutes after the emergency department physician first determined that the medications were not opening the boy's airway. *Turner v. US, 2008 WL* (M.D. Fla., July 1, 2008) (the defendant in this case was the United States as the incident occurred in a military hospital).

Glossary of Terms

Abuse—billing for excessive charges, services not provided or not medically necessary, or undocumented care.

Administrative law—where the body of law is made by administrative agencies that have been granted the authority to pass rules and regulations and render opinions, which explain in more detail the state status on a particular subject. *Common law* is a type of law that includes decisions made by judges in court cases, or established by rules of custom and tradition.

Burden of Proof—The plaintiff has to prove that the incident occurred.

Case Law—composed of the decisions rendered in court cases by appeals courts.

Civil Actions (Torts)—a civil wrong or injury resulting from a breach of a legal duty that exists by virtue of society's expectations regarding interpersonal conduct or by the assumption of a duty inherent in a professional relationship (as opposed to a legal duty that exists by virtue of a contractual relationship).

Common Law—a type of law that includes decisions made by judges in court cases, or established by rules of custom and tradition.

Constitutional Law—refers to the rights, privileges, and responsibilities that are stated in, or have been inferred from, the U.S. Constitution, including the Bill of Rights. States may not pass laws or institute rules that conflict with these constitutionally granted rights or rules because the Constitution is the highest law of our country. Examples of these rights are freedom of speech and religion. The right to privacy is a right that is inferred from the Constitution.

Criminal Actions—occurs when an individual has done something that is considered harmful to society as a whole. These cases involve a trial with a prosecuting attorney, who represents the interests of the state or the United States (the public), and a defense attorney, who represents the interests of the individual accused of the crime (defendant). These actions can usually be identified by the title, which will read "*State v. (name of the defendant)*".

Defendant—the person accused of the crime.

Expert Witness—the most common method to establish the duty owed by a nurse is by the testimony of an RN, with training and background similar to yours. The expert nurse will testify regarding what a reasonable nurse in the same or similar circumstances would be expected to do, and that you did not do it. Testimony by experts is an essential ingredient in malpractice cases for both the plaintiff and defendant, in lawsuits involving nursing care issues.

Felonies— serious crimes that result in the perpetrator being imprisoned.

Fraud—"the intentional deception or misrepresentation that an individual knows to be false or does not believe to be true and makes, knowing that the deception could result in some unauthorized benefit to himself/herself or some other person" or agency (CMS).

Intentional Tort—a deliberate invasion of someone's legal right. In a malpractice suit involving an intentional tort, the plaintiff doesn't need to prove that you owed him or her a duty. The duty at issue (for example, not to touch an individual without his or her permission) is defined by law, and you are presumed to owe him or her this duty. The plaintiff still must prove that you breached this duty and this breach caused him or her harm.

Malpractice—refers to a tort committed by a professional acting in a professional capacity. Malpractice law deals with a professional's liability for negligent acts, omissions and intentional harm.

Misdemeanor— a crime that results in a fine with no jail time.

Nurse Practice Act— probably the most important guideline for what nurses do. Most acts outline the activities, or scope of practice, that the nurse can legally perform within the jurisdiction. These tend to be described in fairly general terms. Things that are considered unprofessional conduct are generally more specific. A violation of any of these acts means that you have fallen below the standard of care set by the state for nurses. It can also mean that you risk action against your license.

Plaintiff—the injured person in the lawsuit.

Qui Tan Whistleblower Statute—In 1998 "as part of its Medicare fraud-busting campaign, [CMS] launched a program … that enlists the country's 39 million Medicare beneficiaries. As the program's 'eyes and ears in the field,' … seniors can report a suspected case of fraud to the agency and collect a bounty of up to $1,000. The money comes from funds recovered from providers" (Haugh, 1999, p. 16). This is called the "qui tan whistleblower statute." This law allows private individuals to sue on behalf of the U.S. government when they become aware of fraudulent activities. The private citizen bringing the suit obtains a reward—usually 15% to 30% of any amounts collected by the government.

Res Ipsa Loquitur **(The Thing Speaks For Itself)**—a type of malpractice case in which an expert is not required.

Reasonable Nurse—a nurse that practices within the scope of practice and upholds the standards of nursing practice.

Respondeat Superior—means that the employer is responsible for acts of the employee.

***Stare Decisis* (Precedent)**—when a decision is reached by an appeals court, a record of the court's opinion and reasoning is recorded, the result is the legal principle of *stare decisis*. This means that if an issue has been decided, all other cases concerning the same issue should be decided the same way. This is also known as a *"precedent."*

Statutory Law—the most common type of law that affects nurses. Statutes (laws) are documented rules that govern living in your state (state laws) or the United States (federal laws) that are passed by state legislatures and Congress. Statutes cover the rules for our relationships with each other and can be viewed as the ethics of our society written down. The most important part of a statute is the section on definitions. Here the authors of the statute explain what they meant when they use a certain word.

Unintentional Tort—a civil wrong resulting from the defendant's negligence.

References

Aiken, L., Clarke, S., Sloane, D., Sochalski, J., & Siber, J. (2002). Hospital nurse staffing and patient mortality, nurse burnout, and job dissatisfaction. *Journal of the American Medical Association, 288*(16), 1987–1993.

Guido, G. (2001). *Legal and ethical issues in nursing.* Upper Saddle River, NJ: Prentice Hall.

The Joint Commission. (2004). *Comprehensive accreditation manual for hospitals: The official handbook.* Oakbrook Terrace, IL: JCAHO.

The Joint Commission. (2005). *National patient safety goals.* Oakbrook Terrace, IL: JCAHO.

Kohn, L., Corrigan, J., & Donaldson, M. (2000). *To err is human: Building a safer health system.* Washington, DC: National Academy Press.

Lafleur, K. (2004). Tackling med errors with technology. *RN, 27*(5), 29–31.

Lovitky, J.A. (1997). Health care fraud: a growing problem. *Nurse Managers. 28*(11), 42–45.

Mohr, W.K., & Mahon, M.M. (1996). Dirty hands: the underside of marketplace health care. *ANS Advanced Nursing Science. 19*(1), 28–37.

National Practitioner Data Bank. (2004). *2004 Annual report.* Washington, DC: U.S. Department of Health and Human Services.

Page, A. (2004). *Keeping patients safe: Transforming the work environment of nurses.* Washington, DC: Institute of Medicine.

Sullivan, G. (2004). Does your charting measure up? *RN, 17*(3), 75–79.

Tahan, H.A., (1999). Home healthcare under fire: fraud and abuse. *JONAS Healthcare Law Ethics Regulations. 1*(1), 16–24.

Thomas, H. (1990). *Effects of scheduled overtime on labor productivity: A literature review and analysis.* Document 60. Austin TX: Construction Industry Institute.

Wunderlich, G., Sloan, F., & Davis, C. (1996). *Nursing staff in hospitals and nursing homes: Is it adequate?* Institute of Medicine Committee on the Adequacy of Nurse Staffing in Hospitals and Nursing Homes. Washington DC: National Academy Press.

Zerwekh, J., & Claborn, J. (2006). *Nursing today: Transition and trends* (5th ed.). St. Louis, MO: Saunders Elsevier.

PART IV

Healthcare and the Economy

Many times nurses do not understand how the healthcare economy affects their practice. They complain about all the administrative budget cuts or talk about the insurance companies as being the "bad guys," yet they do not realize why all this is happening to them. Thus, here in Part IV, we present an economic background that helps nurses to understand how we got here. Hopefully, we can now more effectively deal with all our current problems.

Chapter 9, How We Got to Where We Are, shows how we became a tertiary care, illness-based system that often does not meet the needs of our population lucky enough to have health insurance. Historically, when most people were ill someone in the home cared for them. Amazingly, we are moving back toward that model again. Meanwhile, one can see how insurance companies surfaced; how Social Security, Medicare, and Medicaid coverage emerged as the most prominent player in healthcare; how legislation like the Hill-Burton Act drove the healthcare industry in a certain direction; and how prospective payment has affected the care given. This has led to an ineffective healthcare system, which probably will not be able to pay for itself in a few years. The healthcare industry fiber is further strained as the high cost of drugs, combined with healthcare personnel shortages and an aging population, are having a profound affect on all of us.

Chapter 10 is concerned with the five stakeholders in healthcare: consumers, providers, payers, suppliers, and regulators. All are interrelated, and this chapter gives one a better understanding of each. Our current dilemma is that we have not figured out how to achieve all three healthcare needs at once: universal coverage, paying for it, and containing costs.

Chapter 11 is about microeconomics. This chapter identifies four major forces that healthcare facilities face today: competition, regulation, the profit motive, and quality patient care. These key forces are examined from a microeconomic and cost accounting perspective for the nurse administrator.

CHAPTER 9

How We Got to Where We Are!

Janne Dunham-Taylor, PhD, RN
Joellen Edwards, PhD, RN

> In ancient Asian cultures, citizens paid their doctors to keep them well. If people got sick, it was the doctor's responsibility to take care of them for free (Gottlieb, 2001, p. 23).

How Did We Get Into This Mess?

Presently, healthcare is a wonderful, complicated economic quagmire and a lot needs fixing. The term "health" care is a misnomer; it is really "illness" care that we most frequently address. We use the term "healthcare" in this book but only because it is the common nomenclature for our illness system. Historically, in this country we have pursued treating illness rather than studying and implementing what brings about good health. Research on promoting and achieving health is happening, but there are much larger amounts of money being spent on such things as treating cancer, heart problems, and strokes—the leading causes of death—*after* they occur rather than on *how we can achieve health and avoid illness*. Are we seeing the glass half empty rather than half full? Perhaps if we could get beyond the causes of death (or, rather, concentrate on what happens as we live because we will all die anyway), we would be better off. *Quality of life* is what matters.

We know that our present piecemeal approach to "illness" care has many serious problems. Throughout this last century, there have been a number of both unsuccessful and partially successful attempts to fix the healthcare system through the development of policies at all levels of government. In our country's approach to governance of healthcare issues, we tend to create policies that address specific, isolated problems rather than develop policies that promote a well-coordinated system that makes healthcare accessible and affordable to everyone. Our dubious position as the only highly developed nation that fails to provide basic health services to all its citizens creates unacceptable disparities in the health of our population and persistently maintains a fragmented approach to provision of healthcare. So how did we get into this quagmire? Examining our path will give us a better understanding of the present situation and unresolved dilemmas and offer us some idea of what may come next. Hopefully, we will use systems thinking (defined in Chapter 3) on a national level and learn from our past mistakes. Here's how we got to where we are.

Foundations of Healthcare: Early Days of Our Country

Early in this country's history, medical care was provided by women in the family who took care of relatives in the home. There was no formal education or training for these women. Instead, women relied on their personal knowledge and experience, and if they got any education or training at all, it was from other family members or neighbors who were "healers" themselves or, if they could read, from books.

Physicians, if available, were consulted in more complicated or extreme medical situations. Formal medical education was not accessible until the 1800s. A person could become a physician by apprenticing with another practitioner, and little scientific basis for the profession existed. There was no mechanism for testing competence; anyone could hang out a shingle.

Healthcare was a private matter, paid for by patients or their families with cash or barter. There was no regulatory interference from governments or supportive services from governments to protect and improve people's health. As our nation matured, governmental regulation of many aspects of health-related issues occurred. Over time, local, state, and federal governments became more and more involved in ensuring public well-being through regulations about health professions education and licensing, especially for physicians and nurses; the direct provision of healthcare through agencies and hospitals; and the promotion of sanitation and prevention of epidemics through formal public health departments. Eventually, governments became involved in the regulation of payments for healthcare services, creating a direct connection with the current economics of healthcare.

The development of the public health system serves as a good example of gradually increasing governmental regulation of health-related issues. Public health activities first began in larger cities in the early 1800s. The main focus was sanitation and prevention of epidemics for such things as smallpox, typhoid fever, and diphtheria. Regulations were concerned with waste removal, swamp drainage, and street drainage. If epidemics occurred, they would quarantine homes or ships. Later, as immunizations were developed, public health officials got involved with administering them. The first state board of health was formed in 1869 in Massachusetts. By 1900 each state had a board of health that worked on the above issues with local boards of health. Today, a myriad of public laws and regulations affect people's health, and departments of health at national, state, and local levels assess health needs, monitor compliance with health regulations, and implement programs to improve the public's health.

Collectively, the rules and regulations that define who gets which healthcare services, who can deliver them, and how those services are paid for are the core of the health policies that continuously affect every citizen's well-being. *Health policy* can be defined as the entire collection of authoritative decisions related to health that are made at any level of government through the public policymaking process. These decisions include those of the executive, legislative, and judicial branches of government (Longest, Rakich, & Darr, 2000). Healthcare policies in the United States have in the past and currently continue to attempt to address three specific aspects related to public health concerns. These concerns are *access to* healthcare services, *cost and cost control* of healthcare services, and the *quality* of healthcare available to the population. The remainder of this chapter examines the development of healthcare policies, developed over time in our nation's history, that address access to, cost, and quality of healthcare, issues of constant concern to nurse administrators.

Policies Addressing Access to Care

Access, or the *availability of care*, is a huge issue for the U.S. healthcare system, and one that is growing rather than shrinking. Access can be defined as the use of personal health services in the context of all factors that impede or facilitate getting needed care (Andersen & Davidson, 2007).

Our system is unique in the developed world in that we do not systematically provide basic healthcare services for the entire population. One key factor in gaining access to services in this country is the ability to pay for them.

Medicare and Medicaid, federal and state programs discussed in this section and in Chapter 10, pay for various kinds of care for 27.0% of our citizens. The Indian Health Service offers basic healthcare to Native Americans living on reservations. Private insurance, most commonly obtained through employers with costs shared between employers and employees, covers 59.7% of the U.S. population, although many find themselves "underinsured" when it is time to pay the healthcare bills. Still, more than 47 million individuals have no healthcare coverage at all, leaving them to pay healthcare bills directly, in the old-fashioned way, from their own pockets or to seek care through safety net providers such as free clinics, rural health clinics, or federally qualified health centers (DeNavas-Walt, Proctor, & Smith, 2007). An increasing number of individuals *face bankruptcy* every year due to healthcare bills they cannot pay.

Access is not just about cost, however. Access also includes effective and efficient delivery of healthcare services, meaning that the services need to be culturally acceptable and geographically accessible, as well as delivered at a cost the user can afford.

Access to Direct Services: Hospitals and Beyond

Access to care beyond that available in the home was addressed by creating hospitals, nursing homes, and in-home care by trained nurses. Hospitals and nursing homes existed in the early 1800s but in those days existed on voluntary charitable contributions and served the indigent; were quarantine hospitals, opened and closed sporadically by public health officials to deal with epidemic diseases such as smallpox, yellow fever, or, later, tuberculosis; or were for the wealthy who could pay for the services (i.e., hiding a family member with a psychiatric illness in an insane asylum). By the mid-1800s instruments such as the stethoscope, thermometer, sphygmomanometer, and microscope were introduced; air was viewed as a disinfectant so good ventilation became important; antiseptic procedures were introduced; better ways had been discovered to manage pain in surgery; and, later, the x-ray was invented.

As all this developed, the wealthy started coming to hospitals for treatment because of the technology available there. This changed hospital design. After World War II, wards were replaced with semiprivate rooms, and thus the numbers of nurses needed to care for patients increased. Hospital financing was dramatically increased and resulted in more hospital construction. The matrons became nurse administrators. Nursing homes—supported by a community fraternal or church group—were also established for the poor or for populations that were difficult to manage in the home, including those experiencing mental illness, impaired children, and frail elders.

In the early 1900s visiting nurse agencies were started, especially in larger cities, to make healthcare more accessible for primarily poor residents. If able, clients paid a small fee for services provided. The visiting nurse agency board raised funds to support their work with the poor. Public health departments broadened to include maternal and child services and, in the slums of large cities, to detect tuberculosis (which had become the leading cause of death) and to control venereal disease. This drew opposition from physicians who thought this was within their practice domain, but health policy decisions supported and expanded access to care through these avenues. For instance, in 1935 federal monies were made available to local and state health departments for these purposes, thus strengthening the public health departments significantly.

Social Security Act

A major societal shift occurred that dramatically affected healthcare in the midst of the Depression: In 1935 the Social Security Act was passed. Until this event, local and state governments and individuals and families had been responsible for services for the poor. In a landmark legislative effort, the Social Security Act shifted that responsibility to the federal government. Although not specifically intended to provide healthcare services, the Social Security Act provided funds for health-related programs for the poor in areas such as public health, maternal and child health, crippled children's programs, and benefits for the elderly and disabled. This act started the era of *entitlement*. Perhaps Peter Drucker summarizes this best:

> During the last fifty years, society in every developed country has become a society of institutions. Every major social task, whether economic performance or healthcare, education or the protection of the environment, the pursuit of new knowledge or defense, is today being entrusted to big organizations, designed for perpetuity and managed by their own managements (1974, p. 3).

The Social Security Act of 1935 also dramatically affected the nursing home industry. This Act specified that money be given to private nursing homes and excluded—later repealed—public institutions. Thus for-profit and proprietary nursing homes (privately owned) proliferated to serve the welfare patient. These homes gave first priority to paying patients because the government reimbursement was substantially lower. Sound familiar? A 1948 Amendment made construction grants available to private and nonprofit nursing homes. Later, the proprietary homes did succeed in getting Congress to make Federal Housing Authority (FHA) construction grants available for investor-owned facilities.

Healthcare Access Changes After World War II

Our healthcare system, as we know it today, emerged post-World War II. Hospitals were built as anesthesia agents, medicines, and technologies—along with government money to build hospitals through the 1946 Hill-Burton Act—became available. National legislation now emphasized secondary/tertiary care—highly technical hospital-based care—rather than primary care—defined as preventive, restorative, or medical treatment given while the patient lives at home. Hill-Burton funds focused especially on building hospitals in rural areas, creating geographical access to services that had not previously been available. Hill-Burton also required state-level planning for healthcare services.

Psychiatric treatment also changed dramatically. With the advent of psychotropic medications, more psychiatric patients could be treated in outpatient settings. In 1963 the federal government established community mental health centers for this purpose. Thus many psychiatric patients who had been hospitalized for years were able to leave the hospitals and function in the community setting. Unfortunately, those who were more severely mentally ill suffered greatly, as less money was available for their care. Funding for community mental health centers has continued to decline.

Medicare and Medicaid: New Forms of Access

Until 1965 the federal government financed little in the way of direct healthcare services, concentrating only on some public health issues and providing services for military personnel and Native Americans. State and local governments established and supported special facilities for mental illness, mental retardation, and communicable diseases such as tuberculosis. Less than half of the elderly and disabled Americans had health insurance.

Then in a wave of entitlement programming, the federal government really became enmeshed in healthcare by establishing Medicare and Medicaid. Naturally, this Social Security Act Amendment (Titles XVIII and XIX) benefitted the elderly and the poor and gave them more access to healthcare, but providers—hospitals, other healthcare organizations, physicians, and even suppliers and the building industry—benefitted as well. Medicare often became the largest source of revenue for healthcare providers, resulting in more hospital and long-term care building programs. As more personnel were needed for all the expansion and new building, additional federal programs were funded to supply more physicians, nurses, and allied health professionals.

Although Medicaid was (and is) particularly fraught with tension between federal regulators and states (where the plan is administered), both Medicare and Medicaid opened previously unavailable access to the elderly, the disabled, and the poor. Both Medicare and Medicaid pay for hospital and long-term care, primary care, and some preventive services.

Medicare induced significant changes in long-term care. The federal government redefined who was eligible to care for Medicare patients—skilled nursing facilities (SNF) and intermediate care facilities (ICF)—and set standards for the care that was delivered.

> A skilled nursing facility (SNF) is a nursing home that has been certified as meeting Federal standards within the meaning of the Social Security Act. It provides the level of care that comes closest to hospital care with 24-hour nursing services. Regular medical supervision and rehabilitation therapy are also provided. Generally, a skilled nursing facility cares for convalescent patients and those with long-term illnesses.
>
> An intermediate care facility (ICF) is also certified and meets Federal standards and provides less extensive health-related care and services. It has regular nursing service, but not around the clock. Most intermediate care facilities carry on rehabilitation programs, but the emphasis is on personal care and social services. Mainly, these homes serve people who are not fully capable of living by themselves, yet are not necessarily ill enough to need 24-hour nursing care (Raffel & Raffel, 1994, p. 183).

Medicare and Medicaid also infused the home health industry with the money to expand both agencies and services. Where there had been about 250 home health agencies in 1960, by 1968 there were 1,328 official agencies providing home health services. Federal funding over the next 20 years gradually refocused home health on postacute services. Unfortunately, money became less available for the chronically ill client needing longer term services. Services also changed in the home health industry as home health funding began to include rehabilitative services—physical therapy, occupational therapy, speech therapy, and social work services. This continues today.

In 1980 the Omnibus Budget Reconciliation Act aided home care by expanding the Medicare benefits to 100 visits per year with a $100 deductible. Previously, a 3-day hospitalization had been required before giving home care. This requirement was lifted. For the first time, for-profit home care agencies could become Medicare-certified providers. In addition, advanced technology, such as ventilators, renal hemodialysis, and infusion therapy, originally found only in hospitals, all moved into the home, expanding the need for a home care nurse. This need was coupled with prospective payment for hospitals and resulted in earlier discharges and greater use of home care. The number of home care agencies increased exponentially.

In response, in 1984 the federal government restricted home care significantly by limiting home care services to consumers who were home bound and only required "part-time" and "intermittent" home care. (The "and" changed to "or" in 1989.) The need for home care had to be documented in the patient record. This resulted in a *Duggan v. Bowen* court ruling requiring Centers for Medicare and Medicaid Services (CMS) to clarify its eligibility criteria for home care. So in 1989 CMS redefined and eased home care eligibility.

In 1965 the Older Americans Act mandated and funded Area Agencies on Aging (AAA). These agencies fund a wide array of services for the elderly: senior centers with nutrition and recreation programs, health promotion and screening programs, mental health evaluation and treatment, respite care, case managers to plan care for elders so they can stay in their homes rather than be institutionalized, and services to the homebound such as meals, homemaker service, chore service, and transportation.

As Medicare standards required hospitals to renovate and rebuild in the 1970s, for-profit hospitals, like many other businesses, had publicly traded stocks. Stockholders expected these hospitals to make a profit so stocks would both increase in value and provide good dividends. In this arrangement, hospitals had to pay attention to stockholder interests. These interests might not always be what was ethically best for the patient. Actually, not-for-profit hospitals made profits too—using the profits for pay increases, new equipment or building projects, and investments—but called it *excess of revenue over expenses* rather than profit. Investor-owned nursing homes and home care facilities also increased, creating access for those with private or public insurance.

One of the most recent changes to Medicare legislation is the Medicare Pharmacy and Modernization Act of 2003. Using elaborate eligibility and use criteria, this act provides Medicare participants with access to coverage for prescription drugs through private stand-alone prescription drug plans or Medicare Advantage prescription drug plans administered by approved insurance companies. Coverage actually started in 2006. Today, more than 25 million Medicare beneficiaries are enrolled in drug plans, with the majority in stand-alone plans. Before enactment of this legislation, beneficiaries had no prescription drug coverage associated with their Medicare benefits. With the plan, the private companies administering the coverage can, within the framework of CMS requirements, charge varying premiums, use different formularies, and apply differing utilization management rules.

Since 2006 beneficiaries have seen their premiums and copays rise (Kaiser Foundation, 2008) and have experienced tighter utilization management. Although Medicare drug legislation has certainly provided relief for the costs of drugs, especially for lower income beneficiaries, all beneficiaries experience a gap in coverage, often called the "doughnut hole." When Medicare recipients reach a level of spending on prescriptions ($2,250 in 2006, adjusted yearly), coverage stops completely and resumes when the individual has spent a ceiling amount ($5,100 in 2006, with yearly adjustments). This means that beneficiaries with limited income or no *gap insurance* may have limited access to needed drugs for a substantial portion of the year, with higher spending (sicker) beneficiaries reaching their spending cap earlier (Stuart, Simoni-Wastila, & Chauncey, 2005).

Safety Net Providers

Because our system still has gaps in care, such as services for underserved and uninsured rural and inner city populations, non-English-speaking immigrants, homeless, and migrant workers, modest efforts at providing what is termed *safety net* healthcare services have gradually emerged. Two examples of legislated support for the poor and uninsured can be found in the clinics and services targeted toward these populations.

The Rural Health Clinic Act (RHC), passed in 1971, established higher rates of Medicare and Medicaid payments to rural primary care practices provided that they employ a nurse practitioner or physician assistant and meet the qualifications for federal approval as a rural health clinic. Rural health clinics can be free-standing clinics or can be associated with a rural hospital or nursing home. Although there are no specific requirements to provide care to the uninsured, most rural health clinics do, strengthen the rural safety net beyond just Medicare and Medicaid patients.

The Community Health Center (CHCs) Act, passed in 1965, provided funds for comprehensive health and supportive social services to be provided through clinics established to make primary care available to specific types of populations in the clinic's service area. Community health centers are funded through federal grants available through the U.S. Department of Health and Human Services (DHHS) and operate under specific rules and conditions. They are required to provide services to anyone who needs access regardless of their ability to pay.

As the movement toward advanced nursing practice gained momentum, schools and colleges of nursing established primary care and nursing practice centers and community health services, collectively known as *nurse-managed care*. Community nursing centers (CNCs), community nursing organizations (CNOs, and nursing health maintenance organizations (HMOs) have been sponsored by local communities, community groups, and churches and by university schools and colleges of nursing who provide the majority of these access points. Most nursing centers provide care to poor and underserved population groups (Harris, 1997). Many of these centers are also partially supported on the federal level by the Division of Nursing located within the DHHS, Health Resources and Services Administration, Bureau of Health Professions.

Policies Addressing Cost

Cost, and controlling the cost of providing care, is one of the most perplexing issues facing the U.S. healthcare system today. The *cost* of healthcare can be defined as *the value of all the resources used to produce the services and expenditures* and refers to the amount spent on a particular item or service (Andersen & Davidson, 2007). Both are important concepts, but expenditures are more easily measured and tracked and thus are more commonly used to analyze financial aspects of the healthcare system. Consumers and third-party payers have seen consistently higher rises in healthcare costs and expenditures than in other segments of the economy, with rates of increase of more than 7% per year for the past few years (Rice, 2007; Rice & Kominski, 2007). Insurance companies, employers, federal and state governments, and users of direct healthcare services are all vitally interested in payment systems and cost control.

Blue Cross/Blue Shield: Setting Trends in Paying for Care

The emergence of health insurance was a significant change in healthcare financing, moving payment for healthcare from personal business transactions to a third-party mediator. Initially, insurance coverage was created either to provide healthcare for people involved in rail or steamboat accidents or for mutual aid where small amounts of disability cash benefitted members experiencing an accident or illness, including typhus, typhoid, scarlet fever, smallpox, diphtheria, and diabetes.

In 1929 Justin Ford Kimball established a hospital insurance plan at Baylor University in Dallas, Texas. He had been a superintendent of schools and noticed that teachers often had unpaid bills at the hospital. Examining hospital records he calculated that "the schoolteachers as a group 'incurred an average of 15 cents a month in hospital bills. To assure a safe margin, he established a rate of 50 cents a month.' In return, the school teachers were assured of 21 days of hospitalization in a semiprivate room" (Raffel & Raffel, 1994, p. 211). This was the beginning of the Blue Cross plans that developed across the country. Blue Cross offered *service benefits* rather than a *lump-sum payment—indemnity*—benefit that had been offered by previous insurance plans. If people having Blue Cross wanted a private room, the plan, which paid for a semiprivate room, would pay the semiprivate rate and the person would have to pay the rest themselves.

Following the success of Blue Cross, in 1939 the California Medical Association started the California Physicians Service to pay physician services. This became known as Blue Shield. In this plan doctors were obligated to provide treatment at the fee established by Blue Shield, even though the doctor might charge more to patients not covered by Blue Shield. Blue Shield was in effect for people who made less than $3,000 a year. In one of many unsuccessful attempts at national healthcare reform, physicians designed and agreed to this plan *to prevent the establishment of a national health insurance plan.*

Blue Cross was quite successful. Blue Shield was not. As inflation occurred and patients made more money, the base rate was not changed, so fewer people were eligible for the Blue Shield rates. "Blue Shield made the same dollar payment for services rendered, but because the patient was above the service-benefit income level, the patient frequently had to pay an additional amount to the physician" (Raffel & Raffel, 1994, p. 213). Even when Blue Shield responded and changed the rates, the plan did not work well because inflation continued. There were also problems as radiology, pathology, and anesthesiology physicians moved out of the hospital and established their own billing. Blue Shield did not cover their expenses, yet Blue Cross could not pay the expense because it was no longer a hospital charge.

> Both Blue Cross and Blue Shield faced similar situations in later years as new, often expensive, technology developed. If they paid for equipment, it would encourage hospitals to… [average] the new equipment with all other costs, [increasing hospital charges]. If Blue Cross covered such items, it would eventually force a rate increase, and if there was a rate increase, then competitors would gain an advantage. The pressures on both Blue Cross and Blue Shield became even more acute as they acted as fiscal intermediaries (the agency handling the payments) for Medicare. The federal government, bitten by rising costs, sought to pressure the Blues (a frequently used word for the Blue Cross/Blue Shield movement) and others to stem rising costs; pressure also came from state governments, which were bitten by the rising costs of Medicaid (Raffel & Raffel, 1994, pp. 214–215).

In many states after World War II, private insurance companies proliferated and offered health insurance policies both to individuals and to employers. Large employers were expected to offer employees healthcare benefits. Unionization played a major role. Health insurance became an entitlement. Soon private insurance companies (third-party payers) enrolled more than half the U.S. population. The McCarren-Ferguson Act of 1945 "gave states the exclusive right to regulate health insurance plans…. As a result the federal government has no agency that is solely responsible for monitoring insurance" (Finkelman, 2001, p. 188).

Federal Role in Cost Containment

To administer the multiple Medicare and Medicaid programs that had been established, the federal government started the Health Care Financing Administration (HCFA), now the called Centers for Medicare and Medicaid Services (CMS), within the Department of Health and Human Services (DHHS). Payment for Medicare and Medicaid services was based on the *retrospective* cost of the care—figured and billed to the government by healthcare organizations and by physicians seeing patients. This fee-for-service system did not limit what providers could charge for their services, and initially there was no systematic approach to fees—providers charged what the market would bear. In the 1970s, faced with escalating healthcare expenditures, states began controlling the amount they would pay to a provider for a particular service. The rationale for setting rates that would be paid was to encourage providers to voluntarily control the costs of the care they delivered.

The federal government, along with states, was spending a tremendous amount of money on healthcare. In fact, the *gross domestic product (GDP)* for healthcare has grown from 6% when Medicare and Medicaid were introduced to more than 16% presently. To find money to support these programs, the government was faced with increasing taxes, shifting money from other services such as defense or education, or curbing hospital and physician costs. Curbing costs was the first choice for policymakers. Legislators chose to continue to support tertiary and secondary care rather than less expensive primary care and prevention.

One of the first efforts to control costs was the 1965 amendment of the Social Security Act to establish *utilization review (UR)* for Medicare patients, and 2 years later utilization review was started for Medicaid patients. Hospitals receiving Medicare "were required to certify the necessity of admission, continued stay, and professional services rendered to Medicare beneficiaries" (CMS). Health systems planning, to eliminate duplication of services (and thus unnecessary expense), was initiated at the federal level, although it was discontinued in 1983.

Hospital Prospective Payment: A New World for Hospitals and Providers

The next direct step by the federal government to control healthcare costs, particularly those generated in hospital settings, was the implementation of a *prospective* pricing system for Medicare patients. Before this time, hospitals and providers simply billed Medicare for their services and were paid in full. In 1983, then-Health Care Financing Administration implemented a plan to pay a set price to each hospital for each diagnosis regardless of how much the facility actually spent to provide the care; this payment strategy was called *diagnosis-related groups (DRGs)*. If hospital staff could provide care for a patient with a hip fracture, for example, at less than the DRG payment, they could keep the money and, in a sense, make a profit. If the cost of care for the patient went above the DRG payment, the hospital lost money. DRGs required hospitals to become more efficient and aware of costs. Yet, the requirements of the DRG policy induced providers to release patients from the hospital as quickly as they could and to shift costs to other third-party payers who did not engage in prospective payment, leaving doubt as to the "bottom line" in cost savings to the healthcare system overall.

Prospective payment was expanded in 1989 to include physician services outside the hospital with the introduction of the *resource-based relative value system (RBRVS)*. This policy applied the same concept as hospital DRGs to the outpatient setting, through Medicare Part B legislation. Two of the goals of RBRVS were to control costs and to put more emphasis on primary care and prevention.

Health Maintenance Organizations

In another attempt to hold down healthcare costs, the Health Maintenance Organization Act of 1973 provided federal grants to develop *health maintenance organizations (HMOs)*. This Act required employers with more than 25 employees to offer an HMO health insurance option to employees. HMOs had a good track record of bringing down healthcare costs because they had traditionally been serving younger, healthier populations. (Traditional insurance plans serving a wider range of people were more expensive.) Thus starting more HMOs sounded like a way to cut healthcare costs. This Act provided a specific definition of what an HMO was and gave the states oversight (or licensing) responsibility.

The concept of *managed care*, as delivered by HMOs, has taken hold in the public sector as well. Both Medicare and Medicaid (in many states) have taken their own steps to promote managed care by contracting with private insurers or HMOs to take on the primary care of groups of people enrolled for healthcare coverage and to serve as gatekeepers to specialty services. These measures were intended to control healthcare costs to federal and state governments and to improve the quality of care. In actual practice results have been mixed as the costs of healthcare continue to climb.

The Health Insurance Portability and Accountability Act of 1996 (HIPAA)

The Health Insurance Portability and Accountability Act (HIPAA) addresses several significant issues. These issues touch access, quality, and cost, yet major portions of HIPAA address the financing of healthcare. This act "establishes that insurers cannot set limits on coverage for preexisting conditions,… guaranteed access and renewability [of health insurance],… [and] addresses issues of excluding small employers from insurance contracts on the basis of employee health status.… In addition the law provided for greater tax deductibility of health insurance for the self-employed" (Finkelman, 2001, p. 192).

HIPAA started the *medical savings accounts*, a tax-free account provided by employers. Here the employee can annually set up an account and pay in the amount of money the employee expects to have to pay for health coverage for the year. The money paid into the account takes place before taxes are taken out by the employer. At the end of the year, if the money is not spent it goes back to the employer.

A major portion of HIPAA, and one most familiar to health professionals, mandated patient privacy procedures. This is the aspect of HIPAA that most consumers identify as well. This can vary from state to state as long as the minimum federal requirement is met (see www.hhs.gov/ocr/hipaa.). HIPAA ensures confidentiality and privacy of paper, oral (telephone inquiries and oral conversations), and electronic (computer or fax) patient health information to or from any source. The following three standards must be met:

- *Standard One:* This set governs the proper use and disclosure of personal health information (PHI) by the facility, its workforce, and certain business associates such as lawyers, auditors, consultants, and other third parties who handle PHI.
- *Standard Two:* This set allows patients to request access to their PHI, request reasonable amendments to it, and receive an annual written report of all of the facility's uses and disclosures of their PHI that they didn't authorize in writing. The patient may request certain restrictions regarding disclosure of PHI to certain third parties such as family members.
- *Standard Three:* This set requires facilities to complete several administrative tasks, including appointing a privacy officer, making the various written changes to its operating procedures, educating its workforce about these changes, and establishing an effective method for patients and others to communicate complaints, questions, and concerns about its privacy practices (Ziel, 2002, pp. 28–29).

Balanced Budget Act of 1997(BBA)

The Balanced Budget Act (BBA) significantly lowered payments for psychiatric care, rehabilitation services, and long-term care. Because ambulatory services, skilled nursing facilities (SNFs), and home care services were rapidly expanding and costing more healthcare dollars, the idea was to curb spending by placing these services under prospective payment. *Prospective payment* means that the payer determines the cost of care before the care is given; the provider is told how much will be paid to give the care. Thus the government could limit provider reimbursement. For instance, an *ambulatory payment classification* system was established, giving a fixed dollar amount for outpatient services diagnoses, skilled nursing facilities experienced prospective payment through the *resource utilization group (RUGs)* system, and home care was regulated via the *Outcome and Assessment Information Set (OASIS)* system. Even physician services changed to payments based on an RBRVS, described previously. Hospitals, already experiencing prospective payment, had major, mandated payment reductions limiting DRG and RBRVS payment rates. BBA reduced capital expenditures, graduate medical education, established open enrollment periods and medical savings accounts for Medicare recipients, increased benefits for children's healthcare, and created new penalties for fraud.

One positive aspect of BBA was the creation of the Children's Health Insurance Program, also known as CHIP, that "expands block grants to states increasing Medicaid eligibility for low-income and uninsured children, establishing a new program that subsidizes private insurance for children or combining Medicaid with the private insurance" (Finkelman, 2001, p. 398).

BBA had a major impact on healthcare, causing a number of hospitals, long-term care facilities, and home care companies to fold. A direct result of BBA has been to erode profit margins of hospitals and make cost shifting very difficult. For example, in 1997 it recommended no pay increases. Whereas hospitals averaged a 6% profit margin in 1997, in 1999 the profit margin was 2.7%. Rural hospitals were most drastically affected, and hospital bond ratings have been downgraded due to this Act. This means that it is harder to get credit, and interest rates are higher. BBA had such profound cost-cutting effects that in December 2000, Congress passed relief legislation providing additional money for hospitals and managed care plans.

If hospitals hadn't already been *outsourcing* services like housekeeping, food service, and grounds keeping, this Act encouraged more of this to occur (Contract Management Survey, 2001). "The basic premise of outsourcing is that a specialist organization can perform a particular service more efficiently than can internal operations because a specialist organization has an inherent advantage in producing and delivering a service" (Roberts, 2001, p. 241). Outsourcing has been around for a long time. Instances include contracting with physicians to staff a hospital emergency room, contracting with anesthesiologists to staff an operating room, contracting with pharmacies to provide pharmaceuticals for long-term care patients, and contracting with companies to provide patient satisfaction measurement. Now outsourcing is happening with many healthcare functions and services.

BBA had a major impact on the nursing profession. Under BBA, nurse practitioners (NPs) and clinical nurse specialists (CNSs) practicing in any setting could now be directly reimbursed for services provided to Medicare patients at 85% of physician fees. This occurred to both better serve populations not receiving medical care and to save costs as studies had determined that nurse practitioners could deliver as much as 80% of the medical care at less cost than primary care physicians. This federal legislation overrode state legislation that, in some cases, required nurse practitioners to work under direct physician supervision with reimbursement being made only to physicians.

Policies Addressing Quality

Throughout the historical development of our healthcare system, the quality of care has been assumed to be the business of individual providers (such as physicians and nurses) and specific delivery institutions (such as hospitals, long-term care facilities, and home health agencies). The blame for errors and the praise for cures were held to be between the provider or agency and patient. Outcomes of care were not collected or measured by any external, governmental organization. This is not the case today, however. The quality care movement began in the 1980s but took a strong hold in the 1990s. In 1999 the Institute of Medicine released a shocking report, *To Err s Human: Building a Safer Health System* (Kohn, Corrigan, Donaldson, 1999; Richardson & Briere, 2001). This report, which identified multiple systematic failures in the process of delivering care, was followed in 2001 by a second hard-hitting report, *Crossing the Quality Chasm: A New Health System for the 21st Century*, that provided specific recommendations for improvement of quality and safety. These two documents confirmed what quality experts had been saying: *In spite of the enormous cost of healthcare in the United States, thousands of patients are injured or die due to errors in the process of receiving care.*

Quality in healthcare can be defined as "the degree to which health services for individuals and populations increase the likelihood of desired health outcomes" (Andersen, Rice, & Kominski, 2007, p. 185). Quality of care, measured in patient or population outcomes, is now considered to be the result of the entire system of care. In many cases, aggregate results of care are public information and are readily available on the Internet (see, for instance, www.HospitalCompare.gov). In the case of quality, a mix of public policymakers and private foundations and organizations are concerned with promoting and monitoring quality across the healthcare system. The quality movement goes much further than specific physical outcomes, such as those around outcomes of cardiac surgery, although these are critically important. Outcomes of personal, emotional, or social importance to patients are also developing, such as *patient satisfac*tion or *quality of life indices.* Policy decisions at the federal level have shaped current efforts to ensure that the highest quality of care possible is provided in our healthcare system.

Governmental Agencies Concerned With Quality

The Department of Health and Human Services (DHHS) is the over-arching federal administrative agency concerned with monitoring the quality of healthcare in the United States. Several components of the DHHS infrastructure assume national leadership and focus on quality issues. For instance, the Agency for Healthcare Research and Quality (AHRQ) engages in the testing and reporting of safety improvement strategies and makes significant research awards to determine the best evidence for safe and effective practice guidelines that use the best clinical evidence available for a treatment of action in a particular disease condition or preventive strategy. Another activity of the AHRQ is the reporting of disparities in health services based on race, ethnicity, and socioeconomic status. AHRQ also houses the National Clearinghouse for Quality Measures, where standards and processes for measuring healthcare outcomes can be found. The AHRQ website (http://www.ahrq.gov/qual/measurix.htm) offers a wealth of information on measures used to assess quality in healthcare. AHRQ issues two reports annually to describe the quality of healthcare in the United States, the "National Healthcare Quality Report" and the "National Healthcare Disparities Report," both available at the AHRQ website.

The Centers for Disease Control and Prevention (CDC) is also concerned with safety and quality. One focus of the CDC is the promotion of health information technology systems to reduce human error. Another is the collection of disease surveillance data that tracks both chronic and acute infectious diseases in the private sector and in health departments. Much of the quality data is housed in the Division of Healthcare Quality Promotion, whose mission is to protect patients and healthcare personnel and to promote safety, quality, and value in the healthcare delivery system. This Division has three branches that are directly linked to quality: the Epidemiology and Laboratory Branch, the Prevention and Evaluation Branch, and the Healthcare Outcomes Branch. The CDC website provides substantial information at www.cdc.gov/ncidod/dhqp/about.html.

The U.S. Food and Drug Administration promotes quality and safety outcomes through improving regulations for packaging and labeling of drugs and by maintaining strict reporting requirements. In addition, they are responsible for the regulation of biologics, cosmetics, medical devices, radiation-emitting electronic products, and veterinary products.

The CMS plays a significant role in collecting, monitoring, and reporting patient and process outcomes of the healthcare system. Although hospitals technically "volunteer" in reporting critical quality outcomes, most participate. A financial incentive is offered through the Medicare program to those hospitals who report their outcomes on 10 quality measures on a public Web site (www.cms.gov). A financial disincentive is levied against eligible hospitals that choose not to participate and contribute data. CMS publishes hospital outcomes on its website http://www.hospitalcompare.hhs.gov/, as well as outcomes from nursing homes. Other agencies and organizations publish data on health plan outcomes, medical group outcomes, and selected outcomes by individual physicians. A recent CMS ruling introduces what is commonly termed "pay for performance" strategies. Hospitals are now expected to prevent the development of iatrogenic conditions such as pressure ulcers. Medicare will not pay for extended hospital stay or treatment for preventable complications. Nurses are in a key leadership role in this quality endeavor.

A Look to the Future

Issues of access, cost, and quality will remain driving forces in the healthcare world for years to come, and perhaps forever. *Ever-tightening governmental regulations*, such as the "pay for performance" movement, will force healthcare providers and institutional leaders to pay attention to patient outcomes in ways that have never before been expected. One exciting development presently is the emerging interest in examining patient outcomes resulting from various treatments. *Outcomes research* is rapidly developing in sophistication. It will be exciting to see where this leads us as the research results provide us with more effective answers for care. Now that more outcomes data are available, especially through Medicare and Medicaid data, quality report cards can provide performance information about healthcare organizations, linking staffing with patient outcomes. In fact, CMS is not paying for "never" events, or adverse outcomes caused by the facility. Performance data (discussed in Chapter 4) is becoming available to the general public. In fact, sometimes the patient is better informed about this than the provider.

Our *aging population* of baby boomers, now rapidly retiring, will increasingly strain our healthcare system in both private and public sectors. Shortages of healthcare professionals (such as nurses and physical therapists) to care for them will continue as a problem to be reckoned with. "The number of elderly will double in 20 states between 1995 and 2025" (Lanser, 2003, p. 7). At the same time we are living longer. This means that even though the elderly are becoming healthier, there are more elderly needing healthcare services, especially for chronic illnesses. Women especially feel the impact as they live longer and as they face possibly living at the poverty level in their older years. Today, women in the workforce—and 92.5% of nurses are women—continue to be paid 75 cents to every dollar a man makes. Retirement incomes will continue to reflect this problem. In addition, women at retirement are usually paid lower monthly annuity benefits because they live longer than men. Thus incomes for older women actually average 55% of what older men make. This problem could be further compounded if there is not enough money to pay Social Security benefits. "It is estimated that by 2032, payroll taxes will cover only 70% to 75% of promised benefits" (Meier, 2000, p. 168). To make matters worse, Medicare continues to raise premiums, and Medicare eligibility may be raised to 67 years or more.

Alternative therapies generally focus on health promotion. In the midst of all the cost-cutting in our illness care system, by 1999 "alternative medicine visits (629 million), including those to chiropractors and massage therapists, now outstrip visits to primary care physicians (427 million)" (Hospital and Health Networks, April 1999). Studies indicate that two of every five Americans use some form of alternative medicine. Alternative therapies have been enjoying increased popularity with the American public even though consumers most often pay "out of pocket" for the services. As patients visit physicians and receive medications for diseases, they often discover that this does not cure the problem. In many cases, the medications cause other medical problems. Alternative therapies provide a way to stay healthy as well as to treat disease, and bring comfort, without producing as many side effects and as much pain.

Consumers are more frequently purchasing vitamins and herbs as adjunct therapy for their health and illness conditions. This has brought about changes in the traditional illness care industries. For instance, physicians and the pharmaceutical industry have realized that they have missed a great deal of income as more people take vitamins and herbs. In fact, the pharmaceutical industry has increased their own market share in the vitamin/herb industry and has asked the Food and Drug Administration (FDA) to control vitamin/herb production. The FDA has developed a number of regulations for this industry.

Although most medical schools predominantly teach illness care, medical and nursing education programs have now added more about health in their curriculums. Because many of these health activities are relatively new to Americans, more research is needed to determine their efficacy. The National Institutes of Health (NIH) has funded some initial research examining various alternative therapies. Achieving health has been pursued in various other countries, such as use of herbs in China and homeopathy in Europe. Presently, this movement is bringing together the best information and practices from many cultures worldwide. This global yet personal interest promises to keep alternative therapies on the healthcare scene for the foreseeable future.

Another issue impacting our future in healthcare is that electronic capabilities are changing the face of our healthcare system. As telehealth capabilities increase, healthcare is expanding so that a clinician does not need to actually be present to treat a patient (Greenberg & Cartwright, 2001), opening the door for increased access to care for selected populations. *Electronic medical records* have great potential for increasing patient safety and the efficiency of care yet hold the ethical challenge of protecting patients' personal health information. In addition, the Internet has vastly improved clinician information on *evidence-based practice*. (See Chapter 5, written by dedicated librarians, showing how easy it is to access information at the point of care, to determine the best way to treat a specific patient or to identify better administrative leadership.) Consumers continue to access the Internet, both about their specific illnesses and to determine which providers are most effective. They use this information to evaluate how effectively their provider is determining their care (Meadows, 2001) and will continue to do so with even more frequency in the future.

The science of *genomics* adds a new dimension to healthcare that will have an ever-increasing presence in the future. "While genetics is the study of inherited traits, genomics is the study of the complete set of human genes, the way genes are assembled (sequence), how they are expressed (what they do), and the relationships between different sequences" (Larson, 2000, p. 77). Presently, scientists have joined forces with private companies who supply enormous funds to map genes. With commercial enterprises involved, it has created great ethical implications, as business leaders believe this information can produce future profits. Enriquez and Goldberg (2000) stated the following:

> Optimism reigns that we are on the cusp of a wholly new style of medicine. Ever since Hippocrates, curative regimens have been one-size-fits-all. Until recently it simply wasn't possible to truly dispense custom cures that had been designed for this person, right now. However, suddenly medicine is becoming "personalized medicine" where cures are concocted in line with an individual's genetic makeup. Computer simulation will let medical scientists see exactly what will happen when this person is administered that dose of a medicine. The upshot will be pinpoint cures. When will this genetics-based medicine be widely available? Scientists are not making hard predictions, but the whispered word is that we will benefit from personalized medicine probably before this decade ends. And that just may rank as the biggest revolution in medicine in the last couple millennia (McGarvey, 2003, p. S1).

On one side of the U.S. healthcare landscape are people with excellent insurance, high levels of computer literacy, and life situations that allow them to seek the best care available, wherever it occurs; they will be able to obtain the "personalized medicine" coming to us through genetic break-throughs. On the other side of the landscape are the uninsured and those who are losing benefits, such as retirees, who may lack access to such sophisticated technologies. The growing numbers of uninsured and underinsured, as well as the documented disparities the health status of racial and eth-nic minority populations and all populations living in poverty, will eventually force our legislators to address the inequalities of access and quality of care in our system. At the time of this writing, the American public finds healthcare cost and access concerns second only to their concern over the economy.

Another contributor to changes in the healthcare system in the future will be the effects of global warming. The impact of the extreme weather events, including heat waves, fires, earthquakes, and storms, are predicted to lead to higher levels of insect and water-borne illnesses and the reduction of food production and safe drinking water. Healthcare providers will need to increasingly address the physical and mental health needs that will arise from these conditions (Blashki, McMichael, & Karoly, 2007). Hospitals and other institutional providers will need to become even more focused on disaster preparedness and to be ready to deal with an increasing number of patients requiring care for illness related to heat exposure and poor air quality (Longstreth, 1999). Drug-resistant organisms are predicted to increase, bringing new challenges in treatment of infectious diseases (Kirk, 2002). These developments require significant adaptation in healthcare delivery and are likely to disproportionately affect children, the elderly, and the poor.

The problem is that healthcare costs are still high, with many individuals and employers finding healthcare unaffordable. Present healthcare dilemmas are captured in this editorial quote from the provider perspective:

- The new reality is that we have to give as little care as we can possibly get away with.
- The new reality is that we have to spend as little money as possible.
- We need to figure out how to give as much care as we possibly can in this new era.
- Our challenge is to promote as much health as possible.
- Our task is to determine how to promote the maximum amount of healthcare for the minimum expenditure of money. The real question is how to accomplish this task rather than how much care to give (Finkelman, 2001, pp. 81–82).

That which is, already has been; that which is to be, already is.

—*Ecclesiastes* 3:15

Discussion Questions

1. How can you, as a nurse administrator or manager, work to identify and reduce disparities in health status among the patient groups you serve?
2. What implications does the CMS pay-for-performance have for nurse administrators and managers? Why?
3. What changes might you anticipate in your employment setting as the effects of global warming become more apparent? How can you, as a nurse administrator or manager, be involved in curb-ing global warming?
4. What implications do the increasing number of elderly and frail elderly hold for nurse administra-tors and managers across settings? What policy changes could be suggested to provide a better care situation for larger numbers of elderly?
5. How has the HIPAA legislation impacted your practice site? What implications do you see for nurse administrators and managers?

References

Andersen, R., & Davidson, P. (2007). Improving access to care in America: Individual and contextual indicators. In R. Andersen, T. Rice, G. Kominski, & A. Afifi (Eds.), *Changing the U.S. healthcare system: Key issues in health services policy and management* (3rd ed.). San Francisco, CA: Jossey-Bass.

Andersen, R., Rice, T., Kominski, G., & Afifi, A. (2007). *Changing the U.S. healthcare system: Key issues in health services policy and management* (3rd ed.). San Francisco, CA: Jossey-Bass.

DeNavas-Walt, C., Proctor, B., & Smith, J. (2007). *Income, poverty, and health insurance coverage in the United States: 2006.* Washington, DC: U.S. Government Printing Office. U.S. Census Bureau Current Population Reports, P60–233. Retrieved June 26, 2008 from http://www.census.gov/prod/2007pubs/p60-233.pdf

Drucker, P. (1974). *Management tasks, responsibilities, practices.* New York: Harper & Row.

Enriquez, J., & Goldberg, R. (2000). Transforming life, transforming business: The life-science revolution. *Harvard Business Review*, 96–104.

Finkelman, A. (2001). *Managed care: A nursing perspective.* Upper Saddle River, NJ: Prentice Hall.

Gottlieb, S. (2001). One doctor: One patient. *Cost & Quality*, 23–24.

Harris, M. (1997). *Handbook of home healthcare administration* (2nd ed.). Gaithersburg, MD: Aspen.

Kaiser/HRET Survey of Employer-Sponsored Health Benefits, 1999–2008. Accessed December 8, 2008 from: http://ehbs.kff.org/

Kohn L., Corrigan J., Donaldson M., eds. To err is human: building a safer health system. Washington, DC: National Academy Press, 1999.

Lanser, E. (2003). Our aging population. *Healthcare Executive*, 7–11.

Larson, L. (2000). Genomics: Medicine's future in our molecules. *Hospital & Health Services Networks*, 75–82.

Longest, B., Rakich, J., & Darr, K. (2000). *Managing health services organizations and systems* (4th ed.). Baltimore: Health Professions Press.

McGarvey, R. (2003). Biotech advances: Transforming ourlives with new drugs, better crops, even personalized medicine. *Harvard Business Review*, S1.

Meadows, G. (2001). The internet promise: A new look at e-health opportunities. *Nursing Economic$, 19*(6), 294–295.

Meier, E. (2000). Medicare, social security, and competitive benefits are neglected nursing issues. *Nursing Economic$, 18*(3), 168–170.

Raffel, M., & Raffel, N. (1994). *The U.S. health system: Origins and functions* (4th ed.). New York: Delmar.

Rice, T. H. (2007). Measuring healthcare costs and trends. In R. Andersen, T. Rice, G. Kominski, & A. Afifi (Eds.), *Changing the U.S. healthcare system: Key issues in health services policy and management* (3rd ed.). San Francisco, CA: Jossey-Bass.

Rice, T., & Kominski, G. (2007). Containing healthcare costs. In R. Andersen, T. Rice, G. Kominski, & A. Afifi (Eds.), *Changing the U.S. healthcare system: Key issues in health services policy and management* (3rd ed.). San Francisco, CA: Jossey-Bass.

Richardson W, Briere R, eds. Crossing the quality chasm: a new health system for the 21st century. Committee on Quality Health Care in America, Institute of Medicine. Washington, DC: National Academy Press, 2001.

Roberts, V. (2001). Managing strategic outsourcing in the healthcare industry. *Journal of Healthcare Management, 46*(4), 239–249.

Stuart, B., Simoni-Wastila, L., & Chauncey, D. (2005). Assessing the impact of coverage gaps in the Medicare Part D drug benefit. *Health Affairs, 24*, 167–179. Retrieved June 30, 2008 from ABI/INFORM Global database.

Ziel, S. (2002). Get on board with HIPAA privacy regulations. *Nursing Management, 33*(10), 28–29.

CHAPTER 10

Healthcare Stakeholders: Consumers, Providers, Payers, Suppliers, and Regulators

Janne Dunham-Taylor, PhD, RN

Key Terms

- ☞ Bonuses
- ☞ Capitation
- ☞ Concurrent Review
- ☞ Covered Lives
- ☞ Direct Service Delivery Plan
- ☞ Disease Management
- ☞ Fee for Service
- ☞ Gag Rules
- ☞ Gatekeeper
- ☞ HMOs

- ☞ Horizontal Integration
- ☞ Managed Care
- ☞ Outcomes-Based Pricing
- ☞ Payer Mix
- ☞ Per Case Rates
- ☞ Per Diem Rates
- ☞ Per Episode Rates
- ☞ Performance-Based Reimbursement
- ☞ PPOs
- ☞ Practice Patterns

- ☞ Preadmission Certification
- ☞ Prospective Payment
- ☞ Provider Protection
- ☞ Relative Value Rates
- ☞ Retrospective Payment
- ☞ Risk Sharing
- ☞ Service Benefit Plan
- ☞ Underwriting
- ☞ Vertical Integration
- ☞ Withholds

The United States has struggled for some time to determine the best way to achieve reasonable equitable distribution of healthcare without losing control of total spending on healthcare and without suffocating the delivery system with controls and regulations that inhibit technical progress. This struggle continues today. Most industrialized countries have chosen to focus on equitable distribution of healthcare by providing universal coverage; however, the United States continues to vacillate between equity and innovative dynamism. The result has been one of limited success on both sides.

A definite result of this struggle has been the development of the medical-industrial complex. Healthcare has changed from a social good to a product. Healthcare delivery has become commercialized, and healthcare professionals, such as hospitals and physicians, have turned more toward business techniques, such as advertising, to survive. The rapid growth in hospitals and other types of healthcare facilities puts pressure on all providers to find patients. This pressure has led to economic problems, increasing costs, and new healthcare delivery approaches. Not all of these factors have been negative: Some changes have resulted in improvement with better management and increased focus on community care (Finkelman, 2001, p. 3).

Healthcare Dilemma

Peter Kongstvedt, a proponent of economic theory, observed three major dilemmas in healthcare: universal coverage (*access*), paying for it (*cost*), and *containing costs*. According to economic theory, it is possible to achieve any two but not the third. For example, if you achieve universal coverage and pay for it, costs will be very high. If you contain costs and pay for it, you will not be able to achieve coverage for everyone (**Exhibit 10–1**).

Proponents of economic theory believe that resources are scarce. Accounting and finance are applied areas of microeconomics. The theory of economics forms the foundations upon which all financial management is ultimately built. The essence of economics is that society has a limited amount of resources, with competing demands for them. The economic system attempts to allocate those resources in an optimal fashion (Finkler and Kovner, 2000, p. 4).

According to the quantum physics theory (discussed in Chapter 2), *what we believe is what we get*. We need to be careful about our thoughts because they can create our reality. I would rather choose abundance—not scarcity—in my thoughts because that is the reality I would rather live in. So believing in *scarcity*, rather than *abundance*, is problematic. On the other hand, if one subscribes to the quantum physics theory, then it becomes important that all of us think, *and believe*, we will be successful in solving all three healthcare dilemmas. Perhaps if we could change to a health perspective (encouraging everyone to think, *I am in perfect health*, not giving thought to fears and to disease), we could avoid many of the present illness costs. As a side note, it would be interesting to see whether we could all fix our societal healthcare problems if we made a massive effort to truly believe that it could be fixed.

Exhibit 10–1 Pick Any Two

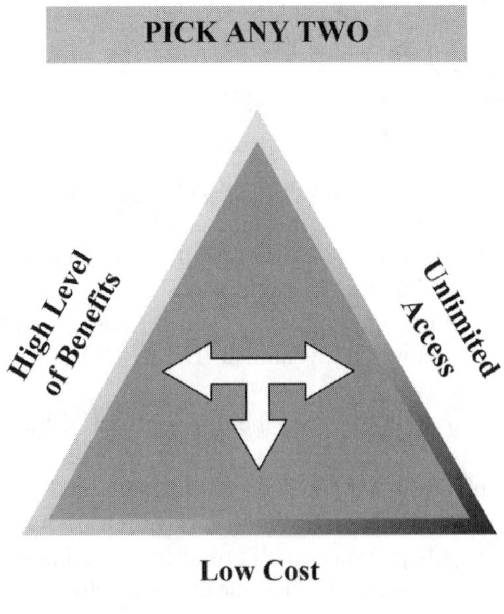

PICK ANY TWO

High Level of Benefits

Unlimited Access

Low Cost

From: Kongstvedt, P., MD, FACP. Capgemini, US, LLC.

Healthcare Expenditures Predominantly Spent for Illness Care

The Departments of Health and Human Services, Defense and the Social Security Administration, and interest on the national debt accounted for approximately 75% of the U.S. government's total net costs in 2007 (see www.gao.gov/financial/fy2007/guide.pdf). In 2006 "total health expenditures reached $2.1 trillion, which translates to $7,026 per person or 16 percent of the nation's Gross Domestic Product (GDP)" (www.cms.hhs.gov/NationalHealthExpendDate/downloads/highlights.pdf). This healthcare total includes expenses from the following, in order of greatest amount received: hospitals, physicians and clinical services, prescription drugs, nursing home care, dental services, other personal healthcare, other professional services, home health, other nondurable medical products, and durable medical equipment (www.cms.hhs.gov/NationalHealthExpendDate/downloads/highlights.pdf). Notice here that *home healthcare lags behind more acute care and that public health service is not even mentioned*.

Five Stakeholders: Consumers, Providers, Payers, Suppliers, and Regulators

To better understand this complicated healthcare system, it is necessary to examine the five key stakeholders, or players, in the healthcare arena: consumers, providers, payers, suppliers, and regulators. Simplistically, *consumers* receive the healthcare, *providers* give the care, *payers* finance the care, *suppliers* provide supplies to the providers, and *regulators* set laws, rules, and regulations that must be followed while giving and paying for the care.

Yet, realistically, these terms are more complicated. First, these players are all integrated together in a healthcare system where actions taken by one stakeholder affect the other stakeholders. So as the federal government passes a law establishing a set of regulations, the providers must make sure they effectively meet the regulations, the payers may be involved in meeting or policing the regulations, the consumers can be affected, and the suppliers may have to change supplies to meet the regulations. Second, at times stakeholders intermingle functions. For instance, the consumer receives the care but is a payer when paying deductibles, the federal government owns the Veterans Administration hospitals (provider) yet is a regulator with the Centers for Medicare and Medicaid Services (CMS) office, and Kaiser Permanente provides insurance (payer) and owns healthcare organizations (provider).

Consumers

Consumers are patients in hospitals, residents in long-term care, clients in home care, enrollees in insurance plans who receive healthcare, or people who pay out of pocket for healthcare. Another insurance term for the consumer is *covered life*. (Don't we have a wonderful way of dehumanizing people?) This concept seems simple enough, but in the U.S. system it is complicated by several factors.

First, who pays for the healthcare? Some consumers pay cash for care. Examples include the wealthy (sometimes) or the Amish. More often, consumers use health insurance. However, even with health insurance, consumers pay up front in several ways:

- By sharing insurance premium costs
- By paying deductibles (the amount of money a consumer must pay before the insurance company will pay for healthcare services)
- By paying copayments (the amount of money a consumer must pay out of pocket for every healthcare service received)
- By paying for any services not covered by the insurance plan such as alternative therapies or plastic surgery

- By paying the amount above what the payer has established as a reasonable and customary charge, such as for outpatient services.[1]
- By choosing to pay cash for a healthcare service so it will not be necessary to go through the insurance company

One advantage for employed consumers is the *medical savings accounts*, using pretax dollars. Most Americans have health insurance through their employers, but employment is no longer a guarantee of health insurance coverage.

As America continues to move from a manufacturing-based economy to a service economy and employee working patterns continue to evolve, health insurance coverage has become less stable. The service sector offers less access to health insurance than its manufacturing counterparts. Further, an increasing reliance on part-time and contract workers who are not eligible for coverage means fewer workers have access to employer-sponsored health insurance.

Because of rising health insurance premiums, many small employers cannot afford to offer health benefits. Companies that do offer health insurance often require employees to contribute a larger share toward their coverage. As a result, an increasing number of Americans have opted not to take advantage of job-based health insurance because they cannot afford it. The National Coalition on Healthcare states the following:

- The percentage of people (workers and dependents) with employment-based health insurance has dropped from 70% in 1987 to 59% in 2006. This is the lowest level of employment-based insurance coverage in more than a decade.
- Millions of workers do not have the opportunity to get health coverage. A third of firms in the United States did not offer coverage in 2006.
- Nearly two-fifths (38%) of all workers are employed in smaller businesses, where less than two-thirds of firms now offer health benefits to their employees.
- Rapidly rising health insurance premiums are the main reason cited by all small firms for not offering coverage. Health insurance premiums are rising at extraordinary rates. The average annual increase in inflation has been 2.5%, whereas health insurance premiums for small firms have escalated an average of 12% annually.
- Even if employees are offered coverage on the job, they cannot always afford their portion of the premium. Employee spending for health insurance coverage (employee's share of family coverage) has increased 143% between 2000 and 2006.
- Coverage is unstable during life's transitions. A person's link to employer-sponsored coverage can also be cut by a change from full time to part time or by self-employment, retirement, or divorce.
- A new study found that 29% of people who had health insurance were "underinsured" with coverage so meager they often postponed medical care because of costs. Nearly 50% overall and 43% of people with health coverage said they were "somewhat" to "completely" unprepared to cope with a costly medical emergency over the coming year (http://www.nchc.org/facts/coverage.shtml).

---

[1] As mentioned previously, this is true for coinsurance deductibles, and what is above the reasonable and customary costs with regular insurance. However, with Medicare Part A and Medicaid, other than billing the deductible and coinsurance, it is illegal to bill the patient for the amount of reimbursement not paid by the government. In Medicare Part B providers can bill up to 15 percent more for services than the cost covered by Medicare.

Most often, employers who do offer health insurance to employees pass the cost of health insurance plans on to employees. Employees pay a set *monthly fee* for the health insurance benefit. If spouses each have an insurance plan, it is necessary to *delineate which plan* would first cover family healthcare needs, with the other spouse's plan picking up uncovered expenses only. In addition, employers offer *cafeteria plans* for employees. In this arrangement an employee chooses the amount and type of healthcare coverage (and other benefits) needed, within certain limits set by the employer. If the employee's spouse had a good insurance plan, it is possible the employee would not require health insurance at all. This saves employers money.

Employers have an additional expense when the Consolidated Omnibus Budget Reconciliation Act of 1985 (COBRA) mandated employers to continue benefits for terminated employees for a certain length of time to ensure healthcare coverage for people who were unemployed or between jobs. Losing a job, or quitting voluntarily, can mean losing affordable health insurance coverage, not only for the worker but also for their entire family. Only 7% of the unemployed can afford to pay for COBRA health insurance (the continuation of group coverage offered by their former employers). Premiums for this coverage average almost $700 a month for family coverage and $250 for individual coverage, a very high price given the average $1,100 monthly unemployment check (http://www.nchc.org/facts/coverage.shtml).

As the price of healthcare rises, consumers are paying more and employers are paying less. Finkelman, illustrates how deductibles and copayments can add up for the consumer. For example, a patient pays the following deductibles and copayments for a hospital stay:

Hospital bill	$20,000	
Patient deductible	−$　　200	
	$19,800	Medical charges after deductible paid
Medical charges after deductible paid	$19,800	
	×　　.20	
	$ 3,960	Medical expenses to be paid by patient/copayment

The deductible must be paid before the insurer will pay its portion.
Patient must pay deductible and copayment.

$　200	Deductible
+$3,960	Copayment
$4,160	Total amount to be paid by patient

So, despite insurance coverage, the patient must still pay $4,160, which is not a small amount (Finkelman, 2001).

Some employer-based plans now have a *maximum out-of-pocket*, or limit, the employee has to pay annually when paying for actual medical costs. For instance, say an employee experiences a catastrophic illness that costs $500,000 during the year. If the plan has specified a maximum out-of-pocket (i.e., the preferred provide organization [PPO] here is $1,300 for a PPO provider and a maximum of $3,900 for a provider out of the PPO network), then once the employee has paid that amount (reached the limit), the employer pays 100% of the medical expenses. *Other plans, including Medicare, do not have this limit.* Thus for the nonworking elderly, healthcare costs, when high, can quickly deplete life savings.

Or, for a bill to see a physician, the patient pays the following change:

Physician's bill for office visit: Bronchitis	$120
Insurer's reasonable and customary charge for this visit	$100
Patient's copayment of 30% ($100 × .30)	$ 30
Uncovered part of bill to be paid by patient ($120 − $100)	$ 20
Patient's total out-of-pocket expenses	
Copayment ($30) + uncovered portion ($20)	$ 50

The $50 represents 41.6% of the total charge of $120.

(Finkelman, 2001).

Let's look at two typical scenarios. An elderly couple, Mr. and Mrs. Oldfield, have a nice savings and own a home. Mr. Oldfield experiences an expensive illness resulting in the savings being entirely depleted—even with insurance and Medicare. What is Mr. or Mrs. Oldfield to do in case either experiences another costly expense or illness? In a second scenario, Mrs. Ancient has lost her husband, is below the poverty level, has no savings, and has no insurance other than Medicare. Mrs. Ancient develops bronchitis. How can she pay for her share of the physician costs (not to mention medication) when her entire monthly income is already spent on food and lodging expenses?

Then there are *uninsured* consumers. Who are the uninsured?

- Nearly 47 million Americans, or 16% of the population, were without health insurance in 2005, the latest government data available.
- The large majority of the uninsured (80%) are native or naturalized citizens.
- The percentage of working adults (aged 18 to 64 years) who had no health coverage was 20.2% in 2006.
- Nearly 90 million people—about one-third of the population below the age of 65—spent a portion of either 2006 or 2007 without health coverage.
- Over 8 in 10 uninsured people come from working families—almost 70% from families with one or more full-time workers and 11% from families with part-time workers.
- The number of uninsured children in 2006 was 8.7 million, or 11.7% of all children in the United States.
- Young adults (aged 18 to 24 years) remained the least likely of any age group to have health insurance in 2005; 29.3% of this group did not have health insurance.
- The percentage and the number of uninsured Hispanics increased to 34.1% and 15.3 million in 2006.
- Nearly 40% of the uninsured population resides in households that earn $50,000 or more. A growing number of middle-income families cannot afford health insurance payments even when coverage is offered by their employers....

How does being uninsured harm individuals and families?

- Lack of insurance compromises the health of the uninsured because they receive less preventive care, are diagnosed at more advanced disease stages, and, once diagnosed, tend to receive less therapeutic care and have higher mortality rates than insured individuals.
- The uninsured are increasingly paying "up front," before services are rendered. When they are unable to pay the full medical bill in cash at the time of service, they can be turned away except in life-threatening circumstances.
- About 20% of the uninsured (vs. 3% of those with coverage) say their usual source of care is the emergency room.

- According to one study, over a third of the uninsured have problems paying medical bills. The unpaid bills were substantial enough that many had been turned over to collection agencies, and nearly a quarter of the uninsured adults said they had changed their way of life significantly to pay medical bills.

What additional costs are created by the uninsured population?

- The United States spends nearly $100 billion per year to provide uninsured residents with health services, often for preventable diseases or diseases that physicians could treat more efficiently with earlier diagnosis.
- Hospitals provide about $34 billion worth of uncompensated care a year.
- Another $37 billion is paid by private and public payers for health services for the uninsured and $26 billion is paid out-of-pocket by those who lack coverage.
- The uninsured are 30% to 50% more likely to be hospitalized for an avoidable condition, with the average cost of an avoidable hospital stay estimated to be about $3,300.
- The increasing reliance of the uninsured on the emergency department has serious economic implications, because the cost of treating patients is higher in the emergency department than in other outpatient clinics and medical practices (http://www.nchc.org/facts/coverage.shtml).

If a patient is uninsured and is unable to pay for care, what should the provider do? Care for the patient anyway and take a loss? Or refuse to care for the patient? What about the ethics of all this? Historically, the Hill-Burton Act, and later COBRA legislation, specified that hospitals receiving money from the federal government for building projects or for Medicare reimbursement must agree to provide care for the uninsured. So hospitals would "cost shift" this expense, charge more to the wealthy or insured patients, and use the resulting profit to pay for the uninsured. Now, as profit margins have been curtailed, most healthcare providers do not have enough "cost-shift" money to offset uncompensated care. Too often, providing care for the uninsured represents a true loss of money to the provider. Because of this, unless it is a life-threatening issue, many providers refuse to provide care unless a patient can pay. This translates into the patient having insurance or paying cash before services are rendered.

Thus *access* to healthcare remains a problem for many in the United States. This reduced access actually can create more expenses in the long run societally because *it is less expensive to provide care based on prevention or early interventions than to let illness progress and become very serious before giving the care.* Presently, there are some trends eroding health insurance coverage:

- Rising premium costs, both for persons who have access to insurance through their employers and for those who buy insurance individually
- An increasing number of temporary and part-time workers, who seldom receive healthcare coverage
- A reduction in explicit coverage, most notably pharmaceutical benefits
- Greater de facto limitations on covered care, especially by health maintenance organizations (HMOs)
- A broad shift from traditional HMOs requiring very low out-of-pocket payments to point-of-service plans and PPOs requiring high payments by patients
- Loss of Medicaid coverage due to welfare reform
- The rising cost of "Medigap" coverage (explained later under Medicare) for the elderly, which leads to substantial underinsurance
- The crackdown on illegal immigrants and the reduction in services to legal immigrants
- The trend away from community ratings of individual insurance premiums, which results in rising costs and, hence, reduced rates of coverage for middle-aged persons (Finkelman, p. 43)

Managed care (more completely defined below under Payers) has had a tremendous impact on consumers. For example, the consumer may have to change providers based on the insurance plan their employer chooses. Or, if consumers experience an acute illness, they are transferred to various units or facilities yet still are not well enough to care for themselves when discharged. If no one at home can care for them, what can the consumer do? (This often becomes a major problem for the provider as well as the consumer. The provider faces the financial and ethical dilemma of discharging the patient vs. providing additional care at a financial loss.)

This problem has resulted in more *uncompensated, untrained caregivers*—most often relatives with no nursing training—caring for the consumer in the home. They need more basic care information on how to appropriately care for their loved ones. They need basics like turning frequently to prevent bedsores and encouraging hydration and better nutrition, which a public health nurse could spearhead in the community if public health programs were more adequately funded.

Along with this problem, as the U.S. population is aging, more people are experiencing chronic illness. If on Medicare or Medicaid, there may be inadequate healthcare coverage for chronic illness. This is where both home health and public health, both drastically underfunded, could make a significant contribution. Often, a consumer must deal with lack of medical care, and this has only worsened with managed care, not to mention expensive drugs, and, if necessary, no one to care for them in the home. More serious illnesses and/or acute admissions to other healthcare facilities that might have been prevented with better home care have also resulted.

Another consistent problem for consumers is *patient education and prevention measures*. Physicians are illness oriented and, with managed care, need to see many patients to make money; therefore patient education does not occur. When patients are acutely ill, have just delivered a baby, or are admitted for immediate surgery, they are so ill, anxious, or exhausted that it is not possible to provide patient education. The good news is that most same-day surgery preoperative programs provide educational information to patients. Other sources are the physician's office, the Internet, the alternative therapist, or the health food store. One obvious answer, used by other countries, is to have the public health department do more population-based education and prevention programs. However, public health continues to be drastically underfunded in the United States.

Aside from the problems with paying for healthcare, *consumer protection* has resulted in various public policy mandates being adopted at the local, state, and national levels. For example, the Health Insurance Portability and Accountability Act of 1996 (HIPAA) is concerned with confidentiality of the medical record (see Chapter 9), the Joint Commission and many states now require organizations to report sentinel events,[2] and the Institute of Medicine's Committee on the Quality of Health Care in America is regularly releasing quality and safety consumer issues and the need for better mechanisms to prevent the reoccurrence of these issues (discussed in Chapter 4).

Providers

Providers are the individuals (nurses, physicians, dietitians, social workers, pharmacists, physical or respiratory therapists, dentists, and other healthcare personnel) and organizations (hospitals, outpatient facilities, long-term care facilities, home care agencies, or other healthcare organizations) providing the healthcare services. Some common provider organizational terms are *managed care*

---

[2] A sentinel event is an unexpected occurrence involving death or serious physical or psychosocial injury, or the risk thereof. Serious injury specifically includes the loss of limb or function. The phrase "or risk thereof" includes any process variation for which a recurrence would carry a significant chance of a serious adverse outcome (www.jcaho.org/sentinel). Examples of such events include patient suicide, infant abduction or discharge to the wrong family, rape, surgery on the wrong body part or on the wrong patient, and unanticipated death.

organization (MCO) or *health services organization* (HSO). Healthcare organizations are groups of people working within an organizational structure to provide healthcare services to consumers. Healthcare services can be provided across the continuum of care, from how to achieve health, such as alternative or preventive care, to treating disease, such as acute, chronic, restorative, or palliative care.

Healthcare organizations are classified in several ways based on profit status:

- *Not-for-profit*, where profit is used by the healthcare organization for additional capital needs, working capital needs, capital replacement needs, or improving services or quality
- *For-profit*, where the profit is paid to owners or investors
- *Sectarian*, affiliated with a particular religious group such as Catholic, Methodist, or Seventh-Day Adventist) as opposed to non-sectarian
- *Governmental or publicly owned*, where cities, counties, states, or the federal governments own, partially finance, or control the healthcare organizations (e.g., a city governs a city hospital, the county runs a health department, the state gives partial funding to a university hospital, and the federal government owns the Veterans Administration facilities)

A healthcare organization can be a single, small, free-standing clinic or long-term care facility or a much larger thousand-bed hospital. It can be multiorganizational where two or more organizations have grouped together in various ways to better achieve delivery of care. The combinations are limitless with multiorganizational arrangements—alliances, cooperative linkages, networks, and joint ventures. They can result from management contracts, umbrella corporations, mergers, and other consolidations. The arrangements may be with other similar organizations or may include a wide range of healthcare services.[3] A single organization may actually be linked in several different arrangements, such as a hospital that has merged with another hospital, which also belongs to Voluntary Hospitals of America, a nationwide purchasing alliance.

Generally, there are three types of multiorganizational arrangements. The first, and most common, is for market transactions. Examples are joining Premier Alliance (to purchase supplies or equipment at lower costs) and having contracts with insurance companies or employers. The second multiorganizational arrangement is where the healthcare organization must participate with another entity. This arrangement might include collective bargaining agreements, federal or state regulatory bodies, bond rating services, and utilization management companies. The third arrangement is a voluntary one. Here a mutual benefit or gain is realized by the organizations in the arrangement. For instance, a rural hospital is linked with a medical center. The rural hospital can then refer patients who need more specific tertiary care to the medical center; the medical center needs "feeder" hospitals for patients.

Healthcare organizations, regardless of category, have an owner or a governing body or board. There are three roles of this governing body: (1) to establish/approve the mission, vision, and strategic objectives of the organization (formulated by the organization's executive senior management group) and the broad responsibility to make sure these objectives are fulfilled (this includes having an appropriate budget to accomplish the objectives); (2) to hire and evaluate the chief executive officer (CEO) of the organization; and (3) to ensure the quality of the medical care.

Choosing board members often becomes a political process. A board member should be familiar with the community, have a good reputation, be familiar with good business practices, have served well in the past or had experience on other boards, and have an understanding of the patient care process. In healthcare often boards are self-perpetuating, meaning that present board members select new board members. At times, the CEO has voting privileges on the board, as do physicians. In a way

---

[3] For more information on multiorganizational arrangements see Longest, Rakich & Darr (2000).

it is a conflict of interest for the CEO or physicians practicing in the organization to be on the board; however, at times they best understand the issues involved with delivering care. (The Joint Commission recommends having physician board members; remember that The Joint Commission was started by physicians.) Compensation of board members is rare, about 20% in all nongovernmental hospitals (Griffith, 1999).

Unless the medical staff is directly hired by the organization, the healthcare organization will have a *medical staff organization* in hospitals, sometimes called a *professional staff organization* in other settings. The medical staff organization is a separate association with its own by laws and governing structure. It has a dotted line responsibility (meaning that the CEO does not have supervisory responsibility for them) to the CEO. Thus the group members are not employees of the organization and are paid independently for their services. Although the medical staff group is mainly physicians, it can also include other professionals such as dentists, clinical psychologists, podiatrists, nurse midwives, nurse practitioners, and chiropractors. To receive *practice privileges* in the facility, the physician has to be recommended by the medical staff organization who examines credentials and competency, the recommendation has to be approved by the governing board, the medical staff organization extends the privilege of membership, and the physician then accepts the bylaws of the medical staff organization. Another title for this group of physicians is *attending physicians*.

Typical functions of the medical staff organization are illustrated by the committee structure often used for hospitals.

- The *credentials committee* reviews qualifications of the membership and recommends practice privileges to the executive committee (and ultimately to the governing board).
- The *pharmacy and therapeutics committee* develops the drug formulary, monitors drug use, and sets drug usage policies.
- The *surgical case review committee* reviews need for surgery and evaluates the pre- and postoperative diagnoses.
- The *medical records review committee* checks on the timely completion and quality of the medical record.
- The *utilization review committee* examines length of stay and use of ancillary services.
- The *quality assessment committee* examines the appropriateness of patient treatment. (This committee can replace the surgical case review and medical records review committees in smaller hospitals.)

Additional committees can include infection control, risk management, safety, blood use, disaster planning, bylaws, and nominating committees. If there are problems with medical staff performance, the medical staff organization deals with the problems. One common problem is that the physician has not completed the medical record in a timely fashion. In this case the physician will not be able to admit patients until getting caught up with documentation. If a serious problem occurs, this becomes an issue, not only for the medical staff organization but for the CEO, the healthcare organization executive group, the governing board (if serious enough), and nurses who deal with this physician.

The *executive group* in a healthcare organization includes the following members: the chief executive officer (CEO), the chief operating officer (COO), the chief financial officer (CFO), the chief nursing—or patient services—officer (CNO), general counsel, and other vice presidents from human resources, plant services, medical officer, and/or information services. Membership depends on the size of the organization as well as on the CEO's and governing board's orientation.

In multiorganizational arrangements, such as strategic alliances, there are a couple governance models used. In the *centralized model* there is one governing board responsible for all healthcare facilities in the alliance. The advantage is that there are not as many stakeholders to deal with, but the disadvantage is that they may not be aware of local issues and differences. The individual healthcare organizations may have an advisory board that has no legal or fiduciary authority. In a *decentralized model* there is a system governing board that shares governance responsibilities with other smaller individual boards within the system. The smaller boards can be set up for specific organizations such as for each individual healthcare facility; for specific functions such as insurance companies, hospitals, or physicians; or for regions. With this model there can be more local autonomy. The disadvantage is that with the many boards, confusion and conflict can result within the system as a whole. In multiorganizational arrangements there is usually a corporate executive, along with a corporate executive team, for the entire system as well as having a CEO, and executive group, for each facility.

Providers generally have several payer contracts and each can pay differently and use different formats for payment. It is necessary to electronically send information to payers. As managed care has expanded, healthcare organizations have responded by using a number of strategies. Providers, such as healthcare organizations and physicians, have merged to serve more patients; they have expanded services—such as hospitals expanding ambulatory and long-term care services, or physicians opening free-standing surgical centers—or organizations have closed and physicians have retired. The hospital often serves regional needs or links with other hospitals to serve regional needs and has survived.

One survival strategy has been to develop an *integrated delivery system* to provide a broad range of services, rather than just to have one free-standing healthcare organization. An integrated system is economically and clinically linked through ownership or by contract.

In *horizontal integration* a facility combines with like facilities. A prime example of horizontal integration has been occurring since the mid-1980s with a number of hospitals in a community merging into multihospital systems or, at least, affiliating with other hospitals in some fashion. Examples of the largest multisystem healthcare groups include Kaiser Permanente, Columbia/HCA Healthcare, and Tenet Healthcare. In long-term care the largest multisystem is Beverly Enterprises, whereas in home care it is Gentiva Health Care. In 1985, 35% of community hospitals were affiliated with a healthcare system, whereas by 1998, 42% (2,142 hospitals) were affiliated with a healthcare system. Presently, this movement has stagnated, perhaps because it now exists in most communities. Other problems with these affiliations are the loss of autonomy and less sensitivity to local community healthcare needs.

Horizontal integration achieves cost savings in several ways. First, services can be consolidated to save money. For instance, only one human resource department or business office is necessary, and policies can be developed or technology can be purchased for the whole system. Second, economies of scale can be achieved when purchasing supplies, saving considerable money. Third, larger organizations have better bargaining positions when negotiating with managed care plans, allowing one person or department to negotiate for all the facilities. Fourth, marketing can occur for all the facilities. Fifth, each facility can benefit the other by broadening available services, that is, "the small rural hospital would provide basic general care; the moderate-sized hospital, more specialized care and equipment; and the regional hospital, the most sophisticated and expensive special types of care" (Raffel and Raffel, 1994, p. 137). Services can be broadened in the specialty areas as well. Let's use cardiovascular services, one of the few remaining profit centers for hospitals, as an example. Between 1985 and 1999, open-heart surgery programs increased by 47% and cardiac catheterization services grew by 70%.

In *vertical integration* an organization integrates as many different healthcare services as possible. Services offered are "womb to tomb," or, to put it another way, they offer a continuum of care—primary to tertiary. The idea behind this strategy is that patients rarely or never have to leave the system for healthcare services and, while there, have convenient accessibility to the care. In addition, it is advantageous to have various care delivery sites in close proximity based on patient needs. For example, it is helpful to have the lab and x-ray departments near the primary care physician or nurse practitioner offices. Or, for same day surgery, to have all the needed pre- and postoperative services near the operating room. The idea is to provide quick, efficient services so patients do not need to spend a whole day just getting needed healthcare services. Services in an integrated system might include

- Acute care
- Primary care
- Specialty ambulatory care
- Acute rehabilitation
- Subacute care
- Home care
- Long-term care
- Traditional skilled nursing care
- Assisted living
- Durable equipment services (Finkelman, p. 64)

Although vertical integration is a popular concept, in reality some of it has been difficult to achieve. "Healthcare organizations poured $5 billion into integration strategies over the last decade, but now those organizations acknowledge that their investments didn't always pay off and say that future integration activities will be sharply reduced" (Haugh, pp. 33–34). There are two examples of unsuccessful vertical integration. The first example is hospitals buying physician practices: "hospital-owned practices turn out to be 50 times less profitable than those owned by medical groups or practice management companies ... the median loss of $47,000 is typical" (Hudson, 1977, p. 26). Now many hospitals are selling off physician practices and restructuring loans. Presently, the best options with physicians seem to be contracting with physician groups for services. Second, some of the large multihospital systems expanded their services by developing managed care insurance lines that could compete with existing insurance plans. Most of these hospital-based plans are losing money and many have closed.

What most healthcare organizations choose to do is to take the middle ground in vertical integration, doing part of the services themselves and outsourcing other services. In making the decision to *outsource* (for such things as billing and housekeeping or the pharmacy in long-term care), it is helpful to evaluate how effective this collaborative arrangement will be.

Within healthcare organizations a consistent, nagging communication problem keeps occurring. Ideally, during an episode of illness, all providers need to communicate well with each other, as well as with the patient and the patient's family, and work as a team to provide the patient care. Unfortunately, this often does not happen. If anything, care has become more fragmented with managed care. Providers often do not communicate, and the quality of care suffers. It is common for a patient to be transferred to several divisions or facilities to receive care. Important information about the patient may not be communicated from one location to another. Most often, the patient experiences new staff members who provide the care. Relationships with care workers, already established, do not continue in the new division or facility. Patients', not to mention healthcare workers', emotional needs, or support connections, are often disregarded. The result is fragmentation of care—even when one has a good insurance policy.

Another problem providers experience is uncompensated care. If a patient is uninsured and is unable to pay for care, what should the provider do? This was discussed extensively under the "Consumers" section. Along similar lines, providers are concerned with *payer mix*. The issue is that different payers actually pay different amounts for services. For example, if most of the patient population served have Medicaid or Medicare payers, it is probable that the provider will lose money as neither will pay the full amount needed to care for the patients. (In fact, they pay less than 50 cents for every dollar spent.) Providers prefer having a majority of private-pay patients who provide better reimbursement. Even with private-pay patients, generally discounts are given to payers, (discounts may be just a flat discount on all services rendered, or the discount may be a sliding scale based on volume); the provider must know whether the true reimbursement amount can still provide a profit or at least cover costs. If the discount is "too deep," losses will be incurred.

Providers face another issue—consumers via the Internet, regulators, and payers are examining provider performance. Here data are collected on patient outcomes—length of stay, readmission rates, adverse reactions, complications, infections, deaths, number of medications per patient, and consumer satisfaction/complaints. (This is discussed further in Chapter 4.) This information is used by payers and consumers.

Payers use the performance data to compare providers' performance and determine who gives the best care and who is less expensive. This is called *performance-based reimbursement* evaluation. Payers use this evaluation before contracting with providers for healthcare services. The contract is for a specified time and for specified services. In addition, the provider is expected to provide evaluation data. Before the contract is renewed, the payer again evaluates provider data. In 2009 provider performance includes Medicare refusing to pay for hospital's mistakes and infections, called "never" events. This has many ramifications (discussed in Chapter 4) but will mean that hospitals will incur additional expense for their mistakes.

With managed care, another provider issue emerged—provider protection. In HMOs there are often rules that physicians are expected to meet to continue working for that HMO. For example, they will not order expensive or frequent diagnostic tests or authorize many patient hospitalizations. The idea behind the rules is to keep down expenses. Often, there are monetary incentives—withholds or bonuses—paid to physicians to ensure costs do not skyrocket. *Withholds* happen when the HMO holds part of the physician or hospital income until the end of the year and pays it back to the physician or hospital based on the physician's or hospital's performance. Withholds may never be paid back to the provider, being used to cover other expenses the HMO is experiencing. *Bonuses* are another method used by payers. Here the provider receives a bonus at the end of the year based on the provider's performance or based on the total plan performance.

Such practices have recently resulted in legislation aimed at either limiting the incentives or revealing the incentives to consumers. Providers need protection for due process in their relationship with payers in these matters, because payers may expect that providers remain quiet about the incentives ("gag rules"). Because of all this, physicians are experiencing "frustration in their attempts to deliver ideal care, restrictions on their personal time, financial incentives that strain their professional principles, and loss of control over their clinical decisions" (Finkelman, p. 103).

Nurses are also providers, though at times they are not treated as such. Nurse practitioners and clinical nurse specialists can bill directly for services within a healthcare organization. However, with the exception of private duty nursing, nursing costs have been bundled into room charges. Only a few organizations have broken away from this model. It is such a problem in long-term care that the therapies receive higher reimbursement, and a higher acuity level, than nursing care gets. It is another example of what is wrong with healthcare reimbursement as it presently exists.

Payers

Payers directly pay for healthcare services (i.e., individuals, employers, insurance companies, or the government). Individuals who directly pay for healthcare services are payers as well as consumers.

Employers are payers when they choose to provide healthcare benefits for employees. They can do this in one of two ways: (1) purchase (or make available) health insurance for employees, in which case the employer is not a direct payer of healthcare services, or (2) the employer can be *self-insured* (usually only larger employers are self-insured), directly paying employee healthcare costs. In this case the employer is the payer and pays an insurance company to administer the insurance plan. The employer sets up the limitations of the plan, including annual limits per employee; provides claim forms for employees; verifies employee claims; and pays providers from the employer budget. Employees can be confused and believe they have insurance, such as Blue Cross, when in actuality their employer is self-insured and Blue Cross is only the intermediary administering the insurance plan. When self-insured, healthcare costs are listed as a line item on the employer budget. This can create the need for huge mid-year budget readjustments for unexpected large costs such as an employee experiencing a catastrophic illness costing the employer $500,000. In this situation the employer must find the additional money to cover the healthcare line item in the budget.

Insurance companies provide individual or group insurance coverage for *covered lives*—the individuals included in the plan—for a contracted amount of time, often a year. The purchaser(s) pays a premium to the insurance company. In group plans the premium payment is shared, or actually paid for, by employees. Generally, individuals, or even small business employers, pay more for insurance premiums than large employers. To counteract this problem, Hawaii established several HMOs for small businesses and aggregated the entire small business population together to get lower rates for small businesses.

Governments are the biggest force in the healthcare payer arena. The *federal government* is a major payer, covering over 50% of the total healthcare revenue. Federal government insurance programs include Medicare, part of Medicaid, the Federal Employees Health Benefit Program (FEHBP), TriCare, and the Civilian Health and Medical Program of the Uniform Services (CHAMPUS). *Thus as the federal government starts some payment strategy, other insurers follow suit.* The state governments, often the state's largest employer, have been responsible for health insurance for state employees, in addition to sharing responsibilities for Medicaid programs with the federal government.

The term "third-party payers," or *insurers*, refers to insurance companies, employers, or government agencies that provide healthcare insurance. The insurance company acts as an administrator of the pool of money collected from all its members, paying, or *underwriting*, the defined illness care coverage to a provider when the consumer has received healthcare services. With insurance there is a risk to the insurance company. What if more people need coverage than anticipated? Obviously, it benefits the insurance company to serve a larger population. This reduces the risk and has the additional benefit of costing less to administer the plan. It is also better to have healthier people in the plan. The federal government, with Medicare, has a problem with this issue because it serves an older population who are more likely to need illness care. To determine the risk, the insurance company uses *actuarial data*—a statistical method that takes into account such factors as the age and sex of enrollees, past use, and cost of medical services—to determine both premium costs and definition of coverage. The purchaser's perception of *risk* is also an issue. Insurance is only worth purchasing if people perceive that they may experience a risk, such as expensive surgery or other care.

RETROSPECTIVE PAYMENT

Historically, the typical health insurance was *indemnity insurance*, where payment occurred after the care was given. This was called *retrospective payment*. Here the consumer chose the provider, the provider determined what was charged, and the insurance company paid it (*fee-for-service*). The insurance contract was with the individual or employer. Except for those who pay cash, true indemnity insurance is largely nonexistent today because health insurance plans use some form of managed care, or financial incentives, to be cost effective.

PROSPECTIVE PAYMENT

Like the name implies, *managed care* refers to any method of healthcare delivery that is designed to cut costs yet provide needed services (i.e., use the least expensive option for delivery of care, only pay for necessary services, control costs by contracting and telling providers what will be paid for services before the services are delivered, and involve consumers in paying for part of their care). In managed care, payers determine the amount they will reimburse for a medical service. Generally, the reimbursement strategy is *prospective payment*, where the payer determines the cost of care before the care is given. The provider is then told how much will be paid to give the care. This is called the prospective payment system (PPS).

SERVICE BENEFIT PLANS

Service benefit plans, an example of both prospective payment and managed care, directly pay providers after negotiating and specifying the prices paid for each healthcare service. In service benefit plans, the patient pays part of the costs with deductibles and coinsurance. Medicare and PPOs, such as Blue Cross, have service benefit plans. (This can be confusing because Blue Cross and Medicare also offer HMOs, a direct service delivery plan, discussed in the next section. In addition, Blue Cross and other insurance companies are the fiscal intermediaries for Medicare.) Because over 50% of our country's population is covered by Medicare/Medicaid, we provide more information on these two plans.

Medicare

Medicare, supported from payroll cash contributions put into the Medicare Trust Fund, pays for healthcare services for Americans aged 65 and older, for some people with disabilities under age 65, and for people with end-stage renal disease. Medicare covers about 75% of the healthcare cost. (Note that Social Security has changed the full retirement age to 66 for anyone born after 1943. Therefore Medicare benefits may not start until a person reaches that age.) Presently, there are approximately 44 million older adults and 5 million disabled people with Medicare benefits. In fact, "Medicare beneficiaries comprise one in seven Americans, and this proportion is expected to grow to one in five by 2030, when the number of beneficiaries will exceed 76 million people" (Longest, Rakich, & Darr, 2000, p. 97). There has been some debate as to whether there will be enough Medicare payroll cash contributions once the baby boomers are all eligible.

Medicare is administered by the CMS, formerly called the Health Care Finance Administration. Medicare usage is monitored by the Medicare Payment Advisory Commission (MedPAC), that independently advises Congress about more effective or less costly ways to manage Medicare. CMS pays an administrative fee to *fiscal intermediaries* to carry out the actual payment system for Medicare. Fiscal intermediaries are other insurance companies who already have experience with processing insurance claims—companies such as Blue Cross.

Medicare divides defined services and payments into four parts:

- Part A covers hospital inpatient services, blood transfusions in hospitals, skilled nursing up to 100 days in a benefit period, some home care and home use medical equipment, and hospice care for those who have less than 6 months to live (see http://www.medicareconsumerguide.com/medicare-part-a.html). Most people receive Part A automatically on their 65th birthday. They do not have to pay a premium because they, or their spouse, paid Medicare taxes while they were working. However, there are deductibles and coinsurance costs for consumers. However, under Part A providers cannot further bill consumers for services.
- Part B covers many services, tests, and preventive treatments that are not covered by Part A (see http://www.medicareconsumerguide.com/medicare-part-b.html). If one has paid Medicare taxes before age 65, one is eligible to sign up for Part B; signing up for Part B is a choice that is

up to the individual. If people choose to sign up, they pay a monthly fee for Part B and pay deductibles and copayments.

- Part C is like a Medicare HMO or PPO, called the Medicare Advantage Plan (see http://www. medicareconsumerguide.com/medicare-part-c.html). Here private insurance companies that are approved by Medicare provide the coverage. It combines Part A and Part B in a lower cost alternative plan and providers usually offer extra benefits and include prescription drug coverage (Part D). Here you must use the doctors or hospitals that belong to the plan, although there is coverage when one takes a trip. Part C has two parts: (1) a high-deductible plan where coverage will not begin until the annual deductible is met and (2) a savings account plan where Medicare deposits money for one to use for healthcare costs.
- Part D provides prescription drug coverage insurance provided by private companies approved by Medicare (http://www.medicareconsumerguide.com/medicare-part-d.html). Part D generally is where one pays a separate premium or yearly deductible, along with copays, coinsurance, or deductible, when one actually uses it to buy a prescription.

Besides what the user is paying, federal tax dollars pay the rest of the costs. Medicare does not provide 100% coverage. This means that additional insurance is needed. *Medigap plans*, sponsored by private insurance companies, can be purchased in addition to paying for Medicare Parts A, B, C, and D. Medigap plans provide supplemental insurance for Medicare consumers. Plans vary. Some Medigap premiums are quite expensive, and many elderly cannot afford them.

Despite the prevalence of public and private supplemental coverage, beneficiaries face substantial out-of-pocket expenses. Medicare covers less than half of older adults' total health spending and is less generous than health plans that are typically offered by large employers. On average, older adults spend 20% of their household income for health services and premiums. "The most vulnerable, ... those with incomes below the poverty level, spend more than 33% of their income; those in fair/poor health spend more than 25%" (Longest et al., 2000, p. 98).

Medicare's *service benefit plan* uses *prospective payment* mechanisms for care that set fixed rates for specific diagnoses. CMS sets the rates. In hospitals these set rates are called *diagnosis-related groups (DRGs)* for medical/surgical and obstetric diagnoses (not for pediatric and psychiatric diagnoses) and are used for reimbursement. *Resource utilization groups (RUGs)* were adopted for long-term care reimbursement. *Ambulatory payment categories (APCs)* were started for ambulatory settings, and *resource-based relative value scales (RBRVS)* were developed for physicians. Home care is regulated using the *outcome and assessment information set (OASIS)*. As CMS has established these prospective payment mechanisms, other insurance companies (Blue Cross, etc.) have also adopted them. Here is how they work, taking DRGs as an example:

> Discharged Medicare patients are assigned to one of almost 500 DRGs based on [ICD] diagnosis, surgery, patient age, discharge destination, and gender. Each DRG's weight is based primarily on Medicare billing and cost data, and reflects the relative cost—across all hospitals—of treating cases that are classified in that DRG. Hospitals that can provide services at lower costs keep the difference. Those exceeding the DRG rate must recoup the difference elsewhere (Longest et al., 2000, p. 71).

The physician is responsible for identifying the principle diagnosis, which has to be the reason for admission, using the *International Classification of Diseases*, 9th Revision, Clinical Modification (ICD-9). Up to four secondary diagnoses can be documented. If the physician does not adequately document all this, payment will not be forthcoming. Outliers occur when either costs or length of stay are longer than expected. Hospitals need to do as much as possible to prevent outliers. The biggest concern with Medicare presently is that it does not adequately reflect severity of illness.

In long-term care, Medicare reimbursement has been based on RUGs, now into RUG-III. "It set 44 reimbursement levels (26 for Medicare, 18 for Medicaid) based on resident condition and use of services. RUG-III uses 300 elements of care to measure a resident's acuity based on differences in ADLs [activities of daily living]; need for specialized therapies, nursing, and ancillary services; and presence of depression" (Longest et al., 2000, p. 72). RUGs "measure resident characteristics and staff care time for various categories of patients. RUGs have seven categories of patient severity. Caregivers derive the classifications from assessments recorded in the resident *Minimum Data Set (MDS)* assessment instrument required for days 5, 14, 30, 60, and 90 during a Part A stay. Facilities must also complete a comprehensive assessment if a patient's condition changes significantly.... To establish payment ... caregivers need to record and code MDS data and use it to assign patients to case mix groups" (Knapp, 1999, p. 14). So in long-term care, reimbursement is determined by how effectively staff complete the MDS data.

APCs have been developed for the whole range of ambulatory services. APCs group thousands of procedure and diagnosis costs into more than 300 categories, with separate classifications for surgical, medical, and ancillary services. Each group includes clinically similar services that require comparable levels of resources. A relative weight based on median resource use is assigned to each classification. Payment for each APC is determined by multiplying the relative weight by a conversion factor, which is the average rate for all APC services (Longest et al., 2000, p. 72).

The resource-based relative value scale (RBRVS), was started in an attempt to even out payments to specialty physicians (who were paid more) compared with family and general practice physicians (receiving less). Presently, physicians are paid for each treatment so there is an incentive to overuse services.

Home healthcare, driven by having to use OASIS, is presently serving patients after acute care episodes. There is no money allotted for chronic illness needs. This is a serious problem in our country because the greatest percentage of Medicare dollars is spent on acute tertiary care instead of health promotion/prevention and primary care.

The problem with all these payment changes is that there may be a tendency to discharge patients too soon. For example, patients might still be medically unstable when leaving the hospital or may not be able to care for themselves and need medical care but have used up their home care allotment.

Medicaid

Medicaid, a cost-sharing program involving both state and federal funds, provides services for medically indigent people, including children, and for people with severe and permanent disabilities who are under age 65—although elderly over 65 receiving welfare are also included in Medicaid. The federal government mandates certain basic coverage—inpatient and outpatient hospital services, physician, midwife, and certified nurse practitioner services, laboratory and x-ray services, nursing facility and home healthcare, early and periodic screening, diagnosis, and treatment (EPSDT) for children under age 21, family planning, and rural health clinics/federally qualified health centers. States can add such things as prescription drugs, clinic services, prosthetic devices, hearing aids, dental care, and intermediate care facilities for people with mental retardation to this coverage. Services and reimbursements vary widely from state to state.

Medicaid predominantly pays for custodial long-term care of more than 100 days, representing 48% of Medicaid expenses. If people need custodial long-term care, they must be at the poverty level, as established by each state, before Medicaid will pay. If people are not at the poverty level, a person can pay cash for care, or if the person has long-term care insurance (including Medigap insurance) that covers custodial care, the insurance plan can pay.

If a person does not have one of these options and is above the poverty level, it is possible to receive Medicaid benefits for custodial long-term care by *spending down* all assets (income, property, and other assets) until the patient is below the poverty level. Then Medicaid benefits will begin. (In this case the spouse is allowed a house, car, and a specified amount of money but the rest must be "spent down.") The other option, used by a significant number of elderly needing custodial care, is to be cared for by a relative in the home. This avoids spending down life savings.

Medicaid is quickly becoming a federal-versus-state rights issue. The federal government has mandated the states to support Medicaid, yet states are struggling to continue to pay their share of Medicaid spending. This is nearing crisis proportions. The situation is exacerbated because of the increased population at the poverty level needing Medicaid services.

Medicaid programs face special challenges. Often, consumers do not have a primary care physician, unless they are in an HMO program where one is assigned. When they need care, a usual practice has been to go to the local hospital emergency room for care. Also, this consumer group may not keep appointments because of lack of transportation or lack of childcare options. Sometimes nurse case managers are assigned to these patients to better, and less expensively, serve them. Some states have increased public health clinic funding to partially deal with this problem.

DIRECT SERVICE DELIVERY PLANS

A *direct service delivery plan* is another type of plan used by *HMOs*. This plan is different because it pays the provider in advance. Generally, there are five types of HMOs:

1. Staff HMOs that employ physicians individually
2. Group model HMOs that contract with one multispecialty group of physicians. A per capita rate is paid to the physician, as specified in the contract
3. Network model HMOs that operate just like group models, except that they contract with more than one group of physicians
4. Individual practice association (IPA) members that include both individual and group practice physicians. The HMO contracts with the IPA for physician services. IPA physician members provide services for the HMO but also treat other patients.
5. More recently, point-of-service HMOs came about more recently. Here an HMO patient can go to a physician or hospital outside the HMO but pays more out-of-pocket expense.

HMOs use capitation as the reimbursement mechanism. The word, *capitation*, comes from the "per capita" (per person) fee the purchaser pays. To purchase HMO services, the employer (or individual purchaser) pays a monthly (capitated) fee to the HMO. The HMO agrees to provide health-care services specified in the contract for no additional costs to the employer or the individual. The HMO either contracts with, or hires, providers who agree to be paid in advance a monthly or yearly fee in return for providing all services enrollees will need for that period.

Under capitation, a provider could lose money if too many services were provided in the covered period; alternately, the provider could make money if fewer services were given to enrollees and the cost was less than the prepaid amount. In addition, physicians are often told they need to see a certain number of patients. All this means that a physician would not want to order too many tests or a hospital would want to quickly transfer an acutely ill patient from intensive care, to a stepdown unit, to a subacute unit, and then to outpatient treatment and/or home care. Capitation established a provider incentive to cut costs.

In addition to capitation, HMOs use another managed care strategy. When consumers need care, they must first see a *gatekeeper* provider, such as a primary care physician or nurse practitioner. The gatekeeper determines if care is necessary and, if so, makes the decision whether the patient should be referred to a specialist. The advantage to the patient is that there is no charge to see the gatekeeper and no insurance paperwork is necessary for reimbursement. In addition, there is no charge for specialty care, as long as the gatekeeper makes the specialty referral. The consumer disadvantage with an HMO is when the gatekeeper does not believe specialty care is needed. In this case, if the patient still wants specialty care, the patient would have to pay for the specialty service or go without.

In the HMO system, gatekeepers are constantly under scrutiny for *practice patterns*. This includes collecting data on such things as *bed days per thousand*, the number of hospital inpatient bed days used by 1,000 health plan members in a year. Capitated payments have forced down patient length of stay, resulting in all healthcare services treating more acutely ill patients. This has created many conflicts and ethical dilemmas, as well as bad publicity, between the various healthcare players.

HMOs use another managed care strategy, *disease management*, with chronic, long-term illnesses. Here the physician, or provider, is given a mandated systematic, population-based approach that defines the patient diagnosis or problem and the specific intervention(s) to take with all patients that meet this definition. The HMO then collects data on the physician practice patterns and the patient clinical outcomes to determine how effectively the physician followed these mandates. "Examples of illnesses that are often targeted for disease management are asthma, arthritis, cancer, diabetes, hypertension, osteoporosis, high-risk pregnancy, congestive heart failure, depression, high cholesterol, and human immunodeficiency virus/acquired immune deficiency syndrome (HIV/AIDS)" (Finkelman, p. 96). Disease management identifies the best practices to achieve fewer poor outcomes or at least to slow down the degenerative aspects of these chronic diseases.

PRICING STRATEGIES

As managed care has developed, various pricing strategies have been used. The terms at the beginning of this section reflect more payer risk, whereas the terms toward the end have shared more risk with the provider. This dispersed risk has been a goal of managed care as it has developed (Smith, 1997, pp. 535–536).

Fee-for-service or *reasonable and customary charges* reimburse the provider a specific amount of money for each service and/or product that is provided. A *discounted fee-for-service* reimburses the provider for the service and/or product but here a discount, either a fixed amount or a percentage, is subtracted from the fee. The discount is specified in the payer-provider contract.

Per diem rates, or fixed rates on a per day basis, cover all the services or products used in that day. *Per case rates* are paid per visit or procedure. *Per episode rates* reimburse the provider for an episode of illness. Examples of this include the DRGs used for hospital reimbursement, the RUGs used for long-term care reimbursement, the APC system, the OASIS system in home care, and the RBRVS for physicians. In these systems, a *relative value unit* is developed where payment is based on the complexity of a procedure. For example, a more complex procedure might be paid the equivalent of two relative value units converted to dollars, as compared with a less complicated procedure where reimbursement is only one relative value unit.

Capitation, already discussed, is used when the provider is paid a per member per month fee. The provider can make money if fewer services are provided but loses money if too many services are given. *Risk sharing* is where the provider shares the cost of care given to a specified risk population. *Outcomes-based pricing* pays the provider a specified amount per case based on expected outcomes.

WHO IS THE BAD GUY?

A common fallacy is to view the third party payers as the "bad guys"—the cause of our societal dilemmas (such as the inadequacy of healthcare coverage, creating limitations on healthcare coverage, paying predominantly for tertiary illness care, and being responsible for the high cost of healthcare.) However, who really is the bad guy? Reviewing the history of healthcare in this country, one sees a much larger societal problem. Employers are spending large amounts of money on illness needs of employees who expect the best tertiary care possible and want someone else to cure all their illnesses. This cost is shared with employees in the form of deductibles and copayments; the majority of the cost then gets passed on to whatever widget or service the employer sells. As consumers purchase the widgets or services, consumers complain about the high costs. Who is really to blame? It turns out that finding the bad guy is really a much larger societal dilemma that holds many implications. This societal dilemma includes us—the general public or consumers, employers, payers, providers, suppliers, and regulators. We all contribute to the problem and all will have to be involved if we ever fix it.

WORKERS' COMPENSATION

Another group of payers cover *workers' compensation* costs, providing healthcare benefits to persons injured on the job. This is a $26 billion healthcare business. State laws vary but generally require employers to purchase insurance to cover workers' compensation. Employers are required to give cash benefits, medical care, and rehabilitation services for work-related injuries. In addition, diseases associated with specific occupations are automatically covered. Employees do not need to supply proof that the employer was at fault. However, in this arrangement employees give up the right of legal action and awards. Employers therefore benefit by having limited liability for occupational illnesses and injury. A current trend with workers' compensation is to have managed care companies take over the insurance. Because state laws differ in this area, it is best to consult the human resource department if an employee is injured on the job. Along with workers' compensation, most employers offer disability insurance to employees. Currently, 55% of all workers' compensation expenditures are for disability costs.

Suppliers

Suppliers—individuals or companies—provide supplies, equipment, and services used by the healthcare providers. Nursing interacts with suppliers in a number of ways. For instance, the product evaluation committee is used to determine the best deal on major equipment or supplies. The infection control nurse can become very involved with equipment and supplies that adversely affect either the patient or the healthcare worker.

In the late 1970s, in response to the importance of cutting costs, nationwide purchasing alliances—Premier Alliance, Voluntary Hospitals of America (VHA), and SunHealth—were formed. The idea was that materials and supplies could be purchased at less cost (many touted a 10% savings) because of the higher volume that could be purchased at once by the alliance. Presently, Premier Alliance and VHA contract volume includes approximately two-thirds of the nation's hospitals. This has caused other issues: Size brings big discounts, but not everyone wants to use the products. From a nursing perspective, it can be an issue when everyone is trained to use one supply, but the purchasing alliance gets a better deal on another similar supply that staff members have not been trained to use properly. The purchase itself may save money; however, staff education may cause the organization to actually spend more on this purchase.

When healthcare organizations join a purchasing alliance, they still must rely on local companies for certain supplies and services such as waste removal, physician contractual services to staff the emergency room, and laundry facilities (if contracted outside the healthcare organization).

Warren Bennis has called the physician group "suppliers" for healthcare organizations. This seems to be the most appropriate term. However, you often hear physicians being referred to as *customers*. Many hospitals market to physicians to be sure there are enough primary care physicians to refer patients to specialty physicians and to make sure there are enough specialists to meet community needs and keep hospital beds filled. At times, the recruitment process also involves providing assistance such as loans for office practices or homes along with a certain amount of reimbursement for relocation expenses to physicians.

Regulators

Regulators are the organizations/agencies that set the rules, regulations, and/or standards that providers must meet to stay in business. This includes many groups, such as the federal, state, and local governments and judicial systems, accrediting bodies, regulators of professions such as medicine and nursing, and professional organizations. The standards used by regulators come from many sources including consumers, providers, payers, professional organizations, and even state or federal laws or executive orders.

FEDERAL REGULATION

In healthcare the federal government, as a regulator, has the overall responsibility for both achieving quality and holding down costs. The Constitution specifies that the federal government has the authority to regulate interstate commerce and provide for the general welfare of its citizens. The main federal healthcare regulator is the CMS, established to administer Medicare and Medicaid and enforce national healthcare regulations. For example, federal legislation, in a 1972 cost reduction strategy, mandated *utilization review*, "a formal assessment of the medical necessity, efficiency, and/or appropriateness of healthcare services and treatment plans on a prospective, concurrent, or retrospective basis" (Finkelman, p. 490). (Most other payers have adopted this strategy as well.) Utilization review is accomplished using several mechanisms:

- *Preadmission certification*—the insurer approves care in advance. If this is required, and certification is not obtained the insurer can refuse to pay for the care.
- *Concurrent review*—Some insurers monitor patients' lengths of stay to ensure the patients are discharged quickly. If an insurer determines that the patient has received all the appropriate tests and treatments, the insurer will not authorize additional care and will refuse to pay for additional days.
- *Discharge planning*—Discharge planning has always been important. However, now it is critical. It is important to keep lengths of stay as short as possible. The discharge plan may include additional care needed by transferring the patient quickly to long-term care, home care, and/or ambulatory care, which is less expensive than the hospital stay.
- *Case management*—More information about case management is in Chapter 18. In this case care plans are developed for complicated patients to provide the needed care in the least expensive way. For example, perhaps a hospitalization can be prevented by providing home care 7 days a week.
- *Second surgical opinions*—For elective surgeries, insurers may require that the patient go to a second physician to determine whether the surgery is necessary. Additionally, the insurer wants to do the surgery in the least expensive way—outpatient is preferred but if hospitalization is needed, this needs to be specified.

Another example of CMS regulation is the special handicap access standards developed by the American National Standards Institute (ANSI) and the federal government. For instance, corridor width needs to be at least 8 feet wide and a bathroom needs to accommodate two certified nurse assistants assisting a resident in a wheelchair. In long-term care, "design principles for the elderly focus on safety, privacy, lighting, texture, color, signage, independence, orienting features, access, and social contact.... For example, it is difficult for an older person to distinguish colors of similar intensity such as pastels and combinations of blues and greens; smooth textures make colors appear lighter; rough textures make colors appear darker" (Mitty, 1998, p. 312).

Another important federal regulator for healthcare is the *Occupational Safety and Health Administration (OSHA)*, implemented to ensure a safe, healthy workplace. OSHA uses Center for Disease Control and Prevention (CDC) standards in healthcare organizations. The CDC's mission is to prevent and control disease, injury, and disability. OSHA regulations are very complicated and change each year. To find more information about either OSHA or CDC current requirements, go to their websites (www.osha.gov or www.cdc.gov). Employers are required to be aware of unsafe conditions (vague wording), are responsible to inform employees about OSHA standards, and are expected to provide safe conditions and appropriate safety equipment for employees. In addition, an employer is expected to accommodate employees who are disabled unless it causes an unrealistic disadvantage on the employer (more vague wording). It is advisable to consult with the human resource department for more details on the disability issue. (Federal OSHA standards can be expanded, but not reduced, by a state.)

Employers violating OSHA regulations can be cited and/or fined, and, if serious enough, a workplace can be closed. OSHA is not well staffed, having fewer than a thousand inspectors for the country. However, they make unannounced comprehensive safety and health inspections, and if an OSHA inspector arrives at the workplace, they have a right to enter and inspect. (Most OSHA cases do not involve an inspector.) Generally, a safety committee at the workplace takes responsibility for meeting OSHA standards. If an employee is injured in the workplace, the safety committee investigates workplace conditions at the site where the employee was injured and evaluates the situation and, if necessary, makes recommendations for changes. The safety committee then has the responsibility to make sure the recommendations have been followed. Safety committee records are to be regularly audited. Most often, accreditation standards include meeting OSHA regulations.

To accomplish quality monitoring, the federal government delegates specific responsibilities to each state's licensure and certification agency. For a facility to participate in Medicare and Medicaid programs, they must undergo this licensure and certification process. States vary as to actual requirements. In addition, healthcare organizations must be accredited to be eligible for Medicare reimbursement.

Other federal regulators affect healthcare:

- The Department of Justice and Federal Trade Commission enforce antitrust issues, which prohibits anticompetitive practices.
- The National Labor Relations Board regulates union organizing and collective bargaining.
- The Food and Drug Administration regulates drugs and medical devices and dietary regulations and inspections.
- The Securities and Exchange Commission regulates how investor-owned healthcare organizations can market, sell, and trade stock.
- The Nuclear Regulatory Commission regulates hazards arising from storage, handling, and transportation of nuclear materials.
- The Equal Employment Opportunity Commission enforces Equal Employment Opportunities (EEO) in hiring, equal pay, civil rights, and age discrimination issues (Longest et al., 2000, p. 74).
- The Judicial system has determined many healthcare regulations. These are discussed in Chapter 8.

STATE REGULATION

When the states delegated certain powers to a federal government and ratified the U.S. Constitution, they retained a wide range of authority known as the police powers, defined as the powers to protect the health, safety, public order, and welfare of the public. Consistent with the police powers, states have enacted legislation to regulate and license a wide variety of healthcare organizations that are required to obtain and retain a license and must submit to inspections and other regulation (Longest et al., 2000, p. 69).

Health and safety issues include radiation safety, sanitation of food and water, and disposal of wastes. States may delegate some of the safety, sanitation, and waste disposal responsibilities to city and county governments. Therefore the states regulate, inspect, and license healthcare organizations on physical plant safety issues and license and regulate various healthcare professionals and nursing education programs. In addition, "each state has an insurance commission. This commission is responsible for regulating both the solvency of insurers and the marketing of insurance.... A particularly important responsibility is the regulation of the level of reserves [savings to cover future claims] that the insurance companies must maintain" (Finkelman, p. 43).

Because states were already conducting annual inspections of healthcare inpatient facilities when Medicare was established, the federal government mandated an annual state inspection of hospitals and long-term care facilities receiving Medicare funding. Home care was added to the list for state licensing if treating Medicare and Medicaid patients. State licensure and certification agencies have a number of responsibilities. First, to be eligible for Medicare and Medicaid funding the healthcare organization must be licensed by the state. For example, in long-term care, the state will "authorize a nursing home to provide certain services when particular criteria are met: minimum staffing levels, personnel qualifications, educational requirements for the administrator, quality assurance systems, compliance with fire and safety codes, service delivery capability, bylaws and administrative organization" (Mitty, 1998, p. 248). After the inspection, the states make recommendations to CMS for Medicare certification.

Second, annual inspections then must occur with organizations treating Medicare and Medicaid patients. Certification is needed each year to receive Medicare reimbursement. Medicaid regulation is shared between the federal government and the states. "Licensure and certification standards may exceed federal requirements but states may not eliminate a standard or requirement or create one in conflict with federal regulations. The federal government has the authority to conduct independent inspections of certified nursing homes to audit the state's certification activities in both the Medicare and Medicaid programs (as a rule, 10% of homes annually)" (Mitty, 1998).

Because of this, each state has designed a different version of Medicaid. This is why Medicaid has different titles in many states, such as TennCare in Tennessee and MedCal in California. Because about 50% of Medicaid funds are for long-term care, the federal government has mandated each state to do a more involved annual inspection of long-term care given to each Medicaid-funded resident. As part of the inspection,

A multidisciplinary survey team must ensure that the care reimbursed with Medicaid funds is necessary, available, adequate, appropriate—and of acceptable quality to maximize the physical and mental potential and well-being of the resident. The review also includes an assessment of [each] resident's continued placement in the home and the feasibility of meeting his needs through alternative institutional or non-institutional services. The survey team looks for evidence that the resident's discharge potential was evaluated (Mitty, 1998, p. 248).

If the facility meets all the federal requirements, the state, representing CMS, then certifies or recertifies the long-term care facility on the day of the survey.

Another important state responsibility concerns individual licensing and certification for various health occupations. Perhaps, as nurses, we are most aware of the *board of nursing.* (In addition, there are other professional boards, such as the board of medicine or the board licensing long-term care administrators.) Each state has a Nurse Practice Act(s) that defines nursing practice and establishes the board of nursing. The professional boards define professional practice, license caregivers (to become licensed a person must show that they have achieved minimum competencies with the board keeping an official roster of all who are licensed), and set standards. Boards of nursing also license licensed practical nurses and nurse assistants. Generally, the practice acts specify that registered nurses can treat patients independently, whereas licensing for licensed practical nurses or nurse assistants specify that licensees are dependent on the orders of a registered nurse or physician. In addition, the board holds regular hearings, regulates practice, determines what is improper professional conduct and takes disciplinary actions when this occurs, introduces legislation to better define professional practice, licenses new nursing education programs, and oversees the quality of current nursing education programs. Most states have mandated that nursing education programs achieve an 85% student pass rate on the National Council Licensing Exam (NCLEX). Having representation on the board of nursing can be an important role in policymaking.

Although it is not a state regulatory body, it is important to note here that there is a National Council of State Boards of Nursing (NCSBN) whose purpose is to provide a national organization where boards of nursing can "act and counsel together on matters of common interest and concern affecting the public health, safety and welfare, including the development of licensing examinations in nursing" (www.ncsbn.org). NCSBN has been involved with several important issues. First, they have developed computerized licensure examinations, the NCLEX-RN and the NCLEX-PN, which are administered by a national test service to all individuals who want to be newly licensed as a registered nurse or licensed practical nurse. Second, NCSBN has established a multistate Nurse Licensure Compact. Presently, nurse practice acts are not uniform in all states. A state legislature can pass a law to become a part of this Compact. Once passed, nurses can practice across state lines, without getting licensed in another state, as long as the nurse follows the practice provisions in place in the state in which the nurse is practicing. One can find the list of states that currently belong to the Nurse Licensure Compact at the NCSBN Web site (www.ncsbn.org/nlc.htm).

CREDENTIALING

Credentialing of healthcare occupations takes place in several ways: licensure, registration, certification, and competency. With *licensure* a person must show that they have achieved minimum competencies to the state licensing board such as the board of nursing. *Registration* is the official roster, kept by the board of nursing, listing all who are licensed. *Certification* is awarded to individual providers by a nongovernmental organization/registry when the individual has met certain educational requirements and passed an examination. For example, family nurse practitioners or certified nurse assistants are certified.

A number of nursing specialty organizations certify nurses (listed at http://medi-smart.com/cert.htm). In turn, these professional certifying organizations are certified by the American Board of Nursing Specialties, a certifier of certifiers (Bernreuter, 2001). Boards of nursing, as well as employers, require that people in certain health occupations are certified (i.e., the nurse practitioner).

Voluntary certification for nurse administrators can be obtained from the American Nurses Credentialing Center (ANCC) and from the American Organization of Nurse Executives (AONE).

Nurse executive certification can also be obtained by admission to the American College of Health Care Executives and for home/hospice care nurse executives through the National Association for Home Care's Executive Certification Program. (Certification can also be given to organizations that have met speci-fied qualifications, such as providers needing Medicare and Medicaid certification to receive payments.)

A component of organizational accreditation includes the standard that employees are properly *credentialed* to do their assigned work. The evaluation process for this standard examines licenses, certification, educational background, and competency (evidence of current, safe practice or performance quality) of personnel, as well as that of the physicians.

Economic credentialing of physician patient volume and practice patterns, including patient outcomes, is now a common practice for hospitals. These factors are considered when renewing physician privileges.

ACCREDITATION

> *Accreditation* is the process by which organizations are evaluated on their quality, based on established minimum standards. There are two major reasons for accrediting healthcare organizations. Healthcare purchasers want objective data to make informed decisions about health plans to support a good return on their investment. Data from accreditation, as well as accreditation status, can supply some of this objective data. In addition, consumers have become more interested in data about health plans as they make their own decisions about which plan to select from the choices available to them. Purchasers and consumers are interested in two critical elements: cost and quality. They want greater accountability for the quality of services (Finkelman, pp. 230–231).

Generally, accreditation involves two steps: reviewing written materials (self-study) and someone from the accrediting body making an on-site visit to determine whether the minimum standards have been met. Personnel in healthcare organizations must have ongoing education about current/new standards to maintain accreditation. There are many healthcare accrediting bodies (see http://gunston.gmu.edu/healthscience/547/MajorAccreditationAgencies.asp).

PROFESSIONAL ORGANIZATIONS

Professional organizations, such as the American Nurses Association (ANA) and the American Organization of Nurse Executives (AONE), continually examine professional scope of practice and professional standards. AONE, ANA, American Association of Colleges of Nursing (AACN), and the National League for Nursing (NLN) have formed a national tri-council on nursing. Together, they represent nursing on certain national issues. In long-term care directors of nursing can belong to the American Association of Directors of Nursing Administration in Long-Term Care or to the National Conference of Gerontological Nurse Practitioners (NCGPN). The American Academy of Ambulatory Care Nursing (AAACN) focuses on ambulatory nursing practice. The National Association for Home Care (NAHC) represents home care professionals.

Nursing Professional Organizations are listed at http://orgs.salisbury.edu/sna/comprehensive%20associations.htm. The authors suggest that the nurse manager belong to both clinical and administrative professional organizations that are appropriate for the area of practice in which one is working. In addition to nursing organizations, there are other professional organizations nurse administrators might want to consider that are pertinent for their work setting, such as the American College of Healthcare Executives (ACHE).

Discussion Questions

1. What would improve our healthcare system? Explain how this could happen.
2. As a nurse manager, how can you and your staff better care for the people you serve?
3. What are the characteristics of the consumers that you regularly see? How could they be better served?
4. What is happening environmentally that is causing more people to go without insurance?
5. What strategies could your healthcare organization adopt that would make them more effective?
6. What is measured for provider performance at your healthcare organization?
7. What is the percentage of various payers in your healthcare organization?
8. What information should nurse managers share with staff regarding payers?
9. What is prospective payment? How does it affect you?
10. Who are the various regulators that impact your healthcare organization?

Glossary of Terms

Bonuses—given to the provider at the end of the year based on the provider's performance or based on the total plan performance.

Capitation—a reimbursement mechanism. *Capitation* comes from the "per capita" (per person) fee the purchaser pays. To purchase HMO services, the employer (or individual purchaser) pays a monthly capitated fee to the HMO.

Concurrent Review—Some insurers will monitor patients' lengths of stay to ensure the patients are discharged quickly. If an insurer determines that the patient has received all the appropriate tests and treatments, the insurer will not authorize additional care and will refuse to pay for additional days.

Covered Lives—individuals included in an insurance plan.

Direct Service Delivery Plan—a plan used by HMOs. Here the HMO pays the provider in advance. The provider agrees to provide certain services.

Disease Management—often used for chronic, long-term illnesses. Here the physician, or provider, is given a mandated systematic, population-based approach that defines the patient diagnosis or problem, and the specific intervention(s) to take with all patients that meet this definition.

Fee for Service—the provider is reimbursed a specific amount of money, *reasonable and customary charges*, for each service and/or product that is provided. A *discounted fee for service* reimburses the provider for the service and/or product but here a discount, either a fixed amount or a percentage, is subtracted from the fee. The discount is specified in the payer–provider contract.

Gag Rules—providers need protection for due process in their relationship with payers because payers may expect that providers remain quiet about the incentives payers give providers.

Gatekeeper—in an HMO when consumers need care they must first see a gatekeeper provider, such as a primary care physician or nurse practitioner. The gatekeeper determines if care is necessary and, if so, makes the decision whether the patient should be referred to a specialist. The advantage to the patient is that there is no charge to see the gatekeeper, and no insurance paperwork is necessary for reimbursement. In addition, there is no charge for specialty care, as long as the gatekeeper makes the specialty referral and the contract specifies that specialty care is available.

HMOs—health maintenance organizations where the plan pays the provider in advance. The purchaser (an employer or an individual) pays a monthly fee to the HMO. The HMO agrees to provide healthcare services specified in the contract for no additional costs to the employer or the individual. The consumer sees a gatekeeper who determines what care the consumer needs.

Horizontal Integration—when a facility combines with like facilities.

Managed Care—refers to any method of healthcare delivery that is designed to cut costs yet provide needed services.

Outcomes-Based Pricing—pays the provider a specified amount per case based on expected outcomes.

Payer Mix—the average percentage of different payers (i.e., Medicare, Blue Cross, self-pay) who paid for services to a healthcare organization over a year.

Per Case Rates—rates paid per visit or procedure.

Per Diem Rates—fixed rates on a per day basis, cover all the services or products used in that day.

Per Episode Rates—reimburse the provider for an episode of illness (i.e., DRGs, RUGs, OASIS).

Performance-Based Reimbursement—data are collected on patient outcomes—length of stay, readmission rates, adverse reactions, deaths, etc.—within a healthcare organization (*provider performance*). Payers use this evaluation before contracting with providers for healthcare services.

PPOs—preferred provider organizations, an example of a service benefit plan. It consists of a group of providers—such as physicians and hospitals—who have agreed to provide services at lower than usual rates to enrollees. The PPO acts as the intermediary between providers and consumers. The PPO pays prearranged fees for services provided. The enrollee incentive is to use the providers in the plan and not have to pay for many of the services provided. If an enrollee chooses to go to a physician not included in the PPO, the PPO only pays part—or none—of the fee, with the enrollee having to pay the remainder.

Practice Patterns—where physicians are under scrutiny about their practice. Data are collected on such things as length of stay and individual physician data is compared with other physician data.

Preadmission Certification—the insurer approves care in advance. If this is required, and certification is not obtained, the insurer can refuse to pay for the care.

Prospective Payment—the payer determines the cost of care before the care is given. The provider is then told how much will be paid to give the care.

Provider Protection—legislation aimed at either limiting incentives offered to providers or revealing the incentives to patients.

Relative Value Rates—payment is based on the complexity of a procedure. For example, a more complex procedure might be paid the equivalent of two relative value units converted to dollars, as compared with a less complicated procedure where reimbursement is only one relative value unit.

Retrospective Payment—indemnity insurance where payment occurs after the care is given.

Risk Sharing—where the provider shares the cost of care given to a specified risk population.

Service Benefit Plan—directly pay providers after negotiating and specifying the prices paid for each healthcare service. In service benefit plans the patient pays part of the costs with deductibles and coinsurance.

Underwriting—an insurance company acts as an administrator of the pool of money collected from all its members, paying, or *underwriting*, the defined illness care coverage to a provider when the consumer has received healthcare services.

Vertical Integration—when an organization offers as many different healthcare services as possible.

Withholds—when an HMO, or payer, holds part of the physician or hospital income until the end of the year and pays it back to the physician or hospital based on the physician's or hospital's performance.

References

Bernreuter, M. (2001). Spotlight on … the American board of nursing specialties: Nursing's gold standard. *JONA's Healthcare Law, Ethics, and Regulation, 3*(1), 5–7.

Finkelman, A. (2001). *Managed Care: A nursing perspective*. Upper Saddle River, NJ: Prentice Hall.

Finkler, S., & Kovner, C. (2000). *Financial management for nurse managers and executives* (2nd ed.). Philadelphia: W.B. Saunders.

Griffith, J. (1999). *The well-managed healthcare organization* (4th ed.). Chicago: Health Administration Press.

Hudson, T. (1977, December). Necessary loses? *Hospitals & Health Networks*, 26.

Knapp, M. (1999, May). Nurses' basic guide to understanding the medicare pps. *Nursing Management*, 14–15.

Longest, B., Rakich, J., & Darr, K. (2000). *Managing health services organizations and systems* (4th ed.). Baltimore: Health Professions Press.

Mitty, E. (1998). *Handbook for directors of nursing in long-term care*. Albany, NY: Delmar.

Raffel, M., & Raffel, N. (1994). *The U.S. health system: Origins and functions* (4th ed.). Albany, NY: Delmar.

Smith, N. (1997). Managed care. In M. Harris (Ed.), *Handbook of home healthcare administrators* (2nd ed., p. 535). Gaithersburg, MD: Aspen.

CHAPTER 11

Microeconomics and Cost Accounting in the Hospital Firm: Competition, Regulation, the Profit Motive, and Patient Care

Mary Anne Schultz, PhD, MBA, MSN, RN

No margin, no mission.

—*Sister Irene Kraus, 1998, former president, Daughters of Charity National Health System, Inc.*

Key Terms

- American Nurses Credentialing Center
- Asymmetric Knowledge
- Bad Debt Expense
- Buyer
- Capitalism
- Competition
- Cost
- Cost Accounting
- Cost-Plus Basis
- Deregulation
- Diagnosis-Related Groups
- Economics
- Economies of Scale
- Expense
- Externalities

- Financial Accounting
- Firm
- Government Intervention
- Health Care Economics
- Incentive
- Liquidity
- Macroeconomics
- Managed Care
- Managerial Accounting
- Margin
- Microeconomics
- Mission
- Motive
- Net Present Value
- Normative Economics
- Nurse Manager

- Operating Expenses
- Perfect Information
- Positive Economics
- Profit
- Profit Margin
- Prospective Payment System
- Regulation
- Risk
- Seller
- Solvency
- Symmetric Knowledge
- Total Compensation Package
- Uncertainty
- Widget

Since the introduction of a prospective payment system (PPS) for health care 25 years ago, hospital services have become increasingly driven by the market forces of price and quality. Rooted in a tradition of caring, hospitals were once seen as places where people could be healed and have their physical needs met—all through the professionalism and trust of health care providers. This was the hospital's *mission*. Today, hospitals are businesses, big and small, where patient care is but one service and patients are no longer the only constituent. The processes are now high technology, caring, curing in some cases, research based, and financially driven serving a number of stakeholders such as physicians, investors, patients and families, and employees such as nurses, to name a few.

Balancing the goals of the players in and supporting the many purposes of a hospital require identification of the pressures shaping its operation. Chiefly, these are (1) competition, (2) regulation, (3) the profit motive, and (4) quality patient care. This chapter examines these key forces from the standpoint of theory and practices in both microeconomics and cost accounting. Recognizing that health care once derived its processes almost solely from mission, we now identify that it is a hospital's *margin* that is first because, without a (profit) margin, the organization, like all businesses, ceases to exist, and hence there is no mission. This chapter in no way provides a comprehensive survey of these interrelated forces but instead offers an explanatory primer, with examples, for a hospital's economic and business behavior. An overview of the disciplines of both microeconomics and cost accounting is provided to acquaint the reader with what is probably an entirely new way of thinking (and talking) about the institution called a hospital. This way, the profession, through the nurse managers and other nurse leaders, communicates with key nonprovider hospital decision makers, such as the chief executive officer or chief financial officer, with the same language and thus on a level playing field.

Microeconomics, Cost Accounting, and Nursing

This section addresses the question, "What is microeconomics (and, in turn, cost accounting) and what has it to do with nursing?" *Economics*, the study of how society allocates scarce resources, can be divided into two categories, macroeconomics and microeconomics. *Macroeconomics* (the prefix "macro" meaning large) is the study of the market system on a large scale. Macroeconomics considers the aggregate performance of *all* markets (so, the performance or outcomes, of *all* companies or firms in *all* industries) and gives us indices or measures ("indicators") of a nation's economy such as stock prices, interest rates, jobless claims, and housing starts. For purposes of this chapter, macroeconomics might serve as a context within which we describe the typical hospital (hospital "firm") behavior with respect to (1) revenue optimization, (2) expense reduction, and (3) production of patient outcomes at an acceptable (not maximal) level of quality. *Microeconomics*, the study of individual consumers in relationship to their markets, is concerned with the choices made by smaller economic units such as consumers or individual (hospital) firms. A key section in this chapter, microeconomics gives us concepts such as profit, profit maximization, price strategy, and nonprice competition to consider.

Cost accounting is an element of financial management that generates information about the costs of an organization and its components. As such, it is a subset of accounting in general and encompasses the development and provision of a wide range of financial management that is useful to managers in their organizational roles. Keep in mind that the goal in generating this information is to provide a basis for decision making. A quintessential question in our field is this: what should the nurse-to-patient ratio be *and* on what basis is this decided? The field of cost accounting, borrowing from financial accounting (information generated by firms largely for external purposes, e.g., the Internal Revenue Service) while encompassing managerial accounting (information generated by firms for their own internal use) affords us tools to address the tough staffing questions such as break-even analysis, profitability

Exhibit 11–1 Relationship of the Accounting Disciplines

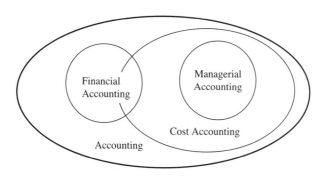

analysis, make versus buy decision making, marginal cost calculations, and cost–quality trade-off analysis. The relationship of the accounting disciplines is depicted in **Exhibit 11–1**. It is the considered opinion of the author that these domains, economics and accounting, were once considered mutually exclusive from the field of nursing. Only as the number of nurses undertaking formal study of these quantitative disciplines, such as in Master of Business Administration (MBA) or Master of Public Health (MPH) programs, increased did our field place itself on equal footing with lay administrators at the top of the hospital hierarchy.

The nurse at the top of the administrative hierarchy, the nurse executive, may have trained with advanced preparation in all three disciplines discussed here, microeconomics, cost accounting, and nursing. The American Organization of Nurse Executives (2005) published its view of the core competencies that the nurse executive should have. Among these are analyses of supply and demand data, analysis of financial statements, articulation of business models based on economics, strategic and business planning, and the development of future business skill sets in leadership team members, all of which are listed under the Business Skills subsection of the document. This is brought to the attention of the reader to dramatize how important it is for current and future nurse leaders to maintain their own skill set in business and financial matters and to massage this process within key leaders in their organizations such as nurse managers. The deployment of nurse resources at the unit level could quite possibly be the most important decision made in hospital care because it is through the provision of nursing care quality that quality patient outcomes are realized.

Today, baccalaureate nursing schools traditionally require one course in leadership, often at the senior level. Most often, this course does not include financial content. Some schools are beginning to offer a separate course in nursing management that does address lower level financial decision making, for example, the use of budgeting and marketing tools for nurse managers on the unit level. All, or nearly all, baccalaureate programs offer a course in health systems that analyzes health care organizations on the macro level, but the core quantitative courses and tools needed to place nursing on equal footing with lay decision makers reside in MBA or MPH programs and only some master's in nursing (MS or MSN) programs in which the volume and type of financial preparation for these future leaders vary.

This does not mean that every baccalaureate or higher prepared nurse must be a manager per se. It also does not mean that the nurse administrator must be a junior chief financial officer. Rather, a nurse executive must possess the financial knowledge necessary to make system-focused decisions that integrate the clinical and business aspects of health care (Lemire, 2000).

Nursing administration, one form of advanced practice (Harris, Huber, Jones, Manojlovich, & Reineck, 2006), is an at-risk specialty given numerous reports of dropping enrollment in graduate nursing administration programs (Herrin, Jones, Krepper, Sherman, & Reineck, 2006); the escalated demand for nurses in the clinical graduate nursing specialties such as pediatrics, geriatrics, and primary care (Furlong & Smith, 2005); a perceived lack of attractiveness of nursing administration as a viable graduate program choice (Rudan, 2002); widespread nurse executive burnout (Rollins, 2008); and the dire situation of the aging nurse faculty workforce (Berlin & Sechrist, 2002). Without this vital specialty, nursing could lose its scientific basis for practice, nurse managers at the unit level might lose recently acquired gains in real autonomy and decision making, and, most of all, research done by nurses on the effectiveness of their measures will continue to be invisible in health care quality, health services research, health policy, and health care finance initiatives (Lang, 2003). This discussion is an appeal to the reader regarding the uniqueness of the nursing administration specialty as well as the special challenges afforded the profession if our critical mass of economic and systems thinkers continues to deteriorate.

Competition

Theory of the firm, the theory of supply and demand, explains and predicts price, quantity of products, and the likelihood of survival of firms in a competitive industry. Before the PPS was introduced into the health care market, hospital firms operated on a cost-plus basis, billing insurers for the total consumption of resources by an individual patient. After 1983, hospitals were switched to a diagnosis-related group basis for reimbursement, receiving compensation for what a typical patient within a medical diagnosis and selected other medical conditions would consume. This departure from the cost-plus reimbursement scheme ended the era of price competition in health care, and hospitals began to compete on a nonprice, or quality, basis, which is when patient outcomes magnified in importance.

For centuries, the relationship of the demand for a product or service to its supply has been thought to be largely due to the intervening variable of price. In the fictional "market for widgets," supply of a product consistently meets the demand for it, given a set of assumptions about the market for widgets. This theory, theory of the firm, explains a lot about the way the world works pending the strength of these assumptions: a large numbers of buyers and sellers, perfect information about the product, absence of barriers to entry and exit as a business entity in the industry, and homogeneity of the product. Note that a full description of all four assumptions as they pertain to markets for health care is beyond the scope of this text, yet a focus on two of the assumptions—a large number of health care buyers and sellers and the existence of good information—is key.

In health care the four assumptions are less clearly visible than in the fictitious market for widgets for a variety of reasons. Among them are the fact that relatively little is known to the buyer of hospital care (the insurance company) about the quality of care purchased from the seller (in our case, the hospital), and the demand for hospital care is a *derived* demand. This is to say that it comes from health insurance companies as the intermediary between hospital care providers like hospitals and the individual consumer-patient. When health care entered the competitive arena, decision makers became highly sensitized to the customary business practices of restricting expenses and maximizing revenue while producing a service of measurable quality whenever possible. (Note that the language "an acceptable level of quality" should not be confused with something time-honored verbalized by nursing such as "the highest possible level of quality." The difference between two such statements is described in a later section, Cost Accounting).

The change from a system loosely concerned with quality of care, through the professionalism and trust of providers, to a system that prices services strategically while competing on quality has resulted in a cost-conscious era unlike that ever seen before. It is widely recognized that as hospitals compete to provide services, they attempt to (1) optimize profit through pricing strategies, (2) reduce expenses through decisions about personnel and equipment, and (3) satisfy recipients of care through both high-technology and caring approaches. This means that hospitals seek to strike a vital balance between cost reduction and quality of care to adapt successfully to external competitive threats to their survival. For example, the ratio of nurses or operating expenses to patient days is a resource input that may influence the output of the system that is the provision of quality care.

Better care provision (a result of wise resource allocation) may result in better patient outcomes (output) and is alleged to be a benefit of an openly competitive, deregulated hospital market. Hospitals that can demonstrate higher quality of care, or even adequacy of care, will win competitions, or bids, for reimbursement plans, more patients, and better-qualified care providers. Over time, "good" hospitals will survive because they have established a pattern of good outcomes. Evidence that this theory, theory of the firm, which explains a lot of how the world works, explains at least *some* things about how the world of hospital care works can be found through such organizations as HealthGrades®, a leading independent health care ranking company (see http://www.healthgrades.com/) or *U.S. News and World Report's* ranking system (see http://health.usnews.com/sections/health/best-hospitals). Both report such measures as risk-adjusted mortality rates and complication rates as patient-population specific measures of comparative quality. Also, hospitals can be designated as magnet hospitals by the American Nurses Credentialing Center (ANCC) (see http://www.nursecredentialing.org/Magnet/ProgramOverview.aspx), which means they meet over 65 process and structural criteria validated by a site visit from the ANCC. Only those hospitals known to be a good place to practice nursing are ranked as such, and the term originally meant that the hospital "attracted" nurses and patients. The inner workings of these organizations and detailed descriptions of their methodologies, too complex to be reported here, can be found at their respective websites. Also, a primer on what risk-adjusted mortality rates means, as an overall general measure of quality or at least adequacy of any one hospital, is discussed in a later section. In summary, the importance of these hospital ranking systems, or stamps of approval as the public might see them, is this: The information about the quality of the product or service of a hospital is accurate enough to be used for comparison ratings. Hence, the information qualifies as perfect information (not to be taken literally).

What microeconomic theory states regarding the eventual number of hospital firms within an industry under long-run equilibrium (hospitals that rival or compete over a long time) is this: Those hospital firms with better products or services will survive, but those with inferior products and services will not. This is due to the perception of quality held by payers and consumers, which, in part, drives the industry's (derived) demand. Unfortunately, relatively little is known about the tenets of competition in health care or variations in the quality of patient outcomes in hospitals. So the usefulness of this theory for the explanation and prediction of future activities in health care remains challenged. This is not to say "well, supply and demand … it just doesn't work in health care!", which is an emotionally charged statement devoid of reason. It is, instead, appropriate to say that predictive power of the theory in health care is limited more than its explanatory power interpreting the how and why of a hospital firm's behavior. Stated another way, all hospitals seek to maximize patient outcomes, especially on those measures that are publicly reported. Most notably, these are mortality rates and complication rates of frequent and costly conditions such as acute myocardial infarction, cardiac surgical conditions, hip fracture, and community-acquired pneumonia. There is, however, no one (or even two or three) composite overall measure(s) of hospital quality that can stand out to represent hospital care throughout one institution, though that topic is much discussed in quality initiative circles.

In the world of competitive hospital management, decision makers continually forecast, or second guess, what their rivals will do when they introduce such novelties as courting new profitable patient populations or programs such as breast centers, cancer centers, symptom-management clinics, and addiction rehabilitation. In short, hospitals must innovate with new programs, new patient populations, or quality initiatives to survive intense competition and hence scrutiny. New sources of (perfect or symmetric) information are continually available on hospital care in both print and electronic media so decision makers must be savvy regarding patient outcome comparisons, making press releases when appropriate to boast their latest claim to excellence. Just as automobiles are rated for gas consumption and airlines for on-time arrivals, payers and consumers contract for hospital care based on price and quality through managed care negotiations.

Regulation and Managed Care

The soaring cost of health care has been one of the most pressing domestic issues for decades. Politicians and pundits speak of how changes in laws could impact this crisis, sometimes provoking a discussion of socialized medicine and cross-country comparison of U.S. versus "other" health care expenditures and outcomes. With no clear answer to this type of health care ill emerging soon, most would agree that although our health care system is among the most market oriented (competitively driven) in the world, it remains *the* most heavily regulated sector of the U.S. economy (Conover, 2004). This author states that the costs of regulation are the benefits we would derive with alternative uses of those resources. After reviewing the literature on 47 different kinds of health care regulations, it was estimated that the net burden of health services regulation on society was $169.1 billion annually. For the novice in economic thinking, let's examine what some of the costs of regulation are said to be. In lay terms, it is the sum total of all expenditures by federal or state regulators that oversee, inspect, supervise, monitor, or award privileges to a health care provider such as physicians, nurses, and hospitals. In just glancing at hospital and nursing regulation costs alone, consider these:

- The Centers for Medicare and Medicaid Services (CMS) utilization reviews of appropriateness
- Office of Safety and Health Administration (OSHA) inspection of workplace safety
- The National Labor Relations Board monitoring of nurse unions
- National Council of State Boards of Nursing licensing exam requirements
- Every state board of nursing, medicine, pharmacy, respiratory therapy, and physical therapy
- American Association of Colleges of Nursing and National League for Nursing accreditation of nursing schools
- National Practitioner Data Bank housing information on practitioners
- Limitations on medical resident or registered nurse (RN) working hours
- Fraud and abuse protections

Each one of these organizations or protections, and scores more of them, have staff, overhead, a place of business to run, and extensive reporting requirements to yet another governmental or quasi-governmental organization. The author makes a convincing case that if health care were deregulated, the cost savings from this could realize gains in health promotion and prevention.

Although in our discussion of rivalry and what hospital firms must do to survive, indeed thrive, a convincing case is made about the benefits of the competitive, or market-driven, environment for hospital care, this is not diametrically opposed to regulatory efforts. This needs to be said because, in essence, a highly competitive market-driven industry is a bit like the polar opposite of one that is highly or completely regulated as is the case in countries with a national single-payer health system. In short, the market for hospitals is not what is known as "purely competitive" as is the market for widgets, far from it. It holds, instead, a complicated mixture of free-market principles, huge regulatory demands, a demand for sick-care services that is derived and not direct, and the most complicated reimbursement scheme known in modern times in any industry.

Managed care, a concept and term invented by Alain Enthoven (1986), was originally intended to reduce health care costs to society through the restriction of resource allocation and improve the overall health of individuals. Now it is a generic term for health care payment systems that attempt to control costs through utilization monitoring: Health maintenance organizations and preferred provider organizations are examples. In the old cost-plus world, physicians as clinicians (not clinicians and business men and women) had free unrestricted aim over treatment plans and resource allocation for their patients. This system, focused on physicians and, arguably, hospitals, involved a complete arbitrariness to clinical decision making and if science (as in evidence-based medicine) was involved, all the better. Imagine a world where the faith and trust in the physician as provider were sacrosanct. Depending on the age of the reader, probably you cannot imagine it, even in your wildest dreams. Also beyond the imagination for some, there was a time that insurance companies paid for resources used without much, if any, review processes for appropriateness of treatment.

Managed care, now considered an economic success and a social nightmare, has, in fact reduced health care costs to society by tying clinical decisions to economic ones that previously were mutually exclusive. In these arrangements, a hospital or group of doctors agrees to provide services in exchange for third-party payment. Managed care networks make available to their members only those providers authorized by the plan. Often, this designation is geographically derived, thereby restricting the individual's choice to go to what they see as the "best" orthopedic or cancer care hospital or doctor if unavailable locally. It is worth mentioning that individuals still have free choice (lots of it)—if they are willing to get out their checkbook! This statement is a positivist (or factual) one amid the rhetoric of concerns from individual patients and physicians about how things used to be or ought to be. The way things "ought to" or "used to" be was inflationary, and there isn't an informed health consumer around who doesn't know this.

In managed care, the provider (physician, nurse in advanced practice, or hospital) provides covered services at a discounted rate in exchange for a steady revenue stream. If the novice reading this wonders why providers would "settle for less" by receiving a discounted rate, consider the alternative. The provider would have an uncertain revenue stream that challenges their abilities to cover the basic costs of doing business (reduces uncertainty) plus there are few, if any, alterative ways of conducting business, generally speaking. Stated another way, consider what is known as *the first rule of finance*: A dollar today is worth more than a dollar tomorrow, due to the time value or opportunity cost of money. That is, any entity that gains revenue in a timely manner not only can retire debt (an asset) but invest; hence the time value of money is realized. Remember that fee-for-service medicine has all but disappeared, taking with it the old model of the solo-practice physician, and patients who pay out of pocket are rare.

Under a per diem rate agreement, the managed care plan pays the hospital a fixed rate for each day of care when in fact nurses are in a particularly strategic position to observe that costs per diem to the institution can be (very) variable for one patient stay. Consider the surgical patient who consumes relatively few resources on the morning of admission for a procedure that afternoon. Once the patient enters the operating room, costs to the institution soar steeply and remain high as the patient travels to the postanesthesia recovery room, not to mention more if intensive care is involved. For a monthly fee, the hospital must provide the specified services to the third-party payer's enrollees such as this patient, who could be those individuals with Blue Shield Preferred Provider health insurance. Under this arrangement, the hospital is ensured money in a relatively timely fashion (based on the average consumption of patients within that diagnosis-related group and other clinical factors) and the patient-consumer knows he or she will be covered for surgeries that are preapproved.

The overall aim of managed care is to make the patient a better health care customer, evaluating if she or he is getting what she or he is paying for (assuming the individual pays health insurance premiums, which most do). Also, the burden of prevention and wellness dramatizes in importance to the patient, and, presumably, physicians and advanced practice nurses share in this responsibility by virtue of recent changes in medical and nursing education. In this system, the patient has less control over selection of the doctor or hospital and may be responsible for higher deductibles and copayments as well as penalties for service done outside the network.

From a positive (or factual) point of view, the real cost savings to the health care system and society at large is through reduction and elimination of *unnecessary* services, tests, and procedures and time delays through the authorization process where untold numbers of individuals drop off, or attrition out of, the care-seeking process. It needs to be said that to the extent that costs are held down by reduction in *necessary* services, tests, procedures, and premature hospital discharge, there are, in fact, real detriments to patients and to society. Many health care professionals and consumers are now claiming that the term "managed care" translates to "discounted care," but adhering to the intent of this chapter, the positive or factual view of health care business operations, the author looks disparagingly upon this rhetorical and editorial change.

Profit Motive and Patient Care

Amid the rhetoric and hysteria regarding hospitals and profit, not enough is said about why a hospital exists. A hospital exists to satisfy the needs of its various stakeholders. Among these are physicians, nurses, and other employees; patients and their families; consumers; researchers; schools of medicine and nursing; and the community at large, to name some. Although many agree that today's hospital exists for the provision of sick care, this is not to say there are no other compelling reasons for it to subsist. It is a business entity and, as such, it responds to many demands from the players, or stakeholders. Among these demands are the volume and morbidity of patients, requests from physicians and nurses in advanced practice for necessary equipment and efficient flow of patients, concerns from patients and families about inefficient or substandard care, training opportunities for students of medicine and nursing, and an outright appeal for more nurses from basically anyone! The profit motive drives all of these.

In an influential book of its time (Gray, 1991), *The Profit Motive and Patient Care*, the author made the previously unexplored claim that two unique accountability factors exist in health care that do not exist in other organizations: the vulnerability of the consumer (patient) being served *and* the absence of payers at the point of service. He goes on to state:

> In many different ways the profit motive—on the part of organizational providers of health care, suppliers of their capital, physicians, employers who provide benefits for their employees, and organizations that administer health benefits plans and monitor the performance of health care providers—has come to shape the behavior of all parties. An ethos that emphasizes trust, community service, professional autonomy, and devotion to interests of individual patients is being replaced with undisguised self interest, commercialization, competition, and the management of care by third parties. For the remainder of the century, these shifts will shape how providers and purchasers of service respond to the two great accountability problems (p. xi).

A cursory reading through these remarks prompts one to believe there is a lament here—perhaps about "the way things *ought* to be." Yet on closer examination, it appears that Gray, instead, is making logical positivist remarks. His explanation of who the important players (stakeholders) are and how they are motivated to perform has far-reaching implications for the overall philosophical *and* business approaches that health care providers, such as nurses, might take. His was among the first credible writings to shake the foundations of why a hospital exists as well as to articulate the important forces shaping the behavior of the stakeholders.

In this section, it is necessary to debunk some myths still prevailing in certain sections of our society, sometimes even among health care providers (some of whom should know better!):

Myth 1: We are a nonprofit entity; we don't *have* profit.
Myth 2: We are here to provide the highest possible quality of care.

These are among the most important misconceptions forwarded by many stakeholders, among them nurses. Replacing what might be our wishes (myths) with factual statements will help us understand the pervasive economic forces shaping our work and provide resolve for nursing research aims and hypotheses.

Getting the Word "Profit" Back

The first myth—that of no profit—has hung around for decades. First, it is important to clarify our terminology. As to profit status, hospitals are now classified as either investor owned (IO), formerly known as "for-profit," or not-for-profit (NFP), formerly known as "nonprofit." All hospitals have profit, *and* each of them chases profit as fast and furiously as the next, period. They may differ on many other factors, chiefly *how* they approach profit optimization as well as descriptive characteristics such as public versus private ownership, urban versus rural, small-margin versus large-margin, safety-net versus non safety-net, high-mortality versus low-mortality, and teaching versus nonteaching, to name some. A number of these factors may, in fact, covary with profit status. For example, major teaching hospitals tend to be NFP hospitals and nearly all IO hospitals are private, but it is thought that the variable of profit status is the prime mover of organizational behavior and may be outcomes.

Profit, loosely defined as the excess of revenues over expenses, is as necessary to hospitals, irrespective of profit status, as oxygen is to the living system. Almost no hospital could survive without it because it could not remain liquid or solvent. Without it, a hospital eventually goes out of business just like any other entity, leaving services unprovided and employees out of jobs. Profitability, as a construct, is measured by these variables: total margin ratio, operating profit margin, nonoperating gain ratio, and return on equity. See Chapter 20, Financial Analysis: Improving Your Decision Making, for more information. As you continue reading the next section on the cost inputs for varying levels of quality, keep in mind that costs to the hospital (what is expensed on the hospital's income statement) relative to revenue (money given to the hospital in lieu of care provided) are nearly synonymous with profitability, at least in the short run.

Finally, an accounting note about the differences in IO versus NFP hospitals. (See Chapter 19 for more specifics on this principle). In lay terms, the key differences between these two sets of hospitals on the matter of profit goes like this: All that matters is where you put it, what you call it, and what you do about it! Restating this old joke another way, the dollar line item of profit is found on the income statement of general funds for NFPs versus the profit and loss statement for the corporation; profit is called "profit" in the IO world versus a "positive fund balance" in the NFP one; and the IO distributes profit (after taxes) at year's end to the shareholders, whereas the NFPs cycle profits back into facility maintenance or expansion after paying no taxes. This partly whimsical look at

Exhibit 11–2 Cost of Higher Quality

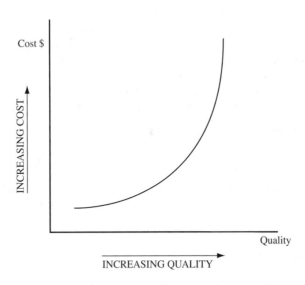

what the terms mean (and do *not* mean) causes this author to conclude "I want the word 'profit' back!" given that although there is a cost–quality trade-off (see next section), there is *not necessarily* a cost–profit trade-off.

Quality of Care: At What Level? At What Cost?

In this chapter's discussion of competition, it was stated that a hospital *is not* in the business of providing the best care money can buy but that a hospital *is* in the business of providing quality of care at a certain acceptable level. It is time to examine why.

Measurement of the costs of providing care quality, long a perplexing problem, is a function of the cost of providing quality *and* the costs of failing to do so. As shown in **Exhibit 11–2**, higher quality is generally associated with higher costs, but to a point. That point, known as the margin, is defined as the point at which a one-unit increment of input (cost) no longer yields a one-unit increase in output (quality). The one-unit increase in cost increment provides *less than* a unit increase in quality, which causes the decision maker to question why that one last unit increase in cost was allocated. In short, a measurable commensurate level of quality was not achieved in spending more. The margin can be found at the top right steep portion of the curve where there is no longer a one-to-one trade-off for inputs in their relationship to outputs. Hence, the hospital has an incentive *not* to raise quality beyond this point because profitability, and thus survival, is threatened.

Lowering quality also has costs to the organization. For example, lowering the quality of care (**Exhibit 11–3**) is related to both declining reputation and rising numbers of malpractice cases (and, remember, reputation *is* an asset). So, as lowering quality occurs, certain costs such as those mentioned above are rising. Further, lower quality of *measurable* care that is reported to public agencies (see next section on Quality of Patient Care) erodes the hospital's competitive position and thus longer term viability. As a balance, or position of homeostasis, on costs and quality, the organization often rests at level B care (**Exhibit 11–4**). This point, the intersection between the marginal curves of cost and quality, is the sought-after acceptable level of quality previously mentioned.

Exhibit 11–3 Costs of Lower Quality

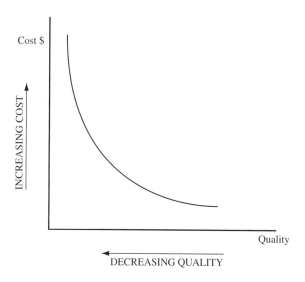

Exhibit 11–4 Costs of Higher Quality

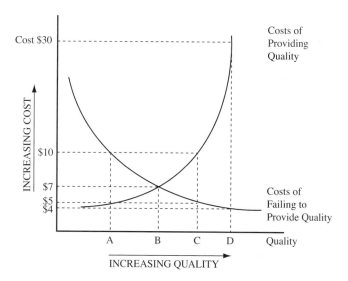

This cost–quality trade-off explains the behavior of firms in every competitive industry, includ-ing the hospital firm in health care. Although seemingly abstract constructs, hospital decision mak-ers use this paradigm as freely as a living system uses carbohydrate for fuel in the cell. An example might clarify the thinking. Suppose that making sure the patient has no known drug allergies is Level A in **Exhibit 11–4**. Additionally, checking for drug interactions, say, by nursing, represents Quality Level B, and Level C represents a double check that the medications dispensed are those ordered. Having the pharmacist visit the division to make sure every ordered medication makes clinical sense is represented by Level D.

If the combined personnel reimbursements for *providing* quality at Level A of care were $5 but the cost of *failing to provide* this care (extensive length of stay or LOS, expensive treatment of adverse drug reactions, lawsuits) is $10, this leaves a wide margin of $5 (the cost difference on providing vs. failing to provide). This position on production of patient care processes is *not* as favorable as the level of care represented by B where *both* the costs of quality and the costs of the failure to provide it are each $7, leaving no discernible margin. The novice economic reader of this reasoning might say "then there seems no leeway for little deviations from the provision of inputs, like nurse-hours, to the quality of care picture." This is precisely correct! In fact, this thinking could explain how narrow the management margin of error on staffing and scheduling is and why nursing personnel seem to have more patients than they can handle, though these conclusions are difficult to demonstrate in actual research.

For a more exaggerated difference on relative positions of these costs, focus on Level of Care D where the costs of high-quality care would have been $30. The costs of failing to provide quality is only $4, leaving an even wider margin of $26 so this position, like A, is also unfavorable, only more so. Note that Level of Care B is only favorable relative to Level of Care D only until such time (in the world of possibilities) that the losses sustained in failing to provide quality (again, prolonged length or stay and/or complications) drops significantly.

In conclusion, what can be said about the profit motive and patient care? That profit, as an incentive, is here to stay. That profit is not a dirty word. Further, that cost–quality trade-offs drive operational (day-to-day) decisions in all organizations in a competitive industry. Also, that cost shifts (costs to the hospital, or expenses) might be borne by the individual, or perhaps the employer, if they are discharged prematurely and too sick to resume employment. That revenues would shift, from one governmental organization such as CMS to another, if they could. And that dramatically changing one variable, such as RN staffing, necessitates significant changes in another, such as expenses for other personnel—something that will prove essentially important to our national debate about hospital staffing.

Quality Patient Care

In this chapter's discussion of profit motive, it was demonstrated how a hospital comes about providing not the best care money can buy but instead an acceptable level of quality. The acceptable level of quality is driven by its cost. Next, the hospital, to compete on a quality of care basis, must report *measurable* aspects of quality of care (not all quality of care is, of course), presumably at an acceptable level, to various governmental (state health departments and federal agencies) and nongovernmental sources such as the Joint Commission on Accreditation of Healthcare Organizations. Through processes such as these, the information about the quality of care in one facility is said to be "perfect information," a cornerstone of a competitive industry. The information can also be characterized as "symmetric" in that both the buyer (the insurer) and the seller (the providers) have access to it. The old quality assurance model, now nearly extinct, was limited in at least two ways: quality cannot be *ensured* and the information, or knowledge, was asymmetric, known to the seller (the one provider hospital) but not necessarily to the buyer. Therefore, under this old model, it was practically impossible for hospitals to modify their care provision processes in a competitive way because they had no information about the performance of their rival hospitals.

Given the preponderance of information-reporting requirements, it is assumed that hospitals have numerous opportunities for improvement—assuming that these many reporting requirements translate to internal care-improvement processes. Next, through the movement now known as "transparency" (symmetric knowledge), hospitals can bid competitively to purchasers boasting superior quality outcomes. A third quintessentially important thing this information preponderance gives us is the *incentive* for public programs (e.g., Medicare) and private insurers (e.g., Blue Shield) to reward quality of care and efficiency. An extensive discussion about Medicare's pay-for-performance program and "never" events is found in Chapter 4. This incentive program has the overall goal of making hospitals pay when they err. At this writing two of the preventable conditions for which it will not reimburse should *never* happen: surgical objects left in patients and blood incompatibility. The remaining events, also preventable, were reflected in at least 500,000 Medicare recipients in 2007. They are air embolism, serious bedsores, fractures, burns, urinary tract infections from catheters, and infection after heart-bypass graft. It is essential to note that it is the *quality and availability of the information* to both buyers and sellers that makes hospital nonprice competition possible. At this writing, there is no consensus on projections for lost hospital revenue due to this program, but the fact that it could have grave implications for a hospital's profitability should be clear.

Information on Quality and the Risk-Adjustment Process

A time-honored claim that hospitals and other providers have made regarding quality measures in general is that their patient populations contain more risk factors than others; hence the appearance of "not looking good" to the state or inspection agency. Granted, patient populations from hospital to hospital (or even from doctor to doctor) will likely always differ on factors other than the care provided, but (arguably) meaningful points of comparison have been devised by clinical and biostatistical experts within many agencies. One such agency is California's Office of Statewide Health Planning and Development (OSHPD). Among the first of the states to develop a database of risk-adjusted quality measures, the California Hospital Outcome Project reported to the public for the first time in 1995 and has continuously updated and improved its risk-adjustment processes ever since. Working first with a common and costly condition, acute myocardial infarction, by reporting risk-adjusted mortality, discharge abstracts served as the basis for data collection for over 400 hospitals representative of over 68,000 patients.

Biostatisticians know that databases this large do, indeed, allow for meaningful points of comparison across hospitals, for reasons to be explained in advanced texts of statistics and econometrics. Generally speaking, risk-adjusted measures of quality of care, such as acute myocardial infarction mortality, are in fact useful tools for the comparison of hospitals on the quality of care it provides, but imperfectly so. Their mortality measure was defined as the observed number of deaths from acute myocardial infarction divided by the number of qualifying persons admitted with this primary diagnosis times the statewide rate. The risk-adjustment process is described in detail in workbooks provided to all by the state (again the information is symmetric) (OSHPD, 1996a, 1996b), and agencies such as this claim to have satisfactorily responded to providers on their claim about disparate findings based on (unmeasured) risk factors by making the process known to all. In fact, the project provides the opportunity for hospital-providers the chance to respond, in writing, as to why their facility "looked worse than expected" in the measures, on a yearly basis, as the press releases come out about new editions of the data. This way, the project measures are refined yearly, in part, on the basis of the responses of participating hospitals. Since inception of this project, the agency has made available other outcome measures, all risk adjusted, that are reflective of common and costly conditions. These include complication rates of cervical and thoracic diskectomy, maternal admissions, hip fractures, and community-acquired pneumonia.

In Microeconomics, Cost Accounting, and Nursing, above, the thought was expressed that for our profession to be seated at the table of quality initiatives in the context of the hospital business entity, we would need expert knowledge of the economic and quality measures being discussed. Further, that societal decision makers and gatekeepers, such as the OSHPD or the CMS, would benefit from nursing representation to make the hospital measures, now used for reimbursement, meaningful. Fortunately, through the years, as nursing acquired a critical mass of administratively prepared nurses, it has become common for nurse executives from hospitals and/or representatives of our professional societies to be invited at such tables where the decisions are made. Because this was not always the case, it could be considered progress of the profession through the acquisition of the same knowledge *and* the same financial language spoken by lay administrators that made this possible.

Healthcare Policy: The Staffing Ratios Debate

The relationship between nurse staffing and patient safety is reasonably well established, especially when considering patient outcomes such as medical-surgical mortality rates (Aiken, Smith, & Lake, 1994), acute myocardial infarction mortality rates (Schultz, van Servellen, Litwin, McLaughlin, & Uman, 1997), community-acquired pneumonia mortality rates (Schultz, 2008), failure to rescue (Needleman, Buerhaus, Mattke, Stewart, & Zelevinsky, 2002), and shorter lengths of stay (Lang, Hodge, Olson, Romano, & Kravitz, 2004), to name a few. How patients fare has long been thought to be due to the number of professional nurse staff available as well as their preparation, visibility, and role as well. Additional organizational variables known to be important are leadership style of the nurse manager, the overall quality of leadership in the institution, whether staffing and other operational decisions are decentralized, physician satisfaction with nursing care, and the nature of the information system used for patient care. As research on hospital characteristics and their relationships to patient outcomes broadens to include these additional variables, it will be interesting to identify which variables are most important in the complex relationships of people and technology relative to quality. It is the opinion of the author that only then will these associations be demystified and contextualized so that clearer policy implications can be delineated.

Mandated minimum nurse-to-patient staffing ratios were legislated in California in 1999 and implemented January 1, 2004 (see http://www.nursingworld.org/MainMenuCategories/ANAPoliticalPower/State/StateLegislativeAgenda/StaffingPlansandRatios_1.aspx). To date, 13 states plus the District of Columbia have similar regulations (Trossman, 2008) (**Exhibit 11–5**), and comparable legislation is being considered in at least 25 other states (Tamara Konetzka, Zhu, Volpp, & Sochalski, 2008) as well as the importance of having patient classification system data to support the appropriate RN staff requirements. Some of the impetus for the movement toward mandating nurse staffing ratios through governmental and scientific imperatives comes from the challenging conclusions offered by the Institute of Medicine's *To Err is Human* in 2002. This report shook both the scientific and lay communities through its most memorable finding, that between 44,000 and 98,000 deaths occur each year as a result of medical errors. Now, there is hardly a scientific journal focusing on these types of organizational studies that does not report the influence of nurse staffing, often in the form of RN hours per patient day or RN to all staff hours.

The beginner to politics and policy might ask "Isn't this a no-brainer.... more nurses, better patient care?" Only a fool would disagree and, certainly, more nurses sound as good as motherhood and apple pie! But so, too, do more police in a neighborhood and fewer pupils per teacher in middle school. In the sections below, the novice nurse–politician is given some food for thought on the potential implications, or consequences, of such legislation in the context of the (1) operation of a hospital within a community or (2) market for hospitals as a whole. The implications can be summarized in four parts: hospital operations including closure, feasibility and the nursing

Exhibit 11–5 States Having Nurse-Ratios Regulations for Acute Care

State	State Nurse-Association Address
California	http://www.anacalifornia.org/
Connecticut	http://www.ctnurses.org/
Florida	http://www.floridanurse.org
Illinois	http://www.nursingworld.org
Maine	http://www.anamaine.org/
Nevada	http://www.nvnurses.org/
New Jersey	http://www.njsna.org/
Ohio	http://www.ohnurses.org
Oregon	http://www.oregonrn.org/
Rhode Island	http://www.risnarn.org/
Texas	http://www.texasnurses.org/
Vermont	http://www.vsna-inc.org/
Washington	http://www.wsna.org/
District of Columbia	http://www.dcna.org/

shortage, political opportunity costs, and costs to society. The implications, economic consequences of legislation addressing what staffing *should be* (normative economics), are couched in positive economics, or *what is*, factually.

Hospital Operations and Closure

As mentioned under the previous section on profit, the health care workforce accounts for at least 50% of a hospital's costs (Kazahaya, 2005). Most of this is nursing personnel costs. Starting with the assumption that some hospitals staff significantly better than the minimum staffing ratios suggest and some staff significantly lower as a baseline, there is a variance around the regulated minimum ratio (also known as "the floor" ratio) on which hospitals vary. Those hospitals staffing well below this floor ratio will experience a rapid rise in operating expenses and a subsequent drop in operating profit margin. This endangers the hospital's liquidity (ability to meet short-term obligations) and solvency (ability to meet maturing obligations as they become due). Those hospitals staffing well above the floor ratio now have an incentive to drop nurse staffing levels depending on the ultimate response of their rivals, that is, whether neighboring hospitals can afford to remain in business after enactment of this law. Finally, those hospitals staffing at about the mandated level may experience no significant change in their financial and, subsequently, business activities, so their staffing may continue as is.

Consider other hospital operations that are disrupted as a consequence of what many nurses thought was a great idea. As reported in *Medical News Report* (2004),

- Elective procedures have been postponed, canceled, or moved to a nearby facility.
- Community hospitals are having a more difficult time transferring patients to tertiary care facilities because beds cannot always be staffed.
- Emergency room (ER) wait times have increased.
- ERs have increasingly switched (or requested to switch) to diversion status.
- Night shifts are nearly impossible to staff.

- There is a huge shift to contract (agency or registry) nursing staff, causing a significant rise in expenses, often tens of millions of (unforeseen) dollars in a year.
- The regulations make the hospital increasingly vulnerable to lawsuits, especially on the occasion when staffing is less than required.
- When the regulations allow for "licensed" nurses in the equation, RN unions block the effort to fill a void with licensed practical nurse hours, thereby inflating union-to-union conflict.

Evidence supporting the view that this mandate was too costly for hospitals to continue operating is seen in the number of them that closed in the years during implementation phase-in of the California law. Twenty hospitals closed (9 in 2003, 8 in 2004, 3 in 2006) (OSHPD, 2006), citing some factors on the revenue side of the profitability equation (drop in inpatient revenue and utilization issues), yet the costs to hospitals of the mandate cannot be underestimated. It is important to note that many forces, both internal and external, cause a business to close and that many of these factors, when occurring simultaneously, push the firm close to the "edge," or, more specifically, to the margin. Usually, a hospital firm that closes had both failing business (patient care processes) *and* economic activities (on both revenue and expenditure sides) in the preceding years that ultimately caused its demise. To date, no one empirical effort has isolated the impact of such a law on a hospital's propensity to close.

Recall from our discussion of profit that when expenses rise in one category, pressure is exerted in the hospital system (or any business) to (1) reduce expenses in another category, (2) make up the expensed activity with an increase in revenue, or (3) both. A guiding principle on hospital profit-maximizing behavior, Needleman (2008) accordingly suggests these questions to consider:

- How much would it cost to increase nurse staffing?
- Would these costs be offset by cost savings from reduced LOS and complications?
- Would the hospital realize these cost savings, or, because of how the hospital is paid, would these savings be captured by payers?
- Can the hospital attract additional profitable patients on the basis of its nurse staffing?
- Are there cost savings other than those achieved via better patient care that might also be realized if nurse staffing is increased?

So, it should be clear that changing a regulation on the most significant personnel expenditure a hospital budget contains, RN hours, has far-reaching consequences for both its business and economic activities. But this subsection looks at the core organizational dynamics of a single hospital, which is a very limited aspect of the staffing ratios laws. Even looking at these activities in all hospitals in a state or the nation offers only part of the view of the consequences of mandated ratios as described here. Read on to see how a hospital's behavior cannot be viewed in such a microcosm because of its essential bond to the other subcategories such as the nursing shortage.

Feasibility and the Nursing Shortage

Hospitals, lawmakers, providers, consumers, and society as a whole are increasingly concerned about the international nursing shortage and its subsequent impact on the quality of care. After implementation of California's safe-staffing law, RN hours per patient day on medical-surgical units rose significantly, perhaps by as much as 21% (Donaldson et al., 2005). Yet the nursing shortage, predicted to be a deficit of 400,000 RNs by 2020 (Buerhaus, Needleman, Mattke, & Stewart, 2002), continued to beg the question of where the nursing hours came from. Over decades, it was a long-standing principle of hospital staffing to "borrow" nurse hours from unit to unit to (a) satisfy short-term patient care demands, for example, a number of new admissions arriving at the same time as intensive care unit transfers, and to (b) satisfy regulatory and reporting requirements. Patient care demands may have been met, whereas regulatory and reporting requirements almost certainly were. In short, a mandate impacting certain nursing units acts as a magnet, drawing resources in the absence of such mandates in the other units.

Many obstacles hinder compliance. Consider these real-world examples from *Medical News Report* (2004):

- Hospitals may start a shift in compliance but not end that shift in compliance.
- Hospitals may start and end a shift in compliance, but the middle of the shift is in question.
- Nurse recruitment efforts have been accelerated, often not associated with the desired result of satisfactory staffing.
- California's law requires nurses to be on standby to cover breaks for bedside nurses, which is practically impossible to implement.
- Penalties exist for noncompliance.
- Nurses increasingly report not taking their breaks, given the lack of coverage while they are to be gone.
- Hospitals could be held *criminally* liable for adverse outcomes in the context of staffing that are less than required by mandate, even in view of evidence of the intent to comply.

These remarks point to "regional shortages" within one hospital carrying yet another set of concerns for patient safety. Chiefly, these concerns are costs associated with noncompliance, nurse recruitment (especially as nurses from outside the country are involved), and legal defense. Also, there are no accompanying changes in the revenue side of the hospitals' profit equation. The examples offered in this subsection highlight merely a few of the difficulties hospitals are having with the mandate. Additional issues include workplace safety, nurse injuries, nurse dissatisfaction, turnover, and propensity to stay in current positions. This subsection, not a comprehensive review for all issues related to a hospital's nurse pipeline, emphasizes some of the more immediate feasibility issues posed by such regulations.

Political Opportunity Costs for Nursing

Highly publicized political wars have taken place, most notably in California and New York, over the staffing ratios debate. Both states had nurse unions that were successful in getting legislation sponsored that evolved into statewide acute-care hospital staffing mandates, but at what political cost? California's 12-year battle (California Nurses Association, n.d.) spanned the reign of two governors, and New York's campaign (Gerardi, 2006) was similarly protracted, both being punctuated by statewide town hall meetings, numerous "call to action" alerts to other professional societies, consumption of resources of nursing associations of all types, and bad press labeling nurses as unyielding and self-serving. In California, such ill will attracted national attention when Arnold Schwarzenegger summarily dismissed both the nurse union's leadership and membership *as well as* nurses in general when calling nurses "a special interest group" who are just angry because "I kick their butt" (Marinucci, 2004).

These campaigns occurred just as the state of the research was judged *not* to categorically support the thesis of better care provision through more RNs in each case. In fact, the research results are mixed (Burnes Bolton et al., 2007), reporting that although a clear and consistent rise in nurse staffing did exist postregulation in California, it was not accompanied by a commensurate rise in quality as measured by significantly fewer falls or pressure ulcers. In a study reported by Mark and Harless (2007), a superior distribution of outcomes (mortality and LOS) with a *lower* level of RN staffing was found. In sum, the evidence points to the prevailing conclusion that there is a strong, but not yet conclusive, case for an impact of nurse staffing on mortality (Needleman & Buerhaus, 2003) and other adverse outcomes. This is not unlike the teacher's union advocating for better teacher-to-student ratios, having to defend the national outcry (and *some* empiricism) that we are a nation of people who lack the necessary reading, writing, and critical thinking skills.

If you believe, as some do, that science drives policy and legislation—and that's a leap—you have now identified a gap between just what we recommend on the matter of staffing mandates (the normative economic view) and a recommendation accompanied by a cogent economic rationale (the positive economic position) and plan. Stated another way, consider the words of Keepnews (2007):

> Ongoing research on the impact of nurse staffing regulation can yield important informa-
> tion that can guide continued staffing policy efforts. Understanding the impact of such
> efforts should include evaluating the outcomes of recent legislation in Oregon and Illinois
> as well as continued examination of staffing ratios in California. Successful efforts will
> need to transcend traditional boundaries between researchers, policy analysts, advocates,
> and organizations (p. 236).

Costs to Society

Social policy is the domain that aims to improve human welfare and to meet human needs for education, health, housing, and social security. It is that part of public policy that has to do with social issues; among them is health. There was a time when "health" was considered "the absence of disease." Couple this limited definition of health with the Hippocratic admonition, "to do no harm," to identify what the public expects from a hospital: to emerge from the experience with an improved state of health, or, at a minimum, to avoid increased morbidity *as a result of* seeking hospital care. Touted as a modern concept, we would do well to review that the Hippocratic admonition regarding harm emerged centuries ago (Hippocrates, n.d./2004). In the previous section (and Chapter 4) on quality, it was noted that, at a minimum, quality care is identified as the absence of adversity or the absence of adverse events.

The costs to society of this adversity are understudied or underreported in modern health services research. The costs to society include, but are not limited to, the alternative use of hospital resources in a community (e.g., feeding the poor, housing the homeless), consumption of a tax basis (in the case of NFP hospitals) for same, the costs of ill health for individuals and employers such as the opportunity cost of lost time and productivity at work, unreimbursed expenses related to caring for the underinsured or the uninsured, as well as the alternative use of people and technology resources in other employment. This subsection briefly lists some questions for further study in the context of the costs to society of mandated staffing ratios with respect to the latter two factors—the function and purpose of safety-net hospitals and the opportunity realized in the operation of a hospital in a community context.

SAFETY-NET HOSPITALS

Defined as those disproportionately serving vulnerable, including financially vulnerable, populations, *safety-net hospitals* also experienced a sustained significant rise in nurse hours after enactment of safe staffing ratios. To assume that a higher nurse-to-patient ratio impacts the financial structure of hospitals the same way across the board is folly. Safety-net hospitals are at-risk institutions, by definition. They have consistently been financially vulnerable organizations when viewed from the revenue side of the profit equation. With large numbers of underinsured or uninsured patients, they have no vantage point from which to compete on price and may not have the resources to compete on the basis of quality. It would stand to reason that although they budget for bad debt expense, this line item varies considerably because it is volume dependent and sensitive to changes in the macroeconomic condition. In short, when the region of its location "has a bad year," this institution, among all institutions there, has an even worse one! It is close to impossible for such a hospital to court more "attractive" (paying) patients not only due to geography but due to poor internal economic conditions, including liquidity crisis.

A study done by Conway et al. (2008) reported that nurse-staffing ratios in California hospitals were relatively unchanged from 1993 to 1999, then showed a sharp significant increase in 2004, the year of the ratios implementation. They reported that hospitals more likely to be below the minimum had high Medicaid/uninsured patient populations and were government owned, nonteaching, urban, and in more competitive markets. Most of these were considered part of the "safety net" that "catches" uninsured and underinsured patient populations, which, presumably, have poorer health outcomes as a baseline. Also, these hospitals are thought to be extraordinarily sensitive to governmental mandates on staffing, with safety-net hospitals reporting significantly fewer professional staff relative to patients in the years after the Balanced Budget Act of 1997 (Lindrooth, Bazzoli, Needleman, & Hasnain-Wynia, 2006).

Having just stated that the competitive position of these hospitals is weak to begin with (less able to compete on the basis of price or quality), it stands to reason that they run a high risk of closure, particularly in view of the fact that the mandate obliges them to spend more on nurse staffing. With this loss of flexibility to vary nursing skill mix comes inefficient allocation of scarce resources and an inability to make trade-offs in other hospital services. The subsequent drop in operating profit margin (and perhaps other measures of profitability) could easily cause negative consequences for patients such as premature discharge, recidivism, and higher complication rates. With the Medicare pay-for-performance structure, it is easy to see the handwriting on the wall for such environments with closure looming in the future.

Nowhere more apparent is the strain felt than in the ER of a safety-net hospital. Long a point of entry for the financially strapped patient, the ER at hospitals such as Los Angeles' Memorial Hospital (Inglewood, California) found it necessary to divert patients to a neighboring hospital, Centinela Freeman, of the same Centinela Freeman Health Care System. Memorial's ER was the 10th to close in Los Angeles County in the 2001–2006 period. Memorial Hospital had lost $30 million in that time frame, and the hospital's executive said the closure was necessary to help the system save money (Quinones, 2006). Meanwhile, Freeman's ER saw a majority of nonurgent cases, approximately 60% of the total clientele, begging the societal questions: Where should those patients have gone to begin with for more cost-effective care? Where will they go now and in the future? Why hadn't the hospital's leadership redirected its activities given the staggering loss of $30 million over 5 years?

As providers, especially safety-net hospital providers, struggle with these enmeshed issues of geographic limitations, a tangible floor in revenue, and dropping profit margins in light of rising bad debt expenses, it is no wonder that the hospital executive has an eye on cash flow relative to debt (cash flow-to-debt ratio) because it is *the* prime predictor of hospital closure. Once again, without a margin there is no mission despite outcries from community leaders in Inglewood and elsewhere that health care is a right—is it? If yes, who is paying for it?

A HOSPITAL FIRM WITHIN A COMMUNITY CONTEXT

Recall that in the subsections on hospital operations and also on the nursing shortage, a number of questions were raised relevant to reducing or delaying services (diversion to neighboring ERs), the potential for a hospital to realize other cost savings as RN hours rise (some economies of scale, perhaps, with nursing duties in common with nonlicensed personnel), and the costs to the hospital of recruiting and retaining nurses—all of which are accentuated in a regulatory climate in which RN ratios are mandated. Here are some questions posed by the author when considering the impact of such a government intervention on small-margin hospitals. Bear in mind that small-margin hospitals include those considered safety-net hospitals or those classified as rural.

- Will there be a drop in the employees' total compensation package, say a reduction in health benefits or a rise in premium prices, in an effort to offset the rise in operating expenditures?
- As the line item for RN hours increases, what happens to the expenditures for nonprofessional nurses and ancillary nursing personnel?
- As these nonprofessional nurse budgets get trimmed, will it be necessary to start outsourcing programs in preparation for layoffs?
- As resources become more constrained, what is the subsequent impact on measurable levels of quality?
- What is the effect of the change in levels of quality on managed care contract negotiations? In short, will the insurer continue to send covered lives to a facility thought or known to be substandard?
- As measurable levels of quality are affected, what is the impact of this on the hospital's creditworthiness?
- As the hospital's creditworthiness is adversely affected, how compromised is the hospital in borrowing, even in the short term, to meet economic obligations such as employee wages and other compensatory line items? How will a hospital's payment to its suppliers be impacted?
- If the hospital does, in fact, close, what is the impact of this event on the unemployment rate in the surrounding community, especially if the hospital is the largest employer around?
- If the hospital closes, what are the costs to society of airlifting or otherwise transporting the most critical of cases to the appropriate environment of care?

As decision makers in small-margin hospitals, including the nurse executive, wrestle with these tough questions, it remains in the mind's eye of the observer whether the charge "well, it's a hospital that *should* have closed anyway" is defensible. These subsections and this chapter do not provide an answer to such normative queries. Instead, the measures (or variables) necessary to construct an individual answer are offered from the logical positivist economic view.

In concluding this discussion of one of the most challenging health care policy questions of modern times, mandated nurse staffing ratios, remember some guiding principles from positive economics, that is, costs shift, revenues shift, and this will *always* be the case. Costs and revenues shift both within and outside the hospital firm. As in the case of "borrowing" nurse hours from unit to unit to "look good" or claim compliance with such mandates, what is the subsequent impact on patient care on the unit from which the "borrowing" occurred? As each hospital chases profit as fast and furiously as the next or neighboring competitor, how long will it continue to play the "shell game" of premature discharge offset by recidivism or shifting ER patient care from one safety-net hospital to another? Finally, as far as costs to society are concerned, how is the health of a region or the nation impacted by the loss of hospitals that fail seemingly from the economic or quality point of view?

The Business Case: Computerized Clinical Information Systems (CCIS) in Hospitals

Although information systems, including the CCIS, is considered essential to the quality and efficiency of our health care system as a whole, the high cost of these systems is prohibitive in successful widespread implementation, especially in hospitals. Vital to daily operations, these systems bring many benefits such as safety, accessibility, retrievability, and convenience. They are a major organizational investment, especially with respect to start-up costs (the initial one-time expenses). This section discusses some costs, some benefits, the relationship of these costs and benefits, and the elements of a successful business case for a hospital's ***computerized patient record (CPR)***. As in the section on mandated nurse staffing policies in hospitals, this section offers the reader some measures (variables) to consider when idealizing that health care systems, especially hospitals, *ought to* have a computerized record-keeping and decision-support system.

Clinical information systems that computerize documentation of physicians, nurses, and other care providers, now nearly 20 years old, hold the promise of numerous benefits—for the health care system or hospital, for the patient, and for the health of the nation. Among them are patient safety, accessibility, legibility, process-adherence evidence, data-mining capabilities (Manjoney, 2004), retrievability, convenience, and a reduction in indirect-care time. Like the previous section on legislative mandates for professional nurse staffing, the desirability of successful CPR implementation in hospitals could be considered a "no-brainer" in that more time could be devoted to bedside care and patient outcomes such as fewer medication errors and increased patient satisfaction would occur. Why then, haven't more hospitals adopted such a system?

Costs for the Hospital

The major costs in acquiring a CPR system include the costs of hardware, software, networking, maintenance, installation, and training as well as opportunity costs (Agrawal, 2002). Direct costs such as training are expensed on the hospital's income statement, and big-ticket items such as the hardware and contracted software are listed as assets on the balance sheet and depreciated over their "useful life." This is a way of spreading out the tremendous cost outlay over time. This is also a way to pair these economic activities with the business or strategic plans the organization might have to determine an asset's future benefits. For example, a CPR is known to be associated with increasing patient satisfaction and with reductions in risk-adjusted mortality or complication rates. It's possible that these improved patient outcomes could be leveraged in a hospital's managed care contract negotiations with insurers. This matching of economic and business activities begins the process of identifying the benefits of the technology relative to its costs.

Other direct costs are for hardware, software, training time, and salary and support fees. Indirect costs, those expenses associated with ongoing operational costs, include those for software maintenance and support fees, salaries for support staff, and the fees related to space and utilities (Nahm, Vaydia, Ho, Scharf, & Seagull, 2007). Note that all costs mentioned thus far are those borne by the health care–providing institution, in this case, the hospital. In the next section, we see that the benefits, however, are shared by more than just this one entity.

Benefits for the Hospital and Patients

Implementation of a system has both tangible and intangible benefits, further complicating a discussion of the dynamics of benefits and costs. Tangible benefits are concrete measurable gains derived directly from the CPR system. They include increased revenue, savings in staff time, and savings in supplies and space. The intangible, or hard-to-quantify, benefits are such things as patient and user satisfaction and safety, increased compliance with federal or state regulations, decreased staff turnover, future leverage derived from the same, and hospital reputation.

Other difficult-to-calculate benefits include reduced resource use (partially from reduced LOS), improved quality through convenient access to information at the point of care, enhanced data capture, enhanced business management, and improved legal compliance with subsequent reduction in claims. In an econometric model making the business case for CPR implementation, Kaiser Permanente justified the costs for an inpatient CPR through such benefits as increased RN and medical records efficiency, decreased RN overtime, reduction in lab expenses, chart review time, and physical therapy wait time along with reduced inappropriate admissions, reduced avoidable days, reduced ER diverts, reduction in forms expenses and medical records supplies, fewer adverse drug events, and redeployment of space (Garrido, Raymond, Jamieson, Liang, & Wiesenthal, 2004). On the revenue side, improved coding accuracy for Medicare risk was mentioned.

Here is where we see a shared-benefit situation. In the case of adverse drug events, the hospital realizes as much as a 2.2-day reduced LOS for those events associated with injury. The patient is spared the inconvenience of the same amount of time plus the reduced opportunity cost of further morbidity from hospital-acquired conditions and, presumably, a shortened recuperation time with subsequent earlier return to work or productivity. At this point, the patient, the family, and the employer begin to share the benefits that resulted from costs incurred by only the hospital in the business case model. Yet if this is in keeping with a hospital or health care organization's mission (as is certainly the case for Kaiser Permanente), then the business model is said to be a successful one.

Cost-to-Benefit Analysis

Many different ways of calculating the hospital's return on investment (ROI), the benefits in relation to costs, exist. Among these are net present value (NPV), payback analysis, and break-even analysis. In each of these, many other influences must be assessed simultaneously, making the ROI analysis, by definition, very complicated. Among these are inflation, deflation, changes in business and strategic goals, shifts in health care management methods, and changes in Medicare reimbursement rates. The implementation team and end users such as nurses are typically not involved in the calculation but should be aware of the implications of the project on which they may team. Of paramount importance is an understanding of the time frame within which the expenses are incurred and the benefits realized. Well beyond the scope of this chapter or this text, econometric models identifying the multiple simultaneous influences on a successful analysis of this sort yield a partial solution for justifying the enormous outlay of costs for such information technology projects as CPR. Executive administration would do well to cost-out both sides of the analysis in the short, intermediate, and long term.

Conventional wisdom leaves little doubt about the ability of information technology to improve clinical outcomes, but equally compelling evidence of the positive financial return of the same has yet to be established. Remember that current provider reimbursement mechanisms do *not* differentiate between good quality and less-than-optimal care. This means that there are currently inadequate incentives for hospitals to act on this important aspect of the hospital infrastructure, especially when many of the benefits are difficult to quantify and forecast. This also means that as incentive programs to reward early adoption of technology or other innovations and quality of care are realized, they will act as a catalyst for the implementation of large-scale CPR projects in hospitals everywhere.

Kaiser's Business Case

In the account of a successful business case for a large-scale multihospital adoption of electronic medical records, Kaiser Permanente is investing $3 billion over 10 years to enhance the quality of care for its members (Garrido et al., 2004). Kaiser Permanente HealthConnect^{TM} is an electronic medical record for both inpatient and outpatient information management. The authors identified 36 categories of quantifiable benefits that contribute to a positive cash flow within 8.5 years.

However, this business case is contingent upon other simultaneous factors, some of which are assumptions: leadership commitment, timely implementation, partnership with labor, coding compliance, and workflow redesign. To be phased in over 3 years, theirs is a system that integrates the clinical record with appointments, registration, and billing. It is a system that includes workflow procedures, charting tools, and decision support rules that will be shared by all Kaiser Permanente regions in 33 hospitals. To calculate NPV, two time lags were accounted for. The first was the implementation lag, the time between installation, training, and actual use. The second was the benefit realization lag, accounting for benefits such as malpractice liability reductions that may not manifest until years after full use is realized.

Net cash flow, the difference between the quantifiable benefits of the system and its costs of implementation and support, was projected for part way through the 8th year of phase-in. Over $2 billion realized cash flow is anticipated from the $1 billion investment over the investment horizon. Projected payback of the system within its 10-year life confirms the potential for it to generate long-term return on investment. Process improvements enabled by the project impact LOS, a key driver of savings where approximately 35% of net benefits are identified. Other significant areas of savings include lower transcription costs, timely delivery of changes in care delivery (e.g., processing of physician orders), 30% to 50% reduction in medical record supplies and non–payroll expenses, and reduction in off-site medical record storage.

The difficult-to-quantify benefits include the adoption of care management protocols and best practices known to improve health outcomes. Again, entities other than the one outlaying the expenses—the hospital—are the patients and their families who benefit from streamlined care delivery and more efficient and informed admission and discharge processes. Although the strategic benefits from these enhancements are significant, the value attributed to them is difficult to measure. These, along with quality improvement, patient safety, continuity of care, and patient-centeredness, are all part of Kaiser Permanente's strategic plan so the business case can account for goals within those plans being met. Kaiser anticipates this system will be associated with higher nurse satisfaction, reduced burnout, and subsequent turnover—so much so that intermediate and longer term nurse recruitment expenses could be reduced. Another yet-to-be-quantified benefit will likely be a related reduction in registry nurse expenses as well as reductions in new nurse orientation, education time, and expense. Finally, a societal benefit is the rich flow of information for clinical, epidemiologic, and health services research. The data could be used for benchmarking, identification of best practices, and clinical outcome studies.

In conclusion, health care information systems play a central role in both the quality of care and daily operations (Nahm et al., 2007). They are extraordinarily expensive, even when the potential benefits are considered. Recalling some of the "lessons learned" in this chapter's discussion of profit seeking, remember that costs shift, revenues shift, and this will *always* be the case. Costs and revenues shift both within and outside the hospital firm, as do costs and benefits, as we have seen. This is the factual view for any big-ticket item (substantially increasing professional nurse staffing or CPR implementation) that a hospital might consider. These subsections and this chapter do not provide an answer to normative queries on whether a CPR system *should be* implemented. Instead, the measures (or variables) necessary to construct an individual answer are offered from the logical positivist economic view.

As each health care organization addresses the issue of widespread implementation of a CPR, it will be increasingly important for decision makers to evaluate the nuances of its own business case for it. Given that many factors obscure the construction of a clear business case for CPR, hospitals are forced to consider the *avoidance of an expense* (e.g., future litigation costs) as parallel with *actual expense reduction*, especially in the short term. Similarly, they are forced to identify benefits that are realized by the hospital as well as those gained by the individual patient, his or her employer, or society as a whole. The propensity of a hospital to invest this way will likely be enhanced by the changing CMS rules on non-reimbursement for selected hospital complications. Forcing a hospital to pay for its own mistakes, such as certain hospital-acquired infections, raises the question of what type of electronic system it will take to capture the processes associated with these adverse outcomes for purposes of both quality improvement and revenue sustainability.

Summary

Hospitals, wrote Lewis Thomas in *The Youngest Science* (1983, pp. 66–67), are "held together, glued together, enabled to function...by the nurses." In this chapter, background was offered to the reader first on the nature of competition and why it is important in the market for hospital care. Moving next to the profit motive and patient care, the reader was asked to join in debunking some myths about why a hospital exists to fulfill its purpose—to satisfy the needs of various stakeholders such as employees, the community at large, as well as patients and providers such as physicians and nurses. The regulatory arena was addressed last in the context of the hospital system as a dynamic microcosm of activity affected, sometimes dramatically, by legislative and societal mandates like safe staffing laws.

The author identifies that some of this monetary analysis is, in fact, a brand new way of thinking for those who have not studied formally in the fields of economics, accounting, or finance from which this chapter is derived. It is hoped that, through this examination of what it takes for a hospital firm to survive competitive circumstances, future cohorts of nurses can preserve the only sustained hospital foundation—the practice of professional nursing. As stated by Buerhaus et al. (2002), "nursing matters greatly in the hospitals' ability to provide quality of care and prevent avoidable adverse outcomes." It is the prevention of avoidable adversity that is going to contribute most significantly to the survival of hospital firms through the coming years.

Most of the statements on hospital conditions and the business activities therein are from the domain of positive economics ("what is" or "what exists"), leaving the reader to draw his or her conclusions in the normative economic ("what *should* be") field of endeavor. Nursing's history, of course, has been to embrace the *mission* of caring, often with less investment in the *impact* of the ideals such as safe staffing on the hospital's *margin*. As our chapter began, the quote, "No margin, no mission" (Langley, 1998), focused discussion on the consequences of nursing's advocacy. This is to say that without a sustainable *margin* of profit, a hospital, like all businesses, fails to provide service, employ personnel, pay its suppliers, or fulfill its *mission*.

Discussion Questions

1. Support or refute the statement, "Well, supply and demand ... it just doesn't work in health care!"
2. Discuss how "margin" and "mission" are related in the hospital environment, or aren't they?
3. Frame arguments for or against the policy of mandated minimum staffing ratios in the positive vs. normative economic dichotomy.
4. Are hospitals competing on the basis of price, quality, or both? Explain.
5. Is hospital care overly regulated? Why or why not?
6. What is health care regulation and what are some of its costs?
7. Why is the provision of sick care (hospital) services said to be a *derived* demand?
8. Should there be minimum safe staffing ratios—from the standpoint of the patient? Why or why not?

9. Should there be minimum safe staffing ratios—from the standpoint of the hospital? Why or why not?
10. Should there be minimum safe staffing ratios—from the standpoint of the profession? Why or why not?

Glossary of Terms

American Nurses Credentialing Center (ANCC)—the world's largest and most influential nurse credentialing organization and a subsidiary of the American Nurses Association. American Nurses Credentialing Center is best known for promoting excellence in practice through its Magnet Recognition Program® and Pathways to Excellence Program™.

Asymmetric Knowledge—a state or condition in which buyers and sellers of a product or service have significantly different sets of information.

Bad Debt Expense—accounts receivable that will likely remain uncollectible and will be written off. It is a line item for which the hospital budgets.

Buyer—one who purchases health care services, often the health insurance company.

Capitalism—an economic system based on private ownership of productive resources and allocation of goods based on the signals provided by free markets.

Competition—effort of two or more parties to gain the business of a third by offering preferably favorable terms.

Cost—dollar value of inputs used in the production of goods and services (output). Types of costs are variously termed and defined. These include direct, indirect, medical, nonmedical, future, intangibles, fixed, variable, marginal, and opportunity. *Not* to be confused with "expenses"; it is a broader term.

Cost Accounting—an element of financial management that generates information about the costs of an organization and its components. A subset of accounting, in general. Encompasses the development and provision of a wide range of financial information useful to managers in their roles.

Cost-Plus Basis—Before the prospective payment system, hospitals and health care firms conducted business on a basis loosely involving costs, expenses (looser still, volume and quality), and a "plus" thrown in for good measure. Variously defined, the "plus" factor was indeed a "dart thrown" by the hospital firm to insurers (payers) of care and remained opaque to consumers for decades, or perhaps since hospitals began.

Deregulation—removal of government controls and/or interventions to allow free and efficient marketplace. Health care was said to be deregulated with the implementation of diagnosis-related groups (1983) and the subsequent prospective payment systems.

Diagnosis-Related Groups—Medicare initiated payment to providers such as hospitals on this basis beginning in 1983. The prices for the groups are updated yearly by Medicare to reflect changes in reimbursement protocols.

Economics—study of how a society allocates scarce resources and goods.

Economies of Scale—also known as "returns to scale," it is the degree to which the cost of providing a good or service falls as quantity (measured by patient-days) increases because fixed costs are shared by the larger volume of units.

Expense—a more exact concept than cost, the exact dollar amount a firm spends on a unit of production. Divided into two major types on a hospital's income statement, there are operating expenses (direct line items for the cost of inputs) and nonoperating expenses (less directly assigned costs, e.g., overhead).

Externalities—an impact (positive or negative) that a transaction has on an entity other than the buyer or seller of a product or service.

Financial Accounting—system that records historical financial information and provides summary reports to individuals outside of the organization of what financial events have occurred and of what the financial impact of those events has been.

Firm—the company, the hospital.

Government Intervention—actions on the part of government that affect economic activity, resource allocation, and especially free choice on the purchase of products or services.

Health Care Economics—a branch of economics concerned with issues related to scarcity in the allocation of health and health care service provision.

Incentive—reward to an organization or individual, for a behavior. Differs from "motive," which is a psychological term describing an inner state.

Liquidity—ability of a firm to meet its short-term financial obligations, i.e., pay bills, as they become due.

Macroeconomics—a branch of economics concerned with how human behavior affects outcomes in highly aggregated markets, such as the markets for labor or consumer products. The behavior of all hospital firms in the health care context.

Managed Care—a system that manages health care delivery with the aim of controlling costs. Typically reliant on a physician or nurse in advanced practice, the clinical activity is paired with the economic activity that is thought to reduce frivolous expenses and moral hazard.

Managerial Accounting—the process of identifying, analyzing, interpreting, and communicating financial information so that an organization can pursue its goals. Differs from financial accounting in that it is an internal process whereas financial accounting focuses on reporting financial activity to an outside source.

Margin—the point at which one more unit of input no longer yields one more unit of output—it yields less.

Microeconomics—a branch of economics concerned with the behavior of individuals and a (hospital) firm. The activities of individuals and businesses with regard to the allocation of resources and the production and distribution of goods and services.

Mission—a health care organization's *raison d'être*; why it *says* it exists.

Motive—internal psychological state of arousal propelling a person (or organization) to approach a goal.

Net Present Value—future stream of benefits and costs converted into equivalent values today. Today's value of an investment's future net cash flow minus the initial investment.

Normative Economics—judgments about "what ought to be" in economic matters. By definition, they cannot be proved "false" because they are based on assessments but they can (and should) be supported by "facts" or positive economics to be most useful.

Nurse Manager—supervisory nurse who has complete operational and financial authority for a unit(s) on a 24/7 basis; her or his practice is said to be decentralized.

Operating Expenses—line-item entries on the income statement traceable to a hospital's day-to-day business, e.g., salaries and bad debt expense. As opposed to nonoperating expenses, e.g., insurance or maintenance of equipment.

Perfect Information—term used to describe a state of complete knowledge about the product of a firm and possibly the actions of other players in it. Not to be taken literally, it is the basis for the purchase of a certain volume of products at a particular price.

Positive Economics—study of "what is" in economic relationships.

Profit—excess of revenue over expenses.

Profit Margin—excess of revenue over expenses divided by total revenue. An index of the amount of profit generated by each dollar of revenue.

Prospective Payment System—introduced by the federal government in 1983, a system by which Medicare reimburses hospitals at a predetermined rate, largely based on discharge medical diagnosis, for its patients. Aimed at influencing hospital behavior through financial incentives that encourage more cost-efficient care, the hospital receives a flat-rate reimbursement for a diagnosis-related group into which each patient falls based on clinical information such as age, gender, and comorbidities for a medical diagnosis, irrespective of actual consumption of services.

Regulation—form of government intervention designed to shape the behavior of an economic entity—organizations or individuals. Health care providers such as physicians, nurses, and hospitals are said to be highly regulated, referring to such things as approval by boards of medicine or nursing and licensure by states.

Risk—state of uncertainty containing possible adversity or undesired outcomes. If quantifiable, this expectation of loss is said to carry a certain probability.

Seller—economic "agents" who are accountable for the production and sale of health care services, e.g., the hospital.

Solvency—ability of a firm to meet its maturing obligations as they become due.

Symmetric Knowledge—knowledge about a hospital's performance (patient outcomes) is possessed by both the health care buyer and seller.

Total Compensation Package—sum total of an employee's payment for services rendered including salary and benefits.

Uncertainty—lack of certainty, either subjective or objective. It differs from *risk* in that it cannot be easily quantified.

Widget—an abstract unit of production.

References

Agrawal, A. (2002). Return of investment analysis for a computer-based patient record in the outpatient clinical setting. *Journal of the Association for Academic Minority Physicians, 13*(3), 61–65.

Aiken, L., Smith, H., & Lake, E. (1994). Lower Medicare mortality among a set of hospitals known for good nursing care. *Medical Care, 32*, 771–787.

American Organization of Nurse Executives. (2005). AONE nurse executive competencies. Retrieved August 26, 2008, from http://www.aone.org/aone/pdf/February%20Nurse%20Leader—final%20draft—for%20web.pdf

Berlin, L., & Sechrist, K. (2002). The shortage of doctorally-prepared nurse faculty: A dire situation. *Nursing Outlook, 50*, 50–56.

Buerhaus, P., Needleman, J., Mattke, S., & Stewart, M. (2002). Strengthening hospital nursing. *Health Affairs, 21*, 123–132.

Burnes Bolton, L., Aydin, C., Donaldson, N., Brown, D., Sandhu, M., Fridman, M., & Aronow, H. (2007). Mandated nurse staffing ratios in California: A comparison of staffing and nursing-sensitive outcomes pre- and postregulation. *Policy, Politics & Nursing Practice, 8*, 238–250.

California Nurses Association. (n.d.). CNA's 12-year campaign for safe RN-staffing ratios. Retrieved August 26, 2008, from http://www.calnurse.org/assets/pdf/ratios/ratios_12year_fight_0104.pdf

Conover, C. (2004, October 4). Health care regulation: A $169 billion hidden tax. Retrieved August 26, 2008, from http://www.cato.org/pubs/pas/pa527.pdf

Conway, P., Tamara Konetzka, R., Zhu, J., Volpp, K., & Sochalski, J. (2008). Nurse staffing ratios: Trends and policy implications for hospitalists and the safety net. *Journal of Hospital Medicine (Online), 3*, 193–199.

Donaldson, N., Bolton, L., Aydin, C., Brown, D., Elashoff, J., & Sandhu, M. (2005). Impact of California's licensed nurse-patient ratios on unit-level nurse staffing and patient outcomes. *Policy, Politics & Nursing Practice, 6*, 198–210.

Enthoven, A. (1986). Managed competition in health care and the unfinished agenda. *Health Care Financing Review, Annual Supplement, 8,* 105–119.

Furlong, E., & Smith, R. (2005). Advanced nursing practice: Policy, education, & role development. *Journal of Clinical Nursing, 14,* 1059–1066.

Garrido, T., Raymond, B., Jamieson, L., Liang, L., & Wiesenthal, A. (2004). Making the business case for hospital information systems—A Kaiser Permanente investment decision. *Journal of Healthcare Finance, 31*(2), 16–25.

Gerardi, T. (2006). Staffing ratios in New York: A decade of debate. *Policy, Politics & Nursing Practice, 7,* 8–10.

Gray, B. (1991). *The profit motive and patient care: The changing accountability of doctors and hospitals.* Cambridge, MA: Harvard University Press.

Harris, K., Huber, D., Jones, R., Manojlovich, M., & Reineck, C. (2006). Future nursing administration graduate curricula, Part 1. *Journal of Nursing Administration, 36,* 435–440.

Herrin, D., Jones, K., Krepper, R., Sherman, R., & Reineck, C. (2006). Future nursing administration graduate curricula, Part 2: Foundation and Strategies [Departments: AONE-CGEAN Collaborative] *Journal of Nursing Administration, 36,* 498–505.

Hippocrates. (n.d./2004). Book 1, Section 2. (F. Adams, Trans.). In *Of the epidemics* (p. 5). Kessinger Publishing, Retrieved August 26, 2008, from http://www.kessinger.net/searchresults-orderthebook.php?ISBN=1419137794

Institute of Medicine. (2002). *To err is human: Building a safer health system.* Washington, DC: National Academy Press.

Kazahaya, G. (2005). Harnessing technology to redesign labor cost management reports. *Healthcare Financial Management, 59*(4), 94–100.

Keepnews, D. (2007). Evaluating nurse staffing regulation. *Policy, Politics & Nursing Practice, 8,* 236–237.

Lang, N. (2003). Reflections on quality health care. *Nursing Administration Quarterly, 27,* 266–272.

Lang, T., Hodge, M., Olson, V., Romano, P., & Kravitz, R. (2004). Nurse-patient ratios: A systematic review on the effects of nurse staffing on patient, nurse, employee, and hospital outcomes. *Journal of Nursing Administration, 34,* 326–337.

Langley, M. (1998, January 7). Nuns' zeal for profits shapes hospital chain, wins Wall Street fans. *The Wall Street Journal,* pp. A1, A11.

Lemire, J. (2000). Redesigning financial management education for the nursing administration graduate student. *Journal of Nursing Administration, 30,* 199–205.

Lindrooth, R., Bazzoli, G., Needleman, J., & Hasnain-Wynia, R. (2006). The effect of changes in hospital reimbursement on nurse staffing decisions at safety net and nonsafety net hospitals. *Health Services Research, 41,* 701–720.

Manjoney, R. (2004). Clinical information systems market—An insider's view. *Journal of Critical Care, 19,* 215–220.

Marinucci, C. (2004, December 8). At tribute for women, Schwarzenegger angers nurses. *San Francisco Chronicle,* p. A1.

Mark, B., & Harless, D. (2007). Nurse staffing, mortality, and length of stay in for-profit and not-for-profit hospitals. *Inquiry, 44,* 167–186.

Medical News Report. (2004, February). New nurse-to-patient ratios present challenges in California. Retrieved August 25, 2008, from http://www.calhealth.org/public/press/Article/107/Medical%20News%20Report.pdf

Nahm, E., Vaydia, V., Ho, D., Scharf, B., & Seagull, J. (2007). Outcomes assessment of clinical information system implementation: A practical guide. *Nursing Outlook, 55,* 282–288.

Needleman, J. (2008). Is what's good for the patient good for the hospital? Aligning incentives and the business case for nursing. *Policy, Politics & Nursing Practice, 9,* 80–87.

Needleman, J., & Buerhaus, P. (2003). Nurse staffing and patient safety: Current knowledge and implications for action. *International Journal for Quality in Health Care, 15,* 275–277.

Needleman, J., Buerhaus, P., Mattke, S., Stewart, M., & Zelevinsky, K. (2002). Nurse-staffing levels and the quality of care in hospitals. *New England Journal of Medicine, 346,* 1715–1722.

Office of Statewide Health Planning and Development. (1996a). *Study overview and results summary.* Sacramento, CA: Author.

Office of Statewide Health Planning and Development. (1996b). *Technical appendix*. Sacramento, CA: Author.

Office of Statewide Health Planning and Development. (2006). Hospital closures in California. Retrieved August 25, 2008, from http://www.calhealth.org/public/press/Article%5C107%5CHospitalclosures.pdf

Quinones, S. (2006, September 22). Closure of Memorial ER is protested. *Los Angeles Times*, p. B4.

Rollins, G. (2008). CNO burnout. *Hospitals & Health Networks, 82*(4), 30–34.

Rudan, V. (2002). Where have all the nursing administration students gone? Issues and solutions. *Journal of Nursing Administration, 32,* 185–188.

Schultz, M. (2008, July). The association of hospital structural and financial characteristics to mortality from community-acquired pneumonia. Paper presented at the Congress on Nursing Research of Sigma Theta Tau International, Singapore.

Schultz, M., van Servellen, G., Litwin, M., McLaughlin, E., & Uman, G. (1997) Can hospital structural and financial characteristics explain the variations in hospital mortality caused by Acute Myocardial Infarction? *Applied Nursing Research, 12,* 210–214.

Thomas, L. (1983). *The youngest science: Notes of a medicine-watcher*. New York: The Penguin Group.

Trossman, S. (2008, March/April). A case for safe staffing: ANA brings together RNs, other stakeholders for summit. *The American Nurse, 40*, 1, 8, 12.

PART V

Budget Principles

Part Five provides the "bread and butter" information on budgeting. It is important that nurse managers, as well as other nurse administrators, have this basic knowledge.

Chapter 12, Budgeting, provides basic budget principles and terminology and gives an explanation of the "break even" budget strategy. Then Chapter 13, Budget Development and Evaluation, adds to the budgeting knowledge base to show a nurse manager how to both evaluate and develop a nursing expense budget. Certain principles should be followed as you develop a budget, including figuring nonproductive time, to be sure enough staff are budgeted.

Another very important budget responsibility for nurse managers, and other nurse administrators, is the ability to evaluate budget variances that occur. These are explored in Chapter 14. Some budget variances are less critical or will have occurred due to circumstances one already has anticipated, such as staff training during the installation of a new clinical documentation system. But some variances can indicate serious problems nurse managers can fix and avoid in the future. Although tracking is presented as an activity to do monthly, the nurse manager will need to perform certain activities on a daily basis to achieve maximum budget savings. Although a number of nurse managers still do not have this kind of budget responsibility, especially in Veterans Administration or long-term care freestanding settings, we recommend that such a process be consistently used all in settings.

Chapter 15, Comparing Reimbursement with Cost of Services Provided, reflects important budget responsibilities that have resulted since prospective payment was implemented. Here the nurse manager/administrator, along with the rest of the administrative group, needs to examine actual reimbursements received and compare them with the actual costs of services provided. Examining reimbursements ensures the facility is not spending more to provide service than the reimbursement amount will pay.

CHAPTER 12

Budgeting

R. Penny Marquette, DBA

Janne Dunham-Taylor, PhD, RN

Joseph Z. Pinczuk, MHA

Key Terms

- ☞ Break Even
- ☞ Budget Variance
- ☞ Capital Budget
- ☞ Cost Center
- ☞ Depreciation or Amortization
- ☞ Direct Labor
- ☞ Direct Materials
- ☞ Fixed Budget
- ☞ Fixed Costs
- ☞ Flexible Budget
- ☞ Indirect Labor
- ☞ Indirect Materials
- ☞ Line-Item Budget
- ☞ Mixed Costs
- ☞ Operating Budgets
- ☞ Overhead
- ☞ Profit Center
- ☞ Program, Performance, Product-Line, or Community-Benefit Budget
- ☞ Realize a Revenue
- ☞ Recognizing a Revenue
- ☞ Revenues
- ☞ Variable Costs

Introduction

There are nurse managers who are not privy to budget information, but most nurse managers are both privy to budget information (at least in their area of authority) and responsible for budgets. Although the extent to which nurse managers are involved in the budget process varies by health care organization, most nurse managers find themselves involved with budget preparation, holding spending to within budget limits, dealing with differences between the budget and actual performance (called budget variances), and identifying budget errors.

For most nurse managers, budget information and activities are involved with *spending*. Having *revenue* information is not as common. On the revenue side, nurse managers may know the breakdown between private pay, Medicare/Medicaid, and paying/nonpaying patients. In some systems the actual reimbursement amount is shared with the nurse manager. Finally, the nurse manager is often involved with the entire area of case management, which involves daily issues of determining whether an insurance plan will pay for services provided. Nurse managers must understand the vital link between the amount of money received from all insurance carriers (including Medicare and Medicaid) and the critical role of charting, which supports the billing documents.

Budgets and Patient Care

Budget responsibility offers an opportunity for the nurse manager to be an advocate for patients. As the level of management closest to the services delivered to patients, a nurse manager with a firm grip on relevant budget information influences patient care, ensuring that the patient receives the best and safest services possible.

All managers are most effective when they are able to make sound decisions and defend those decisions with others in the organization. This is equally true for the nurse manager who needs *the skills and the vocabulary* to determine what financial information is available, acquire that information, and interpret its impact on patient care. Unfortunately, the nurse manager often must "ferret out" the data he or she needs to do this job. Data are often badly organized or even "hidden" from line managers.

Data Systems

Computer systems are becoming the norm in large health care organizations. By system, we mean integrated computer programs that can interface with one another.[1] For example, in an ideal situation, a nurse manager faced with staffing a unit for the coming week would have access to selected data from the finance department, the human resource department, and the nursing department. With data from these sources, the nurse manager could know how much money is available in the budget for the unit, the salaries of cost center personnel, which employees have already worked this month, who has vacation scheduled, and so on. If the patient classification system is also interfaced, the nurse manager would additionally have a description of the patients needing care and the anticipated hours of care needed for each patient. With this information the nurse manager can evaluate whether the present staffing is adequate, too high, or too low to meet patient needs.

There are presently computer programs that do all of these tasks in isolation. The problem has been that the programs cannot "talk to each other." They are isolated programs, not computer *systems*. Although the information may be available, it is not easily retrieved and involves collecting data from many sources.

Charts of Accounts

Within the finance department, to have easy, orderly access to extensive cost information, one needs an organizing device. That device is called a *chart of accounts*. Most charts of accounts consist of two parts. The first is a listing of all units of the organization for which cost information should be gathered. In health care this might include laundry, rehabilitation therapy, infection control, housekeeping, operating room, x-ray, home health, physical therapy, separate nursing units, food service, finance, and others. The second part is a list of those elements of cost that occur in those cost centers. These elements of cost include such things as salaries, various fringe benefits, legal fees, pharmaceuticals, building supplies, grounds repair, equipment repair, oxygen, medical supplies, linen replacement, uniforms, copying, advertising, postage, and so on. Some expenses will occur in only one unit of the organization, but most will occur in several places. By properly organizing our chart of accounts, we can compare similar costs across different units and even compare costs of similar units across different health care institutions.

The typical format of a chart of accounts is a decimal system where a number representing the cost or revenue center of the organization appears before the decimal and the element of cost

---

[1] Interface can mean many different things. At minimum it implies the sharing of data. It can, however, also mean that when one system is changed, all related systems are also updated.

Exhibit 12–1 Chart of Accounts for the Outpatient Clinic

Account Name (organizational unit)	Department Charge Numbers (elements of cost)	
6170 Respiratory Care	.000	Salaries Supervisors
7091 Rehabilitation Services	.010	Salaries - RNs
7010 Laboratory	.020	Salaries - LPNs
	.030	Salaries - Aides
	.160	FICA (Social Security)
	.340	In-Service Training
	.360	Pharmaceuticals
	.420	Oxygen
	.430	Solutions
	.440	Medical Supplies
	.441	Billable Supplies
	.450	General Supplies
	.480	Instruments
	.490	Microfilming
	.491	Minor Equipment

appears after. When such charts are first designed, the numbers are not consecutive. Gaps are left in the numbering so that new departments and new types of costs can be inserted in places where they best belong. For example, you would want to keep all kinds of salaries close together on the chart to help you find things quickly. (Unfortunately, the longer the list, the more likely it is that you will run out of room in logical order and begin adding items to the end of the list.)

Using the chart of accounts recommended by the American Hospital Association (AHA), a brief example may be helpful. Assume an outpatient clinic has three departments: Respiratory Care, Laboratory, and Rehabilitation Services. Their chart of accounts might appear as shown in **Exhibit 12–1**. Using these data, we would have an account numbered 6170.480 to collect the costs for instruments purchased by the Respiratory Care Department. Account number 7091.480 would collect the same costs for Rehabilitation Services.

Comparisons of costs by department can be facilitated by organizing data as shown in **Exhibit 12–2**. Data from the individual cells in this chart represent specific cost elements within specific health care units. These costs form the basis for many of the analytical financial tools used to measure health care entity performance.[2] In addition to the advantage of being able to compare costs across departments within a single institution, using a standardized chart of accounts allows health care entities to compare themselves with similar institutions in their own communities and elsewhere in the country.

Nursing: A Big Budget Item

Nursing department costs often comprise 25% to 30% of the health care organization's budget. Because the nursing budget is so large, it often becomes the subject of close scrutiny. This makes it all the more important for nurse managers to have information available to quickly and

---

[2] One such tool is *ratio analysis* (see Chapter 20), which compares one financial or performance element to another (for example, nursing cost per patient day or in-service training cost per dollar of registered nurse salaries). Another is a management technique called *benchmarking*, where entities are able to compare their costs for an activity to the same costs for other, similar units.

Exhibit 12–2 Cost Comparisons Using a Chart of Accounts

Department Charge Numbers (elements of cost)	Account Name (organizational unit)		
	6170 Respiratory Care	7091 Rehabilitation Services	7010 Laboratory
.000 Salaries - Supervisors			
.010 Salaries - RNs			
.020 Salaries - LPNs			
.030 Salaries - Aides			
.160 FICA (Social Security)			
.340 In-Service Training			
.360 Pharmaceuticals			
.420 Oxygen			
.430 Solutions			
.440 Medical Supplies			
.441 Billable Supplies			
.480 Instruments			
.490 Microfilming			
.491 Minor Equipment			

effectively respond to such scrutiny with documented facts. Some questions to consider are the following:

- Do I have enough information about the nursing personnel? Data the nurse manager might want quickly at hand include starting dates; salaries and salary ranges, including ceilings for different classifications of personnel; sick, vacation, and personal time off available and already taken; hours worked each week; shift(s) worked; and overtime paid.
- Do I have adequate information about the patient population served? Do I have a good handle on the type and severity of illness, length of stay or visit, satisfaction level, and method of payment?
- How productive are the personnel in my assigned area? How can I demonstrate the level of productivity that exists? Could this level of productivity be improved?
- What changes could be made to reduce costs?
- How do selected cost changes impact the quality of service delivered?
- Is my organization and/or my area of responsibility financially viable?

Integrity

As with all aspects of health care, integrity is an essential component of the financial function. In the budget process, the nurse manager is faced with a choice: Does one ask for what is needed or "pad" the budget request, assuming it will be cut later? "Padding" does *not* include reasonable slack. Things never go perfectly as planned. Leaving some slack in the budget is reasonable and prudent. Padding, on the other hand, involves asking for more than you know you will need.

Remember first that your reputation is at stake. Once you have a reputation for padding your budget, every request you make will be examined with a fine-tooth comb. You will never be assumed to be accurate again. On the other hand, if you develop a reputation for prudence and accuracy, that reputation, once established, will support your requests in future years. The authors—representing nursing and finance—unanimously recommend that one choose to be truthful. "Crying wolf" will eventually be recognized. An honest relationship between those involved is always preferable for everyone concerned, including the patient.

Interfacing with the Finance Department

As they deal with their cost center budgets, most nurse managers find themselves forced to interface with their finance department. We say "forced" because there exists an army of reasons why these encounters are generally stressful. Part of our goal in this book is to make those interactions work more smoothly.

Although there are budgeting and financial terms used throughout business, government, and nonprofit organizations, this terminology is not tightly standardized. Terms that mean one thing in a factory mean something at least slightly different in a health care setting. To make matters worse, terminology is not standardized across all hospitals (or any health care facility) and is certainly not standardized across different health care environments. For example, a nurse manager who has worked at one hospital and then moves to another or who moves from a hospital to home care will discover differences in terminology and budget forms.

Finally, the financial people in the health care organization are likely to come from non-health care, business backgrounds. By looking at terminology from both a nursing and an accounting/finance perspective, the nurse manager will learn the links needed to communicate more effectively and maximize mutual understanding of terminology, concepts, and issues when working with financial personnel.

We have one more important instruction before we begin to examine the budgeting process and the dictionary of budgeting terminology. When working with your financial people and you seem to be at an impasse, skip the frustration stage and move on to *defining your terms*. Assume that you may be using a term differently. Once you understand the underlying concepts, you can simply ask, "How are you defining fixed cost? What are you including?" This approach can quickly move you beyond the stage where the finance person is looking at you as though you are an idiot, and you are getting ready to smack him or her with your unit's budget!

The Budget Process

To be most effective, budgeting should be an integrated function within the organization, and all departments should participate. Then, the nurse manager will be an integral part of the organizational whole.

Start with the Strategic Plan

The strategic plan outlines the programs and services to be provided for the upcoming year, including priorities and new opportunities to be pursued. Unfortunately, this process of strategic planning often does *not* include all the managers who need to understand the budget process. The nurse manager may not understand the goals of the organization, may not have seen the strategic plan, or may not have been involved in setting those priorities that specifically deal with the nurse manager's areas of responsibility. When this happens, the resultant budget is not as accurate as it might be. For example, those developing the budget may not know that a surgeon has changed an operating technique, turning an inpatient length of stay into an outpatient procedure. This change (becoming increasingly common with microsurgical techniques) will affect multiple levels of the budget, including most nursing costs. A few years ago, this type of procedural change occurred with gall-bladder surgery. If finance department personnel are unaware of such changes, both the revenue budget and the spending budget may end the year with major differences (called *variances*) between budget and actual.

Strategic plans need to take into account new surgical/medical/diagnostic advances that can require a different staff mix. For example, in long-term care, staff mix formerly included registered nurse coverage for 8 hours a day with 24-hour coverage being provided by licensed practical nurses/certified nurse aides. Now, with the increased complexity of the patient population, the staff mix has changed to 24-hour registered nurse coverage and increased the licensed staff.

Another factor to consider if third-party reimbursement (including Medicare and Medicaid) is using the per diem payment method (explained in Chapter 10) you must know what is included and excluded in the per diem. For example, if per diem includes all medications and the patient is placed on Lovenox bid at $80 to $90 an injection, the budget is affected.

Generally, there are separate budgets for each organizational unit. Units are defined as either *cost centers* or *profit centers*. Profit centers have direct patient billing. These include the operating room, x-ray, laboratory, and outpatient. Cost centers do not bill patients directly; instead, they support the profit centers. Some cost centers have little direct relation to patient care. Payroll, custodial, purchasing, and senior management are examples of such cost centers. Other cost centers do support patient care but do not bill patients directly for their services. These include most nursing services, food service, and medical records.

Cost centers may be identified by their physical location (a floor) or by their function (all cardiology-related costs). Nurse managers are usually responsible for at least one cost center budget. As the manager's organizational responsibilities grow, so will the number of budgets for which the manager is responsible. When a nurse manager moves to a different organization, even at a similar health care entity, it is important to inspect the new budget, line by line, to get an accurate picture of how the budget is constructed. A line item may reflect salaries and benefits at one institution; salaries alone in another; and salaries, benefits, and overtime at a third.

The Finance Department

Often, the budget process begins with the finance department. This process begins at a specified time, perhaps 6 months before the new fiscal year.[3] The finance department generates a budget for next year based on actual spending during the current year. Major differences between the current budget and actual spending are investigated, and anticipated cost changes are factored in for such things as employee raises, supply and pharmaceutical cost increases, and the general rate of inflation. The system should include input from the nurse manager. For example, the nurse

---

[3] In some organizations the fiscal year is divided into 13 months to reflect equal time periods, each 4 weeks in duration. This has some advantages over a 12-month fiscal year where the number of days per month varies in length. With 13 identical 28-day "months," it is easier for a nurse manager to compare staffing costs in February (when the census was up) with July (when the census was down). The combination of fiscal and calendar years can be confusing. Often in health care, different calendar and fiscal years will be used. Usually the budget period will coincide with other financial reporting devices such as managerial reports, balance sheets, and profit-and-loss statements. It is not uncommon, however, to have federal government grants where the fiscal year (and thus the year for grant application, funding reports, and spending deadlines) corresponds with the federal government's fiscal year of October 1 through September 30.

manager's cost center might be experiencing full census when the current budget reflects 80% occupancy. If changes have occurred, the nurse manager must provide changes to finance department personnel.

Although budget figures are generally *annual* estimates divided by 12 (or 13), costs do not flow evenly through the year, and nurse managers should be prepared to explain short-term variations. For example, a clinic may anticipate an increased demand for immunizations in August before school starts in the fall, an orthopedic cost center may anticipate more fractures during ski season, or a psychiatric cost center may have a decreased census during the convention of the American Psychological Association because most of the admitting psychiatrists attend this meeting. Only front-line managers understand these variations, which is another reason why nurse managers should help prepare the budget.

The value of those working *for* the nurse manager should also not be underestimated. This point in the budget cycle is a good time to talk with unit employees about budget issues. Staff can suggest how to provide patient care in a more cost-effective manner while still achieving quality standards. It is also very helpful if administrators *from all departments* can meet and discuss changing circumstances and spending priorities.

Each Unit Submits a Budget to Help Achieve the Strategic Plan

The budget process starts at the top with the strategic plan, but once that is set it moves back to the trenches and the budget is generally built from the bottom up. As each unit submits the costs (and/or anticipated revenue if in the operating room or in a revenue-producing cost center) associated with achieving its portion of the mission, the *finance* or *cost and budget* department aggregates these costs into an overall, entity-wide budget. Clearly, the nurse manager must know what strategic goals are expected of the unit to determine the associated costs.

The Nurse Executive

Once the nurse manager has reviewed the next year's budget and provided feedback on changes, the budget is often sent to the nurse executive for further review. To negotiate successfully with the nurse executive, the nurse manager needs to consider the broader scope of responsibility that the nurse executive holds. Ask yourself what role the nurse executive holds in the organization's strategic plan and how your unit can help fulfill that role.

Developing Budget Numbers

Most budgets are based on the prior year's budget, actual performance, or a combination of the two. It is typical for entities (whether business, government, or nonprofit) to simply take last year's plans, adjust for obvious errors in estimate, add on a little for inflation, and continue on. Called a *line-item budget*, this budgeting program clearly does not start with the strategic plan! Nevertheless, it is simple, and it is the most common approach to budgeting.

There is an opportunity here. If something has changed in the environment, this type of budgeting process allows the nurse manager to take the initiative and seek additional funding when the underlying circumstances have changed. For example, if the strategic plan of the hospital has changed to focus on patients with higher levels of acuity, the opportunity exists to argue effectively for a higher proportion of registered nurses or nurse practitioners. Unfortunately (or fortunately, if you are the one in hiding), activities are often funded long after they fail to support the strategic mission of the organization.

During the Year

Throughout the year the nurse manager must compare the budget (the plan) with actual results. The quality of reporting that supports this work varies from organization to organization. In the best case scenario, the nurse manager will receive regular reports on a pay-period-by-pay-period basis, month-by-month basis, and a year-to-date basis. The year-to-date numbers represent actual and budgeted numbers for the portion of the fiscal year that has passed. For example, if the budget year begins in January and it is now April, the budget report will include the actual and budget numbers for April, along with the actual and budget numbers for the 4-month period that includes January through April. These year-to-date figures help smooth out minor fluctuations and help the nurse manager see if the unit is on target. Additionally, year-to-date numbers also *highlight growing differences between budget and actual numbers that require immediate attention.*

Variance Reporting

In a well-run system each unit receives a regular monthly report showing the actual activity, the budgeted activity, and the difference between the two, called the *budget variance*. This report allows the nurse manager to focus in on those areas where things are not going according to plan.

End of the Budget Year

As the end of the fiscal year approaches, the finance department often asks that purchases for the last month of the fiscal year be completed early in the month so that finance can more accurately reflect yearly expenditures by the end of the fiscal year. In fact, as the end of the budget period approaches, nurse managers are sometimes faced with the unusual problem of wanting to spend more money. Starting 6 months before the end of the fiscal year, nurse managers should begin examining their budgets (including grant budgets) to evaluate their remaining funds. The disposition of unspent funds varies from organization to organization and grant to grant. In the worse case scenario, unspent funds are returned to the administration *and* the following year's allocation is reduced by the same amount. (This is another place where budget "padding" can come back to haunt you.) In the next least attractive situation, the unspent funds are returned to the administration and you are commended for your careful control over organizational resources. In the best case scenario, you are allowed to retain (or roll over) all or a portion of your remaining funds.[4] It is the nurse manager's job to know how unspent funds are handled at the end of the fiscal year and to plan accordingly.

Like our advice on honesty in the budget process, it is best to avoid spending money on things you really do not need. On the other hand, if you have needed new patient beds for 2 years and this year you have money left over, it would be a shame to lose it because you failed to plan ahead.

Fixed and Flexible Budgets

A *fixed budget* predicts a certain level of costs, ignoring the level of activity that occurs.[5] In reality, the cost of nursing services varies greatly with census and acuity. Because the fixed budget is not

---

[4] Even when it is policy to allow a roll-over of unspent funds, it is common for these funds to be "swept up" by the administration in years when financial results are poor.

[5] A fixed budget can be compared with planning the cost of a wedding while ignoring the number of invited guests. Of course, a fixed budget is appropriate for some things. The bride's bouquet, for example, costs the same amount whether the wedding has 50 or 500 guests. Similarly, in a nursing unit with a nurse manager, the nurse manager's salary is the same whether the census is 50% or 100%. Most costs, however, vary with volume.

too useful when activity is shifting, many organizations prepare a *flexible budget*. The flexible budget has different levels of cost based on levels of activity. The nurse manager may plan a flexible budget to cover different scenarios, for example, a 100% census versus a census of 95%.[6]

Some health care systems have computer programs that automatically prepare flexible budgets. Sometimes, however, this is still a manual activity for the nurse manager. But a note of warning: Even when a computer program takes over the number crunching, the nurse manager should evaluate the assumptions underlying which costs change and which stay constant. A flexible budget provides guidance in anticipating cost increases when volume increases in terms of either census and/or acuity.

Optimistic, Pessimistic, or Realistic Budget Estimates

Another approach that many organizations take is to have each manager prepare his or her budget at two or more levels: optimistic (census or department activity levels are very high), pessimistic (census or department activity levels are very low), and realistic (department or activity levels stay the same as the previous year). First, this approach forces managers to consider which costs and services are absolutely essential: What can't the unit do without? Second, it forces the manager to consider the most attractive expansion of costs and services: What would you do if you were rolling in money? Even though these budgets may never be used, the thought process involved in their preparation helps the manager deal with changing realities.

Mid-Year Budget Adjustments

Cash receipts are often less than the amount expected, necessitating mid-year budget cuts.[7] It is best if the nurse manager has a plan for this possibility, rather than being forced to do budget cuts at the last minute.

Everyone Brings Something to the Table

Different groups in the organization have unique information crucial to the overall effectiveness of the budget. Nurses often do not know what revenues were generated last year (which the finance department does know), whereas finance personnel do not understand the myriad problems encountered in taking care of patients (which nursing personnel do know). The most accurate budget predictions are achieved when people from all departments contribute the unique information they have.

Measuring and Adjusting for Inflation

Accountants and finance people adjust for inflation using a *price index*. The price index you are most likely familiar with is the *Consumer Price Index (CPI)*, which measures "the increase (or decrease) in the cost of living for an urban family of four" (U.S. Department of Labor Bureau of Labor Statistics). There are other price indices, including the *Wholesale Price Index*, which measures

---

[6] A flexible budget is sometimes called a variable budget, but this term is not generally used by finance and accounting people. Accordingly, we suggest that the term "flexible budget" be used to describe a budget where costs vary according to volume (level of activity) or acuity.

[7] Shortfalls can be caused by changes in the census, problems with insurance reimbursement, lower-than-anticipated receipts from Medicaid and/or Medicare, or budget shifting, where one unit loses funds to compensate for overspending in others.

price changes in individual industries and sectors of the economy, including a *market basket* of goods and services in health care.

All price indices are in the form of the "to/from ratio":

> Prices in the period we are going "to"
> Prices in the period we are coming "from"

To illustrate all price indices, let's look at the way the CPI is developed. First, a panel of experts (usually economists) decides what items an average urban family of four spends its money on: food, housing, clothing, education, medical costs, entertainment, and so on. For the moment, assume that those are the only items on the list. The panel must now decide how to define one unit of food or one unit of housing. These decisions can be pretty arbitrary *as long as they remain consistent from year to year*. That consistency, however, is actually impossible. How do you compare a unit of entertainment in 1945 with a unit of entertainment in 2009? Most of the things we do for entertainment in the 21st century did not exist at the end of World War II. The panel is simply left to do the best they can.

Generally, the finance department personnel indicate expected levels of inflation for different kinds of equipment, supplies, and pharmaceuticals. They get this information from the market basket index. If contracts for equipment and supplies change, it is important that the correct cost of these items be reflected in the budget.

Basic Cost Concepts: How Costs Are Defined

Cost accounting is an industrial invention. It comes from an environment where things are manufactured. Even today, cost accounting is not heavily applied to businesses that are service entities and provide services instead of goods.

Imagine a business that manufacturers surgical carts. They have certain requirements: a building, insurance, electricity, equipment, materials to make the cart (legs, wheels, shelves, handles, glue, sandpaper, paint), labor to take those materials and shape them into a cart, and, finally, labor to oversee the process and do the paperwork (accounting, payroll, insurance, and taxes). We will go back to this simple example as we "cross-walk" nursing terminology for costs with accounting/finance terminology for costs and try to identify the places where misunderstandings are most likely to occur.

In manufacturing, there are three types of costs: direct materials, direct labor, and overhead. *Direct materials* are those large enough to be identified with a specific product. In the example of the surgical cart, the legs, the wheels, the shelves, and the handles all classify as direct materials. For a patient who comes into the hospital for the surgical insertion of a pacemaker, the pacemaker itself is clearly a direct material.

Indirect materials, on the other hand, are materials that cannot be associated with a specific product *in a cost-effective manner*. These costs may or may not relate directly to the product, but it would be so time-consuming and expensive, there would be no overall benefit. *Indirect materials are part of overhead*. In the example of the surgical cart, indirect materials include items like glue, sandpaper, and paint. For the surgical patient, indirect materials include things like antiseptic swabbing in the operating room, surgical gloves, and surgical masks.[8]

---

[8] Historically, because health care enjoyed "cost plus" billing, health care was far more willing to treat small costs as direct costs. If a cost could be identified with a patient or procedure, the hospital could bill the insurance company and receive reimbursement. Health care treated everything from aspirin to surgical trays as direct costs. With diagnosis-related groups and capitation, the rationale for that type of detailed record-keeping has changed.

Direct labor is the labor that actually turns direct materials (also called *raw materials*) into a finished product. In our surgical cart example, direct labor is the person who puts the cart together. In our hospital environment, floor nurses are direct labor. The physician who inserts the pacemaker is direct labor.

Indirect labor encompasses those persons who do not actually turn direct materials into a finished product. In the industrial example, indirect labor includes the foreman, the person who runs the raw materials storeroom, the accountant, the custodian, the payroll clerk, and others. In our hospital, indirect labor includes all these people, plus the housekeeper, the dietitian, the medical records clerk, and many others. *Indirect labor is part of overhead.*

Overhead is composed of two things, of which you already know—indirect materials and indirect labor. These, however, are a tiny portion of overhead. The main overhead costs are often called the "costs to get ready to manufacture." In our surgical cart example, these costs include the building, insurance, electricity, and equipment. In our hospital example, overhead includes all these costs plus many others: insurance billing, kitchen staff, dietitians, medical records, accounting, billing, payroll, finance, and management.

Basic Cost Concepts: How Costs Behave

The definitions of types of costs (direct materials, direct labor, and overhead) interact with two important concepts of how costs behave: *fixed costs* and *variable costs*. Because health care environments are different from manufacturing environments, this is an area where misunderstandings can easily occur, and one where the nurse manager can play a role in educating finance and accounting personnel about the unique aspects of health care environments.

Fixed Costs

Fixed costs are those that stay the same regardless of the level of activity. The first example of fixed costs are those that would exist even if the organization were "shut down." In a manufacturing environment that would include such things as rent, insurance, taxes, depreciation on (the consumption of) buildings and equipment (although perhaps at a lower or higher rate than if the equipment and buildings were in use), a minimal level of utilities, and so on. Also, fixed are those costs that stay the same whether the organization manufactures 1 surgical cart or 10,000. Many overhead costs fall into this category (manufacturing supervisors, accounting, billing, payroll, finance, and top-level management).

From a nursing administration perspective, fixed costs (including minimum staffing requirements) are the minimum costs that are always paid regardless of the volume of activity.[9] Regardless of patient activity, whether it is measured by patient visits, patient acuity, or patient minutes, hours, or days, certain costs are always present. Examples include a cost center or department secretary working the day shift regardless of patient volume, telephone service, electricity, heating and cooling, staff development, quality assurance, dietary personnel, financial personnel, administration, infection control, and other cost center supplies that do not fluctuate with volume.

There is a subtle difference between the nursing concept of fixed costs and the manufacturing concept. As a profit-focused entity, a business would not consider the cost center secretary a fixed

---

[9] It is important to note that the definition of a cost as fixed or variable would change if, for example, a cost center or an entire institution were closed!

cost (he or she can be laid off), and staff development is certainly not fixed and can be delayed or skipped entirely. Perhaps most importantly, the concept of minimum staffing is alien to a finance or accounting person from a manufacturing background (see Chapter 13). In a health care environment where most financial managers come from a business background, the need to understand the *business* concept of *costs* is increasingly important. If finance department personnel tell you what your fixed costs are, have them explain how they have defined these costs. Generally, the nurse manager or nurse executive will need to educate finance department personnel about minimum staffing. You should be prepared to explain the concept of minimum staffing and present examples of actual minimum staffing requirements for your unit(s).

Variable Costs

Variable costs are those that change depending on the level of volume. In a manufacturing environment it is a simple concept—the more surgical carts we make the more costs we have. *All direct materials tend to be variable costs.* In manufacturing, *direct labor* may also be a variable cost because unneeded workers can be sent home (manufacturing has no concept of minimum staffing). Notice, also, that some elements of overhead are variable, including indirect materials, quantity of utilities used, and the amount of depreciation on buildings and equipment. In a health care environment, volume is a more complex concept. Volume includes not only the census numbers but also patient acuity, patient minutes/hours/days, and patient visits. Variable costs occur *in addition* to fixed costs to yield the organization's total cost:

> *Total costs = fixed costs + variable costs*

Staffing, beyond the minimum, is a variable cost based on the variable patient census. Other typical variable costs are forms used on a per-patient basis, medical and surgical supplies, and both linen and food costs. Although it is important to know these definitions, particularly when planning your budget, be aware that depending on the sophistication of your finance department's software, they may be unable to split out fixed and variable costs with a useful degree of accuracy.

Mixed Costs

Most costs are neither purely fixed nor purely variable. They are what we call *mixed costs*. Utilities are a good example. Even if an organization shuts down, it still needs a minimum level of electricity to light the yard and heat the building in the winter. That level of utilities is a fixed cost. If the organization is up and running, however, it needs more electricity to run the equipment, for lights, and for higher levels of heat or air conditioning. So electricity is actually a mixed cost—part fixed and part variable. Staffing provides a similar example. There may be minimum levels of staffing (fixed cost), but as the census moves upward or the average patient acuity increases, the staffing level rises as well.

In general, we do not attempt to split most costs into their fixed and variable components. Rather, we tend to classify them as either fixed or variable and ignore the area of overlap. In a health care environment, you may be best served by considering minimum staffing as a fixed cost and other staffing as a variable cost. Remember that you may need to explain this unique aspect of health care costing to your finance department.

Exhibit 12–3 Relationship Between Fixed Costs, Variable Costs, Total Costs
(Total Cost = Fixed Cost + Variable Costs)

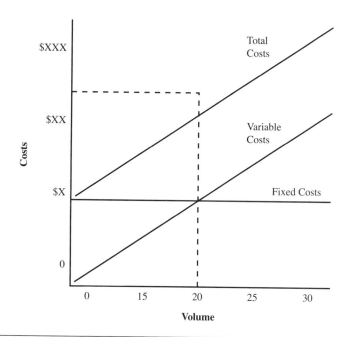

Exhibit 12–3 illustrates the relationship between fixed and variable costs over a *relevant range*.[10] The horizontal axis in Exhibit 12–3 represents activity level.

In our business that could be the number of surgical carts made, whereas in a nursing unit it could be the number of patients or patient days. The vertical axis represents *total* cost. The horizontal line *above the axis* represents fixed costs, staying the same regardless of the level of activity. The slanting vertical line represents the variable costs, increasing as the volume increases. The dotted line shows that at a census of 20 patients, this unit would have an average annual cost of $X dollars. Notice that at shut-down, there would still be costs. Even with a volume of zero, the fixed costs remain.

Exhibit 12–3 not only illustrates the relationship between the different kinds of costs, but it is also a flexible budget. This one diagram (Exhibit 12–3) can provide budget numbers, including both fixed and variable costs, for census levels from zero to 30 patients on a unit. Similar diagrams, or charts that move these numbers into columns for ease of use, can be prepared for many kinds of individual costs and for the overall costs of an organization. The important thing is to remember the names of the costs, the way they behave, and the manner in which they are put together.

---

[10] All financial figures, including cost estimates, rely on the concept of relevant range: the range of activity over which your estimates (particularly estimates of fixed costs) remain reasonable. If, in our manufacturing example, we needed to go to a second or third shift, almost all our fixed cost estimates (particularly indirect labor) change. In a health care environment there is a census or acuity level at which the underlying assumptions of the budget process change. One needs to watch for that point to avoid outcomes that are very different from what was planned.

Break-Even Analysis

To stay in operation, the *minimum* long-run goal of any organization must be to at least *break even*. When one breaks even, the costs of operations exactly equal the revenues. There is no profit and no loss. More revenues result in a profit, and fewer revenues (or more costs) result in a loss. When an entity operates below the break-even point, it must borrow or dip into savings from earlier periods when profits were made. Clearly, these are short-term solutions, and when they are exhausted the entity will be forced to close.

Break even can be shown graphically and calculated mathematically. Both the visual and the mathematical approaches are based on the definitions of costs. Remember that there are two kinds of costs: fixed costs and variable costs. By adding a revenue line to Exhibit 12–3, we create **Exhibit 12–4**, a graphical representation of break even. In Exhibit 12–4 the *fixed cost* line has been eliminated to simplify the diagram. It has been replaced with a shaded area. Notice again that the *variable* costs begin to rise from the base of fixed costs—costs that continue even when activity drops to zero. The new element in Exhibit 12–4 is the revenue line. The revenue line begins at zero—*no activity, no billing*. Thereafter, it climbs at a steady rate toward the upper right corner of the graph. The slope of the revenue line (the rate at which it climbs) is dependent on the rate of billing—bigger bills, steeper climb. Using the same measures on the horizontal and vertical axis as we used in Exhibit 12–3, our revenue slope would be based on the total revenue as it related to the average census or patient day. That is a crude measure, and there are many other measures that could be used. Nevertheless, at best, the break-even chart is a tool that will give you a rough idea of the activity level needed to remain solvent.

Remember, the more detailed your cost analysis is, the better this tool will work for you. A break-even analysis for a procedure will be more accurate than a break-even analysis for a unit or department. Similarly, a break-even analysis for a unit or department will be more accurate than a break-even analysis for an entire health care institution. Unfortunately, at some point, the break-even point for the organization as a whole becomes the issue in question.

Exhibit 12–4 Graphical Break Even

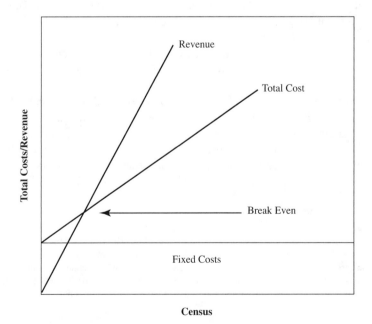

Census

Mathematically, break even is calculated using the formula presented below. It indicates that one breaks even when the revenues equal the expenses. Because both revenues and variable costs are a function of activity level, in this case patient days, *we must know both the average cost and the average revenues as we add patients to the census.* Given that, break even occurs when revenues per patient day equal fixed costs plus variable costs per patient day. The question we want to answer is this: *How many patients do we need in house, on average, to break even?* What is the break even census?

> **Break even occurs when**
> **Revenues/patient day × census =**
> **Fixed costs + variable costs/patient day × census**

Assume the following data:

Revenue per patient day	$ 2,000
Variable cost per patient day	$ 110
Fixed costs per year	$ 1,000,000

> *Revenues/patient day × census = fixed costs + variable costs/patient day × census*
> *$2,000 × census = $1,000,000 + $110 × census (2,000 − 110) × census = $1,000,000*
> *Census = $1,000,000 ÷ 1,890*
> *Census = 529 per year*

You can verify your answer:

> *Revenues/patient day × census = fixed costs + variable costs/patient day × census*
> *$2,000 × 529 = $1,000,000 + $110 × 529*
> *$1,058,000 = $1,000,000 + $58,190*

Your answer may not be exact. First, these are estimated numbers. You cannot be certain that your fixed costs will be $1,000,000, or that your average daily patient revenue will be $2,000, or that your average daily variable cost will be $110. What the break-even analysis has given you is a rough estimate. If, as you move into the year, you find that your estimates of revenues or costs are badly off target, or you find that your average census is only 475, you can go back to the drawing board and change the underlying realities or face a very bleak financial situation.

Similarly, *if your variable revenues do not exceed your variable costs, you can never break even.* If, in this example, the revenues per patient day had been $2,000 but the variable costs per patient day had been $2,001, no amount of activity will result in a break-even situation. You will lose $1 per patient day, and the harder you work, the farther in a hole you will find yourself. This understanding of the fact that variable revenues must exceed variable costs leads to an alternative way to think about the break-even calculation. This is not a change in either the concept or the calculation. It is simply an approach that avoids the manipulation of an algebraic equation and is easier for some people to remember.

Start with your fixed costs. They exist *whether or not* there are patients in the beds. To cover your fixed costs, you must make more revenue on the patients than you have costs caused by the patients. This "extra" revenue can then be used to cover your fixed costs.

Next, think about the revenues and the variable costs. These elements change with activity. In essence, if there were no patient in the bed, neither the revenue nor the variable cost exists. So a patient, in a bed, creates both a variable revenue and a variable cost. The term for the difference between these two is *contribution margin*. Contribution margin is the amount available to *contribute* toward covering fixed costs. When you have just enough contribution margin to cover fixed costs, you arrive at break even:

$$Break\ even = \frac{Fixed\ costs}{Revenues/patient\ day - variable\ costs/patient\ day \times census}$$

$$Break\ even = \frac{\$1,000,000}{\$2,000 - \$110}$$

$$Break\ even = \frac{\$1,000,000}{1,890} = 529\ patients\ per\ year$$

If one approach to calculating break even works, so will the other. Perhaps the most important concept of break even is the understanding that some costs and most revenues are a function of activity. Some costs, however (perhaps most costs in a typical small health care institution), are fixed and continue even after the shut-down point. When you consider actions that will improve profitability or reduce a loss situation, you must clearly identify which elements of cost and revenue you can best affect to improve profitability.

Alternate Ways to Organize the Budget

Thus far we have been using a line item budget. Line item budgets are organized first by a cost center and then by the line items the cost center spends its money on. Line items include things like salaries, supplies, telephone, linen, and copies.[11]

Another approach to organizing the budget is called a *program, performance, product-line,* or *community-benefit budget*. This budget is organized not around a department or unit but around a purpose. For example, a program budget might be organized around a product line in kidney care. The budget could include the transplant program, dialysis costs, outpatient care, and so forth. A program budget for cardiology might include cost center budgets for the operating room, recovery room, coronary intensive care, cardiac step-down, and cardiac rehabilitation services. Although program budgets are conceptually appealing, they are not common. They are difficult to build, difficult to coordinate, and difficult to use as cost-control mechanisms. Perhaps the best way to get a picture of the overall cost of a program budget is to compile the program budget after the line item budgets are complete. A program budget for cardiology might include 100% of the costs associated with coronary intensive care, cardiac step-down, and cardiac rehabilitation services, along with some percentage of the costs for the operating and recovery rooms. Unfortunately, patients do not always fall cleanly within a product line. For example, when a cardiac patient requires kidney dialysis, it is

---

[11] The term *appropriations budget* is used by all governmental agencies, including governmental health care entities such as Veterans Administration hospitals. The "appropriation" (short-hand for an "appropriations budget") has been passed by a governmental, legislative body and represents a legal permission to spend money on specified items. Appropriations budgets are unique in that they are often very detailed in terms of line items. In a private health care institution, the ability to switch money from one line item to another line item (e.g., from full-time salaries to part-time salaries) lies within the organization. With an appropriations budget, on the other hand, the organization may have to petition the legislative body to move money from one budget category to another. The second major difference in governmental budgets is that they almost always recapture unspent funds at the end of each budget period.

unlikely the cost will be picked up. Remember that budgeting is always an estimate; you never have perfect data. When building a program budget, it is important not to miss the less obvious costs associated with such things as counseling cardiac patients and members of their families, training or ongoing education of staff, and recruitment and retention of staff.[12]

The purpose of a community-benefit budget is to identify specific costs allocated to meet social responsibilities in the community. These items include services for the poor and educational or outreach programs that enhance people's health in the community.

Capital Budgeting Versus Operational Budgeting

Budgets can be divided into two major divisions: the *operating budget* and the *capital budget*. Most nurse managers primarily work with the operating budget, which has been the focus of this chapter thus far. Operating budgets cover the day-to-day costs of a unit, including such things as wages for regular and temporary workers, medical and office supplies, equipment rental, repair and maintenance, travel and education, and dues and subscriptions. Like all budgets, operating budgets represent the "best guess" for costs over a coming period.

The *capital budget*, on the other hand, covers the purchase of land, buildings, and long-lived (at least 2 years) equipment.[13] The capital budget is developed separately from the operating budget and is often funded through separate sources such as capital campaigns, designated internal savings, and grants. Nurse managers are most often involved in capital budgeting when they request expensive, long-lived equipment for their units. In most organizations financial rationale must support the request for an item from the capital budget. The following are the most obvious reasons for purchasing long-lived equipment:

1. A necessary item is broken and must be replaced.
2. A newer, better piece of equipment exists that will provide better patient service or equivalent patient service at a lower cost.
3. A new piece of equipment exists that will provide new patient services and help to generate new revenues.

The process of providing a rationale for capital spending is called *capital budgeting*. There are two fundamental differences in the way capital budgeting is approached in business (which may be your finance director's background) and in health care. First, from a *business* point of view, the underlying concept behind capital budgeting is that if the future revenues or the future cost savings from a new project or a new piece of equipment exceed the cost, then this purchase will increase the overall profitability of the organization. From a *health care* point of view, on the other hand,

---

[12] Another term often heard is *zero-based budgeting*. With zero-based budgeting, the manager theoretically begins the budget cycle, not with last year's budget but with a blank piece of paper. Every cost is then created and justified, building the new budget from scratch. Although some variations of zero-based budgeting are used for small units and projects, zero-based budgeting is simply too time consuming and costly to be routinely used. Where you do find true zero-based budgeting is during the creation of totally new programs and services. A hybrid of zero-based budgeting and program budgeting exists when programs are regularly reevaluated to determine whether or not they should continue. This type of analysis, called a *sunset review*, is a practical addition to the line item budget and its tendency is to always assume that last year's programs will simply continue with a slight increase in cost.

[13] Because heavy record-keeping costs are associated with equipment, most organizations set a lower limit on the dollar amount of purchases to be called, and accounted for, as "equipment." This "threshold amount" may be $500 or $5,000. The larger the organization, the higher the threshold is likely to be. When long-lived equipment with a cost below this threshold is purchased, it is treated as "minor equipment supplies" and expensed. Businesses handle low-value equipment in much the same way, generally using the term "small tools." Thus surgical scissors, which may last 5 years but cost only $250, will probably be included as minor equipment supplies in the operating budget.

most capital purchases are based on the requirements of quality patient care. Second, in *business*, if a project is deemed to be profitable, the funds to undertake that project will likely be borrowed if they are not available internally. In *health care*, on the other hand, funds are generally limited and capital projects will compete against each other for available capital funding.

An operating room nurse manager requesting a new autoclave or a new computer system is often faced with a set of forms from the finance department asking for a justification for the expenditure of capital funds. **Exhibits 12–5** through **12–7** are adaptations of the forms suggested by the AHA.

Sometimes when requesting capital funds it is necessary to give further explanation about why such funds are necessary. One possible format is given in **Exhibit 12–6**. Assuming that the department has more than one capital request, the set of requests will be summarized on a capital requests worksheet similar to the one shown in **Exhibit 12–7**.

Exhibit 12–5 Request for Capital Equipment or Services

1. Department _____   Date of request _____

2. Equipment or service requested _____

3. Name of primary requestor _____

4. Type of request:

     ○ Required by regulation or accreditation   ○ Replacement of existing service

     ○ Expansion of existing service   ○ Addition of new service

5. Department priority: Priority number _____ out of _____ requests.

6. Brief description of general specifications (including major components) and possible vendors.

7. Brief description of use and capability.

8. List by name and/or job classification the hospital staff who will operate the requested equipment.

TENTATIVE cost information:

Number of units _____   Personnel cost/year _____

Cost per unit _____   Lease or buy recommended _____

Total equipment cost _____   Estimated useful life _____

Installation cost _____   Supply cost/year _____

Transportation cost _____   Maintenance cost/year _____

10. Optional comments. Describe the present system used to accomplish the same or similar function, why the present system is not adequate, and what other departments and areas will be affected or will support the project. Additional sheets can be used when necessary.

_____   _____
Signature of person completing form   Date

Exhibit 12–6 Problem and Solution Statement

Requesting department _____ Date of request _____

Project title _____ Accountable manager _____

PROBLEM STATEMENT

1. Description of the problem:

2. Which medical and hospital staff have helped define the problem?

SOLUTION STATEMENT

1. Briefly describe the proposed solution to the problem:

2. How will the proposed project resolve the problem?

3. What alternative solutions are available, and why were they rejected?

4. What are the standard uses associated with the project?

_____   _____

Signature of person completing form   Date

Exhibit 12–7 Capital Request Worksheet

For Administrative Use	Referral to Medical Equipment Committee		
	Check Information Needed for Review**	R ☐ P-S ☐ N ☐ I ☐ C ☐ E ☐ F ☐	R ☐ P-S ☐ N ☐ I ☐ C ☐ E ☐ F ☐
Estimated Acquisition Cost			
Unit Cost			
Quantity			
Check Appropriate Box	New		
	Expansion		
	Replacement		
	Required by law or JCAHO*		
Requested month of purchase			
Title of request and brief description			
Department Priority Number			

* If JCAHO standard is the reason for acquisition, complete the Needs Assessment section.

** Letters stand for R = Request Form, P-S = Problem and Solution Statement, N = Need Assessment, I = Impact Assessment, C = Clinical Assessment, E = Equipment Assessment, F = Financial Assessment

The trick to completing these forms is to ask yourself why you need the new equipment. Focus first on patient care needs, then on cost and/or revenue considerations. Remember to look at the "big picture." Failure to fix equipment or failure to acquire new equipment that is faster, more accurate, and/or less invasive may result in patients choosing to go elsewhere for a wide range of associated services and thus a loss in revenue. If a piece of equipment is broken but the patient continues to come for patient services, there are often patient care issues (including possible negative patient outcomes), manpower costs associated with doing without that piece of equipment, and decreased revenues.

When you prepare your request, keep detailed copies of your notes and calculations *whether or not there is room for that amount of detail on the forms and whether or not it is requested.* Remember to

- Make your calculations explicit
- Label everything
- Show every intermediate calculation
- Recopy when you are done and keep your notes where you can pull them up to justify your numbers

Finally, remember to be *specific about your assumptions.* Your work as nurse manager will most likely be reviewed first by the nurse executive, who will set priorities over the full range of nursing services. If the nurse manager requests additional information or clarification, the quality of your notes will be critical in supporting your request.

Generally, you can round your costs and savings to the nearest dollar. Remember that these are estimates, and pennies are not generally accurate or helpful. Larger organizations may have you round everything to the nearest hundred dollars.

Budgeting Revenues

Throughout this chapter we have focused on budgeting for cost control. Most nurse managers work with costs, not revenues. Nevertheless, when you budget revenues, or set your own prices, there are additional things that you should know.

Revenues Versus Cash Flows

First, it is important to understand the difference between revenues and cash flows. *Revenues* are charges made to patients or other clients. When these charges are made, the health care organization believes that it is has earned the payment and that it has a reasonable chance of receiving the money. Accounting (and finance) records a revenue when it is earned, *not* when the cash is received. When the revenue is earned, the accounting department bills the patient (or the insurance company) and records both the fact that the revenue is earned and the fact that the patient is obligated to pay. This step of recording the revenue is called *recognizing a revenue.*

An example may help to clarify the situation. Think of a department store at Christmas. December is a department store's biggest month of the year in terms of both sales (revenue) and expenses (various kinds of costs). *Yet very little money changes hands in December.* Most of the money associated with the Christmas season changes hands in January and February as people pay their charge account bills and the department store pays for the merchandise it purchased for the holidays. Accountants call this *accrual accounting*—revenues are recorded when a sale is made and the seller has done the work, not when the cash is received. Similarly, most expenses are recorded when the organization has an *obligation* to pay, not when the cash changes hands.

Money (cash) is different from revenue. In health care settings, money is received long after the revenue is recorded (recognized). Although some procedures involve direct payment from patients, money generally arrives when the insurance company or Medicare or Medicaid pays the bill. To complicate matters further, when accountants and finance people talk about receiving money, they often say that they *realized* a revenue. To *realize a revenue* is to receive the cash. This situation is not helped by the fact that even accountants and finance people occasionally get these terms backward! For this reason when someone talks to you about revenues, it is often useful to clarify exactly what they mean.

If a health care organization has a very low population of indigent patients, then the difference between revenues and cash flows may be very small. Even in this case, however, the *timing difference* between when services are given and revenues are earned (recognized) and the payment date when revenues are received in cash (realized) may cause difficulties for the organization.

Nurses play a vital role in moving revenues from recognized to realized by charting. Every third-party payer relies on the accuracy and detail of the patient's chart to validate payment. Until the charts are "clean," payment will be withheld. Poor paperwork can be a bottleneck that chokes off cash flow to the entire organization.

When a nurse manager enters any health care environment for the first time, whether that environment is a hospital, home health care, long-term care, ambulatory center, or other, it is important to learn how patient billing works and to develop an understanding of the time lag between submitting patient charges and receiving private insurance or government reimbursement (Dunham-Taylor & Pinczuk, 2006).

Predicting (Budgeting) Revenues

Operating at a profit requires both revenues and costs to be carefully controlled. We attempt to control costs through careful budgeting. We attempt to "manage" revenues through careful price setting and by packaging a set of services that patients want to buy and insurance companies will pay for. Revenues are predicted in the same manner as expenses. First, you examine each major revenue source for the past 2 to 5 years and project the historical trend forward to next year. Next, carefully examine each revenue to decide whether it will behave differently next year than it did in the past. Finally, add any new "revenue streams" coming on line from new goods and services.

Pricing to Cover Your Costs

Pricing is done in several aspects. Beds and physical therapy services, for example, are priced on a per patient per day or per patient per hour basis. On the other hand, procedures such as surgeries and laboratory tests are priced on a per event basis. Last, goods such as pharmaceutical supplies and prostheses are priced on a per unit basis. Regardless of the good or service we are pricing, in the long run prices must cover all costs—direct labor, direct materials, and overhead. Thus to set long-run prices, you must have a good idea of what your costs are. Prices are *not* based solely on costs, but *on average, costs will define the lower bound of pricing.*

For each individually priced good or service, you must try to identify the cost of all the direct materials, direct labor, and overhead associated with providing that good or service and add them together to arrive at the cost—the *lower bound* of the price for that item. Some of these costs are reasonably easy to estimate. Others require enormous estimations. For the examples that follow, let's assume we have a good estimate of our average census for the coming year. We are estimating an average census of 500 patients per day or 182,500 patient days during the year:

> **500 patients per day × 365 days per year = 182,500 patient days per year**

DIRECT MATERIALS AND DIRECT LABOR

Careful cost budgeting can provide you with reasonably accurate cost figures for direct materials and direct labor. Direct nursing labor is generally applied, or added to the cost of a patient day, based on average census figures or patient classification system data. Chapter 13 explains how to determine costs using a patient classification system. If we use only the patient census as an example to arrive at a cost per day per patient for direct care nursing services, we would estimate our total direct care nursing salaries, wages, and benefits for the year and then divide by 182,500 to arrive at a direct labor cost per day. Assume that the labor cost for direct nursing on one unit is $175,000 per year. The nursing cost to be added to each patient's daily bill is then $0.96.[14]

> $$\frac{\$175,000 \; labor \; cost}{182,500 \; patient \; days} = \$0.96 \; labor \; cost \; per \; patient \; day$$

Developing the estimated cost for direct nursing services is a complex problem that involves concepts of minimum staffing, staff mix (i.e., registered nurses vs. licensed practical nurses vs. nurse aides and full time vs. part time), and other elements such as shift differential. Detailed examples of direct labor budgeting are presented in Chapter 13.

Direct materials are easier to budget—the pacemaker is billed to the patient who receives it. Again, the cost of the pacemaker (or the bedside wash kit or the prosthesis) is the minimum charge for that item.

OVERHEAD

Overhead is far more difficult to evaluate and is the reason that pricing is an art, not a science. Let's start with the easiest parts of overhead—indirect labor and indirect materials. Let's assume your *total* costs are calculated as *annual* costs, so you have an idea of the total cost for these items for the year. They can be calculated with some degree of accuracy for indirect labor, and indirect materials can be based on last year's costs. However, even if we knew total costs with absolute accuracy (which we rarely do), we still need to know how to *allocate those costs to billable elements of patient care.*

For example, if I know that a group of supervisory salaries cost $150,000 a year, how do I allocate that cost to patient billings to ensure that the cost is recovered? The unfortunate answer is that you can never be absolutely sure. You can, however, make a very good guess. For example, to spread the supervisory cost we might use our best estimate of patient days. Because we are estimating an average census of 500 patients per day during a 365-day year, we would spread our $150,000 salary cost over 182,500 patient days. Accordingly, we will *attach* $0.83 for this class of supervisory salaries to each patient's daily bill for room and board.

---

[14] With the increased incidence in 23-hour observation patients, we may want an hourly cost. To figure the hourly cost, divide the daily figure by the 24 hours in each day to also get a usable figure for direct nursing cost per hour.

> *Step 1: 500 patients per day × 365 days per year = 182,500 patient days per year*
> *Step 2: $150,000 in supervisory costs ÷ 182,500 patients days = $0.822 per patient day. Let's round to $0.83 per patient day.*

If we are exactly correct in our census estimate, we *distribute* or *allocate* $151,475, and we will recover this cost from our patients and their insurance companies.

> *182,500 patient days × $0.83 per patient day = $151,475*

If our census falls short, we will have *underapplied* this class of overhead. For example, if our census only averages 490, we will apply only $148,446. If we actually spent the $150,000 we anticipated, then we have failed to recover $1,554 in supervisory salaries from our patients.

> *Step 1: 490 patients per day × 365 days per year = 178,850 patient days per year*
> *Step 2: 178,850 patients days × $0.83 per patient = $148,446 recovered from patient billings.*

Alternatively, if our census is larger than anticipated—for example, 505 patients per day—we will have *overapplied* our supervisory salaries by $2,990. In other words, we will have realized an additional $2,990 more than anticipated.

> *Step 1: 505 patients per day × 365 days per year = 184,325 patient days per year*
> *Step 2: 184,325 patient days × $0.83 per patient = $152,990 recovered from patient billings*

When doing this type of budgeting, vary your assumptions and see what happens. Called *sensitivity analysis*, this exercise allows you to check the outcome if your assumptions are wrong (and they always are). In this example, for instance, will you recover the entire $150,000 if your census is 497 instead of 500? How about 495? By testing several alternatives, you can pick a minimum price that provides a reasonable degree of comfort in terms of recovering your costs.

Indirect labor is, perhaps, the easiest example we can provide, although other indirect costs such as linen costs, utilities, and patient meals can be budgeted in a similar manner. Notice that although linens and meals are direct costs in the sense that they directly touch each patient's time in the hospital, they are treated as indirect costs because it is not efficient to allocate them on a per patient basis. Linens and meals are like the paint on our surgical carts. Although not truly "overhead" (like the utilities and supervisory salaries), they are more easily and cost-effectively handled as indirect materials.

For things like surgical supplies we move beyond a per patient allocation and try to associate each kind of supply with the type of procedure that uses that item. We estimate the number of procedures, the quantity of supplies, the total supply costs, and then divide to arrive at a cost per procedure.

ALLOCATING LONG-LIVED ASSETS

The hardest item to allocate is the "using up" of buildings and equipment. Land, buildings, and equipment are most commonly called *fixed assets, fixed tangible assets,* or *plant, property, and equipment.* These are long-lived assets (more than 2 years), and their cost is spread over the asset's useful life. The name of this cost is *depreciation* or *amortization.*[15]

In some cases it might be possible to allocate the cost of a machine directly to patient care. For example, if you knew that a piece of surgical equipment would last through 200 surgical procedures and then be scrapped as no longer reliable, you could divide the cost of the equipment by 200 and *apply* the result to the cost of each surgical procedure. If we can do this, this element of depreciation is treated as a direct cost (one that can be directly associated with a specific element of patient care). Unfortunately, it is rare that equipment can be treated in this manner, and it is virtually impossible to do it with a building. Here we need to make some very *big assumptions.*

Assume we build a $20 million building. We need to recover that cost by charging patients for the building. The question becomes how much to charge per patient per day. If we are lucky, we financed part of the building with grants or a capital giving campaign. Nevertheless, when the building is "used up," we will have to replace it and we cannot be certain that grants and donations will be available when the time comes to do that. Prudence dictates that we try to add the full $20 million cost of the building to patient charges over the building's useful life.

First, we need to estimate the useful life of the building. Assume it is 40 years.[16] Then we need to estimate the volume of activity that will go through that building each year for the next 40 years. Let's stay with our estimate of 500 patients per day. Remember, that was 182,500 patient days per year. In 40 years that is 7.3 million patient days. That is $2.74 per patient per day to recover the cost of the building over its 40-year life.

> **Step 1: 500 patients per day × 365 days per year = 182,500 patient days per year**
> **Step 2: 182,500 patient days per year × 40 years = 7,300,000 patient days over 40 years**
> **Step 3: $20,000,000 building ÷ 7,300,000 patient days = $2.74 per patient day**

Equipment is handled in the same way, but because its life is shorter than a building's, our estimate of useful life is better. Remember, however, that in a high-tech environment like a hospital most depreciation is not caused by physical deterioration but by obsolescence. Our equipment might last 5 years, but if someone comes out with a new piece of equipment that performs the procedure with far less stress to the patient, we'll probably want to replace that equipment long before its 5-year life expires.

Land is not depreciated because it lasts "forever." It is placed on the list of assets and there it remains until you sell it.

What Did We Forget?

Doubtless, you have noticed that we have only scratched the surface. Even when we talk about spreading the cost of buildings and equipment, we are ignoring things like repairs and maintenance. Hopefully, you never find yourself at the "top of the budgeting food chain" until you have had years

---

[15] Technically, this cost should be called depreciation when asset is owned and amortization when the asset is leased. In practice, however, both words may be used interchangeably.

[16] There are published lists of estimates for the useful lives of long-lived assets, such as from the AHA and the American Institute of Certified Public Accountants. Ultimately, the best estimates depend on years of experience in a single environment (e.g., health care).

of experience in health care—years to learn the ropes, budget a unit, budget a clinic, budget overall nursing services—and before you are the person responsible for budgeting an entire entity and possibly setting its prices. But, in the meantime you may have input into price setting, and some of the same ideas that matter in setting prices help you understand the ways in which costs behave.

Discussion Questions

1. What challenge do nurse managers face when dealing with financial data that will help them to make sound decisions and defend that decision with others in the organization?
2. What difficulties exist for nurse managers who must accumulate data from different computer systems?
3. Because the nursing department costs are a large part of the overall budget, what information (documented facts) should the nurse manager be able to retrieve quickly and effectively respond when the budget is scrutinized by administration?
4. Why is it important for the nurse manager to provide a reasonable and fair operation budget?
5. What challenge does the nurse manager face when interacting with non-health care personnel who have only a business background?
6. Why do hospitals have a strategic plan, and why is it important that the nurse manager understands this plan and the goals for the health care organization?
7. Although budget figures are generally annual estimates divided by 12 (or 13), costs will not flow evenly through the year. Why and how should nurse managers be prepared to explain short-term variations?
8. How should a nurse manager prepare to handle minimum staffing requirement costs in the budget process in case this is challenged?
9. Besides a department budget approach, what other alternatives are available in a budgeting process?

Glossary of Terms

Break Even—when one breaks even, the costs of operations exactly equal the revenues. There is no profit and no loss.

Budget Variance—the difference between the projected budget and the actual budget.

Capital Budget—covers the purchase of land, buildings, and long-lived (at least 2 years) equipment.

Cost Center—does not bill patients directly; instead, support the profit centers.

Depreciation or Amortization—the hardest item to allocate is the "using up" of buildings and equipment. Land, buildings, and equipment are most commonly called *fixed assets, fixed tangible assets*, or *plant, property, and equipment*. These are long-lived assets (more than 2 years), and their cost is spread over the asset's useful life. The name of this cost is *depreciation* or *amortization*.

Direct Labor—the labor that actually turns direct materials into a finished product.

Direct Materials—materials large enough to be identified with a specific product.

Fixed Budget—predicts a certain level of costs, ignoring the level of activity that occurs.

Fixed Costs—costs that stay the same regardless of the level of activity.

Flexible Budget—different levels of cost based on levels of activity.

Indirect Labor—those persons who do not actually turn direct materials into a finished product. Indirect labor is part of overhead.

Indirect Materials—materials that cannot be associated with a specific product in a cost-effective manner. Indirect materials are part of overhead.

Line-Item Budget—simply takes last year's plans, adjusts for obvious errors in the estimate, adds a little for inflation, and continues on.

Mixed Costs—most costs are neither purely fixed nor purely variable. They are what we call *mixed costs*. Utilities are a good example.

Operating Budgets—cover the day-to-day costs of a unit, including such things as wages for regular and temporary workers, medical and office supplies, equipment rental, repair and maintenance, travel and education, and dues and subscriptions. Like all budgets, operating budgets represent the "best guess" for costs over a coming period.

Overhead—composed of indirect materials, indirect labor, and the "costs to get ready to manufacture," such as the building, insurance, electricity, and equipment.

Profit Center—bills patients directly.

Program, Performance, Product-Line, or Community-Benefit Budget—a budget not organized around a department or unit but around a purpose. For example, a program budget might be organized around a product line in kidney care. The purpose of a *community-benefit budget* is to identify specific costs allocated to meet social responsibilities in the community.

Realize a Revenue—to realize a revenue is to receive the cash payment from the client.

Recognizing a Revenue—when charges are made to patients, the health care organization believes that it has earned the payment and that it has a reasonable chance of receiving the money. Accounting (and finance) records a revenue when it is earned, *not* when the cash is received. When the revenue is earned, the accounting department bills the patient (or the insurance company) and records both the fact that the revenue is earned and the fact that the patient is obligated to pay.

Revenues—charges made to patients or other clients.

Variable Costs—those costs that change depending on the level of volume.

Reference

Dunham-Taylor, J., & Pinczuk, J. (2006). *Health care financial management for nurse managers: Applications from hospitals, long-term care, home care, and ambulatory care*. Sudbury, MA: Jones and Bartlett.

CHAPTER 13

Budget Development and Evaluation

Janne Dunham-Taylor, PhD, RN

Joseph Z. Pinczuk, MHA

Key Terms

- ☞ Average Daily Census
- ☞ Direct Staff
- ☞ Fixed Costs
- ☞ Flexible, or Variable, Budget
- ☞ Full-Time Equivalent (FTE)
- ☞ Hours Per Patient Day (HPPD)
- ☞ Indirect Staff

- ☞ Length of Stay
- ☞ Loss Leaders
- ☞ Minimum Staffing
- ☞ Nonproductive Time
- ☞ Nursing Hours Per Patient Day (NHPPD)
- ☞ Nursing Workload
- ☞ Occupancy Rate
- ☞ Overhead

- ☞ Patient Days
- ☞ Product Line (Service Line)
- ☞ Productive Time
- ☞ Relative Value Unit (RVU)
- ☞ Staff Mix
- ☞ Unit of Service
- ☞ Variable Costs
- ☞ Vertical Integration

Introduction

Budget responsibilities usually include an evaluation of the adequacy of the budget and, at times, the development of a new budget. It is an important activity because a cost center budget may not have been *totally* evaluated for years. A piecemeal evaluation to add raises or cut the budget may have occurred but is not sufficient in the overall budget evaluation process. What has been appropriate for the last 10 years is not necessarily what is needed presently. This chapter is designed to help the nurse administrator determine whether the overall budget is appropriate and adequate to meet present patient needs.

Budget evaluation needs to occur on both a monthly and a yearly basis. The *monthly evaluation* is concerned with looking at the past month's (or, better yet, the present month, if available) expenditures to determine if budget variances are appropriate. This is discussed in Chapter 14.

The *annual evaluation* is more in depth and provides the nurse manager and nurse executive with data that either demonstrate the budget is appropriate and does not need to be changed or that the budget should be specifically altered to better meet current program needs. This in-depth evaluation process is also appropriate when there is sufficient patient population or volume changes to warrant a budget reevaluation and possible mid-year budget adjustments. In this longer process, question everything:

- Are budget line items appropriate amounts for the patient population being served? Go through line by line and evaluate each category.
- Are we spending less than the reimbursement amount to provide the specified services (discussed in Chapter 15)?
- Are there more efficient ways—staffing, facilities, other resources—to better meet patient needs (see Chapter 6)? For instance, if everyone is working straight 8-hour or 12-hour shifts, chances are the staffing is too heavy for certain times and may be too lean for other times. Or with facilities, would a better physical setup help save staff time? With resources, is there a computerized documentation system in place that helps save staff, especially registered nurse (RN), time?
- Is the staffing plan effective (see Chapter 6)?
- Can staff productivity be improved (see Chapter 6)?
- Is the staff mix appropriate for the patient population served (see Chapter 6)?
- How could the leadership be improved? (If there are leadership problems, these need to be fixed because they cost a lot of money; see Chapter 2.)
- Are there unresolved organizational systems issues that are costing money unnecessarily for the organization? Are there organizational systems that could be streamlined (see Chapter 3)?
- Are there new safety measures, regulatory guidelines, or accreditation standards that impact the budget (see Chapter 4)?
- Does the new budget reflect cost inflation or anticipated raises?
- Are there new innovations or quality improvement strategies that have budget implications?
- What would increase patient—and patient family—satisfaction? Would these measures impact the budget?
- What would improve staff satisfaction and turnover?
- How will Medicare and Medicaid reimbursements, or other reimbursement discounts, impact the budget?

Start a dialogue about these questions with all nursing staff, physicians, other disciplines, and patients and their families. You can obtain invaluable input and find other approaches that better serve patient needs. Include the nurse executive in this process. The nurse manager must always have an accurate picture of the entire organization, understanding how unit issues fit with this larger picture. Many issues need broader organizational involvement. In fact, some issues necessitate the executive team or board action—the nurse executive will be more involved at this level. However, many issues, both on the unit and interdepartmentally, can be fixed by the nurse manager or by the nurse manager working with other department directors.

We would be remiss here not to emphasize the importance of nurse executive expectations of the nurse manager. These expectations are critical to overall organizational success. In the budget evaluation process, the nurse executive should expect monthly variance reports and annual evaluations of each cost center budget from the nurse manager. The reports should include recommendations and rationales for any budget changes needed for each cost center.

The budget calculations presented in this chapter have additional uses. These data provide objective evidence to determine and compare staff workloads to measure outcomes and to provide quality or research data. In addition, these data could be compared with benchmark data from other organizations.

Budget Terminology

Full-Time Equivalent (FTE)

Before evaluating a budget, it is necessary to introduce some additional budget terms that were not introduced in Chapter 12. First, the term "full-time equivalent" (FTE) is used in all health care organizations. A nurse manager is responsible for a specified number of FTEs. An FTE is a unit of measurement that represents one person who works a full-time position. In other words, a person working 40 hours a week works 2,080 hours a year.[1]

> *Full-time equivalent: (FTE)*
> *40 hours a week × 52 weeks a year = 2,080 hours a year*

However, more than one person can fill one FTE. Part-time employees work less than one FTE. To figure out hours worked, let's consider that an employee works 0.8 FTE. How many hours per week does this person work? Looking at this equation below, this employee works 32 hours per week. See **Exhibit 13–1** for a listing of different FTE hours.

> *0.8 FTE × 40 hours per week = 32 hours per week*

Exhibit 13–1 FTE Hours

FTEs	Hours per Week*	Hours per Year*
.1	4	208
.2	8	416
.3	12	624
.4	16	832
.5	20	1,040
.6	24	1,248
.7	28	1,456
.8	32	1,664
.9	36	1,872
1.0	40	2,080

*Based on an 8-hour day—this would need to be changed for a 7.5-hour day.

[1] Occasionally, in certain geographic areas, employees are paid for 7.5 hours rather than 8 hours for a day's work. In this case the workweek is not 40 hours but 37.5 hours; the year is 1,950 hours, not 2,080 hours. If this is the case in your facility, use 1,950 hours rather than 2,080 hours.

A nurse manager responsible for 50 FTEs most likely has 70 to 80 persons reporting directly to him or her. This includes both full-time and part-time staff. An industry standard is that a nurse manager is most effective if responsible for less than 50 FTEs. In fact, ideally a nurse manager should be responsible for 25 to 35 people, or 18 to 25 FTEs. When responsible for more than 50 FTEs, there are too many people on direct report, and the nurse manager will not be as effective. More legal and patient safety issues begin to occur when a nurse manager is responsible for too many FTEs.

Unit of Service

Unit of service is used by health care organizations to measure specific services a patient uses within a specific time frame (i.e., patient minutes, hours, days, visits, births, treatments, operations, or other patient encounters). *Patient days* are the number of inpatients present at midnight. One patient day is given for each day the patient is present on an inpatient unit. Sometimes terms are used such as "average daily census." Average daily census may also be the average number of emergency department/home visits or outpatient treatments for a month or a year.

The patient day is used to determine the length of stay (LOS) or the average length of stay (ALOS). This averages individual patients' lengths of stay within a cost center or facility for a month or a year. Patient days are also used to determine the *occupancy rate*. If a long-term care unit has 50 beds and 40 are filled, a percentage is determined for the number of beds actually filled. So the long-term care unit would have an occupancy rate of 80% (40 filled beds ÷ 50 bed capacity = 0.8 or 80%).

Nursing Workload

Using the various units of service specified here causes a problem in that all patients do not require the same amount of nursing care. For instance, one treatment could take a half hour, whereas another could take 2 hours. Or one patient requires intensive care, whereas another needs only the step-down unit. Or a home care nurse could drive 30 miles to make a visit, whereas other visits require only a 5-mile drive. Therefore further unit of service specification is needed to accurately reflect *nursing workload*, or the volume of work performed by nurse caregivers.

One way to better specify units of service for nursing workload is to use *nursing hours per patient day (NHPPD) or hours per patient day (HPPD)*. NHPPD gives the number of nurse staff hours needed to provide care to an inpatient in 24 hours. NHPPD and HPPD are produced by patient classification systems.[2] NHPPD and HPPD most often have the same meaning; however, at times the definition is different.[3] For instance, if a health care organization uses a patient classification system to measure NHPPD, finance may use HPPD using only patient census data. In this case, the two terms are different and have different measurement. As discussed previously, this is an example where it is important to find out the definition/measurement of either the term NHPPD or HPPD. Because there is not a standardized definition for either term, be sure to clarify definitions.

---

[2] Not all patient classification systems produce NHPPD or HPPD data. Prototype systems usually do not, whereas other task-based or care interaction models usually do (see Chapter 6).

[3] In this chapter NHPPD is used, but HPPD could be substituted.

Another similar term is the *relative value unit* (RVU), used by reimbursement systems. On an inpatient unit, the RVU represents the complexity of a procedure.

The NHPPD, when used as a patient acuity factor in a patient classification system, is produced from descriptors about a patient. In this process the nurse supplies the descriptors about the patient, the descriptors are entered or scanned into the computer, and the patient classification system assigns weights for each descriptor. Then the weight total is given. This weight total places the patient into one of several levels of nursing care needed on a 24-hour basis. Once the level of care is determined, the patient classification system can supply actual nursing care hours (NHPPD) needed that day (see Chapter 6 for additional information).

All levels of direct nursing care staff—RNs, licensed practical nurses (LPNs)/licensed vocational nurses, and nursing unlicensed personnel such as technicians, assistants, aides—are included in the NHPPD. There is no standard for which specific nursing personnel are included in the NHPPD figure.[4] For example, the direct care nursing staff might include RNs and nursing assistants on one unit and have RNs, LPNs, and nursing assistants on another unit. In some hospitals the nurse manager is included. In other organizations the nurse manager is not included or is included only if giving direct care.

Several issues need to be considered when using acuity data. First, the NHPPD is *not* standardized between patient classification systems. Thus there are differences in the hours of care for the same type of patient when using different patient classification systems (Shullanberger, 2000, p. 132):

> Cockerill et al.'s (1993) comparison study of four widely used nursing workload measurement tools (including GRASP) demonstrated that with different workload measurement tools there were significant clinical and statistical differences in estimated hours of (nursing) care. Discrepancies of up to 30% were noted in the costs associated with caring for exactly the same patients.

Second, even within the *same* patient classification system, the NHPPD *measurements* are not always standardized. In the factor evaluation classification systems, the nurse executive can choose the base hours of care given. At one hospital it might be 5.5 NHPPD, whereas at another the nurse executive might choose 6.0 NHPPD. Most likely this number will be higher for a tertiary care hospital or medical center and lower for a smaller, less acute general hospital that sends the more acute patients to the tertiary center. The classification system then uses this base number to compute the hours of care needed for most nursing care areas within that hospital. The acuity number is higher for a critical care area and lower for a rehabilitation floor—all determined by the patient classification database.

Third, it is very important that *reliability* (would two nurses rate the same patient in the same way?) and *validity* (does the tool actually measure the appropriate activities that nurses are doing?) have been regularly evaluated for the patient classification system. The first thing to examine is if the patient classification system has actual reliability and validity established. Some internal patient classification systems do not have reliability and validity established at all—and they may not take into account significant nursing staff time spent on such things as admissions, discharges, and transfers. They also may not include such functions as an IV team.

---

[4] When regulated by NHPPD rather than budget, nurse managers have the propensity to hire all RNs, whether needed or not, because you get more for your money. It is easier to schedule, and it helps if the RN staffing is not sufficient otherwise, but it can be a misuse of RN time if the RNs are expected to do other tasks such as housekeeping.

The second issue with reliability and validity occurs *within* the health care organization. Reliability needs to be evaluated regularly by having a nurse from a different unit rate the patient already rated by unit staff. Evaluation of validity is also necessary annually. For example, the classification system may say that nursing hours for orthopedic patients are 6.0 NHPPD. If the unit is long and narrow with supplies at one end of the unit and charts in another area not as accessible for certain patient rooms, nursing staff may need slightly more than 6.0 hours to complete the care for certain orthopedic patients. Perhaps the system does not take into account that psychiatric nurses spend a lot of time teaching families as part of the RN role. In this case these nurses might be spending more hours of care with their assigned patients than the patient classification system reflects (see Chapter 6 for more details about reliability and validity).

Fourth, *acuity data*, if available, should be used *instead of census figures*, because census figures do not account for the acuity of the patient. If acuity data are not available, one could benchmark with like units.

There is another reason the NHPPD would more closely reflect actual nursing care hours than census data. Census data are gathered at *midnight*. Patients admitted and discharged within the same day may not be reflected by the midnight census at all. The patient classification system generally collects data around 11 a.m. and may be done on a per-shift basis. It is more likely to pick up short-stay patients as well as admissions, discharges, and transfers.

While discussing the census issue, the American Nurses Association supports not using census data. However, this is confusing because in the American Nurses Association (2008) staffing principles it actually says: "There is a critical need to either retire or seriously question the usefulness of the concept of nursing hours per patient day (HPPD) (p. 5)." They further clarify as follows:

> [O]ne size (or formula) does not fit all. In fact, staffing is most appropriate and meaningful when it is predicated on a measure of unit intensity that takes into consideration the aggregate population of patients and the associated roles and responsibilities of nursing staff. Such a unit of measure must be operationalized to take into consideration the totality of the patients for whom care is being provided. It must not be predicated on a simple quantification of the needs of the "average" patients but must also include the "outliers" (p. 5).

This statement seems to really mean using census data rather than acuity-based data.

Overhead

You may see a column named "overhead" on your budget sheets. Overhead items are indirect costs. *Overhead* includes benefits such as health insurance and Social Security, depreciation on buildings or equipment, and nonproductive time (although sometimes this is mixed in with the labor budget figures). Overhead usually includes departments not giving direct care such as administration, housekeeping, maintenance, finance, medical records, and human resources. Overhead can be computed in several ways: Administration costs may be divided by the census and billed to each inpatient unit in a hospital, housekeeping and utility costs can be computed by square footage, and linen computed by the pounds of linen used. Finance traditionally will use the same step-down allocation for overhead as filed with the Medicare and Medicaid cost reports.

In most cases overhead figures on the budget sheet are neither determined nor much affected by a nurse manager's efforts to save costs. Occasionally, such as with pounds of linen, the nurse manager could encourage staff to use linen more expeditiously and thus save on this cost. The overhead figures generally are the responsibility of the executive team and determined by the finance department.

However, the nurse manager should know how the overhead is determined, especially when the nurse manager is checking the budget for accuracy or building a budget from scratch.

Product Lines

Health care organizations may use a term, called "product line" or "service line," that represents total services for a particular group of patients or similar patient diagnoses. For example, typical product lines may be cardiology, oncology, burns, or women's health. The product line can represent operating room, inpatient, ambulatory, long-term care, and home care services for that product line and sometimes can serve as a "profit center" within the accounting system. Usually, when using product lines, there are administrators—including nursing—assigned to each line.

Patients often need treatment in more than one product line. This causes problems, for example, when a patient is admitted into the orthopedic product line for knee surgery but also has diabetes, emphysema, and cardiac arrhythmia. So treatment includes aspects not actually defined, nor costed out, by the product line.

Lost Leaders

There may be services that a health care organization considers a *lost leader*. These services do not make money—in fact, they lose money—but benefit the organization by bringing patients to the organization for services or gain potential patients as they see that hospital personnel are friendly, helpful people. Lost leaders can include such services as the emergency department and women's health programs.

Another unit that often loses money but remains in general service hospitals is the pediatric unit. This establishes the full-service designation for the hospital even though it loses money. It also can help the community if there are no other pediatric inpatient units in the community. Minimum staffing is the issue here—there are so few patients that *minimum staffing* (needing two staff members on at all times) actually *overstaffs* the unit. To deal with this issue some hospitals have adopted strategies where additional patients are diverted to this unit (i.e., short-stay patients, ill children of employees, daycare patients), or hospitals even station pediatric outpatient services there.

Vertical Integration

In vertical integration a hospital might want to add long-term care beds or home care services to increase profits but have additional options to save costs. For instance, it is cheaper to quickly move a postoperative patient into a skilled nursing facility unit—a less expensive option than holding the patient on an inpatient unit for additional day(s). Or the hospital might start a health maintenance organization or preferred provider organization. They could even buy a medical supply company. All these additions are related services that expand the service options of the hospital.

Annual Evaluation of the Cost Center Budget: Building a Nursing Expense Budget

Now we evaluate a nursing expense budget. As we go through this process, we introduce additional budget terminology. Most often, the nurse manager is given an established cost center budget. Yet changes continue to occur (e.g., the patient population changes, the acuity rises, a different staff mix is needed, the location or environment changes, or new reimbursement regulations occur). How does a nurse manager evaluate whether this historical budget accurately reflects current needs?

One way the nurse manager can determine whether the budget is adequate is to build a unit budget from scratch. This provides objective data that can then be used for the evaluation process. Too often, a nurse manager tells the nurse executive, or finance personnel, that budget changes need to be made "for quality reasons" or "the patients are more acute" or "to meet accreditation standards." It is certainly important to meet accreditation or quality standards. And the acuity may have actually increased. However, the nurse manager is more effective when he or she backs up this statement with objective data, when the objective data are available. Building a budget from scratch provides objective data that then can be compared with the actual budget.

The nurse manager and nurse executive may need to either propose different budget amounts that more accurately reflect the services rendered or, within the same budget amount, reallocate how the money is used to better provide the needed services. When a change can be documented with objective evidence, it usually has the best chance of being supported by the nursing executive, the finance executive, and the executive team.

A hospital example is given here. However, examples in long-term care, home care, and ambulatory care can be found in Dunham-Taylor and Pinczuk (2006). Using the hospital example in this chapter, each step is defined in detail in the following sections, with the total process reflected in **Exhibit 13–2.**

Exhibit 13–2 Building a Budget from Scratch by Calculating Direct Care FTEs

Step 1:   Average NHPPD × Patient Census/Year or # of Visits/Year = Average NHPPD/Year.

Step 2:   Average NHPPD/Year × 2,080 Hours = Total Nursing Direct Care FTEs.

Step 3:   Figure nonproductive hours per FTE or get this figure from Human Resources.

Step 4:   2,080 Hours ÷ ____ Nonproductive Hours per FTE = ____ Productive Hours per FTE.

Step 5:   2,080 Hours ÷ ____ Productive Hours per FTE = ____ Actual FTEs.
           (This step figures how many actual FTEs are needed to cover both productive and nonproductive time for each FTE.)

Step 6:   Take Total Nursing Direct Care FTEs determined in Step 2, and multiply times Actual FTEs determined in Step 5.
           (Total Nursing Direct Care FTEs × Actual FTEs = Total Nursing Direct Care FTEs including both productive and nonproductive time.)

Step 7:   Determine the percentage of each nursing staff category to give direct care (staff mix). Then multiply the percentage of each nursing staff category × the total Actual FTEs determined in Step 6, to calculate how many FTEs are needed for each nursing staff category.

Step 8:   Determine the cost of the nursing staff by actually putting in salary [or salary and benefit] amount for each nursing staff category. Total this amount for the total direct care cost for the division.

Step 9:   Determine the percentage of staff that will be appropriate by shift. Divide the number of FTEs needed for each nursing staff category calculated in Step 7 by the percentage of staff needed by shift to determine FTEs in each nursing staff category by shift.

Step 10:   Determine the part-time versus full-time ratio. Divide the FTEs determined in Step 9 by the part-time or full-time ratio. Then adjust the ratios to accurately reflect staffing needs.

Historical Data Sources of Services Rendered

To build a budget from scratch, one needs to collect available historical patient data. Some possible hospital data sources include historical census data (patient days) or visits per year; other volume indicators not on the census such as observation patients; and the NHPPD or HPPD. Admission, discharges, and transfers may be already included in patient classification hours of care data, but, if not, these activities take additional nursing staff time; and the nursing hours per patient day (NHPPD) or hours per patient day (HPPD)—that can be obtained from patient classification data. The patient classification data are most helpful and most accurate if reliability and validity have been established. If there is no patient classification system, or if the system does not have reliability and validity, one may have to use census data. If so, it still can be helpful to establish acuity levels for certain groups of patients by benchmarking with like units. The medical records department may have the most accurate data about short-stay or observation patients. Other sources may include the literature or an actual measurement of the amount of time it takes a nurse to perform certain tasks.

As a nurse manager looks at the available historical data, these data will be totally inaccurate if major changes are occurring that are not reflected in the historical data. For example, perhaps a physician who is a large admitter is retiring and no one is taking his or her place. A nurse manager would then need to use data that would exclude that physician's patients. Or as technology developments occur—such as what happened with knee surgery—it might be possible to do a less invasive procedure that will change the data because the patient stay statistics will now be much lower. In this case the nurse manager would need to find out how many patients came in the previous year for this surgery, find out the care hours they required, and correct the data to reflect this new development.

Let's give an actual example of a nurse manager creating a budget and walk through this evaluation exercise together. You are the nurse manager of 4W, an orthopedic division. The orthopedic unit nurse manager figures the average NHPPD for the year is 6.6 (**Exhibit 13–3**). This means the direct care nursing staff gives an average of 6.6 hours of care in 24 hours to each patient on the orthopedic unit. This figure needs to be compared with the average hours of care for the previous

Exhibit 13–3 Determining the Average NHPPD for the Previous Year

Month	NHPPD
January	6.7
February	6.5
March	6.8
April	6.5
May	6.5
June	6.4
July	6.6
August	6.7
September	6.8
October	7.0
November	6.5
December	6.4
Average for Year	**6.6**

year. If the figures are similar, the current staffing level might be adequate. However, if the average figure is 6.4, the current staffing level might be inadequate.

The NHPPD figure can be further broken down into the individual classifications of nurse direct caregivers (i.e., RNs give 3.4 hours of nursing care, LPNs provide 2 hours of care, and the nursing aides give 1.6 hours of care within 24 hours). The patient classification system specifies such information with established staffing ratios for the orthopedic unit.

Calculating Direct Care FTEs

Average NHPPD × patient census or number of visits = direct care FTEs

Once appropriate historical data have been collected, the nurse manager can begin the calculations to build the cost center budget. First, take the nursing hours worked in 24 hours and multiply by the patient census or number of visits. If patient classification system data are not available, then the nurse manager could actually compute direct nursing care hours worked by employee classification for the past year. Or the nurse manager might want to develop some data: n patients who had 0.5-hour visits this past year and n patients who required an hour visit this past year. In long-term care, the minimum data set could be used.

Now let's go back to being the 4W nurse manager. The census data[5] for 4W shows 6,800 patient days on 4W last year—or an average of 18 to 19 patients each day.

6,800 ÷ 365 = 18.63 patient days
This means there was an average of 18 to 19 patients on 4W each day.

Historically, there is a patient classification system that is reliable and valid on 4W. The acuity data from the patient classification system indicate that

- 50% of the patients are at Level 3 receiving 8.0 NHPPD
- 30% of the patients are at Level 2 receiving 6.0 NHPPD
- 20% of the patients are at Level 1 receiving 4.0 NHPPD.

Going back to the previous equation, to determine the nursing hours worked in 24 hours the 4W nurse manager uses the patient classification system to determine the NHPPD or direct care nursing hours worked in 24 hours. The nurse manager computes the NHPPD as follows (*remember that to multiply 50%, it becomes 0.50 in the equation*):

	50% Level 3 patients @ 8 hours/day*	*= 4.0 NHPPD*	*(0.5 × 8 = 4.00)*
	30% Level 2 patients @ 6 hours/day*	*= 1.8 NHPPD*	*(0.3 × 6 = 1.80)*
+	*20% Level 1 patients @ 4 hours/day**	*= 0.8 NHPPD*	*(0.2 × 4 = 0.80)*
		6.6 NHPPD	
	*For 24 Hours		

---

[5] Make sure the census data include all short-stay patients.

So the 4W nurse manager has determined that the average NHPPD for 4W is 6.6. Now the nurse manager is ready to finish the equation:

6.6 NHPPD × 6,800 patient days/year = 44,880 NHPPD/year

Continuing with this example, the nurse manager is ready to compute the direct nursing care FTEs for 4W. She remembers that an FTE represents 2,080 hours/year. Now she is ready for another equation:

NHPPD/year ÷ 1 FTE = total nursing direct care FTEs
44,880 NHPPD/year ÷ 2,080 hours = 21.58 nursing direct care FTEs

Therefore 21.58 FTEs are needed to give direct nursing care for the 6,800 patient days the previous year. There is a major flaw here. Do you see what it is?

PRODUCTIVE AND NONPRODUCTIVE TIME

The 21.58 FTEs includes *productive* time or actual time worked. This means the budgeted FTEs do not cover anyone taking a holiday, going on vacation, or getting sick. The 4W nurse manager knows that employees receive paid time for eight holidays a year, 10 vacation days a year, and 10 sick days a year.[6] (Another term used in some organizations is paid time off (PTO), which combines sick and vacation time. If actually sick for more than a specified time, such as 4 days, the PTO time reverts to additional sick time.) In addition, staff are given time off to attend two staff development days, so this needs to be included in the 4W nurse manager's budget projection. The term for this is *nonproductive* time or time where an employee is paid but is not actually working.

Usually, the human resource department can give a nurse manager a nonproductive time figure. This figure is often for the entire organization. However, it is possible that this figure is not totally accurate for 4W. For example, if the 4W nurse manager has been an effective administrator and the retention rate is high, the 4W staff members receive more vacation time than the organizational average. In this case the 4W nonproductive time average will be higher than the human resource department number.

For this 4W example, let's say that the human resource department does not have a figure for nonproductive time and, to simplify the equation, that all the direct care nursing staff have the same number of nonproductive days. To calculate the direct nursing staff nonproductive time, the 4W manager uses the following calculation:

2 weeks vacation	*=*	*80 hours/year*
10 sick days	*=*	*80 hours/year*
8 holidays	*=*	*64 hours/year*
+ *2 education days*	*=*	*16 hours/year*
		240 hours/year total nonproductive time

Thus each 4W staff member has 240 hours a year of possible nonproductive time.[7]

---

[6] In some systems different categories of employees may have a different number of vacation days.

[7] This assumes that all part-time and full-time employees receive sick, vacation, or other nonproductive time. If part-time employees do not receive nonproductive benefits, include only their productive time. If employees do not use all their nonproductive time, we recommend that you still compute the full amount because this could possibly be used in the future.

Even though every employee does not always take all this time in 1 year, it is better to figure this total into the equation—unless at the end of employment unused nonproductive time is not paid back to the employee. Then one could use the average number of nonproductive hours taken per year by employees. Even then one has to be careful: If someone has a lot of sick time accrued and suddenly has surgery or an extensive illness, he or she will use much more than the average number of hours for that year. This is another factor that the human resource department will consider with its nonproductive figure: the average number of sick days taken by all employees for the year.

Because each FTE represents 2,080 hours a year but part of these hours (240 hours in the 4W example) are nonproductive time, the next step the nurse manager needs to compute is how many actual FTEs are needed, taking the nonproductive time into consideration. One way of calculating this is

2,080 hours (1 FTE) − 240 nonproductive hours per FTE = 1,840 productive hours per FTE

This means that of 2,080 hours paid to a full-time employee each year, on 4W direct care staff will actually work only 1,840 hours annually.

Next, the nurse manager needs to divide one FTE by 1,840 productive hours to determine the actual number of FTEs needed for the year:

2,080 hours ÷ 1,840 productive hours = 1.13 actual FTEs
(2,080 hours = 1 FTE)

This shows that for every 2,080 patient care hours, it is necessary to actually have 1.13 FTEs. One can translate the 1.13 figure into percentages—100% of the FTE (1 FTE) plus 13% of another FTE.

Usually, nonproductive costs are included in the division budget. This may include a factor for funeral leave or other such benefits where staff members are actually paid for nonworked days.

BENEFITS

Other benefits such as social security, health care insurance, and workers' compensation are not included here because these cost extra money but do not affect actual work hours. Such benefits—and sometimes sick and vacation time are included with these figures—may be 20% to 25% additional cost for a full-time employee. Such benefit costs may be included in a cost center budget or may be included in a different cost center such as a special human resource budget. Once again, there is not a standard for benefit costs and what cost center to put them in.

$40,000 × 1.25 = $50,000
(1.25 = 125%)

Both nonproductive time and benefits can be expensive for the organization to provide. For example, for an RN making $40,000 a year, if 25% of the salary is needed for benefits, in addition to the actual salary, then the organization is actually paying $50,000 for each full-time RN.

This means that an additional $10,000 a year is spent for the benefits for this RN. Thus if writing a proposal for a new RN position, one needs to take into account that the actual cost for a new RN is $50,000—even though the actual budget statement shows only $40,000. The remaining $10,000 for benefits will be reflected in another cost center budget—most likely, human resources.

In the 4W example, the 240 nonproductive hours for the RN making $40,000 a year actually costs $4,615.20 a year.

> *$40,000/year RN salary ÷ 2,080 hours/year = $19.23/hour*
> *240 hours/year nonproductive time × $19.23/hour = $4,615.20*

OTHER PERSONNEL COST FACTORS

Other personnel costs factors that need to be considered before having actual personnel costs are holiday pay, shift differential, charge differential, overtime, on-call pay, cost of staff temporarily transferred to this cost center, as-needed staff used including sitters, funeral leave, jury duty, orientation, or education costs, tuition reimbursement—if not already included in the cost center budget—and other costs such as differentials for having a bachelor of science in nursing degree, for specialty or other certification, and for a specialty area such as critical care or operating room. Tuition reimbursement is another cost, although this often is allocated to the human resource cost center.

A common practice in times of nursing or other interdisciplinary shortages is to pay extra to the staff experiencing a shortage. For example, one decides to pay a critical care differential. The message given to other nurses is that they are not as valued as a critical care nurse. Also, once a differential is started, the personnel involved will be very upset if this is ever taken away. Once a shortage is resolved, it can be tempting for administrators to dispense with the extra pay. One should really *think carefully about the implications if additional pay is given to a specific group based on a shortage.* Quick fixes usually do not work and may end up being permanent. (See the discussion surrounding *The Fifth Discipline* by Peter Senge in Chapter 3, Feedback Issues.)

DIRECT CARE STAFF FTES NEEDED

Our 4W nurse manager knows that the budgeted direct care FTEs must include both productive and nonproductive time. To compute actual direct care staffing FTE needs for 4W, the nurse manager needs to multiply the productive FTEs by 1.13 FTE, which takes into account the nonproductive time. This figure, 24.4 FTEs, takes into account both productive and nonproductive hours of staff.

> *21.58 FTEs × 1.13 FTE = 24.39 or 24.4 direct care nursing staff FTEs needed on 4W*
> *(40 hours/week = 1 FTE based on an 8-hour day)*

Determine the Staff Mix

Now another issue confronts the 4W nurse manager: What direct care staff mix is appropriate for 4W? The term "staff mix" is a marketing term that specifies what kind of direct care staff will provide optimum care within the available budget dollars. Because this is a medical-surgical division with a 6.6 average NHPPD, there is a need for an appropriate RN ratio. (See Chapter 6 for additional information as well as for the importance of setting up a staffing plan.)

When making staff mix decisions, start with the patient care requirements. In the 4W example, the patients are acute, postsurgical, orthopedic patients, and therefore a higher ratio of RNs is preferable. Other things to consider include nursing delivery system practices as well as structure and organizational issues. For instance:

- What is the division size?
- How are assignments made?
- What is the layout of the nursing division?
- Are there delivery system practices such as unit staff accompanying patients to x-ray, an IV nurse, or other off-unit responsibilities?
- What is the nursing department structure?
- Are additional support staff available, such as an orthopedic technician or a float pool? (Sometimes the orthopedic technician is on another budget, i.e., an operating room cost center budget.) If so, these people need to be included in the staffing for the appropriate number of hours worked on 4W. Benchmarking data on staffing for other orthopedic units might be helpful as well.

In our example, the 4W nurse manager chooses to have a staff mix of 70% RNs and 30% nursing assistants. Thus for the 24.4 FTEs of direct care nursing staff needed on 4W, the nurse manager determines that 17.1 FTEs will be RN staff. We continue to use this figure in this example. Fralic (2000) advocates creating a staffing plan based on a slightly lower number, such as 7.3 NHPPD or 7.4 NHPPD if the actual NHPPD was 7.5, to give some additional flexibility to the nurse manager. Then, if the average NHPPD suddenly goes above 7.5 NHPPD, a staff member could be added on a shift without going over budget. In addition, this strategy could save money if less staff were actually needed on a shift.

24.4 FTEs direct care nursing staff × 0.70 RN staff = 17.1 RN FTEs

The remaining FTEs will be used for nursing assistants.

24.4 FTEs direct care nursing staff − 17.1 RN FTEs = 7.3 nursing assistant FTEs
OR (It is always best to double check your figures.)
24.4 × 0.3 = 7.32 or 7.3 (The 0.3 is from 30% nursing assistant staff mix.
It is always best to round to the nearest tenth.)

Indirect Nursing Staff

In the preceding section the direct care nursing staff requirements were computed. Now we determine the *indirect* FTE requirements. Here one decides what indirect staff members are necessary for optimal functioning of a cost center. Still using 4W as an example, the nurse manager knows that two unit secretaries are needed for each day and evening shift. (Staff work 8-hour shifts on 4W.) To compute the unit secretary FTEs, how many FTEs are needed to fill a 7-day-a-week position? If the unit secretaries work 8-hour shifts, then

> *8 hours × 7 days/week = 56 hours/week*
> *56 hours/week ÷ 40 hours/week = 1.4 FTEs per shift*
> *(40 hours/week = 1 FTE based on an 8-hour day)*

To cover both day and evening shifts, the 4W nurse manager would need 2.8 unit secretary FTEs.

As previously noted in the section Direct Care Staff FTEs Needed, the 2.8 FTEs only reflect productive time worked. If there is a mechanism to replace the unit secretaries while they take vacation or sick time, such as a hospital-wide pool, costs for the nonproductive time could be charged to 4W when someone from this pool is actually used on 4W.

Another option to cover the nonproductive time is to hire part-time unit secretaries that are willing to work extra shifts when the other unit secretaries are sick or on vacation. A budgeted amount reflecting up to 0.4 additional unit secretary FTEs would be added to the budget to cover this additional time worked.

> *2.8 productive unit secretary FTEs × 1.13 productive and nonproductive time = 3.2 unit secretary FTEs*
> *(3.2 unit secretary FTEs − 2.8 productive unit secretary FTEs = 0.4 unit secretary FTE nonproductive time)*

Another choice that can be made is to not replace the unit secretaries when nonproductive time is taken. This presents a problem because the division may have no unit secretary 13% of the time. This can be costly because the other RNs and nursing assistants will have to do the unit secretary duties—answer the phone, do the required paperwork, greet visitors—in addition to their regular duties. This can mean that expensive RN time is spent completing clerical functions. With the current nursing shortage, this is a waste of licensed staff time. Perhaps a better option is to specially train certain nurse aides, who are paid at a slightly higher level, to also complete the unit secretary work.

Occasionally, the unit secretary hours are considered under direct care hours. The advantage to putting the unit secretary in the direct care hours is that when the census is low the nurse manager could replace the unit secretary with a caregiver. The disadvantage of this is that the unit clerk could be counted into the NHPPD as a direct caregiver, thus decreasing caregiver hours. We recommend the unit secretary not be considered in direct care hours.

While considering indirect nursing personnel, the nurse manager FTE needs to be included. Going back to the 4W example, the nurse manager had responsibility only for 4W so one FTE would be allocated to the nurse manager position. An industry standard currently is that when the nurse manager takes sick or vacation time, no additional FTEs are allocated to cover this time. Often, the assistant nurse mananger/charge nurse will cover the unit.

There are additional indirect nursing costs for the division. Indirect unit personnel costs might include staff development, clinical specialist time, and/or assistant nurse manager time, if not included in the direct care staffing. Often, staff development and/or clinical specialist time are found on other cost center budgets.

Total Cost Center FTEs

Continuing to use the 4W example, the nurse manager has now figured the total FTEs for the cost center personnel budget:

	1.0	*Nurse manager FTE*
	17.1	*RN FTEs*
	7.3	*Nursing assistant FTEs*
+	3.2	*Unit secretary FTEs*
	28.6	*Total FTEs for 4W*

Dividing FTEs into Shifts

The nurse manager now needs to determine the percentage of FTEs on each shift. As a general rule of thumb, because the patients are more acute, staff are more evenly distributed across shifts. Using 8-hour shifts on a general care division, the industry standard is that most direct care nursing staff are allocated to the day shift (40–45%) with a bit less for the evening shift (35–40%) and the fewest for the night shift (20–35%). A lot of this is determined by the actual patient population needs on the unit. Using 12-hour shifts, the industry standard is that most direct care nursing staff are scheduled for days (50–60%) with the rest of the staff working the night shift. There is no absolute industry standard for shift allocations. This distribution relies on the judgment of the nursing staff and nursing administration.

On 4W the nurse manager determines that there will be 40% of the direct care nursing staff working day shift, 35% on the evening shift, and 25% on the night shift. This decision was made because the majority of medications happen on days and evenings, and most surgical procedures are scheduled on days. Also, days and evenings experience the most admissions and discharges. Now the nurse manager can determine the FTE distribution for each shift:

	Day Shift	*Check Your Figures*	
		RN	*NA*
17.1 RN FTEs × 0.40 = 6.84 or 6.8 RN FTEs		6.8	
7.3 RN FTEs × 0.40 = 2.92 or 2.9 NA FTEs			2.9
	Evening Shift		
17.1 RN FTEs × 0.35 = 5.98 or 6 RN FTEs		6.0	
7.3 RN FTEs × 0.35 = 2.55 or 2.6 NA FTEs			2.6
	Night Shift		
17.1 RN FTEs × 0.25 = 4.27 or 4.3 RN FTEs		4.3	
7.3 RN FTEs × 0.25 = 1.82 or 1.8 NA FTEs		+	1.8
		17.1	7.3

To check your figures, add them together. They should total 17.1 RN FTEs and 7.3 nursing assistant FTEs.

Determine Part-Time versus Full-Time Ratio

After determining the FTE distribution by shift, the nurse manager has another decision to make: *What percentage of staff should be part time versus full time?* One needs to make a thoughtful decision here because too many part-time staff means a lack of continuity on the division. On the other hand, if there are too many full-time staff, it will be impossible to cover weekends with adequate staffing. Ideally, a ratio of about 60% full-time personnel and 40% part-time personnel, or 65% full time and 35% part time, is preferred. It allows for some flexibility in staffing yet achieves continuity.

Going back to the 4W example, the nurse manager decides to use the 60:40 ratio and figures the FTEs for both classifications of nursing personnel, checking the figures:

	Day Shift	*Check Your Figures*	
		RN	*NA*
6.8 RN FTEs $\times$ 0.60 = 4.08 or 4.1 full-time RN FTEs		4.1	
6.8 RN FTEs $\times$ 0.40 = 2.72 or 2.7 part-time RN FTEs		2.7	
2.9 NA FTEs $\times$ 0.60 = 1.74 or 1.7 full-time NA FTEs			1.7
2.9 NA FTEs $\times$ 0.40 = 1.16 or 1.2 part-time NA FTEs			1.2
	Evening Shift		
6.0 RN FTEs $\times$ 0.60 = 3.6 full-time RN FTEs		3.6	
6.0 RN FTEs $\times$ 0.40 = 2.4 part-time RN FTEs		2.4	
2.6 NA FTEs $\times$ 0.60 = 1.56 or 1.6 full-time NA FTEs			1.6
2.6 NA FTEs $\times$ 0.40 = 1.04 or 1 part-time NA FTEs			1.0
	Night Shift		
4.3 RN FTEs $\times$ 0.60 = 2.58 or 2.6 full-time RN FTEs		2.6	
4.3 RN FTEs $\times$ 0.40 = 1.72 or 1.7 part-time RN FTEs		1.7	
1.8 NA FTEs $\times$ 0.60 = 1.08 or 1.1 full-time NA FTE			1.1
1.8 NA FTEs $\times$ 0.40 = 0.72 or 0.7 part-time NA FTE		+	0.7
Total		17.1	7.3
(NA = nursing assistant)			

Now another challenge emerges as the nurse manager computes the full-time calculation. Several of the full-time FTE numbers are a fraction. A full-time person fills 1 FTE, not a fraction of an FTE. So the nurse manager must change several calculations. This first occurs on the day shift with both the RN FTEs and the nursing assistant FTEs. There are 4.1 full-time RN FTEs and 2.7 part-time RN FTEs. Here it is best to take the leftover 0.1 full-time RN FTE and add it to the part-time RN FTEs. There are 1.7 full-time nursing assistant FTEs—one can either have 1 or 2 full-time nursing assistants. In these cases one must think of the implications. The nurse manager could decide to have 2 FTEs be full time, with a resulting 0.9 FTE for part-time nursing assistants on days. Alternately, the nurse manager could choose to have 1 full-time nursing assistant and 1.9 part-time nursing assistant FTEs.

There is no right answer to this dilemma: One must consider the implications of each. There probably will be less continuity with the second option, but it offers more flexibility with scheduling. The author, however, would choose to go with the first option due to availability of personnel. It can be very difficult to find nursing assistants who want to work part time. Because the nursing assistant salaries are lower than other nursing personnel, they would prefer to have a full-time job with benefits.

Looking at the RN FTEs on the evening shift, the same problem occurs. Here there are 3.6 full-time RN FTEs. So the nurse manager must choose between three or four full-time RNs. In this case it may be best to choose to have four full-time RNs rather than three, because if the RNs have every other weekend off, there will be two full-time RNs on every weekend. When one RN goes on vacation or is sick, there will still be continuity with another full-time RN available. So the nurse manager will plan to have four full-time evening RN FTEs and two part-time evening RN FTEs, which totals six evening RN FTEs.

As one changes the budget figures, keep an ongoing tally of the changes as one adds or subtracts FTEs. In the end the tally should add to zero. In the following 4W example, the nurse manager changes the FTE designations as follows and keeps a tally:

Had	Change To	Day Shift	Tally RN	NA
4.1 to	4 full-time RN FTEs	[4.1 − 4 = +0.1]	+0.1	
2.7 to	2.8 part-time RN FTEs	[2.7 − 2.8 = −0.1]	−0.1	
1.7 to	2 full-time NA FTEs	etc.		−0.3
1.2 to	0.9 part-time NA FTE			+0.3
		Evening Shift		
3.6 to	4 full-time RN FTEs		−0.4	
2.4 to	2 part-time RN FTEs		+0.4	
1.6 to	2 full-time NA FTEs			−0.4
1.0 to	0.6 part-time NA FTE			+0.4
		Night Shift		
2.6 to	3 full-time RN FTEs		−0.4	
1.7 to	1.3 part-time RN FTEs		+0.4	
1.1 to	1 full-time NA FTEs			+0.1
0.7 to	0.8 part-time NA FTE			−0.1
17.1 RN FTEs and 7.3 NA FTEs or 24.4 Total FTEs			0	0
(NA = nursing assistant)				

Once again, the nurse manager can double check the numbers. The part-time and full-time numbers should add up to the total FTE number for that position classification; the total direct care staff FTEs should still add up to 24.4.

The last action of the nurse manager, if using these numbers to actually staff the division, is to determine the number of actual part-time staff to hire. Using the 4W example, there are 2.8 RN part-time FTEs on Day Shift. To staff for weekends, it is probably best to have at least four employees in part-time positions—two for each weekend if everyone gets every other weekend off. So the nurse manager could choose to make a couple positions 0.7 or 0.8 FTEs and two positions for less time. One option is to have two 0.8 FTE positions and two 0.6 FTE positions. Gear this decision by part-time staff availability and preferences. And be flexible and change the FTE designations if new staff members prefer different numbers of work hours. The main goal is to stay within the 17.1 RN FTEs and the 7.3 nursing assistant FTEs.

There is no industry standard here. The FTE part-time designations are a result of personal preference, availability of potential employees, and good judgment. For example, if one had 2.6 part-time FTEs for a shift, one would not want all the part-time employees to be 0.4 FTE only working 2 days each week. Continuity would really be an issue if this were the case. On the other hand, if one only has 0.8 part-time FTEs for a shift, it might be preferable to have two different people hired to allow more flexibility in staffing.

Calculate Nursing Care Hours Needed per Day

Now that we have figured productive and nonproductive time, let's go back to the 44,880 NHPPD given the previous year. Assuming that the average number remains the same for this current year, we can divide the 44,880 NHPPD by 365 days to determine the actual number of nursing care hours needed each day, or 122.96 hours.[8] In the box provided one can see that on the day shift the nurse manager should have 34 RN hours and 15 nursing assistant hours; on evenings 30 RN hours and 13 nursing assistant hours; and on nights 22 RN hours and 9 nursing assistant hours. Full-time and part-time staff scheduled to work each shift should add up to these numbers.

4W Nursing care hours needed per day

44,880 NHPPD ÷ 365 days = 122.96 nursing care hours needed each day

Skill mix

122.96 hours × 0.7 RN = 86 RN hours needed over 24 hours*
122.96 hours × 0.3 NA = 37 NA hours needed over 24 hours*
*(*Rounded to an even hour)*

Shifts

86 RN hours × 0.40 day shift = 34 day shift RN hours*
37 NA hours × 0.40 day shift = 15 day shift NA hours*
86 RN hours × 0.35 day shift = 30 evening shift RN hours*
37 NA hours × 0.35 day shift = 13 evening shift NA hours*
86 RN hours × 0.25 day shift = 22 night shift RN hours*
37 NA hours × 0.25 day shift = 9 night shift NA hours*
*(*Rounded to an even hour. NA = nursing assistant)*

If 4W has a staffing plan, the nurse manager could evaluate the staffing plan by comparing it with these numbers of staff per shift. In other words, when 4W has 18 to 19 patients with an average acuity of 6.6 NHPPD (these were the averages for 4W the previous year), the staffing plan should agree with the hours per shift designated previously.

Figure Actual Personnel Costs

To calculate actual personnel costs, one needs either actual salary costs of the personnel or average salaries for different personnel categories (i.e., nurse manager, RNs, LPNs, nursing assistants, nursing technicians, and ward clerks). Usually, this information can be provided by the department or by finance personnel. If available, use actual salaries and computer software programs or finance

---

[8] This assumes that the census and acuity remain at the average level determined by last year's figures. If you know other information that would change these numbers, use those figures. Increases or decreases in census or acuity need to follow a staffing plan based on these numbers, as discussed in Chapter 6.

Exhibit 13–4 Calculate Actual Personnel Salary Dollars

1.0	Nurse Manager FTE (average Nurse Manager salary)	×	$36.00/hour	× 2,080 hours*	=	$74,880.00
17.1	RN FTEs (average RN salary)	×	$26.00/hour	× 2,080 hours*	=	$924,768.00
7.3	NA FTEs (average NA salary)	×	$12.00/hour	× 2,080 hours*	=	$182,208.00
3.2	Unit Secretary FTEs (average Unit secretary salary)	×	$10.00/hour	× 2,080 hours*	=	$66,560.00

Total Salary Dollars Needed $1,248,416.00

*2,080 hours/year = 1 FTE

(Note: This calculation does not include additional benefits, differential, or bonus dollars.)

department programs to generate these data for the nurse manager or nurse executive. Additional costs such as shift differential, charge pay, on-call pay, and other costs discussed earlier in this chapter may need to be included in this equation.

Other factors affecting personnel costs on a unit are such functions as an IV team, escort service, sitter, or orderly. Often, these services are located within the centralized overall nursing department budget under a different cost center than the unit center. In some systems when these services are used by a cost center, the employee costs for that shift or service are billed to that cost center. If such functions exist and are regularly used on a unit, these costs would need to be added to the unit personnel costs. The same is true when regularly using replacement staff from another cost center.

Thus, using the 4W example, the nurse manager could calculate the actual salary costs as illustrated in **Exhibit 13–4**. In this example no other unit personnel have been identified. If such personnel exist and are necessary for the appropriate functioning of the unit, it would be important to include them in this budget.

There will probably be additional costs to figure into this equation. For instance, perhaps shift differential is paid for both the evening and night shift, holiday time is paid when employees actually work holidays, and on-call pay is given. Pay raises or premiums are other possible costs. If per diem or traveling staff will be used, they should be added to the budget.

Overtime—often meaning one is paid time and a half (1.5)—is another factor. One would assume that some overtime will be used. The industry standard is that overtime should not exceed 2%. One could look at what was actually used the year before and determine if this amount was reasonable under the circumstances. For example, if one nurse is on sick leave and two others leave their positions, accruing additional overtime could be a reasonable way to staff the unit to deal with this temporary situation. However, if overtime is consistently used by all the nurses to chart, other solutions may be necessary. Perhaps the workloads or skill mix needs to be adjusted. Maybe a computerized charting system would really save RN time. Maybe the nurse manager leadership needs to be examined because there is so much turnover on the unit. If additional money is paid for other reasons, be sure to add them to the budget if they seem realistic and reasonable.

The nurse manager may or may not have to include fringe benefits into these costs. Fringe benefits include health insurance, Social Security payments, and other benefits. At times these costs are shown on the nurse manager's cost center budget, but often they are not and instead appear on the human resource budget. These are significant costs—20% to 25%—so the executive team always needs to include this expense when determining labor expenses.

Information Systems Technology

It is best to do budget calculations, as well as staff scheduling, using a computer program. Some programs can schedule staff based on patient classification data, give staffing and variance reports, and compare what was actually spent with what was budgeted.

If such programs are unavailable, the next step is to ask personnel in the finance department if they are using an existing program that could compute these data. Another option is to use an existing spreadsheet software program. Dunham-Taylor and Pinczuk (2006) provide examples of spreadsheet systems.

Minimum Staffing

When evaluating the budget, you must understand another concept: *minimum staffing*. When the patient volume reaches a certain low level of service, it becomes a liability because more staff must be present than are actually needed to take care of the existing patients. This is because there are minimum staffing issues. Minimum staffing is a fixed cost. Remember from Chapter 12 that fixed costs are those costs that stay the same regardless of the level of activity.

To figure minimum staffing let's begin with an inpatient example. For an inpatient cost center staying open every day of the year, the industry standard is that two personnel are available to care for patients regardless of the number of patients. Minimum staffing for an inpatient cost center is pictured in **Exhibit 13–5**. Note that it is best not to include unit secretary time in the minimum staffing or fixed cost section of the budget, because this allows for more budget flexibility for the nurse manager.

You may need to determine the actual salary dollars involved for your cost center. See **Exhibit 13–6**, assuming an average salary amount per staff classification. Often, the human resource department or finance department personnel have determined the average salary for each personnel category. Although this salary amount could be used to determine the fixed cost of minimum staffing, it may not be as accurate. For instance, if most staff RNs in a cost center have been there for many years, most may be at the top of the salary range. The human resource average staff RN salary figure may be lower. So it would be preferable to use the actual salaries rather than the human resource figure in this example.

Exhibit 13–5 Inpatient Unit Direct Care Minimum Staffing for 24 Hours

Day Shift	**Evening Shift**	**Night Shift**
8 hours = 1 RN	8 hours = 1 RN	8 hours = 1 RN
8 hours = 1 Aide/tech/LPN/RN	8 hours = 1 Aide/Tech/LPN/RN	8 hours = 1 Aide/Tech/LPN/RN
16 hours	**16 hours**	**16 hours**

Add the hours from each shift:
16 hours + 16 hours + 16 hours = 48 hours/day

Exhibit 13–6 Inpatient Unit Direct Care Minimum Staffing Cost/Day

Day Shift	Evening Shift	Night Shift
(8 hours = RN—Amy) @ $28/hour* = $224/day*	(8 hours = 1 RN—Bill) @ $26/hour* = $208/day*	(8 hours = 1 RN—Carol) @ $27/hour* = $216/day*
(8 hours = 1 NA—Robert) @ $12/hour* = $96/day*	(8 hours = 1 NA—Sue) @ $12/hour* = $96/day*	(8 hours = 1 NA—Tom) @ $12/hour* = $96/day*

Add the salary rate from each staff member:

$224 + $208 + $216 + $96 + $96 + $96 = $936/day* (minimum staffing cost per day)

$936/day × 365 days = $341,640/year*

*Benefits and shift differential not included.

NA = nurse aide.

So far our minimum staffing example has included only the actual direct care nursing staff. Minimum staffing on an inpatient cost center also includes the nurse manager and other consistent cost center/department employees such as the cost center secretaries. To determine the fixed cost per day for the nurse manager, let's assume that the nurse manager is responsible for one cost center. Because the daily cost is based on 7 days in the week, the actual daily rate for the nurse manager would be the nurse manager's hourly salary multiplied by 5.7 hours a day (a fixed cost per day).

> *Nurse manager*
> *40 hours/week ÷ 7 days/week = 5.7 hours/day*
> *5.7 hours/day × $36/hour = $205.20/day*

If a cost center secretary is always present on the inpatient cost center for a 12-hour shift, this would be added to minimum staffing. In this case the hourly rate of the cost center secretary is multiplied by 12 hours per day.

> *Unit Secretary*
> *12 hours/days × $10/hour = $120.00/day*

Thus the minimum staffing actually costs $1,261.20 per day or $460,338.00 per year (**Exhibit 13–7**). So actually looking at the staffing budget for that unit, $460,338.00 would be a fixed cost.

The financial personnel may determine the fixed costs within the nursing cost center budget differently. Usually, they understand neither what minimum staffing is nor how to measure it. If the finance staff tell you what your fixed costs are, be sure to have them define how they have determined these costs. Usually, the nurse manager or nurse executive will need to educate finance department personnel about minimum staffing. The nurse manager/executive should both explain and show financial personnel actual minimum staff examples.

Exhibit 13–7 Total Inpatient Unit Direct Care Minimum Staffing Cost/Day

Direct care staff = $936.00/day*

Nurse manager = $205.20/day*

Unit secretary = $120.00/day*

Total = $1,261.20/day*

$1,261.20/day × 365 days = $460,338.00/year*

*Benefits and shift differential not included.

After determining the fixed cost of staffing—minimum staffing—the rest of the staffing budget is then variable staffing costs. See **Exhibit 13–8** (minimum staffing and variable staffing) to see how this might actually look for a unit. Variable costs are those costs that change (vary) depending on the level of activity or volume. So staffing over and above the minimum staffing is a variable cost. Variable costs occur in addition to fixed costs. Thus the staffing needed above and beyond minimum staffing would increase or decrease as the patient volume increases or decreases. The volume determining the staffing would be related to the number of patient minutes/hours/days, patient acuity, or patient visits.

If a nurse manager were asked to prepare a flexible, or variable, budget (discussed in Chapter 12) giving alternative plans for different levels of spending, the nurse manager would have to figure both minimum staffing and variable staffing at different volume levels. Dunham-Taylor and Pinczuk (2006) provide an example of a flexible budget presented on an Excel spreadsheet.

Systems differ when using a flexible, or variable, budget. In some systems this just means that there are two or more levels of spending (several fixed budgets at various occupancy levels) determined for different volumes of patients. In some systems variable budgets change as the volume of patients and the acuity of patients change. For example, this budget could vary as the patient population changes throughout the day. A nurse manager in such a system could see what budget amount was available for the upcoming shift based on the current patient population. If there is a variable budget, the nurse manager must discuss how finance department personnel determined the gradations in the variable budget.

As the budget changes, it is important for the nurse manager to decrease variable costs in relation to the decrease in volume. When the census or acuity falls below the minimum staffing pattern, the nurse manager and nurse executive might consider closing/consolidating cost centers or assigning patients in a manner that maintains a census on several cost centers that cover the fixed costs of minimum staffing.

Equipment and Supply Costs

The nurse manager also needs to examine equipment and supply costs. These costs often include such items as education, travel, standard office and medical supplies not used by specific patients, telephone costs, equipment lease/rentals, equipment repair, uniform allowance, books, and consulting charges.

Once again it is important to look at the historical data. If these data were accurate and reflected what is anticipated for another year, there is no need to change the data. However, most often the costs in these categories existed for years and may not be totally accurate for present patient needs.

Exhibit 13–8 Fixed (Minimum Staffing) and Variable Staffing

(Average HPPD = 6.5)

Patients		Days			Evenings			Nights		
		RN	LPN	NA	RN	LPN	NA	RN	LPN	NA
25		4	2	1	3	2	1	2	1	1
20		3	2	1	2	2	1	2	1	1
14		2	1	1	2	0	1	1	1	1
		1	1	1	1	1	1	1	1	1
9		1	0	1	1	0	1	1	0	1
8										
7										
1		1	0	1	1	0	1	1	0	1

Column labels (vertical): Variable Direct Caregivers; Fixed Direct Caregivers; Minimum Staffing

RN = registered nurse
LPN = licensed practical nurse
NA = nurse aide
UC = unit clerk

Past experience can be helpful when looking at these data. If nurse managers have been regularly going over budget variances each month, it is often quite obvious that certain budget categories are insufficient to cover supply costs for the present group of patients, whereas other budget categories may not be used as much or at all. It is important to make sure that supplies are expensed to the proper line item to reflect adequate expenditures. If these expenditures are accurate, they may need to be adjusted each year to better reflect actual use. If they remain accurate, the nurse manager may not need to do much with these data.

In addition to the historical data, the nurse manager must anticipate what might change for the coming budget year. Will the unit purchase new equipment that requires a change in supplies? Are physician practice patterns changing? Are there anticipated inflationary costs to consider? How these are determined were discussed in Chapter 12.

For the evaluation process, the nurse manager needs to consider all changes that have occurred, or are expected to occur, on the unit that might result in more or less being spent in equipment and supply costs. The nurse manager needs to provide additional documentation as to why the amounts need to be changed in certain budget categories. For example, if the cost center is treating a different kind of patient, the nurse manager might need to provide the number of such patients anticipated for the next year and document typical supply needs required. Additionally, the nurse manager should specify any equipment and supplies that might be used less frequently. Chapter 17 gives additional information to consider for saving costs on supplies.

Determining Variance Between Historical and Newly Figured Budgets

Now that an accurate budget has been completed, it is time for the nurse manager to compare these data with the current historical budget. Do they agree? If so, the nurse manager can proceed with the budget planning process, knowing that the data are accurate. However, if there is a discrepancy—or variance—between both budgets, the nurse manager will need to do some additional work. The first step is to discuss this issue with the nurse executive or with the nurse manager's supervisor if the nurse manager does not directly report to the nurse executive.

By having computed the budget from scratch, the nurse manager has objective data to use when defining the problem and suggesting solutions. It gives the nurse manager actual objective data; finance department personnel are more likely to listen when presented with such data. It is easy to argue that additional staffing is needed for "squishy" reasons, such as this is needed to improve quality or to meet accreditation requirements. However, having *objective evidence* provides better documentation of actual patient needs, and the executive team will be more likely to hear it. After all, it is the nurse manager who best understands and represents actual patient needs. Patients benefit—and the nurse manager has more success—when actual numbers can be presented to verify patient needs.

If the patient acuity/volume is higher, this provides actual data that verify additional staffing needs. Perhaps if the patient volume is higher, the nurse manager will suggest a different staff mix to better meet the needs of these patients. The nurse manager may propose opening a swing unit, available at times of peak census, or possibly the problem is that more staff are needed because nonproductive time was not taken into account.

If the patient volume has decreased within a cost center, other strategies can be considered. First, current staffing levels may need to be decreased. However, current staffing levels can only be decreased to the minimum staffing level. If below the minimum staffing level, other strategies could be to increase the patient volume on the cost center such as merging cost centers; alternately, one could close the cost center and send the patients to a similar cost center not at full patient capacity. This action is complicated by other issues such as medical patients with infections not being a preferable patient to divert to a surgical unit or labor and delivery area and by staff cross-training issues.

Be creative in thinking through the most appropriate strategy. Things do not need to be done the same way! After thinking through such issues and discussing them with the nurse executive, it may be necessary for the nurse manager to write a thoughtful proposal or business plan clearly defining the problem as well as discussing one or more potential solutions. See Chapter 17 for further information on business plans.

Other Ways Actual Cost Data Can Be Used

Cost data can be used in additional ways:

- *Assignment comparability*: If these concrete cost data are available, when a staff member questions having a heavier load than other staff, the nurse manager can actually compare the acuity levels for assigned patients. These data can also be used for staff evaluation. If one staff member can safely care for a higher volume of patients, this staff member might deserve additional merit pay. Or a staff member might need to be mentored and/or counseled as to how to safely care for a higher volume of patients.
- *Intraunit comparability*: Using our 4W example, the nurse executive or nurse managers on similar cost centers within this health care organization could compare staffing, skill mix, and budget information. For example, two medical cost centers with similar acuity ratings could be compared (**Exhibit 13–9**). Here 6E and Tower have fairly similar NHPPD. However, Tower has a higher number of patient days, whereas 6E has fewer patient days. Each unit could be costed out to determine whether there was comparable staffing on each of these units.

- *Benchmarking*: The cost data can also be used to compare with other similar services across the country using available benchmarking data such as the Premier or VHA data for hospitals. Premier or VHA can give extensive data on skill mix, labor costs, overtime used, wages paid certain types of employees, and even provide the nurse manager a vehicle to network with peers from similar units nationally. When using such data, it is important to make sure one is not comparing apples and oranges—one may believe one is comparing like categories yet may not be. For example, skill mix for a pediatric unit is totally different from the skill mix on a critical care unit. It is important to get definitions of what is actually included for that category. To do this, we recommend that you contact a person at the facility to verify like activities.
- *Skill mix issues*: Skill mix could be an issue. One could compare skill mix on similar units or with benchmarking data. The acuity could dictate the skill mix (i.e., an intensive care unit with higher acuity is generally staffed with more RNs than a general care unit). So it would be important to make sure that the units one is benchmarking are actually serving the same degree of patient acuity.
- *Full-time/part-time ratios*: The ratio of full-time staff to part-time staff must also be evaluated. It is possible that there are constant staffing problems on weekends because the ratio of full-time staff is too high. Or, if a lot of part-time staff work 1 to 3 days a week, it may become impossible to keep all staff informed as to changes as well as to continuity of care being challenged. The cost data can provide helpful information to determine whether the part-time-to-full-time ratio is appropriate.

Exhibit 13–9 Personnel Budget Sheet

General Hospital Personnel Budget
FY 20XX

Medical Cost Centers	NHPPD	Days	Direct FTEs	Indirect FTEs	Total FTEs
4W	6.6	6,800	24.3	3.8	28.1
6E	5.8	6,200	22.2	3.8	26.0
Tower	6.2	7,300	30.4	3.8	34.2

- *Establishing a staffing plan or flexible staffing model*: Another strategy for nurse managers is to establish ideal staffing levels—a staffing plan—for different volumes of patients when there are wide variations in patient acuity and/or numbers of patients served. When the volume is low, perhaps part-time staff or specific full-time staff work fewer hours, or staff are floated to other cost centers. If volume is high, this is reversed. Part-time staff work more hours, full-time staff earn overtime, a float pool is available to supply additional staff, or additional agency staff are hired. It is always best to carefully plan various strategies that can be implemented when a certain volume of patients is present. Additional staff training is needed when staff are expected to work at different clinical sites. Planning for several scenarios ahead of actual happenings can help to eliminate stress for both staff and administrators and maintain a continuity in quality of care. If staffing needs change, this staffing plan can be used as a flexible staffing model where a computer system—or the staffing personnel—automatically set appropriate numbers of staff at the designated staff mix.

Thus an annual evaluation of the budget can be helpful not only to determine that the allocated budget dollars are appropriate but for other staffing and supply/equipment issues as well.

Discussion Questions

1. Nurse managers have many responsibilities when it comes to the development of the budget. What issues would be considered most important for the nurse manager in this process? Who should be involved?
2. This chapter deals with specific units of service for nursing workload requirements. What role should the nurse manager play and how should the manager interact with the finance department for a standard definition for measurement?
3. How should a nurse manager use a patient classification system to justify NHPPD measurements for various units for budget purposes that would be understood by the finance department? How would nursing prove that the patient classification system is consistent in measuring the patient acuity for the various patient areas?
4. Generally, the finance department provides the overhead allocations for the nursing units. If your department is considered a revenue department for budgeting purposes, why is it important for you to know how overhead expenses are allocated to your unit?
5. As a nurse manager, you have to set up a new patient service budget. What sources of information do you need to build that budget?
6. Why is it important to have a patient acuity classification system to calculate minimum staffing needs?

Glossary of Terms

Average Daily Census—average number of inpatients present at midnight for a month or a year. May also be the average number of emergency department/home visits or outpatient treatments for a month or a year.

Direct Staff—staff that give direct care to patients.

Fixed Costs—costs that stay the same regardless of the level of activity. In staffing, minimum staffing is the fixed cost.

Flexible, or Variable, Budget—gives alternative plans for different levels of spending.

Full-Time Equivalent (FTE)—unit of measurement that represents a person or people working 40 hours a week and 2,080 hours a year. One person who works a full-time position is one FTE, whereas part-time employees work less than one FTE.

Hours Per Patient Day (HPPD)—gives the number of nursing staff hours needed to provide care to an inpatient in 24 hours. NHPPD and HPPD most often have the same meaning; however, at times the definition is different. For instance, a health care organization uses a patient classification system to measure actual hours of care needed (NHPPD), whereas finance may use HPPD using only patient census data. In this case, the two terms are different and have a different measurement. As discussed previously, this is an example where it is important to find out the definition/measurement of either the term NHPPD or HPPD. Because there is not a standardized definition for either term, be sure to clarify definitions.

Indirect Staff—those staff (including the nurse manager) that do *not* give direct care to patients.

Length of Stay—an individual patient's length of stay within a cost center or facility for a month or a year. The number of patient days one patient is in the facility.

Loss Leaders—services that do not make money—in fact lose money—but benefit the organization by bringing patients to the organization for services or gain potential patients as they see that hospital personnel are friendly, helpful people. Loss leaders can include such services as the emergency department and women's health programs.

Minimum Staffing—needing at least two staff members on duty at all times to staff a unit.

Nonproductive Time—time where an employee is paid but is not working, such as holidays, sick time, vacation time, and/or paid time off (PTO).

Nursing Hours Per Patient Day (NHPPD)—gives the number of nursing staff hours needed to provide care to an inpatient in 24 hours. NHPPD and HPPD most often have the same meaning; however, at times the definition is different. For instance, a health care organization uses a patient classification system to measure actual hours of care needed (NHPPD), whereas finance may use HPPD using only patient census data. In this case, the two terms are different and have a different measurement. As discussed previously, this is an example where it is important to find out the definition/measurement of either the term NHPPD or HPPD. Because there is not a standardized definition for either term, be sure to clarify definitions.

Nursing Workload—the volume of work performed by nursing caregivers. One way to better specify units of service for nursing workload is to use NHPPD or HPPD.

Occupancy Rate—Patient days are used to determine the *occupancy rate*. If a long-term care unit has 50 beds and 40 are filled, a percentage is determined for the number of beds actually filled. So the long-term care unit would have an occupancy rate of 80% (40 filled beds ÷ 50 bed capacity = 0.8 or 80%).

Overhead—indirect costs, including benefits such as health insurance and Social Security, depreciation on buildings or equipment, and nonproductive time (although sometimes this is mixed in with the labor budget figures). Overhead usually includes departments not giving direct care such as administration, housekeeping, maintenance, finance, medical records, and human resources. Overhead can be computed in several ways: Administration costs may be divided by the census and billed to each inpatient unit in a hospital, housekeeping and utility costs can be computed by square footage, and linen by the pounds of linen used. Finance traditionally uses the same step-down allocation for overhead as filed with the Medicare and Medicaid cost reports.

Patient Days—number of inpatients present at midnight. One patient day is given for each day the patient is present on an inpatient unit.

Product Line (Service Line)—represents total services for a particular group of patients or similar patient diagnoses. For example, typical product lines may be cardiology, oncology, burns, or women's health.

Productive Time—actual time worked.

Relative Value Unit (RVU)—term used by reimbursement systems. On an inpatient unit, the relative value unit represents the complexity of a procedure.

Staff Mix—marketing term that specifies what kind of direct care staff will provide care.

Unit of Service—used by health care organizations to measure specific services a patient uses within a specific time frame, i.e., minutes, hours, days, visits, births, treatments, operations, or other patient encounters.

Variable Costs—those costs that change (vary) depending on the level of activity or volume. In staffing, variable costs are those that are over and above minimum staffing.

Vertical Integration—a hospital might want to add long-term care beds or home care services to increase profits in order to have additional options to save costs. For instance, it is cheaper to quickly move a postoperative patient into an SNF unit—a less expensive option than holding the patient on an inpatient unit for additional day(s).

References

American Nurses' Association. (2008). *Principles for nurse staffing with annotated bibliography*. Kansas City, MO: Author. Retrieved August 2, 2008 at http://www.nursingworld.org/MainMenuCategories/HealthcareandPolicyIssues/Reports/ANAPrinciples/NurseStaffing.aspx

Dunham-Taylor, J., & Pinczuk, J. (2006). *Health care financial management for nurse managers: Applications from hospitals, long-term care, home care, and ambulatory care*. Sudbury, MA: Jones and Bartlett.

Fralic, M. (Ed.). (2000). *Staffing management and methods: Tools and techniques for nursing leaders*. Chicago: AHA Press.

Senge, P. (2006). *The fifth discipline: The art & practice of the learning organization*. New York: Doubleday Currency.

Shullanberger, G. (2000, May–June). Nurse staffing decisions: An integrative review of the literature. *Nursing Economic$, 18*(3), 124–148.

CHAPTER 14

Budget Variances

Norma Tomlinson, MSN, RN, CNA

Key Terms

- ☞ Benefit Expense
- ☞ Nonproductive Man-hours
- ☞ Payroll Reports
- ☞ Productive Man-hours
- ☞ Reported Revenue
- ☞ Revenue and Usage Report
- ☞ Variance Analysis
- ☞ Variance Report

Introduction

Budgets are usually created several months before the beginning of the fiscal year. Annual budgets are based on assumptions about the types and volumes of patients that will be cared for over the coming year and the resources required to provide that care. The difference between the budget and actual performance is the *budget variance*. Well-researched and analyzed budget variance becomes a powerful tool in controlling cost while ensuring safe, effective care.

A nursing unit or department is a *cost center*. Data comparing budgeted dollars to actual dollars are usually provided on a monthly basis by the finance department for each cost center. It normally shows data for the month and year-to-date (YTD). It is important, therefore, to be aware of the beginning of your fiscal year. If your fiscal year begins with January and it is now February, the data for January and YTD are the same because both include only 1 month's data (January). If your fiscal year begins July 1 and ends June 30, in February the YTD will include 7 months of data (July through January).

The *cost center report* compares the actual costs with the budgeted amount. Often, these reports show the percentage of the difference, or variance, between what was budgeted and what actually was spent. If it does not, you can calculate the percentage of variance by taking the difference between the actual and the budget and then divide that number by the budget. For instance, using **Exhibit 14–1**, multiplying the difference between the budget and actual by 100 gives you the percentage of variance. Therefore the actual budget amount was 25% greater than the budgeted amount.

Often, an operational report will show the data for the prior year for the same time frame that gives you an additional perspective to gauge if you are doing better or worse than the same time last year.

Exhibit 14–1 Comparing Budgeted Amount with Actual Amount Used

Budget = $200

Actual = $250

$200 (budget) − $250 (actual) = −$50 variance

The difference between the budgeted amount and the actual amount is $50.

$50 (variance) ÷ ($200 (budget) = 0.25

0.25 × 100 = 25 percent (To get the percentage, one multiplies this amount by 100.)

Therefore the actual amount was 25 percent greater than the budgeted amount.

Types of Variance

The statistics, or types of variance, discussed here include the volume or units of service, revenue, man-hours, information about salary expense, benefit expense, and non-salary expense.

Expense Budget

In an expense budget, units of service for inpatient cost centers are often broken into patient days for patients admitted and observation hours when the patient time on the unit was short enough that it did not qualify to become an admission. *It is important to capture all of your unit activity.*

If your report does not delineate these two types of patient days, it is very important to determine if the statistics include both. The man-hours to care for a patient in observation status can actually be more time intensive per day, because admission and discharge activities have to be done within the same day (23-hour patient) or the next day. If the unit experiences many outpatient or observation days and these are not included in the statistic for patient days, your data are skewed. It can appear that your hours of care per patient day as well as other costs are very high when benchmarked against other comparable nursing units that count all activity (see **Exhibit 14–2**).

If you are responsible for a unit that does not keep patients 24 hours per day, your volume statistic will be different. For example, if you are responsible for an operating room, an endoscopy suite, or a postanesthesia care unit, your volume statistic will be patients or procedures. It is very important to understand which is being counted because a single patient may have several procedures done during the same visit.

- In obstetrics the volume statistic may be patient days, both mother and baby, or it may be births. In obstetrics the volume of outpatient tests must be captured as well. That volume can involve a significant number of man-hours.
- In the emergency department, the usual volume statistic measured is the number of visits. However, in these days of overcrowding, when patients can be held in the emergency department waiting for beds for more than a day, it is important to capture those hours beyond the time that the patient could have been admitted to an inpatient bed.
- Long-term care normally counts patient days.
- Some home-care organizations weight visits for productivity based on greater weight for opening or reopening a case because of the extensive documentation required to meet regulatory requirements.

It is very helpful when operational reports also provide data about full-time equivalents (FTEs), average hourly rate, and a breakdown of data per unit of service. When looking at the data, you need

Exhibit 14–2 Example of a Monthly Report of Statistics for a Surgical Nursing Unit

Department Operations Report
For the period ending 11/30/200_
Main 7

| MONTH | | | | | YTD* | | | |
Actual	Budget	Var%	Prior	Statistic	Actual	Budget	Var%	Prior
735	655	(12.2)%	665	Unit Patient Days	3,662	3,354	(9.2)%	3,356
15	14	(7.1)%	16	Observation Days	68	68	0.0%	75
750	669	(12.1)%	681	Total Units	3,730	3,422	(9.0)%	3,431

YTD = Year-to-Date

to understand the meaning of parenthesis. In the examples provided in this chapter, negative variances (bracketed data) for *statistics* and *revenue* are favorable. Negative variances (data in parenthesis) on *expenses* are unfavorable.

In **Exhibit 14–2**, actual volume for patient days for both the month (735) and year (3,662) is higher than that budgeted (655 for the month and 3,354 YTD) and higher than what was experienced in the prior year (3,356). The actual observation days (15) for the month were higher (by one) than the budgeted days (14) but lower (by one) than the same month last year (16). Year-to-date the observation days are right on target for what was budgeted (68) but lower than last year (75). When combined, the total units, or total patient days, for both the month (750) and YTD (3,730) are higher than what was budgeted (669 for the month and 3,422 YTD) and what was experienced in the prior year (681 for the month and 3,431 YTD). The positive (higher) volume variance of 12.1% for the month and 9.0% YTD becomes very important later when analyzing the resources used to care for that volume of patients.

Revenue Budget

Revenue is as important to monitor as expense. Looking at a revenue and expense budget, managers might believe their department is generating a very high profit margin, *even when it really is not.* Reported revenue reflects *charges* generated for the month and YTD by the department, *not actual dollars received for that care.*

In areas with a high population of Medicaid, self-pay, and managed care as the source of payment, the percentage of charges captured can be less than 50%. By multiplying the total revenue by the percentage of charges captured, you can identify the approximate amount of collectible revenue that will result from the care provided and billed. Subtracting the total expenses, which are actual dollars expended, usually does not leave a high profit margin, if any.

Total revenue × percentage of captured charges = approximate collectible revenue
Approximate collectible revenue − actual expenses = net revenue

For example, the annual revenue budget for Main 7 is $4,119,257. That is the total amount of expected charges to be generated by Main 7 for the year. The budgeted annual expense is

$1,816,255. Net revenue is those dollars remaining after expenses are subtracted from revenue. If the hospital received 100% of charges, the net revenue is

$$\$4,119,257 - \$1,816,255 = \$2,303,002.$$

However, if the true capture of charges is 50%, then half of $4,119,257 or $2,059,628.50 is all that will be collected. The net revenue then becomes

$$\$2,059,628.50 - \$1,816,255 = \$243,373.50.$$

$4,119,257	*Annual revenue (from expected charges)*
− $1,816,255	*Budgeted annual expense*
$2,303,002	*Total revenue (from expected charges)*

When charges were actually 50% of what had been anticipated:

$4,119,257 × 0.50 =	*$2,059,628.50*	*Actual revenue*
	− $1,816,255.00	*Budgeted annual expense*
	$243,373.50	*Net revenue*

That leaves a *small* margin for unexpected additional costs such as greater overtime dollars required or the unanticipated cost of new sharps safety devices.

Before becoming depressed, keep in mind that other departments such as Pharmacy, Laboratory, Radiology, and Surgery normally show much higher positive revenues for the same patients. Those departments would not see higher profits if those patients were not receiving care on your unit.

Just as volume is reported for both inpatient and outpatient, the corresponding revenue is reported in the same manner (**Exhibit 14–3**). In the example shown in Exhibit 14–3, just as with volume, actual inpatient revenue is higher for the month ($355,501) and YTD ($1,794,790) than that budgeted ($318,724 for the month and $1,632,062 YTD). It is also higher than that experienced in the prior year ($286,985 for the month and $1,488,463 YTD). Outpatient revenues for both the month ($5,469) and YTD ($23,482) are less than the budgeted amounts ($5,860 for the month and $28,464 YTD) and less than that experienced in the prior year ($4,436 for the month and $26,991 YTD).

Exhibit 14–3 Example of a Monthly Report of Statistics for a Revenue Budget

Department Revenue Report
For the period ending 11/30/200_
Main 7

MONTH					YTD			
Actual	Budget	Var%	Prior	Statistic	Actual	Budget	Var%	Prior
(355,501)	(318,724)	(11.5)%	(286,985)	Inpatient Revenue	(1,794,790)	(1,632,062)	(10.0)%	(1,488,463)
(5,469)	(5,860)	6.7%	(4,436)	Outpatient Revenue	(23,482)	(28,464)	17.5%	(26,991)
(360,970)	(324,584)	(11.2)%	(291,421)	Total Revenue	(1,818,272)	(1,660,526)	(9.5)%	(1,515,454)

Outpatient or observation charges are usually not reimbursed at a very high rate. Therefore the shift to higher inpatient charges when the patient stays long enough to convert to an inpatient stay, and experiences less outpatient charges, is positive.

Total revenues for both the month ($360,970) and YTD ($1,818,272) are greater than the budgeted amounts ($324,584 for the month and $1,660,526 YTD) and more than that experienced in the prior year ($291,421 for the month and $1,515,454 YTD). So this reflects the same pattern (increased amounts) as the volumes.

Man-hours Budget

Because staffing is usually the most expensive resource in the provision of care, the amount and type of man-hours expensed to a nursing unit is very critical. The monthly operations report usually does not break down the man-hours by job classification such as registered nurse (RN), licensed practical nurse (LPN), nursing assistant, and unit clerk. That information is normally provided in biweekly reports that show individual employee hours and/or man-hours or FTEs by job classification (**Exhibit 14–4**).

Although biweekly reports may not correspond to the exact days, or the month, covered by the operations report, they provide good data to monitor if your mix of staff corresponds to that budgeted. Man-hours are usually broken down into contract, productive, paid time off (PTO), overtime, education, orientation, and other.

Contract labor is usually the most expensive man-hours. Contract staff can be through local agencies or the more expensive "travelers" who are agency personnel assigned for several weeks or months at a time and usually live in local temporary housing. Although they may provide for better continuity of care than local agency staff, their costs include at a minimum hourly rate, rent, food, travel, and car rental.

Productive man-hours are those hours where employed staff members provide care for patients. In the case of direct caregivers such as RNs, LPNs, and patient care technicians, it is the time they are assigned on the nursing unit actually providing hands-on care to patients. For indirect caregivers such as unit clerks, it includes the time they spend on the nursing unit providing their specific indirect services, such as entering orders from the charts into the computer.

Nonproductive man-hours include PTO, such as vacation, holidays, jury duty, sick time, and any other time off where the employee is paid by the organization but does not actually work during that paid time. It is an employee benefit. PTO may be expensed (charged) to the cost center at the time that it is earned or at the time that it is taken.

The time at which PTO is expensed is important to know when analyzing the unit costs for the month. If it is expensed to your department *at the time it is earned*, you will see it charged as an expense against your department based on the hours worked during that month. In this case it goes into a "bank" that the employee draws against when it is taken. Your department is not charged for it again when the employee takes the time off because it was already expensed to you once. You will see it in the detail of what was paid to the employee on your biweekly report.

However, those dollars are not added to the total on your monthly report. If you need to replace the employee to cover the man-hours required to care for the volume of patients, then you will be charged only for the hours worked by the replacement employee. If, on the other hand, PTO is charged to your budget *only when taken* by the employee, you will see it included in the total on the monthly report. If, because of volume, you had to replace the employee to cover the man-hours required to care for the volume of patients, you will be charged for that employee's hours, as well.

In most organizations PTO is earned based on the hours worked. If you use part-time staff members more than their allocated FTE, they will earn PTO on those hours, as well. That will increase the nonproductive time and dollars expensed to your department.

Exhibit 14–4 Example of a Biweekly FTE Report

*Pay Period 0_   1/13/0_–1/26/0_*

Name	Classification	Productive FTE	Nonproductive FTE	Overtime FTE	Total FTE
T. Moore	Manager	1.0	0	0	1.0
Subtotal	**Manager**	**1.0**	**0**	**0**	**1.0**
A. Todd	Charge RN	1.0	0	0.1	1.1
S. Shaw	Charge RN	1.0	0	0	1.0
Subtotal	**Charge RN**	**2.0**	**0**	**0.1**	**2.1**
R. Barry	RN	1.0	0	0.2	1.2
J. Brown	RN	0.45	0.45	0	0.9
C. Collins	RN	0.9	0	0	0.9
R. Dix	RN	0.9	0.1	0	1.0
E. Fisher	RN	0.6	0	0	0.6
J. Robinson	RN	0.9	0	0	0.9
R. Smith	RN	0.45	0.45	0	0.9
Subtotal	**RN**	**5.2**	**1.0**	**0.2**	**6.4**
J. Edwards	LPN	0.9	0	0	0.9
R. Falls	LPN	0	0.9	0	0.9
E. George	LPN	0.9	0	0	0.9
T. Hall	LPN	0.6	0.3	0	0.9
Subtotal	**LPN**	**2.4**	**1.2**	**0**	**3.6**
J. Adams	PCT	0.9	0	0	0.9
N. Coates	PCT	0.6	0	0	0.6
T. East	PCT	0.9	0	0	0.9
Subtotal	**PCT**	**2.4**	**0**	**0**	**2.4**
A. Thomas	Unit Clerk	1.0	0	0	1.0
S. Vender	Unit Clerk	1.0	0	0	1.0
Subtotal	**Unit Clerk**	**2.0**	**0**	**0**	**2.0**
TOTAL		**15.0**	**2.2**	**0.3**	**17.5**

Note: These are fictitious names.

Overtime is that time worked over 40 hours in a week if on a 40-hour workweek. It can include, at the discretion of the organization, hours worked over a scheduled 8-, 10-, or 12-hour shift *even if less than 40 hours are worked in a week*. It can also include time designated as overtime at the discretion of the organization, such as any hours called in and hours worked when on-call. Although discretionary overtime pay can be a positive retention tool, it is also an added expense. It is important to know what the policy is in your organization regarding the designation of overtime.

On-call pay is a minimal hourly rate paid to staff who are not at work but who have committed to be available to work on short notice. It is important to know if in your organization on-call pay hours stop when the individual is called into work. Some organizations stop on-call pay at the time the employee clocks into work. In this case, if they clock out before the end of their time on-call, the on-call pay picks up again when they clock out. Some organizations continue to pay the on-call pay in addition to any hours worked while on-call.

Education and orientation hours are those spent learning and meeting the competencies required for the employee's position. With the Health Insurance Portability and Accountability Act (covered in Chapter 9) and other new regulatory rules, many hours of mandatory education are being added to the cost of staffing to ensure that all employees are educated about the rules.

In **Exhibit 14–5** the data demonstrate a large increase in contract labor that has been utilized both for the month (344 hours) and YTD (1,840 hours). Year-to-date in the prior year shows only 284 hours of contract labor was used for the month.

Note the following:

- The budget of 1,575 hours YTD shows that the shortage of employed nursing staff was recognized and plans were made to use agency staff. However, due to the volume of patients and the shortage of regular employed staff, 16.8% additional contract hours were used in addition to what had been budgeted.

Exhibit 14–5 Example of a Monthly Report of Man-hours for a Surgical Nursing Unit

Department Man-hours Report
For the period ending 11/30/200_
Main 7

	MONTH					YTD*			
Actual	**Budget**	**Var%**	**Prior**	**STATISTIC**	**Actual**	**Budget**	**Var%**	**Prior**
344	315	(9.2)%	258	**MAN-HOURS CONTRACT**	1,840	1,575	(16.8)%	284
5,759	5,267	(9.3)%	5,291	**MAN-HOURS PRODUCTIVE**	28,469	26,893	(5.9)%	26,860
611	570	(7.2)%	573	**MAN-HOURS PTO**	2,883	2,912	1.0%	2,988
192	270	28.9%	363	**MAN-HOURS OVERTIME**	1,117	1,380	19.1%	1,627
764	750	(1.9)%	667	**MAN-HOURS ED/ORIENT/ETC**	3,392	3,825	11.3%	3,933
7,670	7,172	(6.9)%	7,152	**TOTAL MAN-HOURS**	37,701	36,585	(3.1)%	35,692
44.86	41.95	(6.9)%	41.83	**TOTAL FTES**	43.24	41.96	(3.1)%	40.94

YTD = Year-to-date

- Productive hours were higher than budgeted for the month (5,759) and YTD (28,469) as well.
- PTO was over by 7.2% for the month but 1.0% lower than budgeted YTD.
- Overtime was less than budgeted.
- Education/orientation hours and other hours such as on-call were over for the month but under YTD.
- The total man-hours for the month were 6.9% greater than that budgeted for the month.
- The man-hours were 3.1% greater than budgeted YTD.
- The FTEs are based on conversion of the man-hours worked into FTEs (2,080 hours per year = 1.0 FTE).

Salary Budget

Salaries are normally the largest expense for a cost center. Salaries are broken down into the same categories as man-hours. The percentage of variance in salaries not only reflects the number of man-hours used to care for a particular volume of patients, but it also reflects the mix of staff providing that care, such as RN, LPN, nursing assistant or patient care technician, and unit clerk. Salaries for the department usually include the unit manager. If nursing education is decentralized, it may include a nursing educator for the unit. If the unit has a clinical nurse specialist, that salary may be charged to the unit, as well.

In **Exhibit 14–6** productive salaries are higher for the month ($85,670) than budgeted ($76,243), with the variance percentage being 12.4% over budget for the month. The same is true YTD ($424,059 actual against a budget of $381,320 and 11.2% over budget).

Exhibit 14–6 Example of a Monthly Report of Salaries for a Surgical Nursing Unit

Department Salary Report
For the period ending 11/30/200_
Main 7

MONTH					YTD			
Actual	Budget	Var%	Prior	SALARY EXPENSE	Actual	Budget	Var%	Prior
85,670	76,243	(12.4)%	80,107	SALARIES PRODUCTIVE	424,059	381,320	(11.2)%	399,027
9,125	7,601	(20)%	8,567	PTO	43,208	38,826	(11.3)%	42,621
4,547	6,701	32.1%	9,611	SALARIES OVERTIME	22,283	34,237	34.9%	42,610
18,319	8,734	(109.7)%	13,939	CONTRACT SALARIES	95,318	43,670	(118.3)%	15,357
900	2,070	56.5%	251	SALARY/LUMP - SUM/RETENT	1,982	5,988	66.9%	3,251
8,279	9,184	9.9%	7,119	ED/ORIENT/ ON-CALL/ETC	39,699	46,838	15.2%	48,424
126,840	110,533	(14.8)%	119,594	TOTAL SALARY EXPENSE	626,549	550,879	(13.7)%	551,290

Note the following in this example:

- PTO salary is 20% higher for the month ($9,125 actual against a budget of $7,601) and 11.3% higher YTD ($43,208 actual against a budget of $38,826), reflecting the additional PTO earned for the hours worked above budget.
- Overtime is under budget by 32.1% for the month ($4,547 actual against a budget of $6,701). YTD overtime is under budget by 34.9% ($22,283 against a budget of $34,237).
- The ratio difference between the variance percent of contracted man-hours-to-budget for the month of 9.2% in Exhibit 14–5 is very different from the variance percentage of contracted salary-to-budget for the month of 109.7% in Exhibit 14–6. This reflects the extremely high cost of contracted labor. This is explored further in this chapter when variance analysis and variance reporting are discussed.
- The salary–lump sum/retention is 56.5% below budget for the month ($900 actual against a budget of $2,070) and 66.9% under budget YTD ($1,982 against a budget of $5,988). This could reflect less use of this benefit by the staff in filled positions, or it could reflect open positions.
- Education, orientation, and on-call costs are under budget for the month by 9.9% ($8,279 against a budget of $9,184) and under budget YTD by 15.2% ($39,699 against a budget of $46,838). This could reflect less orientation and/or less regular staff able to use the education dollars budgeted for the unit.

The percentages of the total salary expense line compared with the total units line (in Exhibit 14–2) can provide a "big picture" view to determine if your use of staff is in line with the volume of patients cared for during the month and YTD. In this case for the month, Main 7 was 12.1% above budget on volume of patients (from Exhibit 14–2), whereas salary expense was 14.8% greater than budget. YTD Main 7 was 9% above the budget for volume of patients but 13.7% over budget for salary expense.

When budgeting for the year, you should calculate each expense line based on one unit of service. This budget often is based on the cost per unit of service for the same expense line item from the previous year, plus information about changes that would impact that item. For example:

> *If last year the total cost of productive salaries was $941,757 to care for 8,488 patient days, the cost per patient day was $941,757 divided by 8,488 = $110.95 per patient day.*

If this year it is anticipated that salaries will increase 3% and that staffing mix and hours of care per patient day will remain the same, the expectation is that the productive salary per patient day will be 3% higher than last year or $110.95 × 1.03 = $114.28 per patient day. This becomes an indicator to use each month as you evaluate your costs. In this specific instance:

> *$110,533 budgeted salary expense for the month ÷ 669 budgeted units for the month =*
>   *$165.22 budgeted per patient day (from Exhibit 14–2)*
>
> *$126,840 actual salary expense for the month ÷ 750 actual units for the month =*
>   *$169.12 actual expense per patient day (from Exhibit 14–2)*
>
> *$165.22 budgeted per patient day − $169.12 actual expense per patient day = −$3.90*
>
> *The negative number means it actually costs $3.90 more per patient day than had been budgeted for the month.*

The same can be done YTD:

$550,879 budgeted salary expense YTD ÷ 3,422 budgeted units YTD = $160.98 budgeted per patient day

$626,549 actual salary expense YTD ÷ 3,730 actual units YTD = $167.98 actual expense per patient day

$160.98 budgeted per patient day − $167.98 actual expense per patient day = −$7.00

So it actually costs $7.00 more per patient day than had been budgeted YTD.

This tells me that so far this year it has cost an additional $7.00 per patient day for salary above what was budgeted to care for patients on Main 7. However, during the current month the $7.00 has been reduced to an overage of $3.90 per patient day. Although not back to the budgeted salary expense, the salary expense to care for patients on Main 7 is improving from that experienced in previous months.

Benefit Expense

Benefit expense includes retirement, group health, flex benefits, and Federal Insurance Contributions Act, or FICA (**Exhibit 14–7**). Group health is the employers' portion of the cost for health insurance that can include dental, vision, life insurance, and disability. Flex benefits can be called many things, including special benefits such as dollars returned to employees who maintain specified health habits and physical parameters as an incentive to reduce health insurance costs. FICA is the law that covers Social Security and Medicare. The employer is responsible to pay half of the bill for the employee, and it is charged to your department. Keep in mind that because FICA is based on earned income, if your salary budget is over or under budget, FICA will be over or under budget as well.

Non-salary Expenses

Non-salary expenses can include, but are not limited to, purchased professional services, patient nonchargeable supplies, instruments, implants, intravenous solutions, drugs, medical supplies, food

---

Exhibit 14–7 Example of a Monthly Report of Benefits for a Surgical Nursing Unit

Department Benefits Report
For the period ending 11/30/200_
Main 7

| | MONTH | | | | | YTD | | |
Actual	Budget	Var%	Prior	Benefit Expense	Actual	Budget	Var%	Prior
4,104	2,674	(53.5)%	3,011	**Retirement**	18,655	13,535	(37.8)%	15,212
10,342	11,533	10.3%	14,112	**Group Health**	51,174	58,551	12.6%	65,960
1,297	1,022	(26.9)%	1,007	**Flex Benefits**	6,977	5,172	(34.9)%	5,092
6,778	5,800	(16.9)%	6,325	**FICA/Taxes**	32,078	29,353	(9.3)%	32,099
22,521	21,029	(7.1)%	24,455	**Total Benefits**	108,884	106,611	(2.1)%	118,363

service, department supplies, forms and paper, minor equipment, freight, maintenance contracts, repairs, equipment rental, dues and memberships, certification and recertification, books and publications, and travel.

Purchased professional services can include fees paid to physicians contracted to provide services. This could include fees for medical director administrative services such as those paid to the medical head of a psychiatric department. It can also cover fees paid to other professionals who are not employees but who provide services where the hospital both submits charges and receives the reimbursement. An example is for a contracted group of psychologists who provide services to patients where the hospital bills for those services and keeps the revenue. There can also be purchased professional services paid to a physician specialty in short supply that does not receive adequate reimbursement for the services they provide. If these services are critical to the operation of the hospital, the hospital can, using fair market value to ensure compliance with legal parameters, provide a level of compensation in addition to what that specialty collects for billed services. Frequently, anesthesiologists are compensated in this manner in addition to what they bill and collect. This charge is usually budgeted under the anesthesia cost center.

Patient nonchargeable supplies include items that are necessary to care for the patient but cannot be charged directly to the patient, such as admission kits and syringes. It is important to know which supplies can be charged to the patient and which cannot. Usually, chargeable items have stickers or bar codes indicating they can be charged to the patient.

The instrument expense can be very large in an operating room based on the cost of reusable instruments that wear out and require replacement on a regular basis. This would not be the case on a medical-surgical unit.

Implants can be a very large expense for items in the operating room such as joints for total knee and hip replacements or for the cost of cardiac stents in a cardiac catheterization lab. This cost has become an even greater issue with the higher cost of drug-eluding stents.

Intravenous solutions may be expensed to the department or may be expensed to the pharmacy. Usually, intravenous solutions without medications added are expensed directly to the nursing units. Intravenous solutions with medications added are usually expensed to the pharmacy.

Drugs are usually charged to the nursing unit only when patient charges have not been made and when floor stock is used. The same occurs with medical supplies.

Be very aware of the expense your unit incurs for lost charges. That is, if patient chargeable items such as drugs or supplies like catheterization kits are not charged to the patient, when the drug or kit is replaced, it is charged to the unit. If the staff are not careful about entering charges for patient chargeable supplies, expensive and unnecessary costs occur. More and more organizations have invested in drug and supply vending equipment that requires patient data to be entered before the door can be opened to get the drug or supply. This results in automatic charging of the item and provides automatic data to ensure inventory replacement to maintain par levels in the drug and supply vending machines.

Food service is not patient meals but includes those items that are stocked on the nursing unit for patient use in addition to meals. This includes such items as sodas, crackers, sandwiches, and fruit. This is an item to watch carefully. If your kitchen is very easily accessed, visitors may be consuming food for patients. Although staff are usually aware that the food is for patients, staff may consume these as well. If you have special celebrations on your unit and have the dietary department provide the food, the cost of the food will be expensed to this subaccount.

Department supplies include office supplies such as ink cartridges for the printers, pens, and pencils. It also includes hand soap, paper towels, and other items that are necessary to care for patients but are not used specifically on a patient.

Forms and paper can be a significant expense. In departments such as obstetrics and gynecology, there may be use of copyrighted nursing documentation forms from an outside vendor. Preprinted physician orders and clinical pathways need to be updated as evidence-based practice changes and the forms must be changed to match. When policies change, the forms documenting the activity affected by those policies must be changed to match the new policies. Old printed forms may be wasted, or the organization may choose to wait months while stockpiles of the old forms are used before implementing the new policies. At the same time, the setup and printing of new forms can be a significant cost. Many organizations are moving to computerization of their forms and have put the forms online to be printed as needed. The forms are updated without waste of paper.

Minor equipment includes equipment that costs less than the level set by the organization to capitalize the equipment. It can include items such as ophthalmoscopes, video equipment, sphygmomanometers, and chairs. It is important to know when budgeting if the items you anticipate replacing or purchasing fall into minor equipment or capital purchases. It is not unusual to find that an item with a cost close to the line between minor equipment and capital that was put into the capital budget ends up costing less than anticipated. If it falls below the line for capital, it goes into the minor equipment subaccount even though not budgeted for it.

Dues and memberships include those that are paid for by the organization. An example is payment for the manager of an operating room to belong to the local, state, and/or national Association of periOperative Registered Nurses.

Books and publications include *Physicians Desk Reference*, other drug references, textbooks, and journals specific to the nursing care provided on the specific unit. Computer-based learning programs may also be included in this category.

Travel is a non-salary expense that can vary widely. This line item covers all expenses incurred when staff travel to educational programs and includes airfare, car rental, hotel, and food. It also includes reimbursement for mileage when staff travel between locations on the job such as to attend a meeting at another hospital within a system. In home care this can be a very expensive line item because staff members drive between patients' homes. It is very important in home care to teach staff to set up their route for patient visits on a given day based not only on services tied to specific times, such as drawing fasting blood sugars, but also on the proximity of patient homes. Unnecessary mileage can be cut and staff productivity raised by shortening the time spent driving between patients.

Other expense is a line item (subaccount) that should be used as little as possible and only when the item does not fit the description of any other subaccount. Most non-salary expenses will fit into one of the other line items and should have been budgeted accordingly. Expense charges to your department should be reviewed for accuracy. If a charge that was budgeted in one subaccount is charged to another subaccount, it is important to recognize and put the item into the correct subaccount. Otherwise, one subaccount may appear under budget whereas another appears over budget. Also be sure that all charges to your department belong to your department. Many people enter charges to your department and errors can easily happen. By identifying and reporting errors, credits are made and should be noted on the report the following month. Keep track of this month-to-month when reviewing your reports to ensure that credits have been posted properly.

Freight may or may not be a line item that is allocated to the nursing unit. Freight charges can be minimized with appropriate planning. The operating room, for example, may have high freight costs if needs are not well anticipated. Overnight charges for implants or supplies significantly increase the cost of freight. Some organizations expense freight directly to the nursing unit that special orders or uses an item. Some allocate freight charges according to a predetermined percentage of total charges to specific nursing units. Others keep freight charges as a single item in the purchasing department budget and charge it accordingly. Ask how freight charges are handled in your organization so you will know how to respond to the data.

Exhibit 14–8 shows the following:

- No purchased professional services were budgeted or used by Main 7 during the month. However, YTD $250 was actually charged to this subaccount in a previous month, although no money was budgeted for this purpose.
- The patient nonchargeable subaccount was over for the month by 160.9%. The actual YTD expense was $30,934 against a budget of $11,858. YTD this subaccount was over by 52.4%. The actual expense was $92,458 against a budget of $60,656.
- The subaccount for drugs was 100% positive for the month because no expenses were charged to the subaccount and $32 was budgeted. The same is true for YTD with no expenses charged to the subaccount but $165 was budgeted.
- Food service was over budget for the month by 23.4%. Actual expense was $975 against a budget of $790. YTD food service was over budget by 21.8%. Actual expense was $5,252, although $4,313 was budgeted.
- Medical supplies, like drugs, were 100% positive for the month. No expenses were charged against the account, although $68 was budgeted. YTD medical supplies were also 100% positive. No expenses where charged to the account, but $349 was budgeted.
- Department supplies were over budget for the month by 9.2%. The actual expense for the month was $2,038 against a budget of $1,866. YTD department supplies are 1.3% over budget with an actual expense of $9,668 against a budget of $9,546.

Exhibit 14–8 Example of a Monthly Report of Non-salary Expense for a Surgical Nursing Unit

Department Non-salary Expense Report
For the period ending 11/30/200_
Main 7

| | *MONTH* | | | | | *YTD* | | |
Actual	Budget	Var%	Prior	Non-salary Expense	Actual	Budget	Var%	Prior
0	0	0.0%	0	Purchase Professional	250	0	0.0%	0
30,934	11,858	(160.9)%	14,338	Patient Nonchargeable	92,458	60,656	(52.4)%	59,995
0	32	(100.0)%	0	Drugs	0	165	100.0%	0
975	790	(23.4)%	1,068	Food Service	5,252	4,313	(21.8)%	4,736
0	68	100.0%	0	Medical Supplies	0	349	100.0%	0
2,038	1,866	(9.2)%	2,472	Department Supplies	9,668	9,546	(1.3)%	6,429
197	245	19.6%	264	Forms and Paper	1,024	1,254	18.3%	1,204
959	1,134	15.4%	47	Minor Equipment	5,148	5,670	9.2%	1,529
0	216	100.0%	0	Equipment Rental	0	1,080	100.0%	0
0	1	100.0%	0	Dues & Membership	0	5	100.0%	0
136	46	(195.7)%	0	Books & Publications	225	46	(389.1)%	40
228	207	(10.1)%	470	Travel	567	1,058	46.4%	1,325
0	82	100.0%	0	Other Expenses	0	410	100.0%	37
35,467	16,545	(114.4)%	18,659	Total Non-salary Expense	114,592	84,552	(35.5)%	75,295

- Forms and paper were under budget for the month by 19.6%. The actual expense was $197 against a budget of $245. YTD forms and paper were under budget by 18.3%. Actual expense was $1,024 against a budget of $1,254.
- Minor equipment was under budget for the month by 15.4%. The actual expense for the month was $959 against a budget of $1,134. YTD minor equipment was under budget by 9.2% with actual expense of $5,148 against a budget of $5,670.
- Equipment rental was 100% positive to budget for the month with no expenses charged against a budget of $216. YTD was also 100% positive with no expense charged against a budget of $1,080.
- Dues and memberships was 100% positive for the month with no expense charged to a budget of $1. YTD the budget is also 100% positive with no expense against a budget of $5.
- Books and publications was 195.7% over budget for the month due to the expense of $136 against a budget of $46. YTD books and publications was 389.1% over budget with the expense of $225 against a budget of $46.
- Travel was over budget by 10.1% for the month due to the expense of $228 against a budget of $207. YTD travel was under budget by 46.4% with the actual expense of $567 against a budget of $1,058.
- Other expenses were 100% positive for the month with no expense charged against a budget of $82. YTD other expenses were also 100% positive with no expense charged against a budget of $410.

The total of salary (Exhibit 14–6), benefit (Exhibit 14–7), and non-salary (Exhibit 14–8) expenses is listed below the expense budgets in **Exhibit 14–9.**

Exhibit 14–9 Total Monthly Salary and Non-salary Expenses for a Surgical Nursing Unit

Total Department Expense Report
For the period ending 11/30/200_
Main 7

MONTH					YTD			
Actual	Budget	Var%	Prior	Total Expense	Actual	Budget	Var%	Prior
126,840	110,533	(14.8)%	119,594	**Total Salary Expense**	626,549	550,879	(13.7)%	551,290
22,521	21,029	(7.1)%	24,455	**Total Benefits**	108,884	106,611	(2.1)%	118,363
35,467	16,545	(114.4)%	18,659	**Total Non-salary Expense**	114,592	84,552	(35.5)%	75,295
184,828	148,107	(24.8)%	162,708	**Total Expenses**	850,025	742,042	(14.6)%	744,948

Note in review of the subaccounts under Non-salary Expense that one line item, patient non-chargeables, accounts for almost all of the budget overage both for the month and YTD. As with the total salary expense line, to get the "big picture" of non-salary expense, the total non-salary expense line should be compared with the total units line for both the month and YTD. In this case Main 7 was 12.1% (Exhibit 14–2) above budget due to volume of patients for the month. Total non-salary expense was up 114.4% for the month. YTD Main 7 was 9% above the budget for volume of patients and 35.5% above budget for total non-salary expense. This sounds terrible! However, before coming to this conclusion, further analysis is needed.

The *budgeted* non-salary expense per unit of service is the total budgeted non-salary expense for the month ($16,545) divided by the budgeted total units for the month (669 from Exhibit 14–2) = $24.73 per patient day. The *actual* total non-salary expense YTD ($35,467) divided by the actual total units YTD (750 from Exhibit 14–2) = $47.29 per patient day. The difference between the budgeted non-salary expense per unit for the month ($24.73) and the actual ($47.29) is $22.56.

> *$16,545 (budgeted total non-salary expense for the month)*
>   *÷ 669 (budgeted total units for the month)*
>   *= $24.73 per patient day*
>
> *$35,467 (actual total non-salary expense for the month)*
>   *÷ 750 (actual total units for the month)*
>   *= $47.29 per patient day*
>
> *$24.73 (per patient day) − $47.29 (per patient day)*
>   *= −$22.56 per patient day*
>
> *So the non-salary expense is significantly over at $22.56 per day more than what was budgeted.*

This is quite a significant overage and requires appropriate analysis. The budgeted non-salary expense YTD ($84,552) divided by the budgeted YTD total units (3,422) = $24.71. The actual total non-salary expense YTD ($114,592) divided by the actual total units YTD (3,730) = $30.72 per patient day. The difference between the budgeted non-salary expense per unit YTD ($24.71) and the actual YTD ($30.72) = $6.01 per patient day.

> *$84,552 budgeted non-salary expense YTD*
>   *÷ 3,422 budgeted YTD total units*
>   *= $24.71 per patient day*
>
> *$114,592 actual total non-salary expense YTD*
>   *÷ 3,730 actual total units YTD*
>   *= $30.72 per patient day*
>
> *$24.71 per patient day − $30.72 per patient day*
>   *= −$6.01 per patient day*

This tells us that the $22.56 non-salary budget problem for the month is atypical because YTD the overage per patient day is $6.01. Although not as significant as the problem for the month, it still requires understanding and a plan for correction if at all possible.

Variance Analysis

Variance analysis includes finding all the pieces of the puzzle, putting them together, and understanding what the data are telling you about your operations. The pieces of the puzzle include all the various reports you are sent by the finance, materials management, and human resources departments, as well as unit-specific reports of daily or weekly activity that you create and track. These reports are uniquely named by the organization but include specific types of information. From finance you should receive a monthly *distribution register*. This lists accounts payable payments made for your department. This can include items charged to your department by personnel in your department as well as from personnel in other departments. For instance, supplies required to repair broken equipment on your unit may be charged to your department by facilities management.

It is important to communicate effectively with support departments so that there are no surprises on this report. It will also save you time when preparing your variance report if you have made note during the month of special charges that will appear on your department's report. An *accounts payable accrued but not invoiced report* identifies items received on a purchase order but not yet invoiced. An example is dollars you anticipate to be billed for "traveler" agency staff used during the month. Why not just wait until the bill arrives next month and explain it then? The reason is that you want to link expenses as closely as possible to what happened during the time frame that your variance report covers, which is this particular month. If you know that during the month you will be using 160 hours of traveler agency RN staff because of increased patient volume and open RN staff positions, you want the expense for that to show in the month where it happened. If you wait until the bill comes the following month and the volume is down during the following month, or you have filled the positions and are not using agency staff during the following month, it is much harder to reconcile and explain the expenses that appear to belong in that following month. It is better to tell finance to accrue for the services you estimate will be used during the current month. When the actual bill arrives, it will be applied against what was accrued and already be explained.

A *revenue and usage report* identifies charges by financial class and charge code. Financial class tells us if the patients were Medicare, Medicaid, private insurance, or self-pay. Charge code tells us how many charges were made for specific services. In the case of a surgical unit, there should be charges for admitted patient days and observation patient days. In surgery there will be charges for the initial minimum time for using an operating room.

Additional charges under a different code will show for additional increments of time beyond the basic charge. It is important to review this to see that it matches the activity in your department. If on a surgical nursing unit you know that you had 15 observation days but no charges show for those days, you will want to follow up to determine why those charges did not get posted. These become lost charges unless caught before the patient bill is completed and sent out by finance. It is important to find out from your finance department how many days post patient discharge late charges can be added so that the charges are not lost. Lost charges can be minimized if the daily department log is reviewed on a daily basis and reconciled.

The *daily department log* is an excellent tool to ensure that input errors are rectified before a patient's bill is completed. By reviewing this log, you can tell if a patient in obstetrics and gynecology was charged for 10 deliveries instead of 1. Likewise, if you review the daily department log against the log showing births, there is an opportunity to identify lost charges for a delivery that occurred in the last 24 hours that does not appear on the daily department log. The charges can then be input within a time frame that allows for capture.

The *period inventory expense report* lists expenses from material management. This is an important report to review to determine both if supplies are being used effectively and if your unit was charged appropriately for what was ordered. If you note an increase in the number of intravenous catheters being used per patient day, you will want to investigate. Do you have a bad lot of intravenous catheters resulting in multiple attempts by staff to start intravenous lines? Did the hospital just change to a new safety intravenous catheter and the staff is in a learning curve? Did you order a certain number of boxes of intravenous catheters and get charged for that number of cases of intravenous catheters rather than boxes? Unless someone is checking this report, the problem would go unnoticed. By noting and investigating, you not only explain the variance but prevent it from continuing. If it is a bad lot, material management may be able to get free replacements. If it is a change in product and a learning curve, select staff members may need reeducation. If it is a charge for cases rather than boxes and it is reported, you will receive a credit for it the following month, bringing your YTD into line.

Payroll reports are biweekly reports that reflect hours by type being paid to each employee. These should reflect the hours worked by staff and should match the daily staffing plan actually worked. Regular hours, overtime hours, shift differential, education hours, and PTO should be listed for each employee. Any special pay-by-type should appear as well. This could be added pay for being a preceptor for new employees or other unique special pay categories. If you use an automated system for clocking in and out, you may receive individual employee reports from that system that allow you to make manual corrections prior to payroll being cut. Review of these data can identify if staff did not clock in or out appropriate to the hours the worked-unit-staffing plan reflects. It can also identify other errors that can be corrected to accurately reflect staff worked or productive time. Recognize that biweekly reports do not exactly match to the hours worked, and charged, to a department during a given month.

For instance, as shown in **Exhibit 14–10**, if your workweek is Sunday through Saturday and the month begins on Monday of the second week of a pay period, that pay period will include 8 days from the previous month as well as the first 6 days of the current month. The 7th through the 20th will make up the next biweekly report. If it is a 30-day month, the 21st through the 4th of the following month will make up the next biweekly report.

How then can you compare these reports with the hours and dollars charged to your department for the month? You can't. The important work is to ensure that the hours and dollars charged to your department each pay period are accurate. Finance accrues expenses for the days that have not been covered in the current month and reverses them the next month. The important information to know is how the hours and dollars charged to your department for the full month compare with budget. If you are watching the biweekly reports closely, you will not have many surprises.

Unit productivity reports are important to watch as well. Many organizations use national productivity products that compare the productivity of hospital departments with those in comparable hospitals throughout the country. It is crucial to ensure that the specific operations of your department are specified when building the base of organizations for comparison. If your surgical unit cares for orthopedic patients, be sure to identify the type (orthopedics) to determine your comparison group. That is, if your unit cares for patients post–joint replacement and post–spine surgery, the base

---

Exhibit 14–10 Calendar for Sample Month

Sun	Mon	Tues	Wed	Thurs	Fri	Sat
31	1	2	3	4	5	6
7	8	9	10	11	12	13
14	15	16	17	18	19	20
21	22	23	24	25	26	27
28	29	30	1	2	3	4

of hospital nursing departments you are being compared with should care for the same type of patients. If they care for some post–joint replacement, general surgery patients, and no spine surgery patients, the comparison may not be valid. You may have some unique differences that need to be added to the equation to have a valid comparison. For example, if your department includes a decentralized nurse educator, add it to the equation. The comparison groups may not have that position in their departments. Also determine if the productivity tool includes all man-hours or if education and orientation hours are excluded. Once you have validated that your comparison groups are comparable, this becomes a very helpful tool for benchmarking.

National comparative productivity tools normally report data in quartiles of productivity. The budget should reflect the FTEs the hospital expects to be achieved for the quartile of productivity. For example, the FTEs budgeted for Main 7 are set for the 50th percentile of productivity compared with other comparative hospital units throughout the country. The staffing patterns scheduled should reflect that required to meet the productivity levels budgeted. One of the benefits of using a national productivity tool is that you have the ability to contact staff at other hospitals in your comparison group to network for ideas to improve productivity.

Turning to **Exhibit 14–11**, let's examine productivity measurement. Note the following:

- The volume corresponds to the actual patient days identified for the month for Main 7 in Exhibit 14–2.
- The paid FTEs of 44.86 for the month and 43.24 for YTD correspond to Exhibit 14–5. Productive man-hours include man-hours contract (344) + man-hours productive (5,759) + man-hours overtime (192) = total productive man-hours (6,295).
- "Mid" stands for the comparative midpoint of productive hours per unit of service for the 50th percentile for comparative hospitals, derived from the national productivity tool.
- The actual productive hours per unit of service for the month were total productive man-hours (6,295) ÷ total volume (750) = 8.393. This is lower than the national midpoint.
- The actual productive hours per unit of service YTD were 8.425, also below the national comparative goal of 8.791 hours per unit of service.
- The 9% for education/orientation hours and earned PTO hours has been extrapolated from those identified as productive because these hours are not direct patient care hours.
- The next column reflects FTE variance from the comparative midpoint for the month is (2.2). This means that 2.2 less FTEs were utilized to provide direct patient care based on the units of service than the goal for the month.
- The next column reflects FTE variance from the comparative midpoint YTD is (1.9). This means that 1.9 less FTEs have been used to provide direct patient care based on units of service than expected YTD.

Exhibit 14–11 Example of a Monthly Comparison of Actual Productivity Performance to Comparative Midpoints for Actual Volumes Report

Main 7
Productivity

Name	Vol	Paid FTE Month	Paid FTE YTD	Mid	Actual Month	Actual YTD	Ed/Or % YTD	FTE Month	FTE YTD	Prod Index Month	Prod Index YTD
Main 7	750	44.86	43.24	8.791	8.393	8.425	9%	(2.2)	(1.9)	104.7	104.3

- The productivity index for the month shows that the staff worked at a productivity level of 104.7% compared with similar hospitals and 104.3% YTD. The productivity index is calculated by dividing the national midpoint (8.791) by the actual productivity for the month (8.393) = 104.7%.

From a financial standpoint this is a very positive level of productivity both for the month and YTD. Review of patient satisfaction data and other quality data for the unit will reflect if this level of productivity is positive from a quality standpoint, as well.

If you do not use a national productivity tool to compare your department with others, then compare your monthly productivity with your budget by determining your budgeted and actual hours of care per patient day:

1. Subtract from the total man-hours those hours that are not used for direct patient care. This includes PTO, education, and orientation.
2. Then divide the man-hour number by the total budgeted units of service.

Now we give an example comparing actual with budget. This example uses the information for the month from Exhibit 14–2 and Exhibit 14–5.

Use your productivity data to understand your variance. If your productivity was less than budgeted for the month, determine the reason. Did you have many staff in orientation but did not get their hours posted to the education subaccount? This would result in education hours being allocated to productive hours. Did you have many days with volumes that forced staffing to minimum levels? An example is an oncology unit with a census of only four patients for 5 days. For patient safety it is still required that two staff members be present on each shift, thereby resulting in a much higher number of hours of care per patient day than required for care of oncology patients. Understanding these data will help you to not only create the variance report for the month, but also will help you and your staff identify areas to explore for changes to improve productivity while ensuring quality of care.

Budgeted hours for PTO (570) + budgeted hours for education/orientation (750) = 1,320.

Total budgeted man-hours for the month is 7,172 − 1,320 (PTO/education/orientation) = 5,852 (direct patient care hours for the month).

The total budgeted units of service for the month are 669 patient days.

Divide the total budgeted direct patient care hours (5,852) by the total budgeted units of service (669) = 8.75 budgeted hours of care per patient day.

Compare budgeted hours of care per patient day with actual hours of care per patient day.

Actual hours for PTO (611) + actual hours for education/orientation (764) = 1,375.

Total actual man-hours for the month is 7,670 − 1,375 (PTO/education/orientation) = 6,295 (direct patient care hours for the month).

The total units of service for the month are 750 patient days.

Divide the total direct patient care hours (6,295) by the total units of service (750) = 8.39 hours of care per patient day.

Then subtract the actual hours of care per patient day from the budgeted hours of care per patient day (8.75 − 8.39 = 0.36).

This is less hours of care per patient day than budgeted, so it becomes a positive variance.

Variance Report

The variance report is a summary of the major exceptions to the budget that are experienced during a given time frame and an explanation of why the exceptions occurred. Most organizations expect these reports on a monthly basis. This important report identifies opportunities to understand and control the exceptions, or variances, to the budget. It is important not only for the manager to understand but also for the manager to help staff understand and become a part in controlling costs. Managers can use the monthly variance data to involve staff in identifying and planning the activities needed to make midstream corrections.

To focus on the items of most importance, only those variances that are large are noted in the report. You need to know what level of variance is expected to be included in your report. For purposes of this chapter, a variance of at least 10% for statistics and man-hours and at least 10% and greater than $1,000 for the month for each line item reflecting dollars is included in the report. YTD information is only referenced to note overall trends for those variances reported on for the month. As a rule, review of the "total" line under each large category such as "total salary expense" or "total non-salary expense" will give you an idea as to the significance of that area's impact on the budget. Line-by-line review will point to specific areas for focused analysis.

Statistics

Refer to Exhibit 14–2. The actual volume of inpatient days for the month (735) was 12.2% above the budget (655), with the total patient days (750) 12.1% above the budgeted total patient days (669). You will use these data in your report to explain variance based on volume. In review of YTD data, actual inpatient days are above budget by 9.2% with YTD total units up 9.0%. In analysis it is determined that the addition of a new orthopedic surgeon has increased the volume of surgeries, whereas the other surgeons are experiencing the number of surgeries expected from them. However, because the new surgeon started practicing at the hospital only 3 months before and has been increasing volume each month, this trend should be noted with a plan to ensure adequate staffing anticipating additional volume throughout the remainder of the fiscal year.

Revenue

Revenue, in ratio to the volume statistics, is also above budget. This information is also used to explain variance for overages in specific line items that are related to the volume and subsequent revenue. Referring to Exhibit 14–3, the total inpatient revenue for the month of $355,501 is higher than the budgeted inpatient revenue of $318,724. Budgeted charges for Main 7 inpatient days can be determined by dividing the budgeted dollars ($318,724) by the budgeted volume (669) = $476.42. The same can be done for observation day charges. Budgeted charges for observations days are $5,860 ÷ 14 = $418.57. Admitted patient days are paid at a higher rate than observation days. Therefore the higher volume in admitted patient days, and one less observation day than budgeted, results in positive revenue for the month of 11.2%, or actual ($360,970) − budget ($324,584) = $36,386. YTD revenue is up 9.5% from budget, or actual ($1,818,272) − budget ($1,660,526) = $157,746. There is a positive variance in revenue both for the month and YTD based on volume.

Man-hours

Analysis of man-hours without analysis of salary expense information can be deceiving. In the example in Exhibit 14–5, the only variance significant enough to report is overtime, which is down 28.9%. That appears very positive. Overtime hours for the month were down by 78 hours from those budgeted (budget 270 − actual 192 = 78). Contracted man-hours were over only 9.2%, not enough to be reported. Contracted hours were over by 29 hours (actual 344 − budget 315 = 29). Productive man-hours were over only 9.3%, or 492 hours (actual 5,759 − budget 5,267 = 492). PTO was over only 7.2%, or 41 hours (actual 611 − budget 570 = 41). Education and orientation hours were above budget by only 1.9%, or 14 hours (actual 764 − budget 750 = 14). The total man-hours were up only 6.9%, reflecting 498 hours (actual 7,670 − budget 7,172 = 498). The total volume was up by 12.1%. The trend YTD is similar with total man-hours above budget by only 3.1%, whereas total units are above budget by 9%. This looks very positive, but is it?

Salary Expense

This begins the line items to review for reporting purposes on the monthly variance report. Referring to Exhibit 14–6, dollars do not correlate in the same ratio to man-hour statistics (Exhibit 14–5). Productive man-hours for the month were up by only 9.3%. The dollars represented by those man-hours were up 12.4% or $9,427 (actual $85,670 − budget $76,243 = $9,427). PTO man-hours were up by only 7.2%. The dollars reflecting those man-hours were up 20.0% or $1,524 (actual $9,125 − budget $7,601 = $1,524). The salary–lump sum retention was under by 56.5%, which sounds positive and very significant. In reality, it amounts positively to only $1,170 (budget $2,070 − actual $900 = $1,170). Education/orientation/on-call was also under budget. That positive variance of 9.9% reflects only $905 (budget $9,184 − actual $8,279 = $905).

Now compare the contract man-hour coverage, which was 9.2% and too small to report, with the contract salary variance of 109.7%. This significantly reflects the high cost of contract labor. The 29 hours over budget for contract labor resulted in a negative variance of $9,585 (actual $18,319 − budget $8,734 = $9,585). Added together, the positive and negative variances in salary expense result in a negative total salary expense variance of 14.8% or $16,307 for the month. This is far worse than the negative 6.9% of total man-hours.

To fully understand the variance in salary expense, it should be analyzed by dollars per unit of service. Referring back to the calculations made under the Salary Budget section of this chapter, the actual salary expense per patient day was $3.90 more per patient day than what was budgeted. In analysis you note that you have three full-time RN positions and two part-time LPN positions vacant. The good news is that you have hired three full-time RNs who will begin orientation in 2 weeks. Also, because you have involved staff in understanding the negative impact that those open positions have on overtime, part-time RN staff has been wonderful picking up additional hours, thus keeping overtime down. The mix in staffing has changed, resulting in RNs covering some of the hours of care per patient day that should have been covered by LPN staff. Contracts are coming to an end for two of the traveler contracted RNs who have been covering open positions, and they will not be renewed. Given the expectation of continued higher volume of patients than budgeted, it will be important to fill the open part-time LPN positions to get the mix of staff back to that budgeted.

Discussions were held with the nurse recruiter to find two part-time LPNs. Although the recruiter currently had no part-time candidates, she had one full-time LPN candidate who has experience on a surgical nursing unit. Given the continued high volume and the fact that one LPN currently on staff is in school and wishes to work most weekends to be off for weekday classes, based on staff discussions you determine you could cover the schedule using a full-time LPN. You have scheduled the full-time LPN candidate for an interview. When this plan is fully implemented, the salary expense per unit of service should get back in line with the budget.

A review of total salary expense YTD is similar to that for the month. YTD total salary expense is over 13.7% or $75,670 ($626,549 − $550,879 = $75,670). An ongoing review of YTD after implementation of the changes being made will be important. Although by the end of the fiscal year, you may not be able to get salary expense per unit of service to meet that budgeted, it should improve significantly from that currently experienced.

Benefit Expense

Although benefits are an expense borne by the department, managers have little control over them. Retirement, group health, and flex benefits are based on choices made by employees. Analysis of benefit expense is useful for future budgeting purposes and to note the impact that it has on the department as a whole.

In Exhibit 14–7, the total benefit expense line shows that overall this category has little negative impact on the budget for the month. The variance to budget is a negative 7.1%, reflecting a negative dollar impact of only $1,492 (actual $22,521 − budget $21,029 = $1,492). Although retirement and group health meet the reporting requirement for a line item by being over or under budget by at least 10% and $1,000, there is normally not an expectation that these will be covered in the variance analysis. Retirement is over budget by 53.5%, reflecting $1,430 (actual $4,104 − budget $2,674 = $1,430). Group health is under budget by 10.3%, reflecting $1,191 (budget $11,533 − $10,342 = $1,191). Flex benefit dollars, although 26.9% over budget, amount to only $275 (actual $1,297 − budget $1,022 = $275). FICA taxes hospital portion, although over budget by 16.9%, reflects an overage of only $978. This overage is due to the increase in patient volume and the subsequent increase in taxed dollars paid to staff. The budgeted benefits per unit of service are actually below budget. This is calculated as for other unit of service categories or line items:

> *Budgeted benefits for the month ($21,029) ÷ the budgeted volume (669)*
> *= $31.43/unit of service.*
>
> *Actual benefits for the month ($22,521) ÷ the actual volume (750)*
> *= $30.03/unit of service.*
>
> *So the actual cost per unit of service was down*
> *($31.43 − $30.03 = $1.40) $1.40 per unit of service.*

A quick review of total benefit expense YTD shows that YTD the negative impact of benefits to help absorb the additional hours used to cover the added patient days has been only 2.1% or $2,273 (actual $108,884 − budget $106,611 = $2,273).

Non-salary Expense Analysis

In Exhibit 14–8, patient nonchargeables are over by 160.9% for the month, reflecting an overage of $19,076 (actual $30,934 − budget $11,858 = $19,076). What is the difference per unit of service?

> *The budget called for $17.72 per unit of service determined by dividing the*
> *budgeted dollars ($11,858) by the budgeted volume (669) = $17.72.*
>
> *Actual for the month was $41.25 per unit of service*
> *(actual dollars $30,934 ÷ actual volume 750 = $41.25).*

This major difference creates a good point to test if the budget was logical based on prior year data. In review it is found that for the same month prior year there was $21.05 per unit of service (prior year month actual dollars $14,338 ÷ prior year month actual volume 681 = $21.05).

To get an even better perspective, you go to the prior year YTD data and do the math:

- The prior year YTD actual dollars spent on patient nonchargeables was $59,995.
- Divide this by the prior year YTD actual volume of 3,431 patient days and you find that the prior year YTD average cost per unit of service for patient nonchargeables was $17.49.
- The budgeted cost per unit of service of $17.72 was somewhat aggressive considering the usual increase in cost of goods from one year to the next and considering the prior year average YTD was $17.49, or 23 cents more than that budgeted for the current year. However, it was known when budgeting that the hospital had engaged a new buying group that committed to reducing the cost of supplies as well as a plan to introduce an automated supply cabinet system.

Looking at recent months (not shown in this chapter), you determine that although the cost had been slightly higher than that budgeted, it was never over the prior year average of $21.03 per unit of service. You know that during the month of November your department converted to an automated supply cabinet system that required switching out many patient nonchargeable items. Review of the last inventory expense report from material management itemized all the supplies added but none of those removed. A phone call to the director in material management finds that the credits, which should amount to $17,547 for those patient nonchargeables removed, were not placed in time to be reflected in the November reports. He assures you that the credits will show in December, bringing the cost for patient nonchargeables back in line with the budget.

Using this new information, you determine what the actual budget should have been if the credits had been placed.

> *The actual for the month ($30,934) − the credits which should have*
> *been applied ($17,547) = $13,387.*
>
> *Therefore, the actual cost per unit of service was revised actual*
> *($13,387) ÷ actual volume (750) = $17.85.*

Although this is higher than budgeted, all the changes with the new buying group have not been put into place. Therefore the total decrease in the cost of goods has not been realized.

There are no other line items that meet the requirements for variance reporting. Armed with the information that you have, you are now ready to complete your monthly variance report for your cost center, Main 7. This will be done on an Excel Spreadsheet (**Exhibit 14–12**).

Summary

The annual budget is based on assumptions based on experiences from the previous year and what is expected to occur in a given department or cost center during the coming fiscal year. The difference between the budget and what happens is called the *variance*. When you compare the budget to what actually occurred each month and YTD and analyze the variance, you have powerful data to understand what is happening on your unit. Given the multiple departments that can charge items to a given cost center, it also allows for review and accountability to ensure that items are charged correctly or credited in a timely manner. This also maintains the integrity of the data for future budgeting purposes.

Exhibit 14–12 Monthly Variance Report

Month and Year: **2-Nov**

Unit #: **7**   Unit Name: **Main 7**   Reported by: **N. J. Tomlinson**

Account #	Description	Budget	Actual	Variance	Variance %	Explanation
1	Salaries Productive	$76,243	$85,670	$ (9,427)	–12%	Total Volume over budget by 12.1% (actual 750 – budget 669 = 81). New surgeon providing higher volume.
4	PTO	$7,601	$ 9,125	$ (1,524)	–20%	Additional PTO earned based on additional hours worked mostly by part time staff to cover volume and 3 FT RN & 2 PT LPN open positions.
9	Salaries Overtime	$6,701	$ 4,547	$ 2,154	32%	OT hours under budget by 28.9% (budget 270 – actual 192 = 78). OT salaries under budget based on 3 FT RN & 2 PT LPN positions being covered by contract labor, relief staff and PT staff increasing man-hours.
10	Contract Salaries	$ 8,734	$ 18,319	$ (9,585)	–110%	Using contract labor due to open positions and volume over 12.1%. Salaries/unit of service are over $3.90 due to use of contract staff. Have filled 3 FT RN positions to start in 2 weeks. Will not renew agency contracts.
	Total Salary Expense	$ 126,840	$ 110,533	$16,307	–15%	Productivity is 104.7% for the month & 104.3% YTD. YTD actual salary/unit of service is $7 more than budgeted. However, during the month that has been reduced to an overage of $3.90/unit of service. With filling positions and eliminating contract staff, this should return to budgeted levels.
26	Patient Nonchargeables	$11,858	$ 30,934	$ (19,076)	–161%	Volume up 12.1%. Credits for $17,547 for automated supply cabinet conversion not credited during month. Will be credited next month. With credits, cost/unit of service would have been $17.85. While not on budget, all changes with new buying group not completed.
	Total Non-salary Expense	$35,467	$ 16,545	$18,659	–114%	With credits the actual cost/unit of service is $17.85 against a budget of $17.72. This should be achieved with use of automated supply cabinet conversion and changes with new buying group.

Budget variance analysis that uses a line-item-by-line-item approach to determine cost per unit of service puts the information into an understandable context. It reflects the impact of volume and staff-mix changes, new technology changes, and other variables experienced throughout the year. Translating and sharing that information with unit staff allows for planning and implementation of measures to creatively manage fiscal resources required for excellence in patient care.

Discussion Questions

1. Why is it important for a nurse manager to understand variance reporting? How does this reporting become a valuable tool?
2. In an inpatient unit, why is it important to determine which statistics are being captured and included to reflect your unit activities?
3. What challenges are present in capturing statistics for the emergency department?
4. What mistake must a nurse manager not make when reviewing the revenue report for his or her department or unit?
5. Because staffing is usually the most expensive resource in the provision of care, what reports would provide you valuable information for this expense?
6. Contract labor is usually the most expensive man-hours. Why?
7. In your man-hour analysis, why is it important to keep track of education and orientation hours?
8. The monthly distribution register for your department should be carefully monitored. Why?

Glossary of Terms

Benefit Expense—includes retirement, group health, flex benefits, and FICA.

Nonproductive Man-hours—include paid time off (PTO). PTO includes vacation, holidays, jury duty, sick time, and any other time off.

Payroll Reports—biweekly reports that reflect hours by type being paid to each employee.

Productive Man-hours—hours where employed staff members provide care for patients.

Reported Revenue—reflects charges generated for the month and year-to-date by the department, not actual dollars received for that care.

Revenue and Usage Report—identifies charges by financial class and charge code.

Variance Analysis—includes finding all the pieces of the puzzle, which include the various reports that you are sent by the finance, materials management, and human resources departments.

Variance Report—summary of the major exceptions to the budget that are experienced during a given time frame and an explanation of why the exceptions occurred.

CHAPTER 15

Comparing Reimbursements with Cost of Services Provided

Patricia M. Vanhook, PhD, MSN, RN, FNP-BC

Key Terms

☞ Balanced Scorecard and Activity-Based Costing (ABC)
☞ Capitation
☞ Charges
☞ "Costing" a Service
☞ Costs
☞ Cost-to-Charge Ratio (CCR)

☞ Operating Payments
☞ Outlier Payments
☞ Payment
☞ Per Diem Approach
☞ Projection of Reimbursement
☞ Volume-Based Measures

Introduction

One very important question the nurse manager needs to answer is *whether the overall unit expense budget falls within the reimbursement amount*. The evaluation activity described in this chapter will help the nurse manager to recognize whether a service line is profitable and to determine areas within the nurse manager's control that influence profitability. To accomplish this, the nurse manager needs to have a clear understanding of the different mechanisms of cost accounting used to reflect both services and reimbursement. This chapter explains and provides examples of cost and reimbursement for acute care, hospital outpatient, ambulatory surgery, skilled care, and home health. It is imperative the nurse manager is well versed on this topic to understand and to respond appropriately to cost and reimbursement questions generated from the departmental operations reports produced by finance.

Reimbursement

Historical Perspective

Over the past 20 years, hospitals, health care agencies, and primary care providers have moved from a cost reimbursement system based on "reasonable costs" (Cleverley, 1997) to a prospective payment system (PPS). Prospective payment is based on median costs with adjustments made based on the local wage index (Sobun, 1999). Under prospective payment, the agency is paid a set fee regardless of the amount of resources used to provide the service (Division of Health Care Finance and Policy, 1998). This type of payment system creates some financial risk for the agency and keeps costs under control for the insurer, while also providing financial rewards for services provided at a lower cost. If the agency can deliver services under cost and under the prospective payment reimbursement fee, the difference equates to profit for the agency. However, if services cost more than the reimbursement amount, it results in a monetary loss. Therefore prospective payment was an attempt to control rising health care costs through improved efficiency within the health care agency.

Payers

Capitation (further explained in Chapter 10) is a mechanism used by insurers to contain costs by establishing a set payment amount for a population served by a defined health care service (Hoffman, 1984). With capitation, rates are negotiated between the provider and the insurer under a contractual agreement for a year (Cleverley, 1997). Reimbursement rates may be for all services offered or for one specific service area, called a "carve out," such as laboratory. Within the health care setting, financial administration under a capitation system requires critical financial management and knowledge of the payers.

Thus it is important that the nurse administrator understands the various health care payers to appreciate the diversity of billing and reimbursement methods. The two types of payers for health care services are public and private. Federal and state are public payers and include Medicare and Medicaid. The insured and uninsured are considered private payers, which are various insurance plans, indemnity insurance, and self-pay.

The reimbursement structure differs between health maintenance organizations (HMOs), preferred provider organizations (PPOs), and point of service (POS) plans. HMOs strive to maintain the health of the participant and provide "gatekeepers" who must authorize the need for additional services. Reimbursement is a set fee for all the participants of the HMO. The goal of the health care agency is to be the only provider of services for the HMO so it has sufficient numbers of inpatients and outpatients to generate revenue. The PPO is a discounted fee accepted by doctors and hospitals to provide care to participants. A POS establishes a "gatekeeper" to manage and direct care, evaluate the appropriateness of care including diagnostic studies, and either approve or not approve reimbursement. Finally, indemnity is a traditional insurance plan in which the member pays a premium and must pay a deductible. When the deductible is met, the insurance pays a percentage of the health care expenses. In general there are not provider restrictions with indemnity (retrieved June 17, 2008, from http://www.healthinsurancefinders.com/indemnity_health_insurance.html).

Reimbursement Sources

The Centers for Medicare and Medicaid (CMS) paid $125,512 million to acute care facilities in 2007. These payments amounted to 62% of the CMS funds and 19.5% of the federal budget (U.S. Department of Health and Human Services, 2007). For those aged 65 years and older, Medicare is the primary payer for acute care hospitalization, accounting for 75.7% of payments for inpatient care (Ezzati-Rice, Kashihara, & Machlin, 2004), The home health or skilled care manager will also note a higher percentage of patients covered by Medicare and Medicaid referred to their services because these patient populations continue to be the highest users of acute, skilled, and home health care. Why is this important? It means the government sets the trend for reimbursement for other payers. The nurse administrator must understand the drivers of payment and how this affects the overall revenue for the unit and for the health care organization.

This payment pattern is further complicated because the mechanisms of reimbursement vary between acute care, long-term care, skilled nursing, and home health. Payment to the hospital and a long-term care facility is determined by the reimbursement structure the payer uses. It is important to note skilled care may be performed in a long-term care facility and is reimbursed by Medicare. However, Medicare does not pay for the services of long-term care. The residents' care is reimbursed predominantly by Medicaid and a few private payers (van der Walde & Choi, 2003b). Different reimbursement mechanisms for services provided may be based on a per diem (specified daily) rate from private insurance carriers, a negotiated fee from managed care (HMO) or PPOs, a PPS by assigned diagnosis-related groups (DRGs) or resource utilization groups (RUGs) from Medicare, or the patient who is classified as self-pay. Therefore *payment is not standardized and varies by the type of reimbursement structure*. The payment amount can differ within these structures as well. For instance, a different negotiated discount could be given to one PPO versus another PPO. The nurse manager can obtain a breakdown of payer categories and reimbursement amounts for the patients served from the finance or billing department.

An increase in the use of skilled nursing facilities is occurring as the population ages. Payments to skilled nursing care were $21 billion in 2007 (U.S. Department of Health and Human Services, 2007). Medicare reimbursement for skilled nursing care (prospective payment) is by assignment of the patient to one of the 44 RUGs (van der Walde & Choi, 2003b). The concept of RUGs is that there are conditions that require similar resources and services and therefore reimbursement can be calculated based on the resources used by the skilled nursing facility patient. Routine services such as room, board, administrative services, nursing care, and therapy services are the three components of the RUG that are summed to determine the reimbursement. In addition, the CMS do a "market basket analysis"[1] (explained in Chapter 12), and the reimbursement is adjusted annually based on the inflation of prices of goods and services incurred by the facility (van der Walde & Choi, 2003a). Later in the chapter, a case study is presented to demonstrate how RUGs determine reimbursement.

Medicare payments for home health care are $14.2 billion in 2007 with 8,618 agencies providing services (U.S. Department of Health and Human Services, 2007). Reimbursement for home health varies by service. Each payer has fee schedules for the various visits as well as fee schedules for durable medical equipment and for respiratory and infusion therapy services. Van der Walde and Lindstrom (2003) report $33.2 billion[2] was spent on home health care in 2001 with 51.2% generated from Medicare and Medicaid. Under home health care the prospective payment reimbursement is determined by the standardized assessment tool, outcome and assessment information set (OASIS), or negotiated fees from private insurance and HMOs. OASIS is mandated by Medicare. The tool was designed to measure quality of care and to ensure appropriate reimbursement (van der Walde & Lindstrom, 2003). Again, *under prospective payment, neither intensity of services nor supplies can be applied as additional charges*. Instead, the agency must try to maintain costs within the reimbursement schedule. In 2004 each 60-day episode of home health care received $2,230 base payment per patient from the federal government.

Medicare established a PPS, called ambulatory patient category (APC), for hospital outpatients: "The composition of the APC groups is based on two premises: the procedures within each group must be similar clinically, and the procedures must be similar in resource and costs" (U.S. Department of Health and Human Services, 1998, pp. 47,562).

Why do differences in reimbursement exist? *Different payers use different strategies for payment of claims*. Therefore a health care agency's reimbursement varies according to negotiated contracts

---

[1] Market basket is an economic term used to indicate a measure of inflation.

[2] This figure does not include respiratory care and infusion services.

and standard fees from Medicare or other insurers. Insurance companies and managed care organizations negotiate reimbursement with health care entities that provide services for their patients. Contracts are established for a period of time and are renegotiated by the executive management team at contract end. Increases in cost of care for the patient population during the contract year are usually non-negotiable (Cleverley, 1997). The largest hospital payer, Medicare, reimburses by an assigned DRG code or an assigned RUG, with a fixed dollar amount for all services provided during the hospital or skilled care stay. Therefore knowledge of patient and payer mix is essential to understand the variation in reimbursement. Again, the nurse manager may automatically receive this information or may have to request it from the finance department.

Costs

Cleverley (1987) compared the costing of hospital care with that of manufacturing. Consider the patient as the process of manufacturing a car. The patient progresses through stages beginning with admission to discharge, much as a car begins with a frame and is complete at the end of the assembly line. The patient discharge is the *outcome* of the hospital stay. This is not to say each and every patient receives the same services or that each and every disease process is the same (Cleverley, 1987). The nurse manager uses this thought process to identify all areas involved with the patient, including administration, registration, laboratory, radiology, diagnostics, pharmacy, dietary, housekeeping, maintenance, materials management, physician, building and utilities, and nursing with each contributing to the cost of the hospital, skilled care, or long-term care stay.

Hospital cost determination mirrors other businesses and industries with the exception that hospitals have high fixed costs (administration, depreciation, utilities, maintenance, etc.) and must attempt to cover these costs by increasing inpatient volume, adding services, using stringent contract management, and investing in capital to attract more business (van der Walde & Choi, 2003a). Costs are calculated as direct or indirect and fixed or variable. *The nurse manager should consider him- or herself as both the chief executive officer and chief financial officer of his or her nursing unit or department and develop a good understanding of costs and revenue.* Chapters 12–14, as well as this chapter, present how to determine nursing unit costs and manage the budget.

Skilled nursing care costs vary between hospital-based and freestanding facilities. The freestanding skilled facilities continued to decrease their costs after the introduction of prospective payment, whereas the hospital-based costs continued to rise (U.S. General Accounting Office [GAO], 2002). The GAO determined that the increased cost for hospital-based skilled units was related to a higher acuity of patients and historical allocation of overhead costs plus an increased number of Medicare and Medicaid patients compared with the freestanding agency. The freestanding skilled facilities were able to offset Medicare and Medicaid losses by passing the costs on to the private insurers (van der Walde & Lindstrom, 2003).[3]

Hospital outpatient service payments, under the APC, were based on historical average costs. Here, relative payment weights were assigned by calculating the APC median cost of a mid-level cardiovascular clinic visit (that was found to be the most common outpatient service) and assigned a numerical value of 1.0. The assignment of each APC group relative payment rate was determined by dividing the median cost of each APC by the median cost for the mid-level cardiovascular visit.

There are two significant items the nurse manager must understand from this discussion. First, comparison of relative relationship of one APC to another, by knowing the median payment weight is 1.0 and understanding the reimbursement will be less or greater, is based on the variation from 1.0. Second,

---

[3] Further detailed information explaining the RUGs system can be found in Dunham-Taylor and Pinczuk (2006).

the hospital is reimbursed separately for each APC billed. Therefore a patient may have radiological and endoscopy procedures on the same day with each procedure reimbursed independently.

Home health cost determination varies somewhat from inpatient services. The home health agency manager considers different types of visit costs that are provided by a service line that includes nursing care, therapy services, and nursing assistance. The average cost per visit is calculated, much the same as acute care, by applying direct and indirect costs and allocating for special fees such as accreditation services and other intermittent expected fees. The costs are averaged for the Medicare Cost Report and charges are set at an amount greater than the costs to recoup costs from high level care patients and to provide an established level for contract negotiations for private carriers that ensure costs are reimbursed.[4]

Clarifying the Cost Issue

Defining Costs, Charges, and Payments

According to Finkler (1994), many published studies have used the terms "cost" and "charges" interchangeably. Costs and charges are not interchangeable terms, and the nurse manager needs to understand the difference. *Costs* are determined by the organization's financial accounting system, which takes into account actual costs of supplies, manpower, facility, and administration for services provided (Cleverley, 1997). *Charges* are determined by the allocation of costs to the revenue-producing centers and then projecting an amount needed to recover all the costs (Cleverley, 1997). Finally, *payment* is the amount the health care agency receives for the services provided. All payers pay differing amounts for the same service depending on the type of payer and the contractual agreement between the agency and the insurer (Lane, Longstreth, & Nixon, 2001).

Projection of reimbursement is calculated by a payment-to-cost ratio that indicates the percent of costs that are covered by reimbursement. Medpac (2003) reported to Congress the Medicare payment-to-cost ratio was 99.4%, Medicaid 98%, uncompensated care 12.2%, and private payers 113.2%. Hospitals use the private-payer reimbursement as a cushion to offset the reimbursement from Medicare and Medicaid (Medpac, 2003) because it does not cover the full cost of the services provided.

The manager must remember that each private payer negotiates fees contractually with the health care agency, and payment *may or may not* cover costs. **Exhibit 15–1** demonstrates a fictional example of charge, payment, and cost of a hospitalization. The hospital calculated the costs of care to be $7,250 and determined the charge to be $9,500 to capture any extended costs that may occur as well as to recoup losses that may be experienced from Medicare and Medicaid reimbursement. Contract negotiations between the hospital and the HMO and PPO agreed on the reimbursement for the hospitalization to be $8,250. The last column represents the prospective payment from Medicare, which equals approximately 99.4% of the actual costs incurred.

Cost of Service Versus Reimbursement

What if more money is being spent on providing the service than is brought in by the reimbursement? In this case the executive team needs to determine an effective way to provide the service yet either cut the overall budget, decide to take a loss on the service, or stop providing the service. It is possible that we cannot answer this question because we do not know how much a service costs and the actual revenue amount that is realized. In this section we provide some helpful suggestions that can lead us to finding some answers.

---

[4] More details about home care reimbursement can be found in Dunham-Taylor and Pinczuk (2006).

Exhibit 15–1 Comparison of Cost to Charge and Payment*

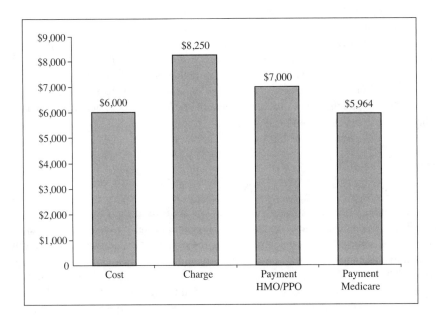

* Y axis represents whole dollars and X axis is the cost, charge, and payment information.

The key financial question is, *are we spending less than the reimbursement amount to provide the specified service?* A "yes" answer is desired. However, if the answer is that we are spending more than the reimbursement amount or, worse, that we do not know, *immediate action* needs to be taken by the entire management group—including the nurse manager.

Calculating the answer to this question is complicated because most often many cost centers—that is, nursing, pharmacy, laboratory, dietary, medical records—have been involved in providing the service. So to answer this question the interdisciplinary team needs to figure all the actual costs expended to provide the specified service. This activity is sometimes called "costing" a service. This costing exercise should take place for all major services provided within the health care organization. Let's break this down into priority levels for the nurse manager. The first issue is determining cost.

COST DETERMINATION METHODS

Four distinct methods of cost determination are used in health care today (Udpa, 2001). The first method is the *cost-to-charge ratio (CCR)*. Medicare specified this method be used to report annual costs. Thus most health care organizations today use this ratio as the primary source of all hospital costs and cost accounting information (Magnus & Smith, 2000). This report, called the *Medicare Cost Report*, is used by the CMS to calculate and update reimbursement rates. Nationwide data are available as public information from the Healthcare Cost Report Information System, or HCRIS,[5] and health care agencies use this information "to benchmark their costs and performance" (Magnus & Smith, 2000).

The information contained in the *Medicare Cost Report* includes CCRs for inpatient, outpatient, departments, and functions such as medical education, utilization data, and financial statement data.

---

[5] The HCRIS can be accessed at http://www.cms.gov

The report is required for all Medicare-certified hospitals, skilled nursing facilities, home health agencies, and renal facilities. The ratio is determined by dividing the costs by the charges. **Exhibit 15–2** demonstrates the CCR calculation. A ratio under 1.0 (equal costs and charges) is positive and indicates that the organization is making money on the service. A ratio over 1.0 indicates the organization is experiencing a loss—the costs are more than the charges (expected reimbursement). In the first example, the service is making money. In the second example, the service is losing money.

Using the CCR, it is assumed that reimbursement (revenue) reflects the intensity of care, and therefore indirect costs (overhead) are assigned accordingly (Udpa, 2001). This method of cost determination does not allow for a full assessment of the true revenue production of a service, because all service areas are considered profitable if the health care agency as a whole is profitable. In addition, this means that the higher the revenue generation, the higher the proportional allocation of overhead regardless of actual resource utilization. The nurse manager should be aware that CCR could lead to misrepresentation of cost when evaluating the profitability of a service (Udpa, 2001).

The second method of cost accounting is *volume-based measures* (Udpa, 2001), which is much like it sounds. Here, the indirect costs are assigned according to the volume (which may be visits, admissions, nursing hours per patient day) or machine hours (in radiology and the laboratory). A typical example of this measure is demonstrated (**Exhibit 15–3**) when the patient volume increases by 15% on a nursing unit and the nursing hours remain the same. The allocation of indirect cost is increased by 15%. Nursing hours did not increase to accommodate an increase of patient volume, yet the department is allocated higher overhead. It is difficult for the nurse manager to

---

Exhibit 15–2 Calculation of Cost-to-Charge Ratio

Cost ÷ charge = cost-to-charge ratio

Examples:

(1) If costs are $50 and charges are $100:
    $50 ÷ $100 = 0.5 cost-to-charge ratio (in the black)
(2) If costs are $100 and charges are $50:
    $100 ÷ $50 = 2.0 cost-to-charge ratio (in the red)

Exhibit 15–3 Volume-Based Cost Calculation

For an average daily census of 18:
- Budgeted direct cost (salaries and benefits) for average daily census of 18 = $18,331
- Budgeted indirect costs (professional fees, depreciation, and utilities) for nursing unit for average daily census of 18 = $5,781

For an average daily census of 21:
- Average unit census per day for month X = 21
- Actual direct costs for census of 21 = $18,331
- Actual indirect costs for nursing unit for census of 21 = $6,648

demonstrate increased productivity under this method of cost assignment. The nurse manager must understand the method of allocation of indirect costs to explain variation.

The third approach to cost allocation is the *per diem approach* (Udpa, 2001). This approach accumulates the indirect costs, divides by the number of patient days to determine per diem costs, and allocates the indirect cost equally to all the nursing units. This method considers all patients the same regardless of intensity of care. In a facility that cares for various types of patients, such as intensive care and obstetrics, this method of costing may also distort departmental costs. For example, in 1 month a 10-bed cardiovascular intensive care unit has 100% occupancy and the 30-bed obstetric unit occupancy rate is 55%. The indirect costs are distributed equally to the units when the per diem method of cost allocation is used. This means the departmental operations reports for the obstetric unit and the cardiovascular intensive care unit have the same dollar amount for indirect expenses even though the obstetric unit had fewer patient days.

The last method, *balanced scorecard and activity-based costing*, became a part of the industry in the 1980s but quickly lost favor due to the resources required to initiate and maintain this process (Easier than ABC, 2003). Over time, the advancement of health care management software technology has allowed health care to use activity-based costing as a means of identifying true patient costs. This method of costing is more closely aligned with the true costs of caring for the patient (Ross, 2004; Udpa, 2001; Young, 2007). Activity-based costing methodology also resembles performance improvement methods as processes and outcomes are evaluated. The complexity of "procedures and tests involved, the intensity of nursing care, the duration of an activity, and the intricacies of operative and postoperative care" identify the true costs (Udpa, 2001, p. 36). In this method all areas and processes of patient interaction are identified and costs are allocated to the activity center.

The balanced scorecard adds the quality dimension to cost and reimbursement data. For instance, cost drivers outside the system, such as patient satisfaction, can be measured and reflected in the overall scorecard (Maiga & Jacobs, 2003). In this example, by combining these tools the nurse manager has an excellent overview of the financial aspects from cost, reimbursement, and patient satisfaction perspectives.

Exhibit 15–4 is an example of a balanced scorecard used by a hospital nurse manager to assess the unit performance against budget and revenue. This type of detail can be obtained from the finance department in a scorecard format if the agency uses this method of analysis. If the agency does not use a scorecard, the nurse manager can create one using information obtained from finance and spreadsheet software. In the example given here, the unit is under budget on expense and over budget on revenue, an excellent position. To truly determine if the unit is financially sound, the manager needs to clarify whether the revenue information is what was billed or whether it was the actual amount received. The nurse manager must remember it is not possible to obtain this information in a timely manner because of delays in both billing and receiving the actual payment from payers.

The following studies have used the activity-based costing method through the hospital cost accounting system to both assess costs and to improve performance and patient care. Lester, Bosch, Kaufman, Halpern, and Gazelle (2001) determined the actual inpatient costs of a patient undergoing endovascular abdominal aortic aneurysm repair. In their study, the direct costs were allocated to the individual units and the indirect costs were spread evenly among all departments. Time studies were performed, and supply costs for each department were monitored. Surgery and radiology comprised 62% of the cost, with nursing contributing 22%, anesthesia 12%, and 4% attributed to an "other" category. The nursing costs reported in the study were allocated to the nursing unit on which the patient received postoperative care. Although nursing costs were noted to contribute only a

Exhibit 15–4 Performance Indicators

a.

St. Mercy Hospital
Somewhere USA

Year: FY 200_
VP: Nancy Nurse
Director: Perry Person
Dept: Medical

PERFORMANCE INDICATORS	NOV GOAL	JUL	AUG	SEP	OCT	NOV	DEC	JAN	FEB	MAR	APR	MAY	JUN	YTD TOT	YTD GOAL	FY04 GOAL
GROWTH																
Total Inpatient Unit	364	401	308	371	364	365								1,809	1,791	4,263
Total Inpatient Unit LYSM	322	361	346	383	377	322								1,789	1,789	4,370
Total Outpatient Unit	29	21	57	28	49	39								194	186	425
Total Outpatient Unit LYSM	47	28	25	37	42	47								179	179	386
Total Unit	393	422	365	399	413	404								2,003	1,977	4,688
Total Unit LYSM	369	389	371	420	419	369								1,968	1,968	4,756
COST																
Total IP Revenue per IP Unit	$506.13	$497.18	$491.94	$494.79	$494.85	$499.62								$495.78	$506.13	$506.13
Total OP Revenue per OP Unit	$324.59	$168.90	$388.28	$344.11	$377.10	$392.21								$356.12	$324.59	$324.58
Total Revenue per Unit	$492.73	$480.83	$475.75	$484.22	$480.71	$489.25								$482.25	$489.05	$489.67
Salary Expense per Unit	$157.61	$182.54	$169.73	$163.36	$158.81	$152.51								$165.44	$158.15	$159.32
Supply Expense per Unit	$9.56	$8.93	$8.46	$8.69	$8.35	$7.65								$8.42	$9.37	$9.16
Non-Salary Expense per Unit	$27.52	$25.50	$32.62	$26.09	$25.76	$25.32								$26.93	$27.50	$27.38
Total Expense per Unit	$185.13	$208.04	$202.35	$189.45	$184.57	$177.83								$192.37	$185.65	$186.70
Gross Margin per Unit	$307.60	$272.79	$273.40	$294.76	$296.14	$311.43								$289.88	$303.40	$302.97
PEOPLE																
Productive Manhour per Unit	8.1767	9.2693	10.3563	9.1105	8.7301	8.9210								9.2534	8.1746	8.1756
Total Manhours per Unit	8.9135	10.0061	10.8079	9.8303	9.4000	9.6263								9.9156	8.9114	8.9124
Overtime Hours	62	91	15	101	133	14								354	314	745
Overtime % of Productive Hours	1.94%	2.34%	0.40%	2.78%	3.68%	0.38%								1.91%	1.94%	1.94%
Total FTE's	19.88	23.97	22.39	23.01	21.98	22.75								22.82	20.26	20.09
Avg. Hourly Rate	$17.91	$20.63	$16.12	$16.69	$16.90	$15.84								$17.21	$17.97	$18.10
Contract Labor Costs	$2,431	$19,168	$468	$32										$19,668	$12,000	$28,705
Contract Labor Hours	44	488	102	17	1									607	217	520
Contract FTE Equivalent	0.25	2.77	0.58	0.10	0.00									0.70	0.25	0.25
VARIANCE																
Productive Manhour Variance		459	797	373	229	301								2,159		
Total Manhour Variance		462	692	366	201	268								2,010		
Productive FTE Variance		2.61	4.52	2.19	1.30	1.76								2.48		
Total FTE Variance		2.62	3.93	2.15	1.14	1.69								2.31		
Productive Salary Variance		$9,469.74	$12,842.59	$6,225.65	$3,870.07	$4,770.04								$37,154.12		
Total Salary Variance		$9,522.00	$11,153.20	$6,112.97	$3,403.53	$4,568.63								$34,583.98		

b.

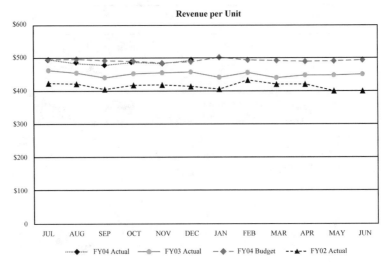

Revenue per Unit

······◆······ FY04 Actual   ─●─ FY03 Actual   ─ ◆ ─ FY04 Budget   ─ ▲ ─ FY02 Actual

c.

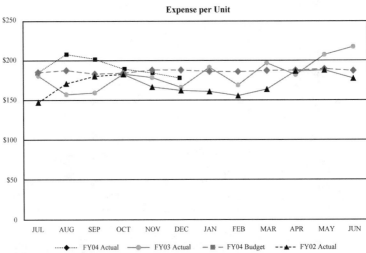

Expense per Unit

······◆······ FY04 Actual   ─●─ FY03 Actual   ─ ■ ─ FY04 Budget   ─ ▲ ─ FY02 Actual

d.

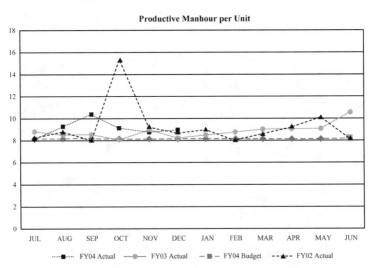

Productive Manhour per Unit

······■······ FY04 Actual   ─●─ FY03 Actual   ─ ■ ─ FY04 Budget   ─ ▲ ─ FY02 Actual

quarter of the costs, the surgical nursing costs were not separated from the total cost of the operative suite. By combining all nursing costs, it is assumed the total nursing costs would have represented a larger percentage than was presented in the study. However, the nursing costs, whether combined or separate, would continue to demonstrate a lesser percentage when compared with all other costs.

Popp et al. (2002) studied the cost of craniotomies to identify factors that affect the profitability of this procedure. The cost allocation method used was from a cost accounting system that used relative value units (RVUs) to assign actual costs. The method to determine the RVU is based on the principle used by Medicare to reimburse physicians. Under physician reimbursement, RVU is the physician's subjective judgment of the time, skill, and resource costs that are required to provide services and procedures. The usual and common time, complexity, skill, and cost are assigned an RVU of 1.0, and all other services have some value above or below this baseline. For example, a weight of 2.0 is considered to be double the work of an RVU of 1.0. By assigning RVUs to tasks, the costs were allocated to different cost centers, which included surgery, radiology, laboratory, pharmacy, anesthesia, physical therapy, rehabilitation, and room and board (nursing). Their findings also supported the research of Lester and coworkers (2001) by identifying 80% of costs for a craniotomy that were allocated into four major areas: operating room, room and board, pharmacy, and anesthesiology. In this study, room and board (nursing) contributed approximately 33% to the overall costs. From the two studies presented, the nurse manager can begin to recognize that although total nursing personnel costs are the highest cost center of a hospital, *the individual nursing unit contributes a quarter to a third of the overall cost of care for a hospitalized patient.*

Nurse Manager's Role in Cost Control

The nurse manager usually has access to information that assists with identification of global agency costs. Cost drivers that increase health care costs include salaries and wages, bad debt expense, depreciation and interest, supplies, and direct fringe benefits (**Exhibit 15–5**). Understanding the relationship of these drivers to the total operating revenue provides guidance for the nurse manager, who can identify cost areas within his or her control. The median cost per hospital discharge in 2002 was $5,619 (Nursing Leadership Academy, 2003). **Exhibit 15–6** demonstrates the contribution of each cost component to the overall total cost for one hospitalization episode.

Kane and Siegrist (2002) reported aggregated cost data for inpatient and outpatient care. *Nursing comprised 33% of the cost for outpatient and approximately 50% of the inpatient cost.* In 2002, salaries of health care workers increased by 6.1% due to workforce shortage (Carpenter, 2003). However, reimbursement rates did not increase to accommodate this increase in cost of providing care. Kane and Siegrist noted that small increases in nursing costs have a tremendous impact on the overall cost of hospitalization. The manager must be aware of this impact and plan the budget to accommodate annual performance evaluation raises.

Is the nurse manager able to control bad debt, depreciation, interest, or liability insurance? Of course not. Areas of cost the nurse manager cannot control need to be understood but are not the nurse manager's responsibility. Instead, the executive team must be concerned with these costs. Utilities, equipment expense, maintenance, and administrative costs are fixed costs that do not change as volume changes. (Of course, if the administrative team decides to take actions that decrease costs in these areas, the fixed cost amounts can change.) During the budget period the manager may be responsible for projecting these costs, or they may be supplied from the finance department. Whether the manager is given this responsibility or the fixed costs are supplied by the finance department, the manager must ensure allocations are made for unusual seasonal or billing issues that may increase or decrease the expense that has been noted by historical data (Nursing Leadership Academy, 2003).

Exhibit 15–5 Health Care Cost Drivers

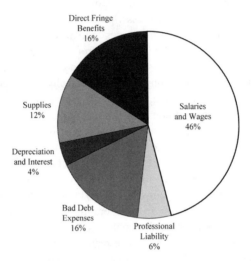

Source: The Advisory Board Company (2003). Nursing Leadership Academy. *The fundamentals of nursing finance: a foundation for financial leadership* (p. 49). (Address: Nursing Leadership Academy, The Advisory Board Company, The Watergate, 600 New Hampshire Ave NW, Washington, DC 20037 202-266-5600 202-266-5700 (fax) http://academy. advisory.com/members.

Exhibit 15–6 Allocation of Cost for One Hospitalization*

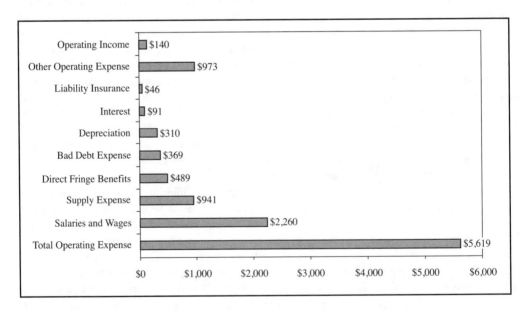

Source: The Advisory Board Company (2003). Nursing Leadership Academy. *The fundamentals of nursing finance: A foundation for financial leadership* (p. 48).

* Y axis represents direct and indirect drivers of cost. X axis represents cost of expense in whole dollars.

Exhibit 15–7 Calculation of Variable Costs

Cost per unit of service equals total variable expense divided by patient days.

($450,000 variable expense ÷ 500 patient days = $900 per patient day)

For example, fees associated with accreditation may occur only once every 2 to 3 years, and the cost of this service may be distributed among the nursing units under professional services. Another example is the expense of rental equipment such as specialty beds. The nurse manager is aware of increased use during the winter months because of the increase of ventilator patients. The astute manager, being a clinician, will not only ensure this information is supplied to finance during the budgeting processes but also will be able to provide sound rationale for the requested increased allocation.

Costs within the realm of nursing administrative control are variable costs. These costs vary in direct relationship to volume. Examples of variable costs include nursing hours, patient care supplies, pharmaceuticals, laboratory, and dietary services. Variable costs per patient day are calculated by dividing the patient days for the month into the total variable expense (Nursing Leadership Academy, 2003). Knowledge of the costs per patient day assists the nurse manager to improve control of the variation and be fiscally astute. **Exhibit 15–7** demonstrates how the nurse manager can calculate the variable (controllable) costs per patient day.

Managing Expenses with a Cost Accounting System

Under prospective payment it is crucial for the health care agency to know the exact costs of care to make responsible and accurate management decisions (Finkler, 1994). The cost of care on a nursing unit may be tracked through a financial cost accounting software system. Cost accounting software was developed after the implementation of prospective payment in the 1980s and has continued to be refined into a useful management tool (Durham, 2000). However, as Durham (2000) reported, less than 30% of health care agencies use cost accounting software because of the constant updates necessary to ensure information is current. The new manager should determine if the agency uses this technology as a means of financial assessment. If this information is available to you, then your job is to diligently manage expenses.

Exhibit 15–8 is a fictitious example of a surgical services report generated from a cost accounting system. The report is for DRG 209, which is "major joint/limb reattachment," and includes hip replacement and fractures that use orthopedic hardware. This summary provides information regarding the number of orthopedic hip surgical cases, cost per case, and hospital charge per case for the operating room for supply items. Note this report does not include personnel costs because the nurse manager only requested supplies to evaluate this area for cost-saving opportunities. For health care agencies with this type of software, the nurse manager can request a report customized to the unit and patient population.

Departmental Operations Report

What if you begin work as a new manager at an agency that does not have a cost accounting system? How do you determine the cost of care on your unit? The most efficient process is to determine the average daily census and review the departmental operations report from finance. **Exhibit 15–9** is part of a departmental operations expense report for November 20XX from nursing unit 5 North.

Exhibit 15–8 Cases/Cost/Charge Summary for DRG 209 Surgical Services

Metrics	Cases	Cost/Case	Charge/Case
Perspective Clinical Summary			
Anesthesia supplies	464	12	63
Anti-embolism hose/devices	359	96	184
Cath lab/angio supplies	1	124	234
Dialysis supplies	1	35	64
GI/Endo supplies	2	60	335
Implants ortho hardware	501	2,620	7,606
Med/surg supplies	522	2,332	9,840
Orthopedic soft goods	212	109	180
Ostomy supplies	39	6	11
Pacemaker/pacing supplies	2	57	130
Pulmonary/endo supplies	1	8	23
Respiratory supplies	494	35	190
Suction supplies	458	35	190
Urological supplies	440	24	45
TOTAL		**5,553**	**19,095**

Exhibit 15–9 Departmental Operations Expense Report

Nov 20XX 5 North	Actual	Budget	Variance	Variance%	Favorable/Unfavorable
Expenses Total	87,121	106,305	−19,184	−18	F
Per unit	229.27	212.61	16.66	7.8	U

How do you, the new manager, analyze this information? This is shown in **Exhibit 15–10**. The actual and budgeted average daily census can be calculated by dividing the actual or budget expenses total amount by the actual or budget per unit amount. The actual average daily census (this might also be called the average patient volume per day) was 12.7, whereas the budget had projected an average daily census of 16.7 patients. Although the total expenses were 18% less than budgeted (−18% variance that was favorable), the cost per individual patient was higher by 7.8% (7.8% variance that was unfavorable). The contributors of these variances may be linked to employee costs, supply costs, and how overhead is allocated to the department. The manager would need to investigate each possible contributing factor to identify opportunities to reduce expenses or to explain the variation that may in fact be due to a higher patient acuity requiring increased nursing staff to provide safe, good quality care.

Now, what if you do not have an operations report? Unfortunately, in many health care organizations costing does not take place at this level of detail. A usual mode of practice is to examine the

---

Exhibit 15–10 Calculation of Average Daily Census from Departmental Expense Report

Actual Expenses Total ÷ Actual Expenses Per Unit ÷ 30 (days in the month)
  = Actual Average Daily Census

  $87,121 ÷ $229.27 ÷ 30 = 12.7 Actual Average Daily Census

Budget Expenses ÷ Budget Expenses Per Unit ÷ 30 (days in the month)
  = Budgeted Average Total Daily Census

  $106,305 ÷ $212.61 ÷ 30 = 16.66 Budgeted Average Daily Census

---

Exhibit 15–11 Comparison of Revenue and Costs of Two Strategic Service Units

Strategic Service Unit	Revenue (actual)	Departmental Cost (actual)	Variance	Variance%	Favorable/ Unfavorable
Cardiology	$706,313	$650,980	$55,333	8.5%	F
Women's Health	$325,987	$309,687	-$16,299	5%	U

---

overall bottom line for the organization or to examine costing of a major service, represented by a product line or group of designated cost centers (i.e., cardiology or women's health). Here, the total reimbursement is compared with the total expenditures. In this case, if there is an over expenditure for one group of patients or services, there needs to be a savings accrued by another group of patients or services because the overall goal is that the bottom line is "in the black" (**Exhibit 15–11**).

The problem with this method is that *the organization may not be aware that one service is losing money and another service is saving money.* Using the hospital example, one DRG may be delivered over cost (losing money), whereas another DRG is costing less than the DRG (profit). So in a time when the reimbursements are not what were anticipated, services may be asked to cut equally, yet services for one DRG has been efficient whereas another has not. The nurse manager, working with the nurse executive, can use these data as an argument as to why cuts should not apply to the unit(s) coming in under costs. The following DRG examples are used to further explain actual costs and reimbursement.

DRG Costing Examples

Let's examine a hospital DRG to determine whether we are spending more or less than the reimbursement amount to provide the specified service. You are a hospital nurse manager/director/nurse executive responsible for an orthopedic cost center. A typical service provided on this cost center is DRG 209: Major Joint/Limb Reattachment Procedure, Low Extremities—No Complications (for Total Hip Replacement) and the Medicare reimbursement for this DRG is $9,269. Do you actually know how much you are expending to provide that DRG?

In this particular DRG there is a further complication: The costs of the prosthesis and direct supplies needed to do the total hip replacement may expend over 50% of the reimbursement dollars. So the amount of money left to provide all other services this patient requires from admission to discharge must be low enough to stay within approximately 50% ($4,600) of the reimbursement amount. The question then is whether the service provided to a patient utilizing DRG 209 is less than $4,600. Or, in providing that service, is the service cost above that amount? If the latter is true, the organization is losing money on each patient having a total hip replacement. *With profit margins as tight as they currently are in health care, it is very important that the nurse manager—as well as the executive team—know actual costs of the services provided.*

Using the total hip replacement example, figuring out costs is further complicated because the reimbursement amount includes services and supplies delivered from several cost centers (i.e., operating room, laboratory, pharmacy, radiology, physical therapy, and orthopedic inpatient unit). So if the orthopedic nurse manager is working on the cost of this DRG, other cost center managers need to provide their departmental costs of service assigned to each hip replacement patient to calculate the total DRG cost.

The following provides a specific example to demonstrate a case scenario for a patient admitted for a total hip replacement.

Jill Anderson is a 78-year-old woman with severe degenerative arthritis of the right hip. She has been evaluated by the orthopedic surgeon who recommends a total hip replacement. Ms. Anderson agrees to the surgery and is scheduled for the procedure 1 week from the office visit. **Exhibit 15–12** is a representation of the hospital costs incurred for a 3-day length of stay for a total hip replacement (DRG 209).

As the manager can see, the cost of providing this service is greater than the reimbursement by $1,668 ($10,937 actual cost – $9,269 reimbursement = $1,668 actual loss), and an average case load of 500 total hips for the year would cost the hospital $834,000. This scenario is supported by Clancy et al. (1998), who concluded a loss of approximately $1,000 per patient occurred for DRG 209 and 210.

How can this procedure be profitable for the hospital? First, the interdisciplinary team must work aggressively to transfer the patient to another level of care, such as skilled care, as soon as medically indicated. The hospital also generates additional revenue from the other services the orthopedic surgeon orders for the patient, such as the surgical procedure, outpatient radiology studies, outpatient physical therapy, and referrals to a skilled nursing unit housed within the facility. By standardization of the hip prosthesis being used, the hospital can negotiate a contract with a supplier to be the vendor of choice and thereby decrease costs. Also, the hospital may opt to purchase a prosthesis that costs less money. In addition, the volume of patients can be an important factor. We know

---

Exhibit 15–12 Costs for DRG 209 Total Hip Replacement

Day	Med surg	OR	Pharmacy	Pharmacy IV	Implants	Pathology	Lab	Supplies	Blood	Physical Therapy	TOTAL
1 (Adm)	480	2,800	253	120	4,600	54	380	217	175	0	9,079
2	480		384				32			175	1,071
3	480		64				21			126	691
4 (D/C)			22	42			32				96
Total	**1,440**	**2,800**	**723**	**162**	**4,600**	**54**	**465**	**217**	**175**	**301**	**10,937**

that excellent patient satisfaction leads to the patient using the facility as his or her hospital of choice. As the manager can see, many global issues are reviewed by management in deciding to provide a service line.

Now, let's take the same patient admitted to the skilled nursing unit. As you recall, the skilled units are reimbursed by RUGs consisting of the costs for administration, room and board, nursing service, and therapy services. The length of stay on the skilled unit for Ms. Anderson is 11 days.

Ms. Anderson's RUG category is "ultra high" because her admission assessment indicated her need for nursing care, physical therapy, and occupational therapy (U.S. General Accounting Office, 2002). In the ultra high category, therapy must demonstrate Ms. Anderson received a total of 720 minutes of services in 7 days (Medicare SNF-PPS Indices, 2003). The reimbursement and cost for the ultra high category is noted in **Exhibit 15–13**. As you can see, the skilled care facility is losing $800 per day of care and services provided to Ms. Anderson. In addition, as her therapy and nursing care requirements decrease as she improves, the reimbursement also decreases. After her 7-day assessment, the reimbursement for her care decreases to $296.15 per day.

How does a health care agency afford to care for patients like Ms. Anderson? Van der Walde and Lindstrom (2003) report that freestanding skilled nursing facilities have fewer Medicare and more private pay patients, whereas a skilled nursing facility in an acute care facility admits a higher percentage of Medicare patients. As their report indicates, the freestanding skilled nursing facilities are profitable, whereas skilled nursing facilities in an acute care setting are not profitable. Many hospitals have closed their skilled nursing facilities because of the continued financial drain on the agency.

The next two examples demonstrate costs and reimbursement for a home health and same-day surgery patient. As you recall, home health came under prospective payment in October 2000 and outpatient surgery also began to be reimbursed by APCs in 2000. The following case scenario was provided by a home health manager as an exhibition of the reality of home care.

Mr. Harold James is a 78-year-old diabetic, hypertensive, African American with new onset atrial fibrillation and survived a right hemispheric stroke (DRG 14). His deficits include left hemiparesis and speech difficulties, and he is discharged from a skilled nursing facility to home with a home health referral. Home health skilled nursing care will include medication management for diabetes and anticoagulation in addition to medication education. The following additional services will be used: physical therapy three times a week, speech therapy twice a week, and certified nursing assistant visits three times a week. As Mr. James continues to improve, the certified nursing assistant visits will be discontinued and occupational therapy will begin services three times a week. Medicare covers 60 days of home health service, and a total of 66 home visits will be made during the 60-day period (www.cms.hhs.gov/manuals/102-policy/bp102c07).

Exhibit 15–13 RUG III Reimbursement for Ultra High Level of Care

Category	Nursing Care	OT, PT, Speech	Room, Board, and Administration	Total Rate per Day
Ultra high*	$142.32	$186.01	$55.88	$384.21
Actual costs	$444.03	$574.30	$165.77	$1,184.10
Difference	−$301.71	−$388.29	−$109.89	−$799.89

* Difference in RUG rates obtained from http://www.cms.gov/providers/snfpps/snfpps_rates.asp. Actual costs calculated from historical data from a skilled nursing facility.

Because home health for this patient is primarily labor intensive, the manager can predict the cost of care by calculating the salaries and benefits for each team member, adding supplies and overhead, then multiplying by number of visits, and finally multiplying this number by two (average hours spent in the home by each caregiver). **Exhibit 15–14** demonstrates this calculation.

Under prospective payment, our patient reimbursement is $6,098. Because the total cost for Mr. James is $6,428.80, the agency will lose $330.80 for this patient (i.e., $6,428.80 [total cost] − $6,098 [reimbursement] = $330.80). For this reason, many home health agencies have limited the complex cases they enroll in their service (van der Walde & Choi, 2003b).

The home health manager is also faced with the issue of the short-term home health admission. For example, a new diabetic may be ordered to receive home health visits for teaching. The visits are limited to three. The cost of admitting the patient to the service is $200 due to the time and intensity of the assessment as well as completion of OASIS. Our previous calculation indicates the cost of the two remaining visits (plus supplies of $25) is $155.10. The payer reimburses only $90 for each visit ($270 total), and the agency again loses $85.10. Although the manager may believe this is a small amount, over time the agency will not be self-sustaining due to losses from complex patients and short-term admissions. Therefore the home health manager must be creative and identify areas of savings such as decreasing supply costs that are not reimbursable and set budget expenditures based on historical data that provide insight into payer reimbursements, as well as the types of patients admitted to the agency.

The same-day surgery patient, under the PPS, receives services reimbursed by APC codes. These are based on RVUs, which are a measure of time and resources that are bundled into 1 of the 750 assigned categories (van der Walde & Choi, 2002). Many outpatient services have benefited from the APC process of reimbursement, more so from the private payers than Medicare. **Exhibit 15–15** shows a comparison of costs and reimbursement for a same-day surgery laparoscopic cholecystectomy. The first example is a 42-year-old woman with private insurance, and the second is a 70-year-old man with Medicare.

From the previous example, the manager has an understanding that the private insurance carriers truly offset the cost of caring for the Medicare patient. The manager, knowledgeable of payer mix, can determine the financial feasibility of the service that is provided by the same-day surgery facility.

Other Factors Contributing to Reimbursement

Reimbursement is a complex issue. The information provided earlier in the chapter is from a broad perspective and can be generalized to health care agencies. Medicare participants are the largest users

---

Exhibit 15–14 Projection of Home Health Care Costs for 60 Days of Care

Salary/hr × benefits (20%) + supplies + overhead × no. visits × average time/visit = costs

RN costs	= ($18.79/hr × 0.2)	+ $37.45	+ $30	× 12	× 2	=	$2,160.00
PT costs	= ($19.50 × 0.2)	+ $0	+ $30	× 16	× 2	=	$1,708.80
CNA costs	= ($8.50 × 0.2)	+ $20.00	+ $30	× 16	× 2	=	$1,926.40
OT costs	= ($19.00 × 0.2)	+ $0	+ $30	× 6	× 2	=	$633.60
Total costs	=						$6,428.80

CNA, certified nursing assistant; OT, occupational therapy; PT, physical therapy; RN, registered nurse.

Exhibit 15–15 Same Day Surgery Cost and Reimbursement for Laparoscopic Cholecystectomy

51.23 Laparoscopic cholecystectomy	Charge code units (RVU)	Charges	Actual payment	Total Direct Costs	Total Indirect Costs	Total Cost
Private Insurance						
1662 Anesthesia	9	$1,658		$240	$77	$317
1665 Same day surgery	29	$4,514		$1,140	$927	$2067
1710 Central supply	6	$264		$131	$34	$165
1715 Pharmacy	12	$352		$96	$21	$117
1720 Pathology	1	$175		$12	$9	$21
1722 Lab	3	$91		$16	$6	$22
TOTAL Private Insurance	**60**	**$7,054**	**$4,573**	**$1,635**	**$1,074**	**$2,709**
Medicare Patient						
1662 Anesthesia	7	$1,384		$201	$64	$265
1665 Same day surgery	28	$4,546		$1,065	$866	$1,931
1710 Central supply	5	$255		$126	$33	$159
1715 Pharmacy	16	$469		$127	$28	$155
1722 Lab	5	$135		$26	$11	$37
TOTAL Medicare Payment	**61**	**$6,789**	**$1,767**	**$1,545**	**$1,002**	**$2,547**

of health care services. In this section additional information is provided that contributes to Medicare reimbursement. The nurse manager can retrieve this information, in addition to the annual market basket updated fees for Medicare reimbursement, from the CMS website (http://www.cms.gov).

Operating payments are additional payments to the base DRG reimbursement and vary from large urban (population over 1 million) to other urban and rural hospitals. In 2009 the reimbursement rate for hospitals will be tied to their quality performance (CMS, 2008). For example, hospitals that have reported successful quality measures for 2008 will receive 3% increase in reimbursement. Those hospitals that do not report successful quality measures will receive only a 1% increase in reimbursement. These amounts are adjusted for the area market basket update.

St. Mercy Example

The following example demonstrates how the operating expense is added into the DRG payment for St. Mercy, a large urban hospital. Capital payments are made for a portion of capital expenditures and are adjusted also according to the local wage index. For fiscal year 2008 the large urban capital payment rate was $413, whereas it was $417 for other hospitals. Calculation of capital payments is the same as in steps 1 and 2 shown in Boxes 15–1 and 15–2 so that 70% of the reimbursement amount is allocated to labor costs and 30% to nonlabor expense; the area wage index of 1.2015 remains the same.

Step 1: *Standardized reimbursement rate for fiscal year 2002 = $4,157*
           (The labor expense is 70%, or $2,910, and 30%, or $1,247, is allocated to nonlabor expense.)

Step 2: *The labor-related portion is multiplied by the area wage index (1.2045) and added to the nonlabor expense:*

           $2,910 × 1.2045 = $3,505

           $3,505 + $1,247 = $4,752

Step 3: *The wage index adjusted amount is now multiplied by the RW (relative weight) of the DRG:*

           DRG 14 (stroke) RW = 1.2065

           $4,752 × 1.2065 = $5,733 (federal rate)

The amount paid to this hospital is $5,733 for DRG 14. However, this is not the ultimate payment.

Step 1: *Capital payment for fiscal year 2002 = $402*
           (The labor expense is 70%, or $281, and 30%, or $121, is allocated to nonlabor expense.)

Step 2: *The labor-related portion is multiplied by the area wage index (1.2045) and added to the nonlabor expense:*

           $281 × 1.2045 = $338

           $338 + $121 = $459

Step 3: *The wage index adjusted amount is now multiplied by the RW (relative weight) of the DRG:*

           DRG 14 RW = 1.2065

           $459 × 1.2065 = $554 (capital payment rate)

The capital payment rate ($554) is added to the federal rate ($5,733) and the reimbursement increases to $6,287:

           $5,733 + $554 = $6,287

Now what if St. Mercy is affiliated with a medical school? Additional dollars are allocated to St. Mercy based on direct medical education (DME) and indirect medical education (IME) to underwrite the higher costs associated with resident training (van der Walde & Choi, 2002). The amount for DME and IME was established in the 1980s and has increased in proportion to inflationary factors. In addition, the amount allocated depends on the number of residents assigned to the facility. With only 1,154 teaching hospitals participating in Medicare, calculation of this amount is left to the finance and education department of those facilities and is not discussed here.

Another component of reimbursement is based on the hospital providing care for the low-income and indigent patient. Hospitals with low-income and indigent care that exceed 15% of their volume are eligible for additional reimbursement and are called "disproportionate share hospitals" (DSH).

Hospitals caring for a large number of Medicaid patients are also noted to have a higher than average indigent patient and uncompensated care population. The DSH program was initiated through the Boren Amendment of the Omnibus Budget Reconciliation Acts of 1980 and 1981 (Coughlin & Liska, 1997). Through this legislation, states that demonstrated high Medicaid enrollment are eligible for federal financial participation dollars. These funds are then given to hospitals that qualify as a DSH provider. The DSH payment is greater than the cost of care for the Medicaid population, so hospitals receive some reimbursement for indigent and uncompensated care. (For more information go to http://www.cms.hhs.gov/MLNProducts/downloads/2008_mdsh.pdf and http://www.gpoaccess.gov/cfr/index.html)

> *Disproportionate share threshold (%) =*
>
> $$\frac{Medicare\ patients\ eligible\ for\ SSI}{Medicare\ inpatient\ days} + \frac{Medicaid\ inpatient\ days}{Total\ acute\ inpatient\ days}$$

The most common additional reimbursement the nurse manager will experience is called *outlier payments*. As you recall, under prospective payment the DRG payments are based on the average cost per case. For the extreme cases of patients with complex disease processes that incur higher costs than the average, Medicare makes additional payments to decrease the hospital's financial burden for caring for this type of patient (van der Walde & Choi, 2002). The outlier payment is calculated by the CCR (discussed earlier in the chapter). To qualify for an outlier payment, the cost must exceed the DRG payment and a threshold is established each year by the CMS (van der Walde & Choi, 2002). CMS then pays 80% of the costs of the case that is in excess of the DRG and the established threshold.

The following is an example of an outlier payment for our hospital, St. Mercy, for a patient discharged with a primary diagnosis of DRG 286—resection of a pituitary tumor. The patient developed complications and incurred hospital charges of over $90,000 with the assigned DRG payment being only $15,200. The Medicare fixed loss threshold for 2003 is $33,560. From this information we calculate the expected reimbursement. The calculations used to determine base reimbursement used in this example are adopted from the appendix of van der Walde and Choi (2002).

This complicated process of calculating outlier payment is done by the Medicare financial intermediary when a facility requests payment for outlier cases. Why is this important for the nurse manager to know? The manager needs to monitor outlier patients and ensure appropriate reimbursement is sought. Without this knowledge, outlier payments may not be sought and the nursing unit is out of budgetary compliance and the organization loses money.

> *Step 1:*   *The provider cost-to-charge ratio (CCR) is 0.78 with 0.72 allocated to operations and 0.06 for capital costs*
>
> *Billed charges = $90,000 × 0.72 = $64,800 (operating costs)*
>
> *Billed charges = $90,000 × 0.06 = $5,400 (capital costs)*
>
> *Total case costs = $64,800 + $5,400 = $70,200*
>
> *Case cost is greater than the assigned:*
>
> *$15,200 (DRG payment) + $33,506 (fixed loss threshold) = $48,706*

continued

Step 2:   *Calculate the DRG payment*

Labor expense = $15,200 (DRG payment) × 0.7 (operations CCR) = $10,640 for labor expenses

Nonlabor expense = $15,200 (DRG payment) × 0.3
= $4,560 for nonlabor expenses

Multiply wage index of 1.2045 for labor: $10,640 labor expenses × 1.2045
= $12,816 labor expenses

Add labor and nonlabor: $12,816 + $4,560 = $17,376 operating expenses

Multiply by relative weight $17,376 × 1.32 = $22,936 total expected DRG reimbursement

Capital payment = $402

Adjusted = $402 × 0.7 = $281 (from labor expenses) × 1.2045 (wage adjustment)
= $339 (total labor expenses) + $121 (nonlabor expenses)
= $459 (total capital payment)

Multiply total capital payment by capital payment rate:
$459 × 1.32 = $606 total capital payment

Add the total expected DRG reimbursement to the total capital payment:
$22,936 + $606 = $23,542 adjusted DRG payment

Step 3:   *Calculate outlier payment which is 80% of the difference between DRG payment and the Medicare fixed-loss threshold*

$33,560 (fixed loss threshold) − $23,542 (adjusted DRG payment)
= $10,018 × 0.8 = $8,014 outlier payment

Step 4:   *Calculate full DRG payment + outlier payment*

$23,542 + $8,014 = $31,538 full payment

Revenue Budget

NURSING SERVICE DOES GENERATE REVENUE

In the health care organization—whether hospital, long-term care, home care, or ambulatory settings—nursing services provide organizational revenue. If you are a nurse manager on an inpatient unit, you may hear a finance employee say your unit does not generate revenue. Technically, on an inpatient unit you probably do not have a revenue account—unless you have oncology services, operating room, or a service that can be directly billed. Instead, nursing services on inpatient units are most often included in the room rate charge, and the finance department keeps the records of revenues. However, nursing care does generate and contribute to the revenue generation for the DRG payment in hospitals and for the minimum data set (MDS) reimbursement, or for other payments, in long-term care. In this example, revenue becomes muddy because so many disciplines are involved in the patient's care. Remember that patients always come to inpatient units because they need nursing care. Nursing services have traditionally been directly billed in home care as a separate line item. Two states, Maine and Maryland, have recognized nursing's contributions and have specified that hospitals take nursing service out of the room rate charge and list it as a separate item on the patient's bill. This could mean that more inpatient units will be considered profit centers and have a revenue budget.

There may be other services or items that can be directly billed, such as operating room procedures, ambulatory services, home care services, drugs, supplies, educational programs, physical or respiratory therapy, consultation services, or wellness programs. In these programs, nurse managers usually have a revenue budget, often called a profit center (profit centers were explained in Chapter 12). In this case, the cost center's services are directly billed to patients. In these settings the revenue budget is used to make sure that the organization/department/clinic remains viable.

Currently, revenues are reported only occasionally on inpatient cost center budgets. If this occurs, the nurse manager must seek information to learn what these figures represent: Are they billed dollars or are these dollars actually received? Are contractual allowances or discounts included in the revenue figures? Is the figure so unreliable that the nurse manager should just ignore it, or does it provide useful data?

When the nurse manager gets a revenue report for billable supplies or services, most often provided by the finance department, the nurse manager should check the accuracy of the figures and then compare costs and revenue. **Exhibit 15–16** is an example of a detailed nursing unit operations report that includes revenues for inpatient and outpatient sources. Revenue in this type of financial report does not equal true reimbursement but is a CCR that is used in the *Medicare Cost Report.* The manager can also note from this report the distribution of payers for the department.

Exhibit 15–16 Monthly Nursing Departmental Revenue Report by Payer

	Actual*	Budget	5 North Nov-0_ Variance	Variance %	Favorable/ Unfavorable
INPATIENT REVENUE					
Medicare	167,519	282,683	−115,164	−40.7	U
Medicaid	22,050	34,802	−12,752	−36.6	U
Managed care	29,578	44,515	−14,937	−33.6	U
Commercial	15,004	9,237	5,767	62.4	F
Self-pay	27,293	5,294	21,999	415.5	F
Other	2,406	3,368	−962	−28.6	U
Total	**263,850**	**379,899**	**−116,049**	**−30.5**	U
per unit	782.94	796.43	−14	−1.7	U
OUTPATIENT REVENUE					
Medicare	16,254	9,624	6,630	68.9	F
Medicaid	5,044	3,994	1,050	26.3	F
Managed care	3,388	6,913	−3,525	−51.0	U
Commercial	627	1,031	−404	−39.2	U
Self-pay	1,533	587	946	161.2	F
Other	627	165	462	280.0	F
Total	**27,473**	**22,314**	**5,159**	**23.1**	F
per unit	639	970	−331	−34.1	U
REVENUE TOTAL	**291,323**	**402,213**	**−110,890**	**−27.6**	U
per unit	767	804	−38	−4.7	U

* The *Actual* column represents gross revenue times the ratio of costs to charges from the Medicare/Medicaid report.

How is this information interpreted? The first column provides the payer source followed by the CCR. Following the reimbursement are the budgeted dollars expected to be collected. The next column is the variance between actual CCR and what was budgeted, or actual – budgeted = variance. Percent variance follows next. This is the percent deviation between the actual column and the budgeted column. The last column shows whether the variance is favorable (F) or unfavorable (U). As you can tell from this report, the revenue total for both in- and outpatient is below the budgeted amount at an unfavorable 4.7%.

The nurse manager must seek information to explain the variation from budget. For this unit, two areas were identified as reasons for the budget variation. First, the census was lower than expected by the budgeted amount, and second, there was decreased reimbursement from contractual agreements that went into effect in the previous month of October. Although nursing management cannot directly impact contractual agreements, nursing does have a strong influence on the census through providing high-quality, safe care the patient and family value as well as by building a trusting relationship with physicians, patients, colleagues, and others in the organization. When everyone acts as an effective team, magic happens.

However, this variance is only a piece of the information the nurse manager has to consider. The manager must also compare the same period last year as well as the year-to-date financials to have the total picture of the unit financial performance. **Exhibit 15–17** provides the fiscal year-to-date financial information for 5 North. This nursing unit is generating 5.2% less than budgeted revenue for the fiscal year to date.

The challenge now is for the nurse manager to be knowledgeable not only of employee and supply expense but also the unit's primary admission and diagnoses, length of stay, complication rates, and reimbursement per DRG. Another area that impacts the financial performance of a nursing unit is the contractual agreements made between the hospital financial management team, a managed care organization, and a preferred price for supplies based on utilization.

The manager should review the DRG historical admission and discharge history of the unit. Then, the nurse manager can evaluate the unit patient population and identify trends or changes in patient base that may require an expansion of nursing knowledge and skills. In addition, the manager should ask for the following information: length of stay by discharge diagnosis, list of secondary diagnosis, and complications. An analysis of this information will guide the manager to identify areas for improving care to decrease complications (which are costly and are not reimbursed), improve efficiency, decrease supply and manpower costs, and thereby improve the financial performance of the nursing unit.

Contractual agreements are negotiations between the health care agency and the health insurer or provider of services and supplies. Contracts may range from the amount paid by the insurer for a specific diagnosis to the amount of supply charges based on utilization. The nurse manager does not have control over contract negotiations but plays a significant role in providing information regarding changes in patient care that influence negotiated reimbursement or prices. In addition, the nurse manager must be aware of the dates of contract renewals to recognize shortfalls during the budget planning process.

Exhibit 15–17 demonstrates an example of how changes in patient payers and contractual agreements impact the nursing units' budget. In this example, Medicare admissions decreased, private insurance decreased contractual reimbursement, and there was an increase in self-pay patients, which often contributes to indigent care services. The key factor that cannot be seen in the example is that the private insurance contract negotiations occurred after the budget had been set and a lower reimbursement was negotiated by management as a means to increase patient volume by this carrier. The manager needs to continually evaluate admissions by payer to identify if the negotiated contract actually increased admissions for the nursing unit.

Exhibit 15–17 Year-to-Date (YTD) Nursing Department Revenue Report by Payer

	Actual*	5 North Budget	FYTD Variance	Nov-0_ Variance %	Favorable/ Unfavorable
INPATIENT REVENUE					
Medicare	1,120,051	1,358,542	−238,491	−17.6	U
Medicaid	205,504	167,253	37,801	22.6	F
Managed care	141,956	213,932	−71,976	−33.6	U
Commercial	67,857	44,392	23,465	52.9	F
Self-pay	50,315	25,440	24,875	97.8	F
Other	12,824	16,187	−3,363	−20.8	U
Total	**1,598,507**	**1,825,746**	**−227,689**	**−12.5**	**U**
per unit	**798.63**	**796.23**	**2.40**	**0.3**	**F**
OUTPATIENT REVENUE					
Medicare	88,162	47,653	40,509	85.0	F
Medicaid	18,805	19,776	−971	−4.9	U
Managed care	32,321	34,229	−1,908	−5.6	U
Commercial	3,615	5,106	−1,491	−29.2	U
Self-pay	5,451	2,907	2,544	87.5	F
Other	4,117	817	3,300	403.9	F
Total	**152,471**	**110,488**	**41,983**	**38.0**	**F**
per unit	**520.38**	**977.77**	**−457.39**	**−46.8**	**U**
REVENUE TOTAL	**1,750,978**	**1,936,234**	**−185,706**	**−9.6**	**U**
per unit	**763.09**	**804.75**	**−41.66**	**−5.2**	**U**

* The *Actual* column represents gross revenue times the ratio of costs to charges from the Medicare/Medicaid report.

Predicting Financial Success

The case mix index has been used by hospital administrators to predict financial success since prospective payment was instituted by Medicare (Adams, 1996). The nurse manager can use this tool to predict financial success at the nursing unit level. DRGs are divided into 25 major diagnostic categories (MDC) that include the following information: DRG number, narrative description, relative weight, geometric length of stay, arithmetic length of stay, and outlier threshold. The relative weight is an assigned number that is an indicator of the amount of resources needed to care for the patient with that particular disease process and includes all costs related to the hospitalization (Adams, 1996). The nurse manager should understand that the higher the weight, the more resources needed to care for the patient. The amount of resources needed to treat a particular disease process is the relative weight. A disease requiring many resources, such as total joint replacement, carries a higher weight than atypical chest pain. Using the DRG relative weight, a simple calculation can be used to determine reimbursement for a specific DRG.

> *DRG relative weight × hospital payment rate = reimbursement*
>
> *DRG 209 with relative weight of 2.2707 × $4,240.54 = $9,629*

The case mix index is an average relative weight over a period of time that indicates the patient's acuity and is used to determine reimbursement from Medicare and Medicaid for all patients admitted to the hospital. Adams (1996, p. 31) uses the following example to demonstrate how the case mix index impacts the overall reimbursement for a six-bed nursing unit:

Doe, John	DRG 89	RW [relative weight] 1.1211
Jones, James	DRG 143	RW 0.5159
Smith, Jane	DRG 127	RW 1.0302
Thomas, Harold	DRG 183	RW 0.5480
Williams, Timothy	DRG 140	RW 0.6312
Young, Mary	DRG 14	RW 1.2065
Total patients: 6	Total weights: 5.0529	CMI = 0.8422

To calculate the reimbursement for the unit, the nurse manager needs to obtain the Medicare median hospital payment rate. Then, this rate is multiplied by the case mix index to get the total expected reimbursement rate for the unit. For example, say the reimbursement rate is $5,200. The total number of patients admitted to the unit for the week equaled six and the case mix index is 0.8422:

> *$5,200 × 0.8422 × 6 = $26,277 (rounded to the nearest whole dollar)*

From this information, as well as knowledge of supply costs and personnel expense, the nurse manager can be proactive in departmental financial management. Further, the nurse manager can alert the nurse executive and finance department about important reimbursement issues (i.e., lost revenues, higher expenses than revenues, etc.). In addition to the case mix index, the nurse manager must realize the hospital's DRG payment rate is also contingent on geographic location, wage index, and patient mix.

The nurse manager should obtain the top 10 DRGs for the nursing unit from the coding department (usually located in Medical Records) and then use the above formula to estimate the reimbursement, and multiply by the number of discharges by DRG for the month or year. This estimates the expected reimbursement. By knowing this information, the manager can influence reimbursement on the unit by assisting staff and physicians to document thoroughly for accurate coding. This then will increase the case mix index (Adams, 1996). The manager may choose to select one DRG that is costing more than the reimbursement, establish a multidisciplinary team to evaluate processes of care that may impact patient outcomes and increase cost, and strategize to determine less costly ways to deliver the care safely and efficiently.

Nursing Management Decisions Impact Financial Outcomes

The nurse manager must be cognizant of unit expenses, including personnel and supplies. These are two key areas that nursing can affect to ensure a positive bottom line. The flow of patients into and out of a service area determines the staffing and supplies needed. Nursing must have financial savvy and be creative to manage within this environment.

In long-term care, reimbursement for Medicaid patients is actually determined by the nurse and depends on how well the nurse has completed the MDS.[6] In addition, the PPS for Medicare exposed the long-term care facilities to an adjusted case mix index (Weech-Maldonado, Neff, & Mor, 2003) as had been done in acute care for many years.

Usually, to accomplish a detailed evaluation of cost versus reimbursement, the nurse manager can facilitate an interdisciplinary management team to determine and compare actual costs of the services provided with the reimbursement amount received for those services. The organization and participation in such a team can help all disciplines within the organization to become cognizant of the importance of rectifying systems problems that can contribute significantly to higher costs if left unidentified and unresolved.

Summary

Cost and reimbursement issues are difficult to understand, because there are many different aspects of how costs are calculated and which payer is paying what amount. Hopefully, this chapter has assisted the manager to have an improved understanding of fiscal management for the nursing unit or department and deems him- or herself as the chief executive officer and chief financial officer of his or her area, now recognizing the power of the position in determining successful patient outcomes and a positive bottom line. Note that this chapter is concerned only with assisting the nurse manager in the financial aspects, not with other quality and ethical factors involved.

Useful Web sites

The Center for Medicare and Medicaid Services http://www.cms.hhs.gov
Social Security Online http://www.socialsecurity.gov
The Urban Institute http://www.urban.org
Agency for Healthcare Research and Quality http://www.ahrq.gov
U.S. Department of Health and Human Services http://www.dhhs.gov
The Henry J. Kaiser Family Foundation http://www/kff.org
Select Quality Care Library (SQC Library) http://www.selectqualitycare.com

Discussion Questions

1. This chapter discusses the need for an interdisciplinary team approach. Why is this important? Which specific areas/departments should be involved?
2. What is a cost-to-charge ratio? Why should a nurse manager understand this ratio and how would he or she use it?
3. What challenge does a unit that provides care for special needs patients have in costing out its service?
4. Why do freestanding skilled nursing facilities function more profitably than skilled nursing facilities in acute care facilities?
5. What source is available for the nurse manager to identify reimbursement for Medicare and Medicaid patients?
6. Finance departments regard nursing units as not being revenue generators. Why do you believe they are inaccurate in their assessment?

---

[6] For more detailed information on the MDS see Dunham-Taylor and Pinczuk (2006).

7. If you were part of the contract agreement negotiations with insurers, what specific contributions would you be able to provide for appropriate reimbursement for services?
8. This chapter hopes to improve your understanding of fiscal management. In your opinion, which factor covered in this chapter would you consider most critical?

Glossary of Terms

Balanced Scorecard and Activity-Based Costing (ABC)—this ratio is more closely aligned with the true costs of caring for the patient. Activity-based costing methodology also resembles performance improvement methods as processes and outcomes are evaluated. The complexity of "procedures and tests involved, the intensity of nursing care, the duration of an activity, and the intricacies of operative and postoperative care" identify the true costs. In this method, all areas and processes of patient interaction are identified and costs are allocated to the activity center. The balanced scorecard adds the quality dimension to cost and reimbursement data. For instance, cost drivers outside the system, such as patient satisfaction, can be measured and reflected in the overall scorecard.

Capitation—mechanism used by insurers to contain costs by establishing a set payment amount for a population served by a defined health care service. Rates are negotiated between the provider and the insurer under a contractual agreement for a year. Reimbursement rates may be for all services offered or for one specific service area, called a "carve out," such as laboratory.

Charges—determined by the allocation of costs to the revenue-producing centers and then projecting an amount needed to recover all the costs.

"Costing" a Service—the interdisciplinary team needs to be able to figure *all the actual costs expended* to provide a specified service. This costing exercise should take place for all major services provided within the health care organization.

Costs—determined by the organization's financial accounting system, which takes into account actual costs of supplies, manpower, facility, and administration for services provided

Cost-to-Charge Ratio (CCR)—a ratio determined by dividing the costs by the charges. A ratio under 1.0 (equal costs and charges) is positive and indicates that the organization is making money on the service. A ratio over 1.0 indicates the organization is experiencing a loss—the costs are more than the charges (expected reimbursement). The report is required for all Medicare-certified hospitals, skilled nursing facilities, home health agencies, and renal facilities. The nurse manager should be aware that CCR could lead to misrepresentation of cost when evaluating the profitability of a service.

Operating Payments—additional payments to the base DRG reimbursement that vary from large urban (population over one million) to other urban and rural hospitals. In 2009 the reimbursement rate for hospitals will be tied to their quality performance (CMS, 2008). These amounts are adjusted for the area market basket update.

Outlier Payments—under prospective payment the DRG payments are based on the average cost per case. For extreme cases of patients with complex disease processes that incur higher costs than the average, Medicare will make additional payments to decrease the hospital's financial burden for caring for this type of patient. The outlier payment is calculated by the CCR. To qualify for an outlier payment, the cost must exceed the DRG payment and a threshold is established each year by the CMS. CMS will then pay 80% of the costs of the case that is in excess of the DRG and the established threshold.

Payment—amount the health care agency receives for the services provided. All payers pay differing amounts for the same service depending on the type of payer and the contractual agreement between the agency and the insurer.

Per Diem Approach—a ratio where the indirect costs are divided by the number of patient days to determine per diem costs and then allocates the indirect cost equally to all nursing units. This method considers all patients the same regardless of intensity of care. The indirect costs are distributed equally to the units when the per diem method of cost allocation is used. This means the departmental operations report for the obstetric unit and the cardiovascular intensive care unit will have the same dollar amount for indirect expenses even though the obstetric unit had fewer patient days.

Projection of Reimbursement—calculated by a payment-to-cost ratio that indicates the percent of costs that are covered by reimbursement.

Volume-Based Measures—a ratio where the indirect costs are assigned according to the volume (which may be visits, admissions, nursing hours per patient day) or machine hours (in radiology and the laboratory).

References

Adams, T. (1996). Case mix index: Nursing's new management tool. *Nursing Management, 27*(9), 31–32.

Carpenter, D. (2003). Soaring spending: No sign of a slowdown. *H & HN: Hospitals and Healthcare Networks, 77*, 16–17.

Centers for Medicare and Medicaid Services [CMS]. (2008). Proposed fiscal year 2009 payment policy changes for inpatient stays in general acute care hospitals. Retrieved June 21, 2008, from http://www.cms.hhs.gov/apps/media/press/-factsheet.asp?Counter=3045

Clancy, T., Kitchen, S., Churchill, P., Covington, D., Hundley, J., & Maxwell, J. (1998). DRG reimbursement: Geriatric hip fractures in the community hospital. *Southern Medical Journal, 91*(5), 457–461.

Cleverley, W. (1987). Product costing for health care firms. *Health Care Management Review, 12*(4), 39–48.

Cleverley, W. (1997). *Financial environment of health care organizations: Essentials of health care finance* (4th ed., Rev., pp. 10–24). Gaithersburg, MD: Aspen.

Coughlin, T., & Liska, D. (1997). *The Medicaid disproportionate share hospital payment program: Background and issues* (Series A, No. A-14). Washington, DC: The Urban Institute.

Division of Health Care Finance and Policy. (1998). Home health: An emerging challenge in health care. *Healthpoint, 3*, 1–4.

Dunham-Taylor, J., & Pinczuk, J. (2006). *Health care financial management for nurse managers: Applications from hospitals, long-term care, home care, and ambulatory care.* Sudbury, MA: Jones and Bartlett.

Durham, J. (2000). Healthcare's evolution in the technological universe. *Health Management Technology, 21*(4) 91–92.

Easier than ABC: Will activity based costing make a comeback? (2003). *The Economist, 369*, 56.

Ezzati-Rice, T., Kashihara, D., & Machlin, S. (2004). *Health care expenses in the United States, 2000.* (AHRQ Pub. No. 04-0022). Silver Spring, MD: U.S. Department of Health and Human Services.

Finkler, S. (1994). Cost allocation: The distinction between costs and charges. In *Issues in cost accounting for health care organizations* (pp. 81–93). Gaithersburg, MD: Aspen.

Hoffman, F. (1984). Prospective reimbursement. In *Financial management for nurse managers* (pp. 193–203). Norwalk, CT: Appleton-Century-Crofts.

Kane, N., & Siegrist, R. (2002). Understanding rising hospital costs: Key components of cost and the impact of poor quality. Retrieved September 23, 2003, from http://www.selectquality.com/PDF/understand...ent%20costs.pdf

Lane, S., Longstreth, E., & Nixon, V. (2001). *A community leader's guide to hospital finance.* Boston: The Access Project.

Lester, J., Bosch, J., Kaufman, J., Halpern, E., & Gazelle, G. (2001). Inpatient costs of routine endovascular repair of abdominal aortic aneurysm. *Academic Radiology, 8*(7), 639–646.

Magnus, S., & Smith, D. (2000). Better Medicare cost report data needed to help hospitals benchmark costs and performance. *Health Care Management Review, 25*(4), 65–77.

Maiga, A., & Jacobs, F. (2003). Balanced scorecard, activity-based costing and company performance: An empirical analysis. *Journal of Managerial Issues, 15*(4), 283–301.

Medicare SNF-PPS Indices [Data file]. Washington, DC: Centers for Medicare and Medicaid Services. Retrieved November 24, 2003, from http://www.cms.gov/providers/snfpps/snfpps_rates.asp

Medpac. (2003). *Report to Congress: Medicare payment policy*. Washington, DC: Medpac.

Nursing Leadership Academy. (2003). *Fundamentals of nursing finance: A foundation for financial leadership* (10889). Washington, DC: The Advisory Board Company.

Popp, A., Scrime, T., Cohen, B., Feustel, P., Petronis, K., Habinak, S., Waldman, J., & Vosburgh, M. (2002). Factors affecting profitability for craniotomy. *Neurosurgery Focus, 12*(4), 1–5.

Ross, T. (2004). Analyzing health care operations using ABC. *Journal of Health Care Finance, 30*(3), 1–20.

Sobun, C. (1999). What does the future hold for Medicare and your reimbursement. *Health Care Biller, 8*(9), 1–4.

Udpa, S. (2001). Activity cost analysis: A tool to cost medical services and improve quality. *Managed Care Quarterly, 9*(3), 34–41.

U.S. Department of Health and Human Services. (1998). *Medicare program: Prospective payment system for hospital outpatient services: Proposed rules* (42 CFR Part 409, et al.). Washington, DC: Health Care Financing Administration Office of Inspector General.

U.S. Department of Health and Human Services: Centers for Medicare and Medicaid Services (2007). *2007 CMS statistics*. (CMS Pub. No. 03480). Retrieved January 26, 2009, from www.cms.hhs.gov/CapMarketUpdates/Downloads/2007CMSstat.pdf

U.S. General Accounting Office. (2002). *Skilled nursing facilities: Medicare payments exceed costs for most but not all facilities* (GAO-03-183). Washington, DC: U.S. Government Printing Office.

van der Walde, T., & Choi, K. (2002). *Health care industry market update: Acute care hospitals* (volume II). Washington, DC: Centers for Medicare and Medicaid Services.

van der Walde, L., & Choi, K. (2003a). *Health care industry market update: Acute care hospitals*. Washington, DC: Centers for Medicare and Medicaid Services.

van der Walde, L., & Choi, K. (2003b). *Health care industry market update: Nursing facilities*. Washington, DC: Centers for Medicare and Medicaid Services.

van der Walde, L., & Lindstrom, L. (2003). *Health care market update: Home health*. Washington, DC: Centers for Medicare and Medicaid Services.

Weech-Maldonado, R., Neff, G., & Mor, V. (2003). The relationship between quality of care and financial performance in nursing homes. *Journal of Health Care Finance, 29*(3), 48–60.

Young, D. (2007). The folly of using RCCs and RVUs for intermediate product costing. *Healthcare Financial Management*, 100–108.

PART VI

Budget Strategies

Budgeting strategies, and especially cost-cutting methods, are widely used today. Budget strategies need to be aligned with a larger issue, strategic management, which is discussed in Chapter 16. Systematic, objective strategic planning, along with the implementation of the plan, drives successful health care organizations. The key to successful planning is to make the process a part of the daily operations of the organization. Strategic management is a continuous process of revisiting the system and restoring balance.

Chapter 16 also describes the strategic management process that includes situation analysis, strategic formation, strategic deployment, and strategic management—which encompasses measurement, evaluation, and performance improvement. Directional strategies, mission, vision, values, goals, and objectives provide needed processes for the organization to define and to implement in order to achieve the desired outcomes.

Strategic management includes performance measurement. We advocate that the best way to conduct performance measurement is to use balanced scorecards. Metrics captured within the organization's balanced scorecard are tied directly to the strategic plan. A primary utility of the balanced scorecard is the tie between strategic management and performance management. Measurement of key financial, quality, market, and operational indicators provide management with an understanding of performance in relation to established strategic goals and graphically displays a snapshot of the institution's overall health. Chapter 16 outlines some common tools and techniques that are useful, such as cost-benefit analysis, break-even analysis, and forecasting models.

Chapter 17 covers a number of budget strategies, each of which works best depending on the setting. Organizational context is an important element because knowing and understanding the differences in parts of the organizational assessment may determine if we succeed in attaining our goals. Chapter 17 also examines the budgeting process and makes suggestions on how to both decentralize and streamline the process: presently, in some organizations it can waste 30% of administrators' time. It is important for a nurse administrator to know how to write a business plan, or proposal, that includes the financial information along with what is needed. Thus at the end of Chapter 17 an appendix includes a sample proposal for a step-down unit.

In Chapter 18 we turn to another budget strategy: case management. According to the American Nurses Credentialing Center, case management is a dynamic and systematic collaborative approach to providing and coordinating health care services in a defined population. It is a process to identify and facilitate options and services for meeting individuals' health needs while decreasing fragmentation and duplication of care, enhancing quality, and achieving cost-effective clinical outcomes. Chapter 18 looks at new models that link within-the-walls and beyond-the-walls models.

Mutual knowing between client and nurse enhances care, including the client's ability for self-care. Chapter 18 describes three key certifications available to nurses and discusses present trends that integrate and coordinate care and increased use of information technologies.

CHAPTER 16

Strategic Management: Facing the Future with Confidence

Sandy K. Calhoun, PhD(c), MSN, RN, CPHQ

Key Terms

- Acquisition Entry Strategy
- Adaptive Strategies
- Alliance Strategies
- Balanced Scorecard
- Brainstorming
- Break-Even Analysis
- Contraction Strategies
- Cooperation Strategies
- Cost-Benefit Analysis
- Culture
- Customers (External)
- Customers (Internal)
- Delphi Technique
- Directional Strategies
- Diversification
- Divestiture
- Divisional Structures
- Enhancement Strategies
- Expansion Strategies
- External Environment
- Focus Groups

- Functional Organizational Structures
- Gantt Charts
- Goals
- Harvesting
- Horizontal Integration
- Internal Development
- Internal Environment
- Internal Ventures
- Joint Ventures
- Licensing Strategy
- Line Graphs/Multiple Line Graphs
- Liquidation
- Maintenance of Scope Strategies
- Market Development
- Market Entry Strategies
- Matrix
- Matrix Structures
- Merger
- Mission

- Nominal Group Technique
- Objectives
- Penetration Strategies
- Performance Improvement
- Product Development
- Purchase Strategies
- Regression Analysis
- Retrenchment
- Scenario Development
- Situation Analysis
- Status Quo
- Strategic Management
- Strategic Planning
- Strategy Deployment
- Strategy Formation
- Values
- Venture Capital Investment
- Vertical Integration
- Vision

Strategic Management

> You got to be careful if you don't know where you are going, because you might not get there.
>
> —*Yogi Berra (The Quotations Page, 2007a)*

Effective decision making is the primary task of management. Seemingly justified by time constraints and the mistaken assessment that issues are minor, nurse managers often make decisions without essential information. By chance, the nurse manager may be successful in the short run, but in the long run the use of intuition—without the benefit of pertinent data, systematic input from stakeholders, and careful planning—often results in calamity. The delivery of health care devoid of a systematic process for planning forces managers to "fly by the seat of their pants" by relying on their own intuition and experience. Contemporary health care systems are complex and require teamwork and collaboration for organizational leaders to make informed decisions and maintain a viable organization.

Strategic planning shifts decision making from intuitive information gathering to systematic and objective investigation. Thus the task of strategic planning is to generate accurate information for decision making. In the midst of chaos, as the volume and pace of change in health care accelerates, managers may declare they have no choice but to spend their time and resources "putting out fires." Notwithstanding, Gelatt (1993) observed that change itself had changed. The author described the chaos found in health care organizations as *white water change*, because change in health care had become so rapid, complex, turbulent, and unpredictable. It is surprising that seemingly well-adjusted individuals are overwhelmed by change after years of colliding with it. Nevertheless, the dynamic and complex nature of health care mandates that managers not forsake planning and strategic management if the organization is to be positioned for long-term success. Strategic management fulfills the need for knowledge of the organization, the market, and the competitive situations health care leaders face and provides for ongoing, dynamic changes in the strategic plan when appropriate.

Mintzberg and Markides (2000) noted that *strategy* is the art of crafting a unique position in the market. Strategy does not need to change often; however, when there is a need to rethink the organization's position, the change should emerge from the ideas and actions of the people in the organization. Nurse managers, situated in the organization between the front line staff and senior leaders, are in a unique position to recognize the need for change. Successful organizations understand the need to modify or change their strategic plan based on feedback from customers. Nurse managers may be the first to recognize when strategies that have been successful in the past are no longer. In addition, innovative ideas are better conceived if everyone in the organization, not just senior leaders, puts their intellect to the task.

Even though everyone in the organization should be encouraged to come up with new strategic ideas, it is the responsibility of senior leaders to make the final choices. Organizational leaders must choose which ideas will be pursued; otherwise, the result is chaos and confusion. Strategic planning allows health care leaders to meet the future proactively rather than responding to the internal and external environment in a haphazard manner. Although strategic planning will not eliminate all challenges, the process can drive innovation, integrate the system, and align resources to enable the organization to face the future with confidence.

Systematic, objective planning is the key to the development and implementation of plans that drive successful health care organizations. *Strategic planning* is a continuous process of revisiting the system and restoring balance. How do organizations get beyond large binders with numbers, graphs, charts, and jargon? Can organizations use this dense document to improve organizational performance? The answer is "yes." Perhaps employees in organizations that do not view their strategic plan as a useful document need to explore the organization's culture related to the strategic planning process. Why do many organizations have separate plans for performance improvement, education, recruitment, and retention? Silo thinking is effective to prepare and sustain war or missile sites, entities that need to stand alone. However, in health care organizations employees from different departments must work together to ensure the long-term success of the organization. The key to successful planning is to *make the process a part of the daily operations* of the organization rather than a task to be completed during the planning cycle in preparation for the budget.

Health care organizations must focus on patient satisfaction as well as patient retention and loyalty. What is the status of the organization's market share? Are new markets emerging? Do available services need to be "repackaged" to attract new or evolving markets? These aspects are key factors in competitiveness, profitability, and success of the organization. Choices made by organizational leaders 5 to 10 years ago may no longer be valid and must be continuously questioned. In the past, being decisive was an essential talent often thought to be reserved for those in leadership positions. The health care environment of today has replaced the skill of making up one's mind with a *new essential skill of the future—learning how to change one's mind* (Gelatt, 1993). Technologies, customer preferences, and competitors are ever changing, and the organization must be flexible. Successful organizations question past choices to determine if change is necessary. The heart of strategic planning is to devise a systematic, well-balanced process that allows the organization to fit in the environment.

Strategic planning must be objective. The necessity for objectivity was cleverly stated by the 19th century American humorist Artemus Ward, who said, "It ain't so much what people don't know that hurts as what they know that ain't so" (Creative Quotations, 2007). Thus the facilitator of the strategic planning process must be detached and impersonal rather than engaged in biased attempts to prove preconceived ideas.

According to Mintzberg and Markides (2000), strategy is nothing more than answering three simple, yet difficult questions:

1. Who should the organization target as customers and who should they not?
2. What should the organization offer these customers and what should they not?
3. What is the most efficient way to do this?

Organizations that do not have clear answers to these three questions drift aimlessly until they eventually fail. Team members need clear parameters to guide their actions; these three dimensions help provide the autonomy they need to focus on the key tasks at hand. Without clarity of these three dimensions, organizational efforts will be disjointed because no common understanding of the strategies, actions, and goals of the business exist.

National and state quality programs outline the essential role of strategic planning within organizations. The 2008 Baldrige National Quality Program, "Health Care Criteria for Performance Excellence," strategic planning criteria category represents a total of 85 points toward a possible 1,000 total points in the award's scoring system that is distributed across seven criteria categories. The strategic planning criteria category stresses patient-focused quality and operational performance improvement (National Institute of Standards and Technology, 2008). These key strategic issues are fundamental to the organization's overall planning. Patient-focused quality and health care performance provide a strategic view of quality, focusing on patient satisfaction, patient loyalty, patient health status, and health care service improvement. The ultimate test of quality is customer satisfaction, and it carries significant weight among the award's criteria—40 points for "Patient, Other Customer, and Health Care Market Knowledge," 45 points for "Patient and Other Customer Relationships and Satisfaction," 100 points for "Health Care Outcomes," and 75 points for "Patient- and Other Customer Focused Outcomes" (National Institute of

Standards and Technology, 2008). Although the term "customer" was not used often in health care until recent years, 21st century health care leaders recognize the primary customer to be the (formally called) patient. Areas to consider are those important to the patient such as speed, responsiveness, and flexibility. Improvement in operations contributes to short- and longer-term productivity, cost containment, and the overall well-being of the organization.

The Tennessee Center for Performance Excellence (2008) is an example of a state quality program. These criteria outline that customers are the judge of the organization's quality and performance. Because strategic planning focuses on operational performance and quality as judged by the customer, we examine first the notion of customer-driven quality. Who are the customers of health care? Customers of health care are both internal and external to the organization. *Internal customers* include patients and families, physicians, visitors, team members, and volunteers. The employment of physicians has changed physicians from external customers (supplier of the patients we served) to both internal (employee) and external (supplier) customers. This dual role may conflict when organizational priorities are unclear or when organizational and personal goals are incongruent.

The primary *external customers* of health care are quite complex and consist of suppliers (insurance companies, physicians, labor markets, and donors), consumers (the general public and research community), and interfacing organizations (medical profession, teaching hospitals, board of directors, health insurances, and drug and supply companies). Additional external influences include licensing, governmental, and regulatory agencies, in addition to other health care facilities (Bennis & Nanus, 1985).

Determining the measures customers use when they assess and judge the quality of health care services is an important process. Health care leaders' perception of quality may be vastly different from customers' perceptions. Nurse managers may believe that zero defects are priority when, in fact, timeliness is what is most important to the customer. Various listening strategies, aimed at assessing how the customer perceives quality, are discussed. Listening to the customer provides baseline knowledge. Once opportunities to improve are identified, leadership, through strategic planning, must assess and drive improvements. Thus the Joint Commission on Accreditation of Healthcare Organizations (The Joint Commission, 2008) holds leadership accountable for strategic planning as well as for performance improvement.

Why do our customers choose particular health care services? Providing quality care does not guarantee success; customers must perceive added value. Health care leaders may have an erroneous perception that the provided services are superior in design and service. When, in fact, the services are inefficient or outdated, lack of innovation and advances in the market will produce customer dissatisfaction with our endeavors. Customer satisfaction is paramount to the success of the organization, and capturing this information encompasses a major expenditure. This is true whether the data are captured internally or through an outside vendor such as Gallup or Press Ganey.

Are patients and families qualified to assess health care quality? The answer is an astounding "yes." The Internet has eliminated the time-honored adage, "We know what is best, after all we have years of education" and has ushered in the age of informed consumers. No longer is it acceptable to lecture the patient, "Just do as I say" or "The doctor knows best." Many patients seek health care services after an extensive Internet search on the diagnosis and/or treatment(s) in question. Patients and families often arrive for care with an array of scientific literature—indeed often better informed than the clinician.

An organization's commitment to performance excellence should not be measured by cost but rather viewed as an *investment*. Organizations purchase equipment to improve processes and cycle times. An organization that makes a similar investment in their team members receives a much higher return. Successful health care organizations recognize and reward team members with an appreciation of the link between team member satisfaction and patient satisfaction—rarely is the latter realized without the reality of the former. If team members are expected to meet the needs of customers, their needs must be met first.

The second notion related to strategic management stressed by the Tennessee Center for Performance Excellence (2008) examines operational performance. What are the short- and longer-term goals of the organization? How does the organization maintain cost competitiveness? Operational capabilities such as speed, responsiveness, and flexibility contribute to the organization's competitive fitness. The strategic plan must align work processes with the strategic direction of the organization by embedding improvement and learning in work processes. This alignment ensures that priorities for improvement and learning reinforce the priorities of the organization. Comprehensive strategic planning establishes the organization's strategy (the plan for achieving the desired end result) and plan of action (what the organization must do to get there). Of key importance is the deployment of the plan of action to all business units and identifying how accomplishments are measured and sustained. The Joint Commission (2008) requires leaders to engage in short- and long-term planning. This includes data measuring the performance of the processes and outcomes of care, treatment, and services.

Although the business sector has successfully used strategic planning for the past 50 years, strategic planning has been used in health care only since the 1970s, and then only sporadically (Zuckerman, 1998). According to Ginter, Swayne, and Duncan (2002), the concept of strategic planning was broadened to strategic management during the 1980s when business transformed planning and budgeting beyond the traditional 12-month operating year and began to understand the importance of strategy implementation and control.

The strategic management process described in this chapter traces the following map: (1) situation analysis, (2) strategy formation, (3) strategy deployment, and (4) strategic management, which encompass measurement, evaluation, and performance improvement. **Exhibit 16–1** outlines the strategic management process.

Exhibit 16–1 Strategic Management Process

Situation Analysis	Strategy Formation	Strategy Deployment	Strategic Management
External environmental analysis: • Opportunities • Threats	Directional strategies: • Mission • Vision • Values • Goals and Objectives	Culture	Goals and Objectives
Internal environmental analysis: • Strengths • Weakness	Adaptive strategies	Structure	Measurement • Balanced Scorecard
• Mission • Vision • Values • Goals	Market entry strategies	Resources	Evaluation standards
	Competitive strategies		Performance Improvement

Situation Analysis

Situation analysis, the initial stage of strategic planning, is the process of determining the current state of the organization. Although historical data are an asset in determining the current state, leaders should resolve to avoid the trap of focusing on the analysis of past performance. Zuckerman (1998) describes this phenomenon as "analysis paralysis," a serious problem that can bog down the strategic planning process. Undue emphasis on past performance can result in loss of focus and momentum. Key players may become disinterested, and buy-in may be lost. Leaders must focus on *results*, not "busy work." There will always be those in the group who insist on more and better data; however, profiling key business drivers for the organization should be captured and analyzed on an ongoing basis, thus negating the need for over-analysis of historical data. Rarely are data needed beyond the past 5 years. *Key issues to consider include which factors are within the control or influence of the organization and how external forces affect the competitive position of the organization.* Understanding and analyzing the current situation is accomplished through three interrelated processes: external environmental analysis, internal environmental analysis, and the development of the organization's mission, vision, values, and goals. These processes are not separate and distinct but rather overlap, interact with, and influence one another.

External Environmental Analysis

The first process, *external environmental*, focuses on determining the current position of the organization within both the general environment and the health care environment. This profile is the beginning of a forward-looking process that considers market trends and forecasts (Zuckerman, 1998). To understand the external environment, the organization must look outside its boundaries (beyond itself) to identify and analyze issues taking place outside of the organization. These issues represent opportunities and threats and assist in identifying "what the organization should do." DeSilets and Dickerson (2008) suggest the following basic questions, "Do you have an area of expertise worth promoting? Are you undercapitalized?" "Is your market growing or shrinking?" (p. 196). Opportunities and threats influence strategy formation and represent fundamental issues that can directly impact the success or failure of the organization. It is insufficient to simply be aware of these issues; health care managers need to understand the nature of the opportunities and threats before they affect the organization. The organization must have an effective method for scanning the external environment for pertinent information. Factors to be considered include legislative/political changes, economic modifications, social/demographic shifts, new technology, and competitive/market changes (Ginter et al., 2002).

Review of legislative, political, and regulatory trends is necessary to determine any major environmental influences that may affect the future performance of the organization. Regulatory and legislative changes in both public and private health care organizations will continue as these entities struggle to ensure health care access, patient safety and privacy, and cost management. Major trends should be profiled for the past 3 to 5 years. Forecasting, using alternative scenarios, should be identified and discussed (Zuckerman, 1998). What should be done to minimize negative impacts? What can be done to maximize potential benefits?

Economic trends and forecasts should be exercised with caution; overanalysis should be avoided. Only the broadest trends and variables that impact the organization should be considered. Nevertheless, shifts in the national economy cannot be ignored, because the impact will be realized at the local level. Although minor shifts in economic performance are of minimal consequences to the strategic planning process, local trend analysis may identify geographic segments with potential for future penetration (Zuckerman, 1998).

Demographic changes, such as an aging population and increased life span, must be considered because these factors directly impact health care organizations. Major population shifts may indicate geographic areas that may be targeted for future market growth. Social trends, such as a more ethnically diverse and better educated population, impact the provision of services as well. Critical shortages of nurses, pharmacists, physical therapists, and other health care professionals necessitate a focus on retention and recruitment efforts.

Technology needs continue to escalate. As health care organizations become "wired," system integration (radiology, nursing, laboratory, pharmacy, and other ancillary departments) become a logistical nightmare. No one system has "one-stop shopping"; whereas one system excels in a key feature, it may be deficient in another. Furthermore, the software competitor probably excels in a different key aspect of an integrated system. To be more efficient, practitioners no longer complete laborious manual record reviews and "paper and pen" documentation. Those facilities that do not keep pace with emerging trends in technology will become dinosaurs in short order. Health care organizations need to leave the chisel and stone technique with comic characters such as Fred Flintstone.

Primary market research is completed by focusing on competitive and market changes external to the organization. This information helps to determine the organization's competitive position in the market. Market research is completed through interviews, focus groups, and surveys. Targets of this research include senior leaders of competitor organizations, community leaders, primary employers, and those knowledgeable of the market situation. The primary task is to generate information, thereby decreasing the uncertainty that comes with the managerial art of decision making. Research means literally to "search again," a process whereby one looks at the data to understand all that needs to be known about a subject (Zikmund, 2003). Although caution must be exercised so that this aspect of the process does not take an undue amount of time and resources and is not overemphasized, leaders must know the market. At times, research reveals information not readily apparent and key to success in the market.

> The secret of business is to know something nobody else knows.
>
> —*Aristotle Onassis (BrainyQuote, 2008)*

A parallel matrix is helpful when examining the external analysis. This matrix allows visualization of competitively relevant threats with external opportunities. **Exhibit 16–2** provides an example matrix.

Internal Environmental Analysis

Available resources, competencies, and capabilities influence success in the external environment. *Internal environmental analysis* involves an extensive review of internal processes, culture,

---

Exhibit 16–2 External Environmental Analysis

Nurse's Heaven Medical Center
Strategic Plan 20XX
Opportunities and Threats

Opportunities	Threats
No competitors offer wound management services.	Increased competition from larger hospital serving the same population.
Physician offices are needed to attract new physicians.	Customers expect specialized care that the organization cannot afford to offer.

structure, and technology to reveal strengths and weaknesses. Strengths are those things that the organization does well, not only from the viewpoint of the organization's employees but from the customer's viewpoint (DeSilets & Dickerson, 2008). Gelatt (1993) offers caution regarding "info-mania." He described info-mania as the idolizing of information. "Info-maniacs" worship facts. There is sure to be at least one member of the leadership team that demands more and more facts even when the team is drowning in information. Exactly how many admissions did Dr. X have 3 years ago? Four years ago? Five? Focusing only on facts leaves little room for innovation. Generating more information than the human mind can process is dysfunctional. Health care leaders must understand the competitive relevance of these issues. Weaknesses require strategies to minimize the vulnerability of the organization, whereas strengths must be optimized to maximize their impact. This information provides a foundation for strategy formulation (Ginter et al., 2002). Plotting strengths and weakness on a parallel matrix (**Exhibit 16–3**) provides a visual for evaluating the competitive advantages relative to strengths and the competitive relevance of weaknesses.

The real voyage of discovery consists not is seeking new landscapes, but in having new eyes.

—Marcel Proust (The Quotations Page, 2007b)

Zuckerman (1998) explains that primary market research serves to gather information regarding the organization's strengths and weaknesses as it relates to its competitors and to involve leadership in the strategic planning process. Leaders should begin by reviewing any recent market research that is available and gathering information through interviews, focus groups, and surveys. Primary target groups for market research include board members, physicians, health professionals, management staff, and other key stakeholders of the organization.

Many organizations use focus groups to solicit stakeholder input (Krueger, 1988; Morgan, 1993). Focus groups incur significant cost (time and money); thus priority is given to key customer groups such as patients, families, team members, community members, and physicians. A focus group consists of a small group of individuals (6–10), usually with similar interests, who participate in an unstructured, free-flowing interview with a skilled facilitator. The facilitator begins by introducing the topic with the goal of uncovering core issues related to strategic planning. A recorder documents key statements for management to consider in strategy development. Caution must be used, however, because focus groups may not represent the entire population.

Drenkard (2001) documented the success of the Inova Chief Nurse Executive team in using large group interventions to convene and engage nurses across a large health care system in northern Virginia. This method involved the entire system and used a key mass of people affected by the change. This critical mass participated in (1) understanding the need for change, analyzing the current state, and deciding what needed to be changed; (2) generating ideas about how to make the

---

Exhibit 16–3 Internal Environmental Analysis

Nurse's Heaven Medical Center
Strategic Plan 20XX
Strengths and Weaknesses

Strengths	Weaknesses
Convenient ground level parking	Resistance to change by many team members
Patient-oriented team members	Lack of well-defined management succession plan

needed changes; and (3) implementing and supporting the change. The Inova Chief Nurse Executive team sponsored six large group events to engage the several hundred nurses in the workforce. These sessions provided time for interaction, development of the strategic plan, and networking for the involved nurses.

Mission, Vision, Values, and Goals

The mission, vision, values, and goals of the organization ultimately affect the strategy that is adopted. According to Ginter et al. (2002), the organization's *mission* is the articulation of the external opportunities and threats and the internal strengths and weaknesses. The *vision* is the view of the future based on the understanding of the forces. Chapman (2003) notes our mission needs to matter. It must not be just tired words framed on the wall. Likewise, health care organizations need volcanic vision statements that eliminate old patterns of mediocrity. He describes three elements of effective mission and vision statements: clear and easy to remember, a call for dramatic improvement in the lives of others, and proclamation by leaders who, through example, demonstrate a passionate commitment to making the statements come alive.

The *core values* (an organization's purpose and core values are explained further in Chapter 3) constitute the fundamental truths that the organization holds dear and reflect the philosophy of the organization. Examples include honesty, integrity, customer service, and commitment to excellence. *Goals* specify the major direction of the organization and provide actionable linkage to the mission. The mission, vision, values, and goals are considered a part of the situation analysis because they are influenced by both external and internal environmental analysis.

Strategy Formation

The first step in the strategic planning process, situation analysis, involves data gathering. *Strategy formation* uses these data for decision making. These decisions are critical to the success of the organization, because they become the organization's strategy. Ginter et al. (2002) describes four types of strategies: directional, adaptive, market entry, and competitive.

Directional Strategies

Although the mission, vision, values, goals, and objectives are part of the situation analysis, they are also part of strategy formation; they provide the broadest direction for the organization— *directional strategies*. Common mission, vision, values, and goals indicate what the organization wants to do. These strategies reflect the critical success factors within the particular service category, in this case, health care. Critical success factors are applicable to all competitors and take into account the external environment. In other words, they define what the organization must accomplish to stay in business. These strategies provide initial direction for the organization and guidance when making key organizational decisions. The reciprocal relationship (adapted from Ginter et al., 2002, p. 177) of directional strategies is shown in **Exhibit 16–4**.

MISSION

The organization's *mission* should articulate the organization's purpose or reason that it exists. It describes what makes the organization distinct and reflects the expectations of stakeholders, those who have an interest in the business. In short, the mission defines the organization and describes what it does. The mission statement must be more than an attractive wall hanging. The mission must be communicated with and lived by all team members in the organization, especially to team members who work directly with customers.

Exhibit 16–4 Directional Strategies

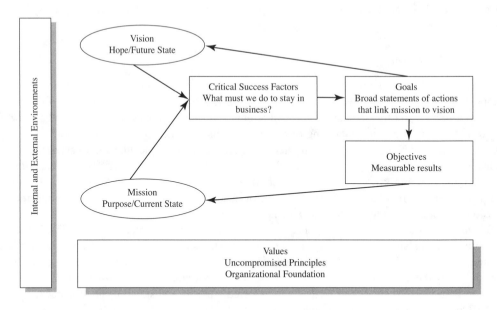

Source: Adapted from Ginter, P., Swayne, L., & Duncan, W. (2001). *Strategic management of health care organizations* (4th ed.). Malden, MA: Blackwell.

VISION

The organization's *vision* describes the optimal future state of the business. The vision should create a mental picture of what the organization will be when leaders and team members accomplish their mission. It describes the hope for the future—what should the organization be 5 years from now? Time and effort link the mission (what the organization is today) and vision (what will it be in the future)? The vision should be stated in clear, simple terms that provide a challenge and leave no doubt as to the importance of the vision. Stakeholders should be able to understand the vision and commit it to memory. The vision should be inspiring and is generally not stated in quantitative terms. Though the vision should stand the test of time, it should be constantly challenged and revised when necessary.

VALUES

Values represent the basic principles, fundamental beliefs, and tenets of team members and define what they deem important to the organization. Values state uncompromised principles that are timeless and do not change with the ever-changing climate of business operations. Some organizations use the terminology "guiding principles" to refer to values. Values guide beliefs, attitudes, and behaviors and provide the foundation for operating the business. Key business decisions should be measured against the values of the organization so the organization never loses sight of its purpose.

GOALS

Goals are more specific than the mission and vision. Nevertheless, goals are broad statements that provide direction for team members and link the mission to actions necessary to reach the desired future state of the organization—the vision. Goals that focus on activities unrelated to the organization's critical success factors have the potential of diverting leadership attention and team member energy. The number of goals should be limited for the same reasons. Goals should be stated in easily understood terms so that team members can readily link what they need to do with the mission and vision for the organization:

- Expand Women's Services to encompass all key aspects of the business
- Position Nurse's Heaven Medical Center as a strong community hospital with a focus on primary care
- Develop a comprehensive health care system including primary care, radiation therapy, skilled nursing facility, home health, and durable medical equipment

For the desired outcome to be achieved, objectives are designed to make each goal operational.

OBJECTIVES

Objectives describe the results to be achieved, when and by whom, and are measurable. Examples of objectives for the above goals are as follows:

- The Director of Women's Health will direct the completion of renovations of the existing unit by December 31, 20XX.
- The Chief Executive Officer will recruit six hospitalists by August 31, 20XX.
- The Chief Nursing Officer will recruit/hire 20 team members for the skilled nursing unit by November 30, 20XX.

Mission, vision, values, goals, objectives, and the external and internal environment present a picture of the situation and provide a basis for strategy formulation.

Adaptive Strategies

Whereas directional strategies provide general guidance, adaptive strategies are more specific and describe the process for carrying out the directional strategies. Directional strategies are the ends, whereas adaptive strategies are the means. Adaptive strategies describe how the organization will expand, contract, or maintain its scope of services (Ginter et al., 2002). These are the strategies most visible to those outside the organization.

EXPANSION STRATEGIES

Expansion strategies include diversification, vertical integration, market development, product development, or penetration (Ginter et al., 2002). *Diversification* occurs at the corporate level when markets outside the organization's core business offer potential for significant growth. Because the organization is venturing outside the core business, diversification is generally considered a risky venture. Diversification is most often seen in health care when there are opportunities in less-regulated markets such as specialty hospitals, long-term care, or managed care.

There are two types of diversification: related and unrelated. In health care organizations, *related diversification (concentric)* includes related products and services such as home health, hospice, or radiation treatment. *Unrelated diversification (conglomerate)* includes businesses in the general environment such as a laundry, restaurant, or office buildings and those within the health care industry such as pharmaceuticals, medical supplies, or insurance. Selecting markets and products that complement one another can reduce risk. Nevertheless, unrelated diversification has been found to be generally unsuccessful in generating revenue for health care organizations.

Vertical integration is the second corporate level expansion of adaptive strategies. The purpose of vertical integration in health care is to enhance the continuity of care while simultaneously managing the channel of demand for health care services. Health care organizations that use vertical integration grow the business along the channel of distribution of core process (Ginter et al., 2002) (refer to Chapter 3 for more information about core values). Vertical integration can reduce supply costs and enhance integration. A successful example would be the inclusion of technical education programs for team members in critically short supply such as nursing assistant and technicians. Vertical integration was the fundamental adaptive strategy of the 1990s. This rapid change was realized as hospitals joined networks or systems in an effort to secure resources, increase capabilities, and gain greater bargaining power with purchasers and health care plans (Ginter et al., 2002).

Market development occurs at the division or strategic service unit level and focuses on entering new markets with existing products or services. The purpose of this strategy is to add volume through geographic expansion of the service area or by expansion into new market segments within the present geographic area (Ginter et al., 2002). Horizontal integration is a type of market development that grows the business by acquiring or affiliating with competitors. Horizontal growth of health care systems in the 1980s and early 1990s created multihospital systems. Many of the expected benefits such as reduction of duplication of services, economics of scale, improved productivity, and operating efficiencies did not materialize, and horizontal integration strategies slowed in the late 1990s (Ginter et al., 2002).

Product development also occurs at the division or strategic service unit level and involves the introduction of new products or services to existing markets. Whereas related diversification is the introduction of a new product, product development refines, complements, or extends existing products or services such as women's health or cancer treatment. Product development may be used when customer requirements are changing, technology is changing, or when there is a need to create differentiation advantage.

Penetration strategies, like market and product development, focus on increasing volumes and market share. Market penetration is an aggressive marketing strategy centered on extending existing services. This strategy is used when the present market is growing and expected revenues are high.

CONTRACTION STRATEGIES

When the organization needs to decrease the size or scope of operations at either the corporate or divisional level, four *contraction* strategies are considered. Divestiture and liquidation occur at the corporate level, and harvesting and retrenchment occur at the divisional level (Ginter et al., 2002).

When a service unit is viable yet a decision to leave the market and sell an operating unit is made, *divestiture* occurs. Generally, the divested business unit has value and will continue to be operated by the purchasing organization (Ginter et al., 2002). This strategy has become common over the past decade as health care organizations carve out noncore business. Examples of noncore health care business that may be divested include pharmacy, laboratory, and radiology. Business units may be divested for several reasons, including industry decline, the need for cash to fund priority operations, or marginal performance. Services too far from the core business may be divested in an effort to focus on business at hand, or management expertise for the particular service may not be available within the leadership group.

Liquidation is the selling of assets of an organization that can no longer operate. In contrast to divestiture, liquidation assumes that the operating unit cannot be sold as a viable operation (Ginter et al., 2002). Some assets, of course, may still have value, such as buildings and equipment. Reasons for liquidation include bankruptcy, the need to dispose of nonproductive assets, the need to reduce assets, or the emergence of expensive new technology that will make the current technology obsolete.

Harvesting occurs when the market has entered long-term decline or there is a need for short-term cash (Ginter et al., 2002). For example, despite a strong market position, revenues are expected to decline industry-wide over the next years. The unit will be allowed to generate as much revenue as possible; however, no new resources will be invested in the business. This allows for an orderly exit from the market by planned downsizing. Harvesting has occurred with many small rural hospitals that could not maintain or improve their financial positions due to the lack of physician and community support, an aging population, and the migration of the young to urban areas.

Retrenchment occurs when the market has become too diverse, and there is a decline in profitability due to increasing costs (Ginter et al., 2002). Although the market is still viewed as viable, costs are too high. Retrenchment involves redefinition of the market if it is too geographically spread out. Costs such as personnel or facility assets that are marginal or nonproductive are reduced.

MAINTENANCE OF SCOPE STRATEGIES

When current strategies are appropriate and few changes are needed, the organization may elect to *maintain* the existing strategies. This does not mean that the organization does nothing but rather pursues either enhancement or status quo strategies (Ginter et al., 2002).

When the organization is progressing toward its vision yet nevertheless improvements are needed, *enhancement strategy* may be used. This may entail quality improvement efforts directed toward improving organizational processes or reducing costs. This is a time for innovation and redesign of timeworn systems. The focus should be on those identified as most important to key customers such as patients and families.

Status quo is based on the assumption of a mature market when growth has ceased. The goal is to maintain the market share. When using the status quo strategy, organizations may attempt penetration or market/product development (Ginter et al., 2002).

Market Entry Strategies

The three major strategies to enter a market include: purchase, cooperation, and development. Market entry strategies are not ends of themselves, but rather the adaptive strategies may be used to bring market strategies to fruition (Ginter et al., 2002).

PURCHASE STRATEGIES

There are three *purchase market-entry strategies*: acquisition, licensing, and venture capital investment. Purchase market-entry strategies allow a health care organization to quickly enter the market. Each strategy places different demands on the organization (Ginter et al., 2002).

When health care organizations purchase an existing organization, organizational unit, or a product or service, *acquisition entry strategy* is used. Acquisition takes place at the corporate or divisional level. The acquisition may be integrated into existing operations, or it may operate as a separate unit. Acquisitions often flounder because it is difficult to integrate existing culture and operations. Often, it takes several years post acquisition to combine two organizational cultures. Despite the difficulties of integrating cultures, the synergy realized by the creation of a comprehensive health care system has demonstrated that acquisition is an effective purchase strategy.

Licensing avoids the time and market risks of technology or product development (Ginter et al., 2002). When licensure is used as a strategy, proprietary technology is usually not purchased and therefore the organization is dependent on the licensor for support and upgrade. Health care organizations frequently use licensing strategies for implementation of clinical documentation systems. This strategy lowers the financial and market risk of technologies outside the core business.

Venture capital investment is a low-risk option whereby health care organizations purchase minority investment in a developing enterprise. This provides an opportunity to "try out" and, possibly later, enter into new technology. Examples include life science portals for bioinformatics, home-based health care services for the elderly, and cardiology arrhythmia management companies (Ginter et al., 2002).

COOPERATION STRATEGIES

According to Ginter et al. (2002) mergers, alliances, and joint ventures—*cooperation strategies*—were the most popular strategies of the 1990s. Cooperation strategies allow organizations to carry out adaptive strategies.

Although similar to acquisitions, in a *merger* two organizations combine through a mutual agreement to form a single new organization (recall that in an acquisition a health care organization purchases an existing organization, organizational unit, or a product or service). Merger strategies are used to accomplish horizontal integration by combining two similar organizations, or vertical integration, by creating an integrated delivery system. Reasons for mergers include to improve efficiency and effectiveness (combine resource and exploit cost reduction strategies), enhance access (broader services), enhance financial position (gain market share), and overcome concerns of survival (endure in an aggressive market). As with acquisitions, the major hurdle is the integration of two separate organizational cultures. Because a new organization is formed, mergers are often more difficult to navigate than acquisitions. In a merger, a totally new organizational culture must be developed. If mergers are to be successful, work groups must be formed to reformulate the mission, vision, and core values of the new organization. Merger of two organizational cultures into one takes years to complete (Ginter et al., 2002).

Alliance strategies entail arrangements among existing organizations to achieve a strategic purpose not possible by any single organization. Alliances include federations, consortiums, networks, and systems. Alliances attempt to strengthen competitive position while the organizations maintain their independence. Health care organizations often form an alliance to achieve economies of scale in purchasing. Examples include Premier and Voluntary Hospitals of America (Ginter et al., 2002). Although not a merger or acquisition, alliances have many of the same issues with conflicting cultures.

Joint ventures are used when risks are too high or the project is too large or too expensive to be done by a single organization. In a joint venture, two or more organizations combine resources to accomplish a designated task. The most common health care joint ventures are

- Contractual agreements
- Subsidiary corporations
- Partnerships
- Not-for-profit title-holding corporations

In a *contractual agreement*, two or more organizations contract to work together toward specific objectives. *Subsidiary corporations* form a new corporation, usually to operate non–health care activities. A *partnership* is a formal or informal arrangement between two or more parties for mutual benefit of the organizations involved. *Not-for-profit title-holding corporations* form tax-exempt title-holding corporations to provide benefits to health care organizations engaged in real estate ventures. The dynamic health care environment mandates that organizations engage in joint ventures to lower costs (Ginter et al., 2002).

DEVELOPMENT STRATEGIES

Organizations may enter new markets through internal resources. There are two types of *development entry strategies:* internal development and internal ventures.

Internal Development

Organizations use *internal development* for products or services closely related to existing products or services. The organization maintains a high level of control through the use of existing resources, competencies, and capabilities. Although internal development presents an image of a growing organization, there is a time lag to break even, and obtaining significant market share against strong competitors is difficult (Ginter et al., 2002).

Internal Ventures

In contrast to internal development, *internal ventures* are most appropriate for products or services that are unrelated to the current products or services. Internal ventures set up separate, relatively independent entities within the organization. An example of an internal venture is a hospital that develops home health care through an internal venture (Ginter et al., 2002). Success of this strategy is mixed, because the organization's internal climate is often unsuitable for the venture.

In the final stage of strategic formation, a *gap analysis* examines the difference in the current state and the desired state, or vision for the future. Gap analysis is the process of examining how large a leap must be taken to meet the vision and what must be done to make the leap. If organizational leaders set their vision too narrow, they will find their current state meets the vision but lacks incentive to aspire for higher and greater things. Their task is accomplished, and the planning process ends. With this in mind, leaders must communicate the vision in a somewhat revolutionary manner. The vision should inspire team members to perform their best—there is no room for mediocrity in health care vision. The desired outcome of the gap analysis is a strategic plan that has a reasonable probability of success. To accomplish this, priorities must be established and resources allocated to narrow the gap between the current state and the desired state. This process establishes the groundwork for the strategies necessary to ensure the desired outcome (Drenkard, 2001).

Planning encompasses stewardship of the organization and its resources. Care must be taken to articulate the core assumptions about the nature of the market, the competitions, and the organization; otherwise, a gap will exist between the aspirations of the organization and the way the organization actually behaves. When what we do day-to-day is in contrast to what we say we do and hope to be, a paradox exists that leads to team member frustration. What does the organization value—creativity or discipline? Is the focus on short-term or long-term goals? Quality or the bottom line? Although conflicts occur in every organization, successful organizations meet the challenge and reconcile aspirations and actions as part of the strategic planning process (Solovy, 2002). Decisions regarding resources must be made with the core value—what does the patient need or value and what is best/safe for the patient—as focal points of the organization. The financial bottom line is a secondary priority to safe care. When the financial bottom line is the priority, money is wasted.

An additional gap can also exist between management's view of the organization and the team members' view. Because team members are closer to the core business (patient care), input from team members must be sought as part of the planning process. A planned process whereby each business unit can share information and seek guidance and clarification facilitates "buy-in" and avoids duplication of efforts. The alternative, top-down, directive approach may result in a high quality strategic plan, but team members who have input into planning more readily accept the expected outcomes and so become more vested in work processes. Thus the process includes a system of notification for team members as to the status of their suggestions—how they were evaluated, or if their ideas were not used, feedback is given to team members as to the rationale.

It is imperative that health care leaders understand and focus on their core business. Focusing on the core business provides a clear strategic vision—the big picture—in contrast to scattered plans that steal time and energy with little to show except charts and graphs. Successful organizations focus their strategy on their core rather than on the industry's competitive factors. One method of assessing the health of the organization's strategic planning process is to consider the time spent focusing on the competition. If more time is spent analyzing competitors than focusing on the core business, the process is off task. What must the organization do well to remain in business? What does the organization do particularly well? Health care dollars are scarce. Across-the-board investing often signals that competitors are setting the organization's agenda. Conversely, when an organization's strategy is formed reactively as it tries to keep up with the competition, it loses its uniqueness (Kim & Mauborgne, 2002).

Strategy Deployment

Failure to implement the strategic plan is the most common flaw in the planning process (Zuckerman, 1998). Zuckerman emphasized that team members may be overwhelmed with managing the day-to-day crises, leaving little time to implement strategic objectives. In addition, if the objectives are not specific, team members may lack the direction needed to meet the established goals. Communication of the strategic plan must be coordinated throughout the entire organization—vertically and horizontally. To provide direction at the work level, goals and objectives must be established for each business unit and ought to link to the overall plan for the organization. This linkage provides guidance and consistency in decision making and allows managers and team members to understand the present and plan for the future. All team members must be able to articulate how "what they do" fits into the overall plan for the organization.

For each goal and objective, *at least one person should be assigned as the primary individual responsible for planning, implementing, and monitoring progress*. This is often a member of senior leadership. Specific target dates are assigned to provide a timeline for expected progress. If realization of goals involves intradepartmental work processes, performance improvement teams may be assigned. Senior leadership should establish specific dates to review progress toward each goal. Accountability is accomplished (and rewarded, or otherwise) through linkage between the goals and objectives of the strategic plan and individual team member evaluation criteria. **Exhibit 16–5** provides an excerpt from a strategic planning matrix.

Exhibit 16–5 Sample of Strategic Planning Matrix

Nurse's Heaven Medical Center　　Strategic Plan 20XX

Goal	Objective	Actions	Measure/ Benchmark	Target Date	Responsible Party
Expand Women's Services to encompass all key aspects of the business	Complete renovations of the existing unit by 12/31/XX	1) Monitor progress daily 2) Facilitate weekly construction progress meeting 3) Facilitate monthly medical staff meetings 4) Facilitate biweekly team member meetings	1) Phase I complete by 08/31/XX 2) Phase II complete by 10/31/XX 3) Complete Phase III by 12/31/XX Benchmark: There Medical Center, Anywhere, USA	12/31/20XX	Director of Women's Health

Culture

The *culture* of the organization includes the shared assumptions, values, and behavioral norms of the group. These assumptions and values remain constant over time, even when the membership of the organization changes, and are the basis for an informal consciousness (Ginter et al., 2002). This is significant in the current climate of mergers, acquisitions, and buy-outs. The shared values of team members may not reflect the values of the organization. When this occurs, the customary way of doing things (behavioral norms) may sabotage the strategic plan. To ensure congruency, shared assumptions (mission—who we are) must support the organizational vision and goals (what we want to accomplish). If the plan is in conflict with the culture, deployment will be a challenge. Unfortunately, if the culture is in significant conflict with the strategic plan and a strong subculture exists, change will be difficult because team members may prefer to "do things the way we have always done them."

To be cognizant of the assumptions, values, and behavioral norms of the work group, successful leaders are involved in the day-to-day operations of the organization. Health care leaders must schedule regular visits to each business unit. In addition, regular visits to all stakeholders are imperative. It is not acceptable to attempt to lead from the office or through computer technology. E-mail, voice mail, and other technologies do not take the place of face-to-face contact, nor do they reflect a complete picture of the culture of the organization. Insights gleaned from involvement with stakeholders and the day-to-day operations of the organization provide vital insight during the situation analysis. Leaders must assess whether the directional strategies are still appropriate and reflect the culture of the organization. *Considering the organizational culture is perhaps the most crucial aspect in the deployment of the strategic plan.*

What can be done to develop a culture that is adaptive to change? Involving stakeholders in the strategic planning process cultivates an environment of trust and respect. "Buy-in" from those involved in the processes and outcomes of care is worth the extra time necessary to glean these insights. This input is especially pertinent during the shaping of directional strategies—mission, vision, values, and goals. Cultural assessment during the situation analysis may determine that additional implementation strategies are necessary to maintain or change the organizational culture. As previously mentioned, the roles of nurse leaders position them to be acutely aware of the "pulse" of the organization. Nurse leaders must feel comfortable to express views different from those in senior leadership. An atmosphere of trust encourages risk taking and is necessary for innovation to occur. If trust is absent, personal safety and security become the priority, and the status quo will be maintained despite an elaborate strategic plan. In addition, time and money may be wasted on endeavors that do not reflect current customer needs.

Maintaining a climate of trust and respect, one that encourages risk taking and innovation, is hard work. Leaders must "walk the talk." Saying one thing while doing another (or, even more critical, rewarding another) creates confusion. The directional strategies, mission, vision, values, and goals must be communicated often, both verbally and in writing. Prominent posting in both common areas and each business unit is essential. Additional successful strategies include having the mission appear on all meeting agendas and minutes, on stationery, and on laminated cards for team members. The key strategy for maintenance of an organizational culture that is adaptive to change is "live it"—as reflected in the daily business of the organization.

Structure

Ginter et al. (2002) describes three basic organizational structures: functional structure, divisional structure, and matrix structure. Similar to organizational culture, structure must not impede the overall strategy.

Functional organizational structures organize activities around mission-critical functions or processes. This is the most prevalent organizational structure for organizations with a relatively narrow focus such as health care. Departments are organized according to their function, such as clinical services, finance, marketing, or information systems. Organizations that are structured around mission-critical functions may consider clinical services as the center of the functional structure with other sections of the organization organized around clinical processes such as registration, radiology, laboratory, and so forth (Ginter et al., 2002).

Health care is highly specialized, and expertise within the specialty is highly valued. Functional structures can foster efficiency; however, this type of structure can also result in silo thinking. Functional structure slows decision making, makes coordination of work difficult, and inhibits communication as each department "looks after its own interest" without the realization of how their processes affect others.

Divisional structures are common in health care organizations that have grown through diversification, vertical integration, or market or product development (Ginter et al., 2002). Divisional organizations attempt to break down larger, diverse organizations into more manageable and focused sections. This division is especially important when structures of the organization are in different geographic locales, thus with a different environment and with unique customers. Divisional structures have difficulty in maintaining a consistent image and purpose. Divisional structures may additionally require multiple layers of management and duplication of services, thus increasing costs. Organizations that choose divisional structures must carefully coordinate strategic business unit activities.

Matrix structures organize activities around problems to be solved rather than functions, products, or geography (Ginter et al., 2002). The nurse manager may have a dual reporting structure, to the vice president of Women's Health (product) as well as to the vice president of Nursing Services (functional). Thus the nurse manager is responsible to the vice president of Nursing for nursing care and to the vice president of Women's Health when working on the women's health product line. In some matrix structures, the reporting relationships follow a project or program, and the relationship ends when the project is complete. Matrix structures foster creativity and innovation; nevertheless, they are difficult to manage because priorities can become confused. Thus matrix structures require expert coordination and communication.

Resources

Deploying the selected strategies uses four key resources: financial, human, information systems, and technology (Ginter et al., 2002). Analysis of *financial resources* was a key factor in the internal environmental analysis. In addition, finance provided key input for strategy formation. Once strategies have been decided, finance is the vehicle to implement them. Leaders should require that major purchase requests be submitted with documented links to the strategic plan. Major projects require capital investment, which generally must be approved by the governing body.

Human resources must be considered before deployment of the strategic plan. There are several questions to consider: Will additional training be required? Are additional team members needed? Will there be a need for team members with different skills and experiences? This is a critical time to complete an organizational learning needs assessment with all team members. This provides a bridge between the strategic plan, education plan, and performance improvement plan. Multiple plans should be consolidated into one master strategic plan. This is less confusing for team members and assists with unified communication of the organization's plan for improvement.

Although *information resources* are crucial to develop the internal and external environmental analysis, they are equally important in the deployment of the strategic plan. As previously mentioned, clinicians can no longer be expected to complete laborious paper documentation. Likewise, leaders must be able to extract data entered into clinical documentation systems with relative ease, thereby negating the need for manual data extraction. A shared drive on the organization's computer system assists in ease of review of the strategic plan. Key business drivers selected as part of the organization's balanced scorecard should also be available on a shared computer system (balanced scorecards are discussed in more detail below). Large binders containing the organization's plans, placed on the highest shelf and never used, are dinosaurs.

The strategies selected drive the needed technologies. *Strategic technology* is concerned with the type of organization, the sophistication of the equipment, and management of the technology used *within* the organization (Ginter et al., 2002). Health care organizations are high technology organizations. Equipment becomes obsolete as quickly as it is installed. This is an area of increasing concern for health care leaders because it represents major expenditures for the organization.

Strategic Management

Goals and Objectives

Exhibit 16–5 demonstrates a sample strategic planning matrix. Senior leaders ensure that team members remain focused by assigning specific dates/times for review of the status of each goal and objective. Someone once said, "People respect what you inspect." Although this may not be an example of transformational leadership, the adage is unfortunately true. Assessment of efforts toward meeting established goals and objectives not only keeps leaders aware of the status of planning efforts, but it also provides team members the opportunity to "show off" their hard work. This personal time and attention by senior leaders demonstrates that the strategic plan is more than a "dusty binder on the shelf" but is rather a working document that ebbs and flows with the organization.

Follow-up reviews can be assigned by target date or minimally twice per year. Typically, quarterly reports are assigned to assess if the work is proceeding as planned or whether adjustments need to be made based on current reality. Assigning quarterly due dates for status reports on alternate months assists in time and agenda management for senior leaders as well as busy team members. Responsible parties should be forwarded a reminder of the date, time, and place of the meeting as well as the report expectations (i.e., verbal, written, visuals, etc.). Presenters should be instructed on the amount of time allotted for their presentation. To assist team members to prepare for the meeting, it is helpful if a general format is established. Beware, however, because being too prescriptive can stifle creativity. **Exhibit 16–6** demonstrates a quarterly report matrix for follow-up of progress toward established goals and objectives.

Measurement/Balanced Scorecard

Kaplan and Norton (1996) of the Harvard Business School developed scorecards (also known as dashboards, instrument panels, and data display devices) in 1991. The utility of the *balanced scorecard* remains unchanged—the provision of a strategic management and performance management

Exhibit 16–6 Sample Goals and Objectives Quarterly Report Matrix

Nurse's Heaven Medical Center
Strategic Plan 20XX
Goals and Objectives Report Matrix

Goal	Jan	Feb	Mar	Apr	May	Jun	Jul	Aug	Sept	Oct	Nov	Dec
A	X			X			X			X		
B		X			X			X			X	
C			X			X			X			X

tool. Measurement of key financial, quality, market, and operational indicators provides management with an understanding of performance in relation to established strategic goals and graphically displays a snapshot of the institution's overall health (Health Care Advisory Board, 1999).

Selection of critical metrics is key because the Health Care Advisory Board (2002) noted in their study of hospital downturns that inadequate performance measurement was the cause of 10% of financial flashpoints—an unexpected, dramatic decline in total margin and cash flow. As organizations grow increasingly complex, it is critical that leaders have easy access to accurate data that provide a view of overall organizational performance rather that being inundated with mountains of disparate reports from the various business lines and departments.

Successful balance scorecard implementations have been documented using the process shown in **Exhibit 16–7** (Health Care Advisory Board, 1999).

Theurer (as cited in Health Care Advisory Board, 1999) recognized that the following pitfalls should be avoided when creating indicators for a balanced scorecard: (1) lack of context (measures should tie to strategic goals and drive organizational strategy and resource allocation) and (2) lack of benchmark data (seeing how the organization ranks against a peer group).

Leadership must empower employees and provide sufficient resources to develop unit-level performance measures. Without sufficient resources, the staff will simply recycle existing measures. Bureaucratic uniformity squelches the individualized nature of each unit and should be avoided so that each unit can be measured based on its unique attributes. Indicators must be used as tools for continuous improvement, not as tools to punish poor performance. Leadership should provide positive reinforcement for improvements realized. The Health Care Advisory Board noted that dashboards should be limited to 15 to 30 standards of measurement. Drill down data should be reserved for situations when a more comprehensive assessment is warranted.

Performance Improvement

Performance improvement is a systematic, organization-wide approach to improving the processes and outcomes of the health care system. Performance improvement shifts the focus from individual performance to the performance of the organization's systems and processes. Although individual performance must be maintained, only those team members who are unwilling or unable to change (a very small percentage of the workforce) are penalized. There are four basic tenets of performance improvement: *customer focus, continuous improvement of processes, team member involvement, and use of data and team knowledge to improve decision making.* To be successful, performance improvement effects must be embraced by senior leaders and involve all departments/team members in clinical as well as nonclinical areas. Performance improvement efforts are a part of the strategic planning process, not a separate function (to comply with regulatory standards).

QUANTITATIVE METHODS

Collecting Data

The process for measurement, assessment, and performance improvement is designed to assist the organization to effectively use resources in the provision of quality patient care. Performance improvement activities focus on interrelated factors, governance, managerial, support, and clinical processes, which affect patient outcomes and the financial viability of the facility. Clinical measurement, assessment, and improvement activities should focus on the flow of patient care and assess how well the processes in which individuals participate are performed, coordinated, integrated, and improved. When a problem or opportunity to improve care is identified, action is taken, and the effectiveness of the action is assessed. Results of performance improvement activities are used primarily to improve patient care processes. When the results of performance improvement activities are relevant to the performance of an individual, the results are used as a component in the evaluation of the individual's capabilities.

Exhibit 16–7 Balanced Scorecard Implementation/25- to 26-Month Process

	J	F	M	A	M	J	J	A	S	O	N	D	J	F	M	A	M	J	J	A	S	O	N	D	J	F
Commitment from senior leadership; senior leadership education before initiation prevents ambiguity	X	X	X	X	X	X	X	X	X	X	X	X	X	X	X	X	X	X	X	X	X	X	X	X		
Strategic planning retreat (critical); involving the entire organization	X	X																								
Select strategic planning committee; identify objectives for each perspective in the balanced scorecard				X	X																					
Strategic planning committee communicates with staff					X	X																				
Revise scorecard based on staff input							X																			
Revised scorecard deployed to staff								X	X																	
Each unit/department and employee develops scorecard that supports facility scorecard								X	X																	
Strategic planning committee reviews departmental and individual scorecards; suggests revisions										X	X															
One-year mark; senior leaders formulate 5-year plan based on finalized scorecard												X														
Departmental and organizational progress reviewed quarterly; identify opportunities to improve													X	X	X	X	X	X	X	X	X	X	X	X		
Evaluation committee assesses staff performance based on the individual balanced scorecards. Based on the results: retention, promotion, salary increases, and rewards																									X	X
Strategic planning committee revises the balanced scorecard and 5-year plan based on results of the metrics																									X	X
Cycle continues in the following years																										

Priority for data collection is given to those aspects of care evaluating the following areas:

1. *High risk*: patients who are at risk of serious consequences or are deprived of substantial benefit if the care is not provided correctly (including providing care that is not indicated or failing to provide care that is indicated)
2. *High volume*: aspect of care occurs frequently or affects large numbers of patients
3. *Problem prone*: aspect of care has tended in the past to produce problems for staff or patients
4. *High cost*: aspect of care is resource intensive
5. *Top money loser*: care provided has been documented to lose money for the facility

Measures are used to capture performance improvement data. A *measure* is a variable relating to the structure, process, or outcome of care. Measures are selected based on the organization's key business drivers (what do we need to do well to remain in the business): identifiers of key quality characteristics and customer satisfaction, strategic management goals and objectives, assessment of performance relevant to functions, the design and assessment of new processes, measurement of the level of performance, and stability of important existing processes. An *operational definition* of each measure must be well defined for ease and reliability of data collection. *Measures of process* are often standards of care or practice. Measures of process include objective criteria based on authoritative sources and supported by the best available clinical and performance improvement literature. Quality control measures are also documented as required by regulatory agencies.

To be useful, data must be transcribed to information through data display, interpretation, and analysis. Tools for analyzing data over time include line graphs, run charts, or control charts. These tools allow the nurse manager to look for trends or patterns in the data (The Joint Commission, 2003).

Line Graphs

Line graphs aid in assessment of trends or changes in performance. These simple graphs indicate whether a process is working and may reveal areas in need of improvement. The data are plotted as the events occur over time. The horizontal axis (x) is used to plot time, for example, days of the week, months of the year, and so forth. The vertical axis (y) is used to plot the observed level of performance. Once the data points are plotted on the graph, lines are drawn connecting from point to point allowing visualization of trends. Line graphs are used when data collection is still in the early stages before sufficient data are available to complete a control chart (usually 24–30 data points). Nevertheless, at least 10 to 12 data points are needed to have a meaningful graph. If it is discovered that a problem occurs at identified times, an in-depth analysis as to the cause and resolution may be undertaken (The Joint Commission, 2003).

The line graph in **Exhibit 16–8** demonstrates data collected for an identified compliance issue for the months of October 20XX through February 20XX. Five data points connected by a line provide visualization of the compliance rate that ranges from 24% to 43%. At this early stage of data collection, visualization for a beginning analysis is possible; however, additional data points are required before construction of more sophisticated graphs.

Run charts are used when the nurse manager requires a more sensitive analysis of data over time than available via a line chart. Although run charts are more sophisticated than line charts, they do not have the benefit of assessment of statistical process control. Typically, run charts are used until sufficient data points are available for assessment of statistical process control (SPC). In addition to the data point connections, an arithmetic mean is calculated and plotted on the graph.

There is "natural" variation in everything. An objective of statistical process control is to analyze this variability and to assign causes. Is the variation "normal" or "abnormal"? This is done by establishing the limits of chance variation. Variation beyond these limits is due to designated causes. Common cause (normal) variation is derived from random, expected differences in the process, whereas special cause (abnormal) variation is outside what is expected and is derived from identifiable reason(s)/change(s) in the process.

Exhibit 16–8 Line Graph

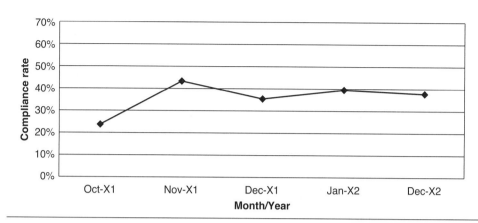

An example of common cause variation related to charting omissions is those due to layout of forms and time constraints of health care workers. Special cause variation is variation due to computer down time (unless, of course, the computer is down as much as it is up) when workers must use paper charting.

Deciding when to follow up on common cause variation depends on the nature of the data. If variation results from common cause, the result of work inherent in complex processes, and the results are satisfactory, then monitoring rather than additional study may be all that is needed. This may be true of charting. Although 100% compliance would be ideal, it is probably not achievable.

Leaders must decide how much variation (i.e., deviation from the mean) in the process is acceptable. This is usually done based on the nature of the process and outcomes deemed key to the organization. Most often health care leaders strive to decrease variation in processes where there is potential for adverse patient care. If significant variation in the process is unsatisfactory, such as medication errors, patient falls, or nosocomial infections, then the process needs to be studied (for example, using a rapid-cycle performance improvement team).

Responding to special cause as if it were common cause can create false alarms and/or increase costs (time is money). The quest for reasons for special cause may lead to blaming individuals for poor results. These investigations often waste resources, create resentment, and may increase variation, for example, targeting one department with low satisfaction scores for one month with the expectation of "improving or else." If the identifiable cause is apparent, there may be no need to "work on the process." Unfortunately, facilities often react to special cause variation due to pressure from regulatory agencies. The best way to deal with special cause variation is to design quality into the process—prevent adverse events rather than study them.

The run chart in **Exhibit 16–9** provides a visual cue of an error rate plotted for 12 months from April 20XX through March 20XX. The mean is documented as 0.42. Two data points are worthy of analysis, May and June 20XX. What is the root of these two data points, both on the upper side of the mean with successive increase—special cause or common cause? Although this run chart provides more information than a line chart, a control chart is constructed to assess for statistical process control. *Statistical process control* is a method for monitoring the "control" or extent of variation in a process or outcome. The goal is to reduce variation, thus increasing the desired result.

Control charts are specialized run charts that also allow visualization of data over time. Control charts are used when the nurse manager wishes to discover how much variability in a process is due

Exhibit 16–9 Run Chart

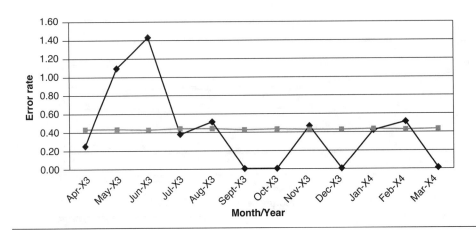

to random variation (process design) and how much is due to special cause variation (unique actions/events) to determine whether a process is in statistical process control. Control charts are borrowed from manufacturing where predictable results are required. In health care, as in manufacturing, there should not be a high degree of variation in the product. In health care the primary product is patient care. Because these are typically called control charts in manufacturing, we use this term here.[1]

A mean (arithmetic average) is established for each data set/chart. Health care organizations typically calculate the upper and lower control limits at three standard deviations above and below the mean. Data points outside of the established control limits are due to a special cause. These data points represent deviations from the way the process normally operates (Goal/QPC, 1988). A fluctuation in the data within the established control limits results from variation in the process resulting from common causes within the system (design, choice).

Criteria for interpreting control charts are as follows:

1. *Outside of the control limits*: a data point that falls outside the control limits on the chart, either above the upper control limit or below the lower control limit.
2. *Shift*: eight or more consecutive points either all above or all below the mean. Values on the mean are skipped and the nurse continues to count. Values on the mean do not make or break a trend.
3. *Trend*: six points all going up or all going down. If the value of two or more successive points is the same, the point is ignored when counting; like values do not make or break a trend.
4. *Two out of three*: two out of three consecutive points in the outer third of the chart (greater than two standard deviations). The two out of three consecutive points could be on the same side or on either side of the mean.

The control chart in **Exhibit 16–10** demonstrates a medication error rate for August 20XX through March 20XX. The mean is 0.90 with an upper control limit (three standard deviations above the mean) of 2.69 and a lower control limit of zero (a negative error rate is not possible). All data points are within the control limits. No shifts (eight or more consecutive points all above or below the mean) or trends

---

[1] In Chapter 3 we recommend finding other words to better express the evaluation process rather than using the word "control."

Exhibit 16–10 Control Chart

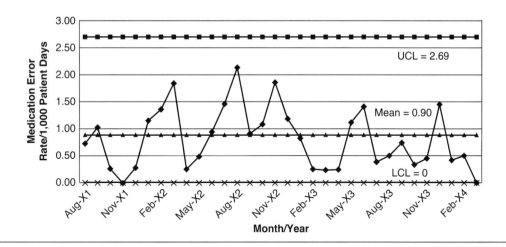

(six points all going up or all going down) are identified. The "two out of three" criteria (two out of three consecutive points in the outer third of the chart) are not demonstrated. Nurse managers needing more in-depth information regarding control charts are referred to Lighter and Fair (2004).

Matrix

A *matrix* is used to show combinations of data. Examples include unit statistics such as admissions, nursing hours per patient day, percent of occupancy, medication error rate, and overall rate of patient satisfaction for an obstetrical unit over a period of months. In **Exhibit 16–11** the months are documented in the matrix heading with the measures listed down the left side. This chart provides the data, but it is not as easy to spot anomalies or trends using this method.

The data in Exhibit 16–11 could be used to assess relationships between data sets, for example, overall patient satisfaction and nursing hours per patient day. Does patient satisfaction decrease as nursing hours per patient day decrease? Yes, in this example. Do medication errors increase when nursing hours per patient day decrease? Yes, in this example. Each data set is compared with a different data set for identification of applicable relationships. Relationships are sometimes difficult to discern using a matrix for comparison. A multiple line graph demonstrates a better visual of relationships between data sets.

Exhibit 16–11 Matrix Chart

OB Unit	Jan	Feb	Mar	Apr	May	Jun	Jul	Aug	Sep	Oct	Nov	Dec
Admissions	650	653	640	600	590	575	555	602	643	670	675	700
Nursing Hours/ Patient Day	5.9	6.0	6.1	6.3	6.6	6.8	7.0	6.7	5.8	5.9	5.7	5.5
Percent Occupancy	.75	.76	.74	.68	.67	.65	.63	.68	.74	.78	.79	.81
Medication Error Rate	1.5	1.0	.75	.54	.45	.16	.05	.50	1.45	1.3	1.7	.10
Overall Patient Satisfaction	.85	.88	.89	.90	.96	.97	.98	.95	.86	.81	.80	.78

Exhibit 16–12 Multiple Line Graph

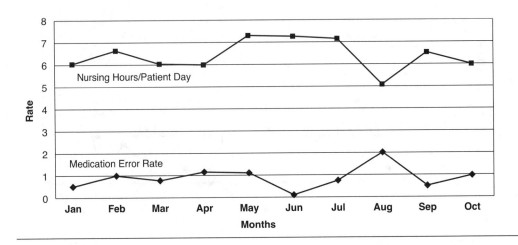

Multiple Line Graph

Relationships of the data captured in a matrix may be better visualized in a *multiple line graph*. What do the data show happens with the rate of overall patient satisfaction when nursing hours per patient day decrease? Does patient satisfaction increase as nursing hours per patient day increase? Are data relationships more readily apparent during certain months of the year? Spreadsheet software can be used to easily convert matrix data to a multiple line graph. Caution should be exercised to not display too many indicators on the same graph, thus making it difficult to interpret. Color coding the lines to correlate with data elements assists in analysis of data relationships.

The multiple line graph in **Exhibit 16–12** allows for easy visualization of the relationship between a decrease in nursing hours per patient day and subsequent increase in medication error (September and October). Each applicable data set from the matrix may be plotted on a multiple line graph to discern relationships.

Cost-Benefit Analysis

Comparison of the benefits and costs of a proposed endeavor is completed through cost-benefit analysis. *Cost-benefit analysis* (cost-benefit and break-even analysis were covered in Chapter 12) is a budgeting technique once used primarily by the government. However, it is becoming increasingly popular as organizations realize the impact their business has on society and the community they serve. Cost-benefit analysis is an analytical technique that compares the social costs and benefits of a proposed program against the costs of the venture under consideration. If the benefits outweigh the costs, a positive cost-benefit is expected, and it makes sense to spend the money; otherwise, it does not. Criteria for evaluation in a cost-benefit analysis include project goals, benefits and costs, discounting cost and benefit flows at an appropriate rate, and completing a decision analysis (Finkler, 2001).

The first step in cost-benefit analysis is to determine the goals of the project—what does the organization hope the project will accomplish? What would the community gain if the project comes to fruition? Identifying goals and objectives clarifies the expected benefit for those we serve. Examples include less travel time for patients in need of cancer treatment or local education resources for high-risk mothers.

Once project goals and objectives have been determined, project benefits must be determined. All losses and gains expected to be experienced by society are included, expressed in dollar terms. Losses incurred to some sections of society are subtracted from the gains that accrue to others. The benefits include only those things that are a direct or indirect result of the project. Alternative strategies are considered so as to choose the option with the greatest net benefit or ratio of benefit to cost (Finkler, 2001). Leaders would not include benefits that are a reality whether or not the project is realized. For example, although cancer treatment may be available at a tertiary medical center 100 miles away, the dollar costs related to the benefit of not having to travel such a long distance are included in the analysis but not the benefits of cancer treatment because it is already available.

Costs must be estimated as part of the cost-benefit analysis. All costs must be considered including opportunity costs, because when a decision is made to do something, other alternatives are sacrificed. For example, an increase in inventory requires extra cash. The cash used will not be available for use somewhere else in the organization (another opportunity). This is a critical consideration in cost-benefit analysis (Finkler, 2001). In our cancer treatment example, the facility may have to forgo a transplant program to finance the cancer treatment program. This opportunity cost should be estimated. These calculations include the time value of money.

Project costs and benefits often occur over a period of years. Money has different value over time. If a project has a $2 million start-up cost that will be paid back through revenue over a 5-year period, the $2 million is worth more today than over the next 5 years. This comparison of benefits and costs over time is referred to as discounting cash flow. *Discounting cash flow* uses an interest rate (discount rate) to convert all cost and benefits to their value at the present time (Finkler, 2001). The methodology for the discounting method is beyond the scope of this chapter. Nurse managers requiring in-depth information related to long-term financing are referred to Chapter 5 in Finkler (2001).

To complete the decision analysis, estimated costs and benefits are compared with each other in the form of a ratio—benefits divided by costs. If the resulting metric is greater than one, then the benefits exceed the costs and the project is desirable. The greater the benefit-to-cost ratio, the more advantageous the project (Finkler, 2001).

Break-Even Analysis

Increasingly, health care organizations must search for projects or ventures in an effort to improve financial stability or to subsidize services for which the organization loses money but still provides based on community need. *Break-even analysis* determines the minimum volume of services that a program or service must provide to be financially self-sufficient. This tool is useful for determining whether a new venture will be profitable. It is used in situations in which there is a specific price associated with the service such as a specific charge or a system of cost reimbursement (Finkler, 2001). A break-even analysis is an essential part of a business ProForma.

This seems like a simple endeavor—if the reimbursement per unit of service is greater than the cost, the new endeavor would be expected to make a profit. On the other hand, if the expected reimbursement is less than the cost, the new endeavor will lose money. However, cost per unit depends on volume. When volume is low, the cost per unit will be higher. As volumes increase, the venture may become profitable. Thus it is imperative that the organization understand at what point *revenues (money expected to be received) will be equal to expenses (cost to provide the service)*. This is the break-even point.

To grasp the steps in calculating the break-even-point equation, key terminology must be understood:

- *Total revenue* is the average price multiplied by the number of units.
- *Total expenses* include fixed and variable costs (both fixed and variable costs were further explained in Chapter 12).

- *Fixed costs (FC)* are costs that do not change as volume changes within the relevant range (range of activity that would be reasonably expected to occur in the budget period).
- *Variable costs (VC)* vary in direct proportion with volume. When calculating expenses, variable cost is expressed in variable cost per unit.

Finkler (2001, p. 107) describes the following calculation, included in the text boxes, to find that break-even point. In this example, 1,000 cesarean deliveries at a total cost of $2,500 per cesarean delivery generate $2,500,000 in total revenue. The break-even point (at cost of $2,500 per case) is 450 cesarean deliveries—the point at which total revenue equals total expenses. **Exhibit 16–13** provides a visual example of the break-even point for cesarean deliveries.

Recall that the break-even point occurs when the total revenues equal the total expenses, thus the break-even point is calculated as follows:

> *Total revenue = P (price) × Q (volume)*
>
> *Total expenses = V (variable costs [VC] × volume [Q]) + fixed costs (FC)*

> *P × Q = (VC × Q) + FC*
>
> *$1,125,000 × 450 cases = $625,000/450 (recall that variable cost is per case)*
>
> *× 450 cases + $500,000*
>
> *($1,125,000 = 450 cases at $2,500/case)*
>
> *($625,000, the variable cost = $1,125,000 total cost − $500,000 fixed cost)*

The next step is to subtract (VC × Q) from both sides of the equation:

> *(P × Q) − (VC × Q) = FC*
>
> *$1,125,000 × 450 cases − ($625,000/450 × 450 cases) = $500,000*

Next, factor out the Q from the left side of the equation:

> *Q × (P − VC) = FC*
>
> *450 cases × ($1,125,000 − $625,000/450 cases) = $500,000*

The resulting formula is as follows:

> *Q = FC divided by P − VC is the quantity (Q) needed to break even*
>
> *450 cases = $500,000/$1,125,000 − $625,000/450 cases*
>
> *Q = 450 cases*

Exhibit 16–13 Break-Even Point

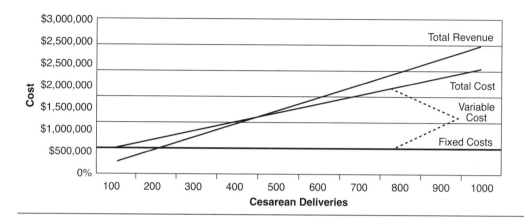

Regression Analysis

Understanding regression analysis is imperative for successful budgeting and strategic planning. Nurse managers must understand how to effectively predict a variable (for example, cost) based on an independent variable (for example, patient days). Without this knowledge, nurse managers are merely "guessing" as to whether their nursing unit can remain financially viable. *Regression analysis* is a statistical technique available via computer software used to forecast the relationship between two variables. The independent variable is typically plotted on the *x*-axis of a scatter graph and the dependent variable is plotted on the *y*-axis. The computer software requires the user to enter the data for the *x* and *y* values. After entering these data, little more than a command to compute the regression is required. It is important that nurse managers not be intimidated by this technique but rather become familiar with its use in the planning process. Guessing is not suitable for professionals charged with meeting the needs of suffering society.

Regression measures the linear association between a dependent (criterion) and an independent variable (predictor). Regression assumes that the dependent variable is predictively linked to the independent variable. Regression analysis is particularly valuable for forecasting because it attempts to predict the values of a continuous, interval-scaled, dependent variable from the independent variable. For example, the number of full-time equivalent (FTE) team members (the dependent variable) might be predicted on the basis of patient days (the independent variable). Forecasting in this manner is crucial to anticipate staffing needs as volumes fluctuate.

Bivariate linear regression investigates a straight-line relationship. This is not as commonly used as multivariate regression. The formula is as follows:

$$Y = \alpha + \beta X$$

In this example, *y* is the dependent variable, *x* is the independent variable, and α and ß are constants to be estimated. The symbol for the *y* intercept (the point at which the regression line intercepts the *y*-axis) is α and ß is the slope (the inclination of a regression line as compared with the base line) coefficient. Slope can best be considered as the increase in the number of units on the *y*-axis divided by the run in units along the *x*-axis (Zikmund, 2003). Although the nurse manager may attempt to simply draw a line through the data points on a scatter graph, this method is not valid and fluctuates based on human error. Finance staff may be called on to assist if bivariate analysis is needed.

Multiple Regression

Multiple regression analysis allows for the simultaneous investigation of the effect of two or more independent variables on a single interval-scaled or ratio-scaled dependent variable. As outlined by Zikmund (2003), the formula is as follows:

$$Y = a + \beta_1 X_1 + \beta_2 X_2 + \beta_3 X_3 + \ldots + \beta_n X_n$$

This method is especially useful when several factors are likely to affect the dependent variable. Nurse managers may seek input from the finance department related to multiple regression analysis.

QUALITATIVE METHODS

Brainstorming

A *brainstorming* session is convened to understand an issue, the impact the issue may have on the organization, or to generate ideas for strategic alternatives. Members of the group present ideas with brief explanations; however, dialogue and evaluation of the ideas are not undertaken at this juncture (Ginter et al., 2002). The ideas are usually recorded on flip charts. Team members are encouraged to verbalize ideas no matter how impossible they may seem at first. According to Brassard and Ritter (1994), there are two methods for brainstorming: structured (each team member gives ideas in turn) and unstructured (team members give ideas as they come to mind). Structured and unstructured brainstorming can be done silently or aloud. Brainstorming enhances communication, generates new ideas and alternatives, sparks creativity, and stimulates innovation.

Focus Groups

Similar to brainstorming, *focus groups* are convened to reach conclusions regarding environmental issues. Focus groups were discussed earlier in this chapter as a mechanism for generating information during the internal environmental analysis. Experts in the areas related to the identified issue provide leadership and the opportunity to discuss important issues. In addition, focus groups provide a venue to gain new insight and fresh alternatives (Ginter et al., 2002). This insight empowers and equips them with ideas for alternative actions if necessary.

Nominal Group Technique

Another problem-identification and -solving method for groups is called *nominal group technique (NGT)*. In nominal group technique, team members independently generate a written list of ideas regarding the issue. After members have been given sufficient time to generate their list, each member takes turns reporting one idea at a time to the entire group. As new ideas are generated, all members record these on a flip chart for consideration. Members are encouraged to build on the ideas of fellow team members. When all ideas have been exhausted, the team discusses the ideas, and then team members privately vote by ranking the ideas in order of preference. After the ideas are ranked, the group discusses the vote, and voting continues until consensus is reached. The advantage of nominal group technique is that everyone has equal status and power, ensuring representation of the group. In addition, nominal group technique eliminates the biases of those in a leadership position (Ginter et al., 2002).

According to Brassard and Ritter (1994), nominal group technique allows a team to quickly come to consensus regarding the importance of issues, problems, or solutions by individual rankings into a team's final priorities. Because all team members participate equally, commitment is built to the team's choice. It is especially useful for reserved team members because it places them on equal footing with more dominant team members.

Delphi Technique

The *Delphi technique* uses a structured group decision-making technique based on repeated use of rating scales to obtain opinions about a decision. Computer software is available that summarizes the results, making the process easier and faster. Members of the group first explore the issue individually and then design a questionnaire for a larger group. The results are tabulated and given back to the group for discussion. The process continues with progressively focused questionnaires. The process is repeated until members of the group reach consensus regarding the issues and a decision is reached.

Alternately, the process may begin in a more free-flowing style with team members initially identifying important issues. This individual brainstorming technique is particularly valuable when team members are unable to meet in a group setting. Key themes are then put into a questionnaire for ranking by team members. After team members rank issues, the questionnaire is sent out again to all members for further input. This process continues as many times as necessary to reach consensus on key issues.

The Delphi technique is particularly valuable for obtaining input from team members during the strategic planning process when face-to-face conversation is not possible but input is valued. An advantage of the Delphi technique is the protection of anonymity, making the technique particularly useful for issues where there is significant disagreement. The technique is particularly useful for groups that have historically failed to communicate effectively. The Delphi procedures offer a systematic method that ensures team member opinions are considered (Gordon, 2002).

Scenario Development–Tree Diagram

To implement an identified strategy, tasks must be mapped for implementation. *Tree diagrams* are used to break broad goals, graphically, into increasing levels of detailed actions so a stated goal can be accomplished (Brassard & Ritter, 1994). This tool encourages team members to expand their thinking while simultaneously linking the team's overall goals. Tree diagrams assist team members to move theory to reality.

The first task is to choose the goal statement. Alternately, the team may have been assigned a goal on which to work. If the team selects the goal, care must be taken to create, via consensus, a clear, action-oriented statement. Team members must have intimate knowledge of the goal topic.

Next, major tree headings, or subgoals, are selected. These subgoals may be established first through brainstorming and then by using the nominal group technique. These subgoals are the major means of achieving the goal statement. The first level of detail must remain broad so it does not jump to the lowest level of task. After working from the goal statement and first-level detail, the team proceeds through the three levels of detail. Some subgoals are simple, whereas others require more breakdown. At each level the facilitator queries the group as to whether or not something obvious has been forgotten. An additional important question for the team is whether these actions result in accomplishment of the given goal or subgoal. Post-it™ notes may be used to create the levels of detail because they can easily be moved around. Lines are drawn when the tree is finished. The tree can be oriented from left to right or top to bottom.

The tree diagram is an effective communication tool. This technique allows for input from direct caregivers. The team's final task is to revise, add, or delete goals or subgoals as deemed appropriate (Brassard & Ritter, 1994). **Exhibit 16–14** is an example of a tree diagram for a health care organization.

Gantt Charts

Project management is critical as new ventures or programs are pursued. Complex projects require that successive activities be completed in a timely fashion. Several commercial computer software programs are available; however, a simple Gantt chart can be constructed with materials at hand.

Exhibit 16–14 Tree Diagram

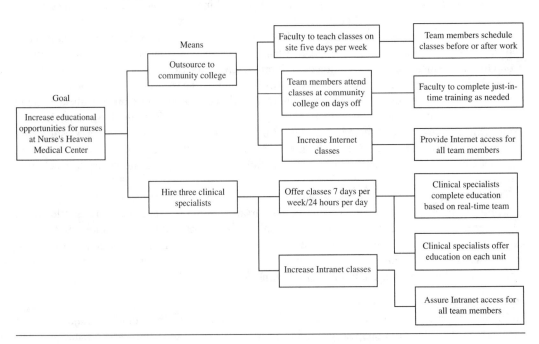

A *Gantt chart* displays activities or goals in a matrix format. The time frame is displayed on the horizontal axis, and the activities to be completed for the project are documented on the vertical axis. If dates are especially important (i.e., when one phase of the project must be completed on a specific date in order for the next phase to begin), project leaders may designate specific dates on the chart. **Exhibit 16–15** shows a sample Gantt chart for a performance improvement team. Gantt charts are also useful as a planning tool for new managers. It is easy for "time to get away," and before a new manager may realize it, evaluations are past due or reports are due the next day without adequate time to prepare. Managers may also use a Gantt chart to "pace" themselves so they do not get overwhelmed—everything cannot be done in a week's time. Planning activities throughout the year decreases stress and the need to "fight fires" on a daily basis. Gantt charts are especially helpful for nursing leaders who are visual learners—you can see what needs to be done and when.

Evidence-Based Information

Empirical research related to the efficacy of the strategic planning process is limited (Kaissi, Begun, & Hamilton, 2008). In Kaissi and coworkers (2008), the sample was limited to hospitals in the state of Texas. Hospitals within the sample reported that 87% had a strategic plan, and most reported that physicians and their board were involved. Responsibility for the plan was assigned to the chief executive officer in approximately one-half of the organizations. Three strategic planning processes were positively associated with financial performance: having a strategic plan, having the chief executive officer responsible for the plan, and involvement of the board. Further longitudinal studies were recommended to evaluate relationships between planning and performance. Kaissi and colleagues provided beginning evidence related to one of the most common practices within health care organizations—strategic planning. It is imperative that hospital leaders use evidence to guide leadership practices and not just maintain practice due to tradition (for more details, see Chapter 5).

Exhibit 16–15 Sample Gantt Chart for a Performance Improvement Team

Activities	Jan	Feb	Mar	Apr	May	Jun	Jul	Aug	Sept	Oct	Nov	Dec
Select process	X											
Charter team	X											
Collect baseline data	7											
Analyze baseline data		15										
Select improvement		28										
Plan the improvement			5									
Do the improvement			10									
Check the results			31									
Act to maintain the improvement				X								

Role of the Nurse Manager

Nurse managers are situated in a unique position to recognize the need for change in the organization. Sandwiched between the front-line staff and senior leaders, nurse managers may be the first to recognize the need for changes in strategy. Nurse managers stimulate their team members by cultivating a positive culture of performance excellence and a corresponding reward system. Their challenge is to define the parameters within which team members can experiment and be innovative. Nurse managers uphold the organization's value system and maintain systems that focus on the core business of patient care. Managers ensure that strategies are in tune with the current needs of customers and are balanced so that one strategy does not suffer at the expense of another. They are sensitive to important changes all the time and inquire of all their customers "Are your needs being met?" Of key importance, nurse managers maintain the system by ensuring issues get picked up quickly and senior leaders are made aware. They do not just herald problems but offer solutions as well. Nurse managers bind the organization together within the internal environment so that team members are galvanized into action. Managing a nursing unit is not an easy task and is certainly not for the faint of heart.

Gelatt (1993) defined the skills needed to continually adapt, innovate, and change: "This 'flexpert' is open-minded, comfortable with uncertainty, delighted with change, and capable of unfreezing and refreezing beliefs, knowledge, and attitudes" (pp. 11–12). "Flexperts" understand that the inability to shift paradigms not only restricts flexibility but causes the individual to become out-of-date, inaccurate, and in need of revision. Culture, communities, experiences, and health care organizations change constantly and make old paradigms dysfunctional.

As nurse managers look toward the future, strategic planning fosters a sense of positive uncertainty that assists team members in the acceptance of change, ambiguity, uncertainty, and inconsistency. As Chapman (2003) states in *Radical Loving Care*, "Our Vision statements need to be engraved in our hearts, not just on plaques" (p. 110). Committed leadership begins with those who make up the majority of caregivers in health care: nurses.

Discussion Questions

1. Because effective decision making is the primary task of management, discuss mechanisms that nurse managers may use to ensure they make the best decisions.
2. Discuss the process of external and internal environmental analysis and then speculate scenarios that may result if these steps in strategic management are omitted or are not done well.
3. Reflect on the mission, vision, values, and goals of a health care organization and provide examples of how individual employees, departments, and work units support all four of these as a foundation for directional strategies.
4. Describe how leaders may positively affect organizational and unit culture in the current health care environment and then consider how the culture affects relationships, learning, change, and innovation.
5. Consider a health care organization and discuss measures that might be selected for a balanced scorecard. Explain the rationale for selection of each measure and describe how leaders could ensure a "balance" of measures. Next, discuss how leaders can remain informed regarding the current status of the organization considering at a minimum volume, financial, quality, and satisfaction measures.
6. Using the measures selected in discussion question 5 above, explain tools and techniques that could be used to display and analyze the data.
7. Qualitative tools and techniques are often dismissed in health care organizations. Select one qualitative method and discuss how the technique could be used to drive improvements.
8. Think about the role of the nurse manager, and discuss the importance of the role to employees and the overall organization.

Glossary of Terms

Acquisition Entry Strategy—when health care organizations purchase an existing organization, organizational unit, or a product or service.

Adaptive Strategies—describe how the organization will expand, contract, or maintain their scope of services (the means). They include expansion strategies, contraction strategies, and maintenance of scope strategies.

Alliance Strategies—entail arrangements among existing organizations to achieve a strategic purpose not possible by any single organization.

Balanced Scorecard—measurement of key financial, quality, market, and operational indicators that provides management with an understanding of performance in relation to established strategic goals and graphically displays a snapshot of the institution's overall health.

Brainstorming—a group is convened to understand an issue, the impact the issue may have on the organization, or to generate ideas for strategic alternatives.

Break-Even Analysis—determines the minimum volume of services that a program or service must provide to be financially self-sufficient.

Contraction Strategies—decrease the size or scope of operations.

Cooperation Strategies—where the organization enters into mergers, alliances, and joint ventures.

Cost-Benefit Analysis—comparison of the benefits and costs of a proposed endeavor.

Culture—includes the shared assumptions, values, and behavioral norms of the group or organization.

Customers (External)—in health care these consist of suppliers (insurance companies, physicians not employed by the organization, labor markets, and donors), consumers (the general public and research community), and interfacing organizations (medical profession, teaching hospitals, board of directors, health insurances, and drug and supply companies). Additional external influences include licensing, governmental, and regulatory agencies, in addition to other health care facilities.

Customers (Internal)—in health care these include patients and families, physicians (when employed by the organization), visitors, team members, and volunteers.

Delphi Technique—a structured group decision-making technique based on repeated use of rating scales to obtain opinions about a decision.

Directional Strategies—provide initial direction for the organization and guidance when making key organizational decisions. They include mission, vision, values, goals, and objectives (the end).

Diversification—occurs at the corporate level when markets outside the organization's core business offer potential for significant growth. Related diversification (concentric) includes related products and services. Unrelated diversification (conglomerate) includes businesses in the general environment.

Divestiture—occurs when one leaves a market and sells an operating unit.

Divisional Structures—attempt to break down larger, diverse organizations into more manageable and focused sections.

Enhancement Strategies—when the organization is progressing toward its vision yet nevertheless improvements are needed.

Expansion Strategies—strategies to expand services.

External Environment—the organization must look outside its boundaries to identify and analyze issues taking place. These issues represent opportunities and threats and assist in identifying what the organization should do.

Focus Groups—convened to reach conclusions regarding environmental issues.

Functional Organizational Structures—organize activities around mission-critical functions or processes.

Gantt Charts—display activities or goals in a matrix format.

Goals—specify the major direction of the organization and provide actionable linkage to the mission.

Harvesting—occurs when the market has entered long-term decline or there is a need for short-term cash.

Horizontal Integration—grows the business by acquiring or affiliating with competitors such as multihospital systems.

Internal Development—uses this strategy for products or services closely related to existing products or services.

Internal Environment—involves an extensive review of internal processes, culture, structure, and technology to reveal strengths and weaknesses.

Internal Ventures—when products or services that are unrelated to current products or services are started within the organization.

Joint Ventures—used when risks are too high or the project is too large or too expensive to be done by a single organization. In a joint venture, two or more organizations combine resources to accomplish a designated task.

Licensing Strategy—when licensure is used as a strategy, proprietary technology is usually not purchased and therefore the organization is dependent on the licensor for support and upgrade.

Line Graphs/ Multiple Line Graphs—aid in assessment of trends or changes in performance (quantitative).

Liquidation—selling of organizational assets.

Maintenance of Scope Strategies—when current strategies are appropriate and few changes are needed, the organization may elect to maintain the existing strategies.

Market Development—focuses on entering new markets with existing products or services.

Market Entry Strategies—adaptive strategies used to bring market strategies to fruition. The three major strategies to enter a market are purchase, cooperation, and development: internal development and internal ventures.

Matrix—used to show combinations of data.

Matrix Structures—organize activities around problems to be solved rather than functions, products, or geography.

Merger—where two organizations combine through a mutual agreement to form a single new organization.

Mission—the articulation of the external opportunities and threats and the internal strengths and weaknesses.

Nominal Group Technique—team members independently generate a written list of ideas regarding an issue. After members have been given sufficient time to generate their list, each member takes turns reporting one idea at a time to the entire group.

Objectives—describe the results to be achieved, when and by whom, and are measurable

Penetration Strategies—focus on increasing volumes and market share.

Performance Improvement—a systematic, organization-wide approach to improving the processes and outcomes of the health care system.

Product Development—the introduction of new products or services to existing markets.

Purchase Strategies—when health care organizations purchase an existing organization, organizational unit, or a product or service.

Regression Analysis—a statistical technique available via computer software used to forecast the relationship between two variables. Multiple regression allows for the simultaneous investigation of two or more independent variables on a single interval-scaled or ratio-scaled dependent variable.

Retrenchment—occurs when the market has become too diverse, and there is a decline in profitability due to increasing costs.

Scenario Development—used to implement an identified strategy where tree diagrams are used to break broad goals, graphically, into increasing levels of detailed actions so a stated goal can be accomplished.

Situation Analysis—the initial stage of strategic planning; the process of determining the current state of the organization. This is accomplished through three interrelated processes: external environmental analysis, internal environmental analysis, and the development of the organization's mission, vision, values, and goals.

Status Quo—the assumption of a mature market when growth has ceased. The goal is to maintain the market share.

Strategic Management—fulfills the need for knowledge of the organization, the market, and the competitive situations health care leaders face and provides for ongoing, dynamic changes in the strategic plan when appropriate.

Strategic Planning—to devise a systematic, well-balanced process that allows the organization to fit in the environment. It stresses patient-focused quality and operational performance improvement. It is a continuous process of revisiting the system and restoring balance.

Strategy Deployment—implementing the strategic objectives. This includes culture, structure, and resources.

Strategy Formation—gathering data and using these data for decision making. There are four types of strategies: directional, adaptive, market entry, and competitive.

Values—the fundamental truths that the organization holds dear and reflect the philosophy of the organization.

Venture Capital Investment—a low-risk option where organizations purchase minority investment in a developing enterprise.

Vertical Integration—grow the business along the channel of distribution of core process such as an acute facility adding home care or long-term care.

Vision—the view of the future based on the understanding of the forces.

References

Bennis, W., & Nanus, B. (1985). *Leaders: The strategies for taking charge.* New York: Harper & Row.

BrainyQuote. (2008). *Aristotle Onassis.* Retrieved July 6, 2008, from http://www.brainyquote.com/quotes/authors/a/aristotle_onassis.html

Brassard, M., & Ritter, D. (1994). *The memory jogger™ II: A pocket guide to tools for continuous improvement & effective planning.* Salem, NH: Goal/QPC.

Chapman, E. (2003). *Radical loving care.* Nashville, TN: Vaughn.

Creative Quotations. (2007). *Artemus Ward.* Retrieved July 6, 2008, from http://www.creativequotations.com/one/1839.htm

DeSilets, L., & Dickerson, P. (2008). SWOT is useful in your tool kit. *Journal of Continuing Education in Nursing, 39*(5), 196–197.

Drenkard, K. (2001). Creating a future worth experiencing: Nursing strategic planning in an integrated healthcare delivery system. *Journal of Nursing Administration, 31*(7–8), 364–375.

Finkler, S. (2001). *Financial management for public, health, and not-for-profit organizations.* Upper Saddle River, NJ: Prentice Hall.

Gelatt, H. (1993). Future sense: Creating the future. *The Futurist,* (9–10), 9–13.

Ginter, P., Swayne, L., & Duncan, W. (2002). *Strategic management of health care organizations* (4th ed.). Malden, MA: Blackwell.

Goal/QPC. (1988). *The memory jogger: A pocket guide of tools for continuous improvement* (2nd ed.). Methuen, MA: Goal/QPC.

Gordon, J. (2002). *Organizational behavior: A diagnostic approach* (7th ed.). Upper Saddle Ridge, NJ: Prentice Hall.

Health Care Advisory Board. (1999). *Balanced scorecards.* Retrieved July 8, 2008, from http://www.advisory.com

Health Care Advisory Board. (2002). *Avoiding financial flashpoints: Foreseeing and preventing decline in hospital and health system fortunes.* Retrieved July 9, 2008, from http://www.advisory.com

Health Care Advisory Board. (2006). *Effective use of dashboards to analyze hospital success.* Retrieved July 8, 2008 from http://www.advisory.com

The Joint Commission. (2003). *Staffing effectiveness in hospitals.* Oakbrook Terrace, IL: Joint Commission Resources.

The Joint Commission. (2008). *Comprehensive accreditation manual for hospitals: The official handbook (CAMH).* Oakbrook Terrace, IL: Joint Commission Resources.

Kaissi, A., Begun, J. W., & Hamilton, J. A. (2008). Strategic planning processes and hospital financial performance. *Journal of Healthcare Management, 53*(3), 197–208.

Kaplan, R., & Norton, D. P. (1996). *Translating strategy into action: The balanced scorecard.* Boston: Harvard Business School.

Kim, W., & Mauborgne, R. (2002). Charting your company's future. *Harvard Business Review, 80*(6), 76–83.

Krueger, R. (1988). *Focus groups: A practical guide for applied research.* Newbury Park, CA: Sage.

Lighter, D., & Fair, D. (2004). *Quality management in health care: Principles and methods* (2nd ed.). Sudbury, MA: Jones and Bartlett.

Mintzberg, H., & Markides, C. (2000). Commentary on the Henry Mintzberg interview. *Academy of Management Executive,* 39–42.

Morgan, D. (1993). *Successful focus groups: Advancing the state of the art.* Newbury Park, CA: Sage.

National Institute of Standards and Technology. (2008). *2008 Baldrige national quality program: Health care criteria for performance excellence.* Gaithersburg, MD: Author.

The Quotations Page. (2007a). *Yogi Berra.* Retrieved July 6, 2008, from http://www.quotationspage.com/wotd.html

The Quotations Page. (2007b). *Marcel Proust.* Retrieved July 6, 2008, from http://www.quotationspage.com/search.php3?homesearch=proust&x=31&y=5

Solovy, A. (2002). The paradox of planning. *Healthcare & Healthcare Network, 76*(9), 32.

Tennessee Center for Performance Excellence. (2008). *Criteria for performance excellence: Traveling the road to success '08.* Nashville, TN: Author.

Zikmund, W. (2003). *Business research methods* (7th ed.). Mason, OH: South-Western.

Zuckerman, A. (1998). *Healthcare strategic planning: Approaches for the 21st century.* Chicago: Health Administration.

CHAPTER 17

Budget Strategies

Janne Dunham-Taylor, PhD, RN

Linda Nash Legg, MSN, RN

It is important that nurse administrators, and all nursing staff, continually identify budget strategies—just as they need to continually identify how services can be improved or changed for the better. *Once all have determined what the patient values (the first priority), the second issue becomes the budget that is available to implement this service.*

As discussed in Chapter 3, the old linear, authoritarian models are not effective and are outmoded. In this model, sometimes finance and nursing personnel do not even discuss issues together. In this model, finance personnel give a nurse manager the same budget amount with a bit more added for inflation or a percentage taken out for a budget cut. The nurse manager is not supposed to question anything. This is *not* an acceptable way of dealing with budget issues.

Instead, systems thinking is preferred with all in the organization understanding the connectedness of each person, action, and service that is happening throughout the organization. There needs to be ongoing dialogue with everyone throughout the organization as part of the budget process. (We start with the actual budget process because it is so flawed.) So in this newer model, the finance personnel are having an ongoing dialogue with nursing personnel about the proposed budget. This means that the players have *equal* importance in the dialogue, not that finance *tells* nursing what the budget will be. Both have key information that, when *shared*, results in better decisions and, ultimately, a better budget being realized.

We cover a number of budget strategies that we believe are important. This list is by no means complete because there are infinite numbers of strategies that can be used. Please add to this list and then share what works—and what does not work—with each other.

When thinking about strategies, it is important to put them into an organizational context. We advocate systems thinking, collaboration between players, and effective teamwork, with all focusing on the core values as the first priority (see Chapter 3). Then, the second issue is budget dollars available and how to best use those dollars to achieve the core values. This also takes into account, and supports, the strategic plan (see Chapter 16), giving priority to those services that are strategically necessary to realize the plan. In addition it takes into account which departments are already more cost conscious and does not penalize those departments by demanding that, when budget cuts are necessary, all equally share across-the-board cuts—that often happen in more authoritarian, linear systems.

Certain strategies work more effectively in one setting but not as well in another, because all our facilities have particular quirks or differences that affect the outcome. Knowing and understanding the differences are part of the organizational assessment, an administrative competency (discussed in Chapter 3). If our assessment is accurate, we can often guess how people in the organization will respond to changes. So it is important, when considering budget strategies, to think about where the organization presently is and to choose strategies based on this assessment. Otherwise, the chosen strategy may result in other more serious, unanticipated side effects.

Budget strategies stay ahead of the competition, recognizing that the competition is much more than just what a similar facility is doing down the road. Competition can come from unlikely sources such as all the public interest in alternative therapies and vitamins, or the advanced technologies that are less invasive to patients, or a stand-alone surgery center.

Budget Cuts

Budget cuts happen regularly in health care. A predominant reason is that government reimbursement for Medicaid and Medicare services gives back only cents on the dollar. This means that the reimbursed amount is less than half of that expended by the health care facility. Other insurance plans follow suit, taking similar measures, asking for larger discounts each year.

Budget cuts can also result from poor business decisions, such as giving too great a discount to insurance carriers, losing contracts with insurance companies such as Blue Cross, rescuing physician offices running at a deficit, providing poor leadership, or operating consistently at a loss yet never taking any measures to improve the situation.

What Is Our World View?

Our cost-cutting strategies are driven by our world view. This view creates silos (**Exhibit 17–1**). Thinking "outside the box" is important for all of us, even when we believe we are at the cutting edge of change!

One silo is that *resources are scarce*. This is not surprising because, as we have discussed in previous chapters, accounting and financial theory are based on scarcity:

> Accounting and finance are applied areas of microeconomics. The theory of economics forms the foundations upon which all financial management is ultimately built. The essence of economics is that society has a limited amount of resources, with competing demands for them. The economic system attempts to allocate those resources in an optimal fashion (Finkler & Kovner, 2000, p. 4).

Correspond this way of thinking with quantum physics theory where the world is composed of energy fields. Using quantum physics, one would say we need to be careful about our thoughts because they can create our reality. If this is the case, we would much rather choose *abundance* than *scarcity*.

Exhibit 17–1 Cost-Cutting Silos

Silos	Reality
• Resources are scarce.	• Resources are abundant.
• Doing things the way we have always done them.	• Change will always happen. We cannot escape it.
• One uses bottom-line thinking.	• The bottom line comes second, behind what the patient values.
• Financial decisions are separate from the rest of the organization.	• Financial decisions need to be made within the context of the total organization.

In fact, perhaps our present cost-cutting dilemmas have been caused by too many people thinking there are limited resources! We probably would make different decisions if we thought resources were abundant! In this book we choose abundance. Many financial people will have difficulty with this concept because their education and their work environment have always emphasized scarcity.

It is easy to get caught up in another box, or silo, as we continue to *do things the way we have always done them*. Staying with what is familiar is certainly more comfortable than change. However, if we never change anything, we will cause the organization's demise. Stasis equates with death. Regardless of our efforts to remain the same, *everything changes*. Thus this effort can lead us into difficulties because change is our only constant. Does everyone in the organization realize this?

A third silo is *bottom-line thinking*. Throughout this book we have advocated that the core value, such as providing what the patient values, comes first with the bottom line being second. The core value(s) is another guide for us when choosing a budget strategy.

Then there is the belief, another silo, that one can *separate financial decisions from other organizational decisions*, when actually any action we take will affect the bottom line. This means that everyone in the organization needs to be aware of, and involved in discovering, budget strategies.

How Do We Choose a Strategy?

What should guide us in choosing a strategy? The first priority is the core value(s). Second, everyone needs to be constantly vigilant as to what each patient values and needs and try to accomplish this in the most cost-effective way while still achieving safety/quality guidelines.

When making budget strategy decisions, it is important to come back to the Institute of Medicine's (IOM) safety/quality guidelines that every health care organization, purchaser, regulator, and educational institution focus on and align their environments toward providing care that is

- Safe: avoiding injuries to patients from the care that is intended to help them
- Effective: providing services based on the best available scientific knowledge to all who could benefit and refraining from providing services to those not likely to benefit
- Patient-centered: providing care that is respectful of and responsive to individual patient preferences, needs, and values and ensuring that patient values guide all clinical decisions
- Timely: reducing waits and sometimes harmful delays for both those who receive and those who give care
- Efficient: avoiding waste, including waste of equipment, supplies, ideas, and energy
- Equitable: providing care that does not vary in quality because of personal characteristics such as gender, ethnicity, geographic location, and socioeconomic status (Shortell & Selberg, 2002, pp. 7–8)

The importance of dialogue between organization staff members cannot be emphasized enough when determining strategies because each of us possesses only a partial answer. The more we can work as a team, and as equal players, the more effective our strategies will be. (In the old authoritarian system the chief executive officer [CEO] or executive group made all the budget decisions even though they were out of the loop on actual care and the issues that staff dealt with every day.) This is why it is so important for all administrators to do weekly rounds, interacting effectively with everyone they are in contact with, as described in Chapter 3. This provides a more accurate picture of what is actually happening in the trenches.

Several major health care systems have achieved national recognition in implementing the IOM recommendations in Health Care in America's 100 Top Hospitals study. For example, Exempla Healthcare—a Denver-based health care system—was named as having one of the top intensive care units in the nation. They implemented the IOM strategies in their strategic plan, making quality their key priority. This achieved improvements in quality and in collaboration with the medical staff by becoming a system-oriented, rather than a process-oriented, institution (Shortell & Selberg, 2002, p. 8).

Exempla first started with a protocol, for example, caring for a surgical patient, and then by using a systems perspective that accounted for both processes and the interdependencies of caregivers, evaluated and redesigned the protocol from admission to discharge. Responsibility was then assigned in this larger entire systems context rather than with just one process within the system. This integrated approach achieved a common framework with a common goal (Shortell & Selberg, 2002, p. 10).

In this example, Exempla's first priority was the patient. The IOM strategies were achieved, but the redesign also achieved a better profit margin. (The bottom line did not drive the change but was an effect of the change.) It is an example of how improved health care quality provides improved outcomes—for the patient, for the organization, and for the bottom line.

The Budget Process: Is It Flawed or Effective?

We need to examine the budget process that is used. In our interconnected world, the best budget process involves *everyone* in the organization—including patients, families, and physicians. This process is participative but extends beyond just participation. The process is most effective when all involved are equal partners, using dialogue (both sharing information and listening to others). This approach is much more effective than an authoritarian, or top-down, method of communication.

Therefore everyone from the housekeeper or nursing assistant through the physician and the board chair is involved in the decision-making process, including the strategic plan, with the patients and their families being the pivotal, or most important, part of this process. Physicians have to be included because physician practice patterns can have a direct effect on increasing or decreasing the budget.

We recommend being *honest* about budgets (see Chapter 12). The problem with dishonesty is that once you have been found out, your believability is gone. Trust, once lost, is extremely difficult to gain again or, realistically, is probably never gained again! Integrity, discussed in Chapter 2, is essential. After all, when integrity is not present, lies beget more lies.

Honesty can become a problem in an organization if everyone is playing games. If you, a manager, have been honest and have been diligent about holding down costs yet no one else has been held accountable, when there are budget cuts you may be expected to cut the same percentage as those who have not been accountable. Your unit then becomes penalized for being more effective! Thus it is very important to stress with your supervisors right from the start that you are holding down costs and ask them to promise that your unit will not be penalized if there is a budget cut. In certain organizations it is important to get this in writing.

> *We recommend being honest about budgets.*

Historically, a *flawed budget process* has been used. This process started in the 1920s when large companies used the process "as a tool for managing costs and cash flows" (Hope & Fraser, 2003, p. 113). Then in the 1960s:

> [C]ompanies used accounting results not just to keep score but also to dictate the actions
> of people at all levels of the company. By the early 1970s, a new generation of leaders

schooled in the finer arts of financial planning had begun to rely on financial targets and incentives—in lieu of such benchmarks as productivity and marketing effectiveness—to drive performance improvement (Hope & Fraser, 2003, p. 113).

This caused serious problems in the 1980s and 1990s when companies started paying more attention to sales targets than to satisfying customers. Suddenly money was running the game rather than supporting it.[1]

Budget Games

When dishonesty is prevalent and allowed to continue, serious problems result throughout the organization. This includes the budget process. Hope and Fraser (2003) report that budgeting can take up to *30% of management's time*! This time commitment becomes even more overwhelming when mergers and reorganization occur. This is expensive time that does not really accomplish much in the way of outcomes. In fact, many harmful games can result. Consider the following from Jensen (2001, pp. 96–97) in the *Harvard Business Review*:

> CORPORATE BUDGETING IS A JOKE, and everyone knows it. It consumes a huge amount of executives' time, forcing them into endless rounds of dull meetings and tense negotiations. It encourages managers to lie and cheat, lowballing targets and inflating results, and it penalizes them for telling the truth. It turns business decisions into elaborate exercises in gaming. It sets colleague against colleague, creating distrust and ill will. And it distorts incentives, motivating people to act in ways that run counter to the best interests of their companies.

> Consider… the recent debacle involving a big beverage company. The vice president of sales for one of the company's largest regions dramatically underpredicted demand for an upcoming major holiday. His motivation was simple—he wanted to ensure a low revenue target that he could be certain of exceeding. But the price for his little white lie was extremely high: The company based its demand planning on his sales forecast and consequently ran out of its core product in one of its largest markets at the height of the holiday selling season….

> The sad thing is, these shenanigans have become so common that they're almost invisible. The budgeting process is so deeply embedded in corporate life that the attendant lies and games are simply accepted as business as usual, no matter how destructive they are….

> As soon as you start motivating unit and department heads to falsify forecasts and otherwise hide or manipulate critical information, you undermine the salutary effects of budgeting. Indeed, the whole effort backfires. You end up with uncoordinated, chaotic interactions as people make decisions on the basis of distorted information they receive from other units and from headquarters. Moreover, since managers are well aware that everyone is attempting to game the system for personal reasons, you create an organization rife with cynicism, suspicion, and mistrust. When the manipulation of budget targets becomes routine, moreover, it can undermine the integrity of an entire organization.

---

[1] For more on this subject, see the book coauthored by Tom Johnson, *Relevance Lost: The Rise and Fall of Management Accounting*.

Another similar perspective is presented by Hope and Fraser (2003, pp. 108–109):

> Budgeting, as most corporations practice it, should be abolished.... Companies... cling tenaciously to budgeting—a process that disempowers the front line, discourages information sharing, and slows the response to market developments until it's too late.... In practice, they marshal the power of computer systems to uncover mind-numbing levels of detail and, using the budget as a benchmark, demand to know why a sales team has rung up higher-than-normal telephone charges, for instance, or why it has underspent the quarter's entertainment allowance. And where is 'all the authority of the chairman' when the team finds it can't meet the budget's sales targets? Fearing the consequences, the team will lean on customers to order goods they have every intention of returning. And if by some chance the team thinks it will exceed its targets, it will press customers to accept delivery in the next fiscal period, delaying valuable cash flows.
>
> In extreme cases, use of the budget to force performance improvements may lead to a breakdown in corporate ethics. [They then discuss several failed companies where, for example, employees had to be 2 percent under budget with nothing else being acceptable.] Other failed companies had tight budgetary control processes that funneled information only to those with a 'need to know.'
>
> A number of companies have recognized the full extent of the damage done by budgeting. They have rejected the reliance on obsolete data and the protracted, self-interested wrangling over what the data indicate about the future. And they have rejected the foregone conclusions embedded in traditional budgets—conclusions that render pointless the interpretation and circulation of current market information.

Bart's research (1988) on gamesmanship found several games that managers played: understating volume estimates, not declaring/understating price increases, not declaring/understating cost reduction programs, and overstating expenses for advertising, consumer promotions, trade-related issues, and market research. These budget manipulations resulted in "'cushion,' 'slush fund,' 'hedge,' 'flexibility,' 'cookie jar,' 'hip/back pocket,' 'pad,' 'kitty,' 'secret reserve,' 'war chest,' and 'contingency' funds" (p. 286). This occurs because usually senior management does not have the time to find the cushions, or because others were not as familiar with the product and did not realize the true costs.

Another game that is played with budgets is the "spend it or lose it" mentality that goes on at the end of the budget year. In this game, a manager knows that any money left in the budget will be lost at the end of the fiscal year. So the manager decides to find things to spend the money on just before the fiscal year closes.

Bart's research (1988) also examined companies where *games were not played*. Here "there was a good deal of trust between senior management and product managers" (p. 290). Honesty was valued. In fact, trust and honesty were so important one manager said,

> The moment I betray my... manager, I've had it in this company. My bosses will be angry with me for being unfair. And [people reporting directly to me] will never take my word at face value again. They'll start to play games with me and I'll have to try and catch them... and that sure can waste a lot of time! (p. 291).

What Can We Do to Solve the Budget Process Problems?

Today, we are using more participative, customer-oriented processes. This results in flatter structures and rapid responses to market changes and stays closer to the customer—emphasizing public relations, empowering workers to make appropriate decisions as they do their work, and sharing information, including information about budget expenses and revenues. All this enhances our systems so employees have all the tools present to do their work more effectively. Yet, if we still use the cumbersome, flawed, historical budget process, we do not achieve any of these objectives.

That is why we advocate different, newer processes that include dialogue and honesty. For instance, we present and discuss three examples.

DO AWAY WITH THE BUDGET

Some companies have done away with the budget and the budget process. Instead, they use the following method:

> Alternative goals and measures—some financial, such as cost-to-income ratios, and some nonfinancial, such as time to market—move to the foreground. And business units and personnel, now responsible for producing results, are no longer expected to meet predetermined, internally selected financial targets. Rather, every part of the company is judged on how well its performance compares with its peers' and against world-class benchmarks.

> In companies using these standards of performance, business units become smaller, more numerous, and more entrepreneurial. Strategy becomes a grass-roots endeavor. The aggregate result of many small teams exploiting local opportunities is a much more adaptive organization.

> But that's not to say these companies abandon their high expectations. They don't naively assume that everyone who is given more autonomy will improve his or her performance. In fact, they require employees to do something much tougher than meet a fixed target. They ask them to chase a will-o'-the-wisp, to measure themselves against how well comparable groups inside and outside the company will turn out to have done in the same period, given the economic conditions prevailing at the time. Because employees won't know whether they've succeeded or by how much until the period is over, they must use every ounce of their energy and ingenuity to ensure that their performance is better than that of their peers. Business units... can measure their progress against comparable units within the company through the use of a few key financial measures. In order to measure themselves against external peers, they can use operational benchmarks based in industry-wide best practices....

> Abandoning budget targets... frees a business to give a wise variety of emerging information its due.... This shifts the emphasis from meeting short-term promises to improving our competitive position year after year. The result is much more accurate interpretation of our results (Hope & Fraser, 2003, pp. 109–110).

REPLACE THE TRADITIONAL BUDGET WITH ROLLING FORECASTS

Hope and Fraser (2003) report that the focus has shifted from detailed budget plans to trend analyses and 3-month rolling forecasts for five to eight quarters. Managers, along with the finance department, are expected to constantly revise the forecasts. Instead of the cumbersome, detailed traditional budget approach, these forecasts include only "key variables, such as orders, sales, costs, and capital expenditures, which means they can be compiled relatively easily and quickly, sometimes by a single person in a single day" (p. 112). This way the budget information is constantly updated and takes the latest economic trends and customer usage patterns into account. Information is open to all in the organization. Playing budget games becomes difficult, and everyone receives more accurate, updated information for appropriate strategic planning information.

Here's how rolling forecasts usually work. Let's say that in the middle of March 2003, a company creates a five-quarter forecast that covers the period from the beginning of April 2003 through the end of June 2003. From the moment it is completed, new data start coming in. Once three months' worth is in hand, the process begins again. A new five-quarter forecast updates the projections for the period covered by the previous forecast and creates a brand-new projection for the quarter farthest in the future, July-September 2004.

Volvo relies on several types of rolling forecasts. Every month, it orders up a "flash" forecast that looks three months ahead, informing managers about current demand and helping them determine whether, for example, price promotions should be introduced or curtailed. Every quarter, a 12-month forecast updates the managers' working assumptions about customer behavior and economic trends. And every year, two additional forecasts—one looking four years ahead, one looking ten years ahead—help managers assess the company's market positioning and determine schedules for phasing out old models and phasing in new ones (Hope & Fraser, 2003, p. 112).

Companies using this approach have discovered that they can *save up to 95% of the time they originally spent going through the historical budget process.* For those of us used to traditional budgets, this can be a difficult change to picture. Instead of anticipating the budget for the next year, longer term goals, often rolling forecasts that project for the next couple years, are identified. Then the manager reviews the forecasts every quarter. The quarterly review helps managers to continually assess the action plan and to change it as new developments occur. Elements measured include both hard and soft performance data such as profits, cash flows, cost ratios, customer satisfaction, and quality. The organizations became *radically decentralized and needed a much smaller corporate structure* to support the front-line managers. Hope and Fraser (2003) describe companies that use this method:

In an empowered organization, people are free to make mistakes and equally free to fix them. Managers have wide discretion in making decisions; as a result, they can obtain resources more quickly than in traditional companies and without having to document need quite so elaborately, partly because they are accountable for the profitability of their units and can therefore be expected to shed any excess in the event that demand falls.... And employees, because they don't require much supervision, don't need the extensive central services that most organizations provide. Eliminating those services has a dramatic effect on a company's cost structure....

Without budget expectations to worry about, staff members can do something with the nonconforming customer and market information they collect—other than hide it. The reporting of unusual patterns and trends as they unfold helps the business avoid shortages or overages and formulate changes in direction. Instead of being imposed from above, strategy seeps up from below (pp. 110–111).

MARGIN MANAGEMENT

Posner reported a similar solution in 1987. Determining that the budgeting process had become too cumbersome, McManus, a CEO, changed the budgeting approach in the company he had started. He found that the final budget, arrived at during a painful, traditional budget process, was "based on assumptions that may or may not bear any resemblance to what will actually happen in the next 11 months" (p. 117). So what could be done about this time waster?

Luther, one of his managers, suggested doing away with the historical budget process and, instead, move to a margin management way of doing budgeting. McManus decided to try it. In a margin management system, of every dollar generated, 15% pays corporate overhead expenses and pretax profits. Then the manager would take over from there, determining how the rest of the money will be spent to accomplish the work. This turned the whole budgeting process around. Managers were careful to only spend money on what was necessary, and all employees began to really watch expenses. Managers were now planning budgets with input from staff based on what was actually occurring and then making the decisions on how the money was spent.

The article stressed how this was a much more effective process than having the CEO make the budget decisions, because the CEO was so removed from the day-to-day issues employees faced. This worked very well for normal business, and they suggested using three guidelines: (1) agree on the overhead amount, (2) empower managers and employees to make the budgeting decisions rather than having the executive group make the decisions, and (3) add incentives for both managers and employees to benefit from revenues they generated. There were two times when this strategy did not work—in new start-ups when people did not have any idea as to actual costs and revenues and with very unstable businesses.

Budget Strategies

Once the budget process is examined, and changed if necessary, other budget strategies can be considered. The first priority with budget strategies is that they support the core value(s) and effectively manage costs yet give safe, quality service. Also, it is important to put the budget strategies into an organizational context because most often the strategies will effect more than one department.

Exhibit 17–2 lists the budget strategies that we discuss in detail below.

Administrative Leadership

A first priority within an organization is to identify and rectify poor administrative leadership. Effective leadership was discussed in detail in Chapter 2. Some clues to look for are issues like administrators who focus too much on the bottom line, those who give lip service to core values yet their actions do not support the values, or those who lead from their own selfish motives, not what is best for others. Another problem that can occur is that an administrator may not realize how various actions or decisions impact others. For example, the president preaches that everyone else

---

Exhibit 17–2 Budget Strategies

- Administrative leadership
- Systems problems
- Environmental issues
- Creating a cost-conscious environment
- Progressive care units
- Benchmarking hospital length of stay
- Employing advanced practice nurses and hospitalists
- "Delight"ful service
- Trend spotting
- Creating ambulatory centers
- Acquiring technology
- Barcoding
- Coding accuracy using ChargeMaster
- Telehealth

needs to be cost effective and make budget cuts but purchases expensive new cherry office furniture. Or, administrators never make rounds, never deal with patients or patient issues, yet continue to make budget decisions and pull big salaries.

As previously noted, poor administrative leadership results in higher direct costs—such as more patient complications and other patient safety issues, an increased need for service or increased length of stay, more expensive staffing, more patient care delivery problems, or patients and physicians choosing to go elsewhere for services. There are also large indirect costs such as high staff turnover with new staff needing to be hired and oriented, more legal fees due to more patient lawsuits, more service that is not reimbursed, and more dissatisfaction on the part of the remaining patients, staff, and physicians. The spiral continues downward.

Contrast this with effective leaders who are doing daily rounds, can identify many issues that can be fixed as they occur, can encourage staff to take action on problems, and have a more realistic picture of the organization—what staff and patients are actually experiencing. In this case, chances are the unit or organization is using effective teamwork, patients are satisfied with their service and may even rave about how helpful certain people have been, physicians enjoy unit staff and know the patients will be taken care of properly, and direct and indirect costs will not get out of hand while revenues continue to come in.

Systems Problems

Besides the leadership problem, incredible cost savings can be realized by examining and fixing systems problems. For example, it is amazing how many things we continue to do that no one really needs to do anymore. Take our admitting procedure. Perhaps there are 120 steps that need to be done to admit a patient and only 75 of them are necessary presently, yet we go on doing all 120. Or on an inpatient service, the bed may not need to be changed daily. Or certain administrators never deal with problematic behaviors with staff or physicians—directly causing more budget costs that could be saved.

Another problem is duplication. For example, we may have five or six people all getting histories and physicals from the same patient. Or, we do not use the history and physical already completed in the facility that just transferred the patient to us.

Staffing issues can cause problems. The largest cost within the expense budget in health care organizations is the employee budget. Because this is a service industry, more people are needed to give the care the client receives. Chapter 6 provided strategies on workload management/staffing. However, one bears repeating here: Budget savings can be realized by hiring a higher number of registered nurses (RNs) rather than hiring a higher number of nursing assistants or licensed practical nurses. For a person oriented to the bottom line as first priority, this may be hard to fathom. You will hear, "But nursing assistant salaries are less than an RN salary. How can this be true?" Chapter 6 showed how expenses are lower using higher RN ratios, having enough support staff present to facilitate the RN function. This is true across the health care continuum.

Another factor with staffing is making sure that the staff is there when needed and not there when there is less to do. For instance, perhaps certain staff members are very busy for a certain period of time but do not have enough to do at other times, but at peak times there are not enough staff. Yet we continue to schedule them in the same way. Effective scheduling is essential.

Actually, we need to get out of the box on this one. Think about how rewarding it would be to see someone in the hospital, follow him or her through a skilled nursing facility unit, and then see that person at home for home care. And the patient would love the continuity. Think of the cost savings achieved with the larger bonus of both patient and staff satisfaction! We need to break down the barriers!

Along with staffing by actual needs, some hospitals have given RNs the responsibility to restrict admissions. One system used at the Mayo Clinic's Luther Midelfort Health System in Eau Claire, Wisconsin, follows:

> At least three times a day staff nurses or clerks on each unit fill out a simple form via the hospital's Intranet indicating the Unit's current patient volume and staffing situation. The computer assigns a numerical value to "anecdotal data," entered by the unit staffer and generates a "traffic light" color—red, orange, yellow, or green—signaling the unit's capacity. The unit's assigned color is posted on the Intranet's "status board" and is immediately available to nursing supervisors. Nurses have the ability to override the assigned color if they disagree with the computer's assessment. Each unit designates its own nurse or nurses to evaluate the computer-generated assessment; very often the charge nurse or another direct-care nurse with a leadership role is given the assignment. The nurses' "capping trust"—the authority the system grants them to restrict unit admissions—cannot be over-ridden by doctors or administrators…. [This] has not only improved throughput… but also contributed to increased job satisfaction among nurses and a percent drop in the hospital's RN vacancy rate (Connolly, 2002).

Martha Jefferson Hospital in Charlottesville, Virginia, implemented a program that provided a nurse refresher program to inactive nurses and then hired them as admission-discharge-teaching nurses to help with this function throughout the facility. This was another win–win situation because the patients got better care, hospital stays were shortened, and staff morale improved (Blankenship & Winslow, 2003). Another cost strategy to reward employees is to either provide a wellness program or to get employee discounts at local facilities that will enhance employee health and well-being.

Huge problems can occur when we, as administrators, implement a quick-fix solution that actually compounds the situation and results in more problems than had previously occurred. Quick-fix solutions were discussed further in Chapter 3. A common example occurs when suddenly the executive team, or the financial officer, determines that drastic cost cuts are necessary. Then everyone gets into the frenzy, and quick-fix cost cuts are made:

- Cut the education budget, travel costs, and positions—and then wonder later why there are more safety issues occurring
- Have every department take the same percentage cut, not taking into account which departments might be more efficient already or which departments need to contract or expand due to environmental changes
- Suddenly restructure—which generally translates into losing some positions with no preplanning

Another strategy is to give the patient care in the least expensive setting, such as moving a surgical patient quickly from the recovery room, to the intensive care unit, to general care unit, to skilled nursing unit, to home with home care. This saves money but can result in less continuity for the patient.

A big time waster is the time spent finding caregivers. For instance, sometimes a nurse will call or page the physician who is unavailable at the time. Then the physician calls the nurse, but it is hard to track down the nurse. Having computerized documentation systems linked between the practice setting and the physician's office can facilitate this communication. Another example is a family member who wants to talk to the nurse but the nurse cannot be found. Some facilities are using a tracking device that the nurse wears so the nurse can easily be found, or the nurse has a cell phone.

For some reason many administrators, when faced with personnel problems, problem departments, systems issues, or budget cuts, resort to reorganizing or reengineering/restructuring. Both reorganization and reengineering were meant to happen in a carefully crafted way, following dialogue and careful planning by all involved. Instead, they are actually quick fixes that then create further problems. Meanwhile, the original issues are not resolved and actually got worse. Is it any wonder that in this frenzy there are additional costs incurred that were not considered?

> It is both obvious and worthy of emphasis that if we are going to improve cost and service performance in [health care organizations], we must begin by looking at how we use our employees—how many there are, what kinds, what we ask them to do, how we organize them, and how in reality they spend their time and the institution's resources.... For [health care organizations], the value added is the sum of all personnel-related expenses.... Not all costs are created equal.... What was needed was a framework that recognized the differences between costs and the different strategies to which each might or might not be susceptible. As a result, operations strategists devised a conceptual model for thinking about costs: the cost performance hierarchy (Lathrop, 1993, pp. 24–27).

This operations performance hierarchy asks three questions (Lathrop, 1993, p. 28):

1. "**What** is done?" Evaluation includes: "census and admission rates; variability of external demand; intensity of care required/severity of illness; quality of care objectives; service offerings; and location."
2. "**How** is it done?" Here one would examine "organizational structure, management processes, operating policies and systems, capacity management, physical size and layout, equipment deployment, and skill mix."
3. "**How well** is it done?" Evaluation includes quality measurements, "productivity levels, work pace, and skill level."

For instance, if one is starting with the basics, at the inherent level, one would ask, "What is done?", and one might measure census or location. If one wanted to find out structural issues, one would ask, "How is it done?", and one might measure skill mix or physical size and layout. And if one were in the execution phase, one would ask, "How well is it done?", and one might measure productivity levels.

Two common ways to restructure or reorganize are inpatient bed consolidation by reaggregation of the patient population with increased outpatient or freestanding facility solutions and/or by downsizing and cutting present staff positions. Either can have drastic effects on both the remaining workforce and on efficiency in general. Most often, the result is inefficiency, realized in elevated costs and other costly short-term and long-term effects.

A short-term effect of redesign is that the "survivors" need an orientation to assume the duties of displaced personnel. This means that a less effective, less efficient staff are not only dealing with the acquisition of new duties—and the resultant creation of more patient safety issues—but are also experiencing "survivor sickness." Burke (2002) describes "survival sickness" as having the following characteristics: "low morale, decreased commitment, and increased cynicism, mistrust, and anger. Affected caregivers may question the effectiveness of their facility's functioning, describe their work environment as deteriorated, and believe that this deterioration threatens patient's well-being" (p. 41). These are the short-term effects. However, it may not stop there.

How well the organization supports staff during times of restructuring directly impacts retention of the remaining staff. So a long-term effect, along with additional costs, may be a subsequent increase in staff turnover rates resulting from restructuring. Sometimes it is easier to be the person who is displaced than to be one of the remaining staff on a unit/department. Based on these facts, it is very important for the nurse leader and other health care organization officials to provide support for the "survivors."

Actually, providing survivor support is a tall order. It is best if administrators are continually communicating with staff about the changes that will take place as well as why these changes were necessary. Once staff trust is lost, it is very difficult to regain. In addition, staff morale will suffer when layoffs or restructuring occur, and teamwork may be affected within and between departments. Burke (2002) advocates taking the following steps to improve staff involvement that will deal more effectively with survivor issues:

- Create focus groups or hold employee meetings to discuss the restructuring, particularly what went right and solutions for what went wrong. (Note here that it would have been better to do focus groups and employee meetings as part of the planning process for redesign in the first place.)
- Develop education programs to help employees adjust.
- Identify employee concerns through surveys (or do rounds!).
- Formulate new communication strategies.
- Reevaluate jobs to better reflect new responsibilities.

There is an important long-term financial effect. People who advocate "slash and burn" cost cutting would do well to heed some research published in the *Harvard Business Review*: "Companies with few or no layoffs performed significantly better than those with large numbers of layoffs" (Rigby, 2002). In addition, the research found that companies with similar growth rates that did not downsize were found to consistently outperform those that did downsize. Aside from all this, there were costs associated with layoffs:

- Severance packages
- Temporary declines in productivity or quality
- Rehiring and retraining costs

Thoughtless approaches are implemented without considering future consequences. This research shows that greater cost savings are realized by dealing with the more knotty organizational and leadership problems and that downsizing and layoffs can actually be more expensive in the long run.

Environmental Issues

Shortell and Selberg (2002) suggest four main environmental areas that should be targeted for improvement:

1. The infrastructure that supports the dissemination and application of new clinical knowledge and technologies. When we are focused on providing evidence-based care, we will significantly improve quality. As nursing executives, we must provide the latest and greatest in tools for clinicians to use to adopt best practices. With the growing number of elderly in the US, which in turn increases the population of patients experiencing chronic illness, healthcare teams with best knowledge and best practices will provide the most improvements in patient care (p. 7).

2. The information technology infrastructure. Automation is a must. From automated drug order entry to the automated patient record, a paperless system with its integrated documentation provides less errors and better quality. When improvements in quality are noted by consumers/patients, The Institute of Medicine committee believes that confidence in the healthcare system will return (p. 8).

3. Payment policies. Financial incentives must be built into the system to provide for the alignment of care based on best practices with the achievement of better patient outcomes. This change in the environment directly affects the budget process. These incentives would be built in up front. The Institute of Medicine is suggesting that "all stakeholders in the system reexamine payment policies to develop methods that provide fair payment for good clinical management of the types of patients seen" (p. 8).

4. Preparation of the healthcare workforce. Today's healthcare workers will need new skills to accommodate the aims of the 21st-century healthcare system as set forth by The Institute of Medicine. Because systems thinking will be a cornerstone of a transformed health system, its workers will need skills to transfer best practices to other parts of the organization. Administrators at all levels must also learn to work closely with clinicians so that there is less separation between medicine and management (pp. 7–8).

Creating a Cost-Conscious Environment

Supply costs, rising daily in health care, also need to be examined. These costs are second only to the cost of staffing. One way to decrease supply costs is by exercising more reasonable use of supplies by nursing staff. Nurse managers responsible for creating and maintaining their unit's fiscal budgets can provide substantial decreases in costs by controlling supply expenditures. An overall decrease in the organization's fiscal budget may be realized as each individual unit's supply budget is trimmed for efficiency.

As we become more conscious of supply costs as managers, it is important to involve staff in this issue.

> We must also communicate to patients, nurses, and physicians that [health care organizations] no longer can afford to give things away. Someone always ends up paying. Nurses are trained to help people, to be generous and giving. For example, a nurse may give a patient a bunch of sterile pads rather than instructing him to go to the local pharmacy. Even those who mean well can put a [health care organization] out of business (Lefever, 1999, p. 30).

Inefficiencies mount up. For unit-based cost savings to occur, staff should be involved in the formulation of the department's fiscal budget and know the overall organization's financial targets. Staff then have a better sense of how they are contributing to either cost inefficiencies, or to cost containment, without compromising quality. After all, practice behaviors can affect the cost of delivering patient care.

Another strategy to maximize efficiency of supply usage by staff is to provide an educational approach to the issue. Krugman, MacLauchlan, Riippi, and Grubbs (2002) report a successful multidisciplinary financial education research project taken by a Western tertiary teaching hospital. In this project nurses, resident physicians, pharmacists, and nursing students integrated fiscal knowledge into practice. This study measured baseline financial knowledge regarding charges, reimbursement, and regulatory issues before implementing several initiatives. The team then developed a variety of initiatives to target knowledge deficits. A logo was created and used as a symbol for identifying financial articles published quarterly in the hospital newsletter. Subcommittees addressed the institution's financial problems. Efforts began with various educational activities, such as videos and the purchase of a financial software program for nursing leadership.

The post-survey showed that the subjects' financial knowledge improved. Targeted educational interventions proved successful. Financial outcomes included an increase in captured patient charges, improved documentation of services rendered, and decreased materials loss/wastage. This study was indicative of the positive effects that can be realized from awareness campaigns and educational activities involving staff and physicians (Krugman, et al., 2002, p. 277). An additional finding was that often nurses had negative attitudes related to cost-effectiveness, associating these with staffing reductions, pay cuts, longer work hours, and diminished resources. Because of these negative attitudes, nurses may not be as cost effective in their nursing practice.

Invisible costs for unused supplies from packs and trays, obsolete and slow-moving inventory, pilferage, giveaways, and uncontrolled usage create waste and are a prime target for nurse managers wishing to correct supply budget variances. First, a nurse manager must determine how and where the major waste is occurring. This may be done by reviewing the unit's present inventory of supplies and determining if there are opportunities for efficiency in areas where practice creates costly waste. An example of this may be when there are supplies requested by physicians who no longer have patients in the department where they are kept. Correcting this waste may be as simple as revising or providing standardization of supplies and of supply usage. Decreasing this type of stock will not only decrease the number of dollars required for the department's supply budget but will also provide more space for pertinent supplies.

As the financial resources available for purchase of supplies, linen, and equipment have dwindled due to low reimbursements, there has been more hoarding of supplies and equipment. Although hoarding provides staff with immediate access to the resources they need for patient care, staff do not realize that they add to their supply and equipment problems overall. Overstocking costs money. Tying up financial resources for purchase of more and more supplies due to stockpiling can actually build to a point where the whole facility is not efficient in the management of materials. For example, hoarding of IV pumps (or linen, monitors, or wheelchairs) only creates the need to purchase more IV pumps for the facility—a big, unnecessary expense. This "lost" inventory would be less costly if left in circulation throughout the health care organization.

In actuality, *the shortage problem is a symptom of a larger systems problem.* Instead of hiding and storing up more inventory for the unit, it is much more cost efficient to bring together a group of representatives from appropriate departments to work out a better solution. The solution needs to have the right numbers at the right times in the right place.

This systems strategy is also a useful way to examine supply and equipment fluctuations as patient volume changes. For instance, if the patient census, or acuity, has decreased, the nurse manager, as well as other appropriate departmental managers, could check to see if the inventory usage has also decreased. A periodic survey and inventory of all nursing units in a facility can help with these issues.

In addition, nurse administrators can periodically review overall monthly budget costs for linen, supplies, and equipment. Sudden variances in this budget could indicate hoarding, creating the need for purchases to counteract the decreases in certain areas. Close interaction with departments, such as the laundry, central supply, and materials management, could shed light on areas of concern. Educating staff concerning supply costs so they can adjust inventories to meet patient demands is extremely important. The staff should realize that they have a direct responsibility to achieve efficiency and, if something is not working, to express their concerns to the appropriate managers so problems can be fixed. Everyone, including the nurse manager, needs to be involved in achieving better efficiencies.

One common purchasing approach has been to only have supplies delivered as they are needed: the *just-in-time* philosophy. The idea behind this is to save money by not stockpiling and to avoid having too much already present at the facility. In health care, a service industry, where one is not making the same widgets every day, it can be difficult to anticipate which patients with which medical or surgical problems will need supplies each day. It is difficult to anticipate emergencies. So it is best to be more moderate with this approach.

Standardization of supply usage can also provide cost savings. For example, the standardization of items placed in sterile trays and packs for labor and delivery procedures on obstetrical units, in emergency rooms, or in surgery departments may be warranted. Meeting with the physicians up front to elicit their input on the design of the new trays is a must. The changes need to satisfy their needs as well as provide efficiency. Otherwise, more waste could occur.

Sales representatives from supply vendors who are providing the most efficient contracts for their supplies may be especially helpful in the design of these new packs and trays. Attending health care supply trade fairs may also provide the nurse administrator with excellent information concerning the newest, and most efficient, items available to be placed in the packs. Price wars from vendors may be your best bet in acquiring the most items of quality for the least amount of money. In other words, cost comparison is a must.

Because the cost of medical supplies and equipment is one of the major costs associated with health care, it is imperative for nurse administrators to be knowledgeable in the latest trends affecting the purchasing of these supplies. Having knowledge and being able to "talk the talk" with purchasing managers is essential for nurse managers to have an influence on the buying practices for their units and the institution as a whole.

Progressive Care Units

Progressive care units, also called swing units, have been established to provide care for patients who are waiting for an available bed for admission (i.e., from the emergency room) or have been in an intensive care unit and are waiting for a step-down bed. It may be an overflow unit or may be designated for certain kinds of patients, such as cardiopulmonary or neurological step-down units. Generally, criteria are established for admission. This prevents the bottlenecks that occur when patients have not yet been discharged but other patients already need these beds (Meyer, 2002).

Benchmarking Hospital Lengths of Stay

As prospective pay and managed care became a reality, it was suddenly necessary to make hospital lengths of stay as short as possible. Inpatient stays were directly linked with resource use. As hospitals benchmarked length of stays for specific diagnosis-related groups with other hospitals, using averages was somewhat useful but did not capture enough information about distributions to make the data as meaningful as it could be. Histograms have proved to be more helpful to picture these data:

> Histograms are bar graphs which employ relative heights of each bar to identify relative numbers of patients generating particular stays. Histograms thus take the form of collections of bars where peaks identify stays with the largest numbers of discharges and valleys indicating stays with the lowest numbers of inpatients. They provide more information than simple median lengths of stay in identifying the compactness of the distribution of stays and more information than mean stays in identifying numbers of outlier cases. Outlier cases are also more clearly pictured with histograms (Lagoe, Arnold, & Noetscher, 1999, p. 76).

Benchmarking has aided hospitals to decrease the length of stay by using multidisciplinary approaches, like case management and critical/clinical pathways, as discussed in the next chapter. For instance, case management departments use benchmark data to identify the costs and efficiencies associated with their care practices. Improvements can then be made to these practices to deal more effectively with outliers.

Employing Advanced Practice Nurses and Hospitalists

Recently, advanced practice nurses have been employed in health care organizations in an attempt to become both more effective and cost efficient. Nurse practitioners are often involved in primary, and less often in tertiary, care roles where they can do an initial assessment and history. They also follow up with chronic or typical acute patients while the physician is involved with the care of more acute or complicated patients. Nurse anesthetists are often found in the operating room, thus achieving a cost savings for less complicated surgeries. Clinical nurse specialists can be found in hospitals helping nursing staff take care of more complicated patients and/or having an education role with nursing staff with a result that patient outcomes improve and length of stay is reduced (Rosenfeld, 2000). In psychiatry, clinical nurse specialists have patient practices in the community. In some states, nurse midwives are delivering babies in both hospital settings and in the home.

Advanced practice nurses can be employed by hospitals, long-term care facilities, physicians, or can freelance on their own. When employed by hospitals, they are credentialed along with the physicians. Some physicians believe that advanced practice nurses help them care for chronic patient conditions, freeing physicians to treat more complicated patients, whereas other physicians believe that advanced practice nurses have a negative impact on physician income. Advanced nursing practice varies in practice act definitions from state to state.

Another recent addition on the hospital scene is to hire hospitalists. *Hospitalists* are physicians that treat inpatients of all ages only during a hospital stay—admission through discharge.

> Managed care and the Balanced Budget Act are propelling the shift to hospitalists, an emerging subspecialty of internal medicine which is devoted to improving the efficiency of care for hospitalized patients. Intensive, on-site care management by hospitalists can produce substantial savings.... Studies show that inpatient specialists can reduce length of stay by more than 30 percent, and hospital costs up to 20 percent.
>
> ... The reasons for these dramatic improvements in costs per case and length of stay are not hard to find:
>
> - No delays of treatment after admission,
> - Volume-based experience of hospitalist enhances diagnostic speed, facilitating earlier start of treatment,
> - Vigilant attention to changes in patient condition on a 24x7 basis, e.g., new lab data, nursing observations,
> - Minimal patient down-time in waiting for care, testing results, or specialty consultations,
> - Continuous, rapid fine-tuning of therapeutics over the course of hospitalization,
> - Ready availability of hospitalist to patient and family improves communication and facilitates their approval for changes in treatment,
> - Hospitalist knows "how to get things done around here" to facilitate timeliness, improve efficiency in use of the hospital's resources,
> - Greater confidence in early discharge from ICU, recovery room, to more appropriate (and lower-cost) levels of care, and
> - Discharge planning begins at start of admission (Coile, 2000, p. 8).

There are downsides to hospitalists. They provide less continuity of care for the patient because the patient returns to the regular physician when discharged. The patient does not know the hospitalist and does not have a relationship with him or her. Also, some primary care physicians want to continue to follow the patient. And finally, at times the hospitalist can order more tests and drive up costs rather than decrease them.

"Delight"ful Service

This occurs when everyone goes the extra mile and "delights" the patient. Disney, Southwest Airlines, and Marriott built their market share on this premise. The only way to achieve patient "delight" is for all staff members in an organization to perform their daily tasks as best they can. On a personal level, it means that everyone is evaluating the patient experience and personalizing approaches to best meet patient needs. On an organizational level, it involves improving environmental processes and enhancing structural capabilities.

Examples of customer delight might include special "helps" that are available to patients such as not having to walk long distances to get to an appointment (this is especially helpful for the frail elderly but is useful for anyone coming to the facility), not having long waits for service, and providing someone to help fill out all the insurance paperwork. The sky is the limit on ideas here.

The most effective marketing that an organization can achieve is the marketing that is done by "word of mouth" from satisfied clients/patients. If processes and procedures are in place to ensure that patient care is delivered in a manner pleasing to the patient and supportive of good patient outcomes, this will speak for itself. Having satisfied clients is much more effective as a marketing tool than all the high-tech market research that can be performed. In fact, much of the marketing budget is wasted if service is poor.

Trend Spotting

Identifying trends occurring in the health care market can be a helpful indicator of possible change.

Creating Ambulatory Centers

Because there is more competition from increasing numbers of ambulatory centers, it can be helpful for a larger facility to start a center(s). The advantage is that facility charges in an ambulatory center are lower than a larger full-service facility.

Acquiring Technology

Achieving complete and accurate documentation is another large expense with a lot of potential cost savings. The upfront cost of purchasing and implementing computerized charting is offset by the cost efficiency it provides. Streamlined documentation is a vital necessity in the overall medical records process to provide accuracy and ease of access to the required records to provide safety checks, to document the time and cost of nursing care, and also to meet regulatory guidelines and justify insurance payments. Take coding, for instance. In a paper system a lot of time is spent searching through mounds of paper to obtain coding information. Computerized charting decreases the turnaround in reimbursement for hospital stays by providing a fast, efficient retrieval of the pertinent coding information.

Another advantage is the growing competition. For example, health maintenance organizations now cover some 67 million Americans. Kaiser Permanente, the nation's largest health maintenance organization, spent $1 billion for information technology that will achieve better care as well as document that the care was given (Schonfeld, 1998, p. 111). Then they marketed this to employers to show that their care would be safer because of this technology. This was prompted when employers, such as General Motors and Xerox, started ranking health plans by cost and quality to give their employees the best possible health care. To give a health maintenance organization the edge in the saturated market, low cost care was not enough. Higher standards and quality of care must also accompany the lower cost.

Information technology also makes it possible to achieve better management decisions and patient safety. Chapter 5 covered more information on the technology available and on Internet links for best practices available to practitioners in real time.

Barcoding

Barcoding is another recent information technology tool implemented by the health care industry. It accomplishes several purposes:

- Decreases the incidence of medication error
- Improves patient identification processes
- Improves medical supply inventory
- Achieves a more accurate charge for treatments and supplies
- Provides for more automation of the electronic medical record

The U.S. Food and Drug Administration mandated that, by the end of 2003, barcoding would be mandated on all single-unit packages of prescription drugs, over-the-counter drugs commonly used in hospitals, vaccines, and biologics such as blood. With barcoding, a three-way match is required before drugs can be administered.

Coding Accuracy Using Chargemaster

Coding[2] has become a part of information technology necessary for prompt patient billing. It is easy to overlook possible charges that could be made and miss out on revenue because of denials from inaccurate coding, missed charges, and incorrect use of modifier codes. It is helpful to standardize costs and provide frequent updates online and in Chargemaster. This can be very confusing because, as outlined in Chapter 10, reimbursement varies depending on the service. Sometimes specific costs can be directly billed, such as in some outpatient and surgical services, but other times, such as with diagnosis-related group and with resource utilization group reimbursements, the costs cannot be billed separately because an overall reimbursement amount is paid for a specific patient stay.

It behooves the nurse administrator to understand how billing should occur for areas of responsibility. If costs can be directly charged, and if no one realizes this, the facility could lose considerable money. Usually, the finance department is cognizant of what can be directly billed and what cannot, but sometimes nurse administrators have discovered that additional items should be billed. So, the nurse administrator needs to have accurate knowledge of billing nuances. Several sources can be very helpful, besides a discussion with the finance department, such as professional seminars or networking with peers across the country who are responsible for similar specialty areas.

---

[2] Coding is explained in detail in Chapter 10 of Dunham-Taylor and Pinczuk (2006).

Telehealth

Telehealth can provide health services more conveniently for patients as well as provide another cost-saving approach. One of the most exciting new uses of telehealth is in the form of telemergency services, including triage services, which bring the benefits of fast and efficient emergency care to underserved rural areas. Electronic or telephone links can connect patients at distant sites with physicians and nurse practitioners for care.

Besides emergency medicine, "telephone health consultation accounts for up to 25% of patient encounters in internal medicine and even more in pediatrics" (Simonsen-Anderson, 2002, p. 117). Phone consultations can save as much as $50 to $240 per member and also save the customer's time. Nurses with physician backup can provide services. Telephone nursing service does not come without a significant organizational cost upfront.

Writing a Business Plan

Because budget strategies can result in making changes, and especially if they alter the way money is spent, the nurse manager must be able to effectively express needed changes in an organized, professional fashion that emphasizes not only what needs to happen but the costs of this change. Thus we have included this section on writing a business plan, or a proposal.

Business plans/proposals may request a needed piece of equipment, explain a different way of implementing patient care, or be more extensive such as designing a new service. This plan/proposal may simply be given to a supervisor, go to the nurse executive or director of nursing, or, after consultation with the nurse executive, it may go to the finance department personnel, the executive team, or even to the board.

The business plan/proposal should present actual data and costs as well as provide a thoughtful rationale for the solutions. It should be readable and concise—executive team members like one-page executive summaries. However, the first step is to prepare a thoughtful business plan/proposal for the nurse executive, and this is what we discuss here.

Generally, a business plan reflects changes in the way services are delivered and involves a shift in the way money is spent. Alternately, the plan/proposal may request that the budget reflect different monetary amounts within certain categories based on changes in the patient population. However, the plan may be more extensive and ask for several different, or more updated, pieces of expensive equipment needed to provide a service—such as new cardiac monitors—or the proposal may request new technology such as a new system for computerized charting for the entire facility or system. And, because nurses are involved with patients, the plan may even suggest a new, innovative service that the nursing staff and the nurse manager have realized is not presently provided.

A business plan/proposal has more credence if it is typed neatly using word processing software and can often be illustrated more effectively using Power Point or other graphic computer programs. The plan needs to be carefully thought out and lead the reader through understanding a problem, provide the reader with the proposed solution to effectively deal with the problem, and present the reasons why this proposed solution is the best way to solve the problem. At times, it may be best to actually present several solutions that may cost different amounts of money, giving the pros and cons of each solution.

Think of to whom the plan will go. What is their perspective about the situation to which your proposal refers? What information will they need to know? What background information might be helpful to include in the plan? Be clear about what is requested and what the impact or effect will be on the whole organizational system. Be organized in the delivery and present a reasonable solution to the problem. Plans should include the following:

- Title—The person's name who wrote the proposal followed by appropriate background information.
- Definition—Define the proposed item, change, service, or program.
- Rationale—Why is it needed? Why is this the best item, or way, to do the service? Here you may need to outline other alternatives you considered.
- Implementation plan—Specify what needs to happen. Provide timelines.
- Costs/benefits—Show the actual costs and, if appropriate, how this will change existing costs. This can often be presented more clearly using a spreadsheet, table, pie chart, or bar graph.
- Evaluation plan—How will you evaluate the effectiveness of this proposed item or service?

Discussion Questions

1. Describe the effectiveness of the budget process where you work. What is very positive about it? What needs to be improved? What could be done to improve it?
2. Name 10 budget strategies that would improve budget effectiveness at work.
3. Take one of the strategies, listed from question 2, and describe how you would introduce it in the workplace. Then map out what would need to happen for it to be implemented.
4. Name five trends that affect your workplace.
5. Write a business plan for something that is needed at work.

References

Bart, C. (November 1988). Budgeting gamesmanship. *Academy of Management Executive, 11*(4), 285–294.

Blankenship, J., & Winslow, S. (2003). Admission-discharge-teaching nurses: Bridging the gap in today's workforce. *Journal of Nursing Administration, 33*(1), 11–13.

Burke, R. (2002). The ripple effect. *Nursing Management, 33*(2), 41–42.

Coile, R. (2000). Hospitalists redefine the future of inpatient medicine. *Cost & Quality*, (4): 8–11.

Connolly, A. (2002, May). Luther Midelfort: Granting RNs authority to restrict admissions streamlines patient flow. *Boston Business Journal.*

Dunham-Taylor, J., & Pinczuk, J. (2006). *Financial management for nurse managers: Applications in hospitals, long-term care, home care, and ambulatory care.* Sudbury, MA: Jones and Bartlett.

Finkler, S., & Kovner, C. (2000). *Financial management for nurse managers and executives* (2nd ed.). Philadelphia: W. B. Saunders.

Hope, J., & Fraser, R. (2003). Who needs budgets? *Harvard Business Review, 81*(2), 108–115.

Jensen, M. (2001). Corporate budgeting is broken—let's fix it. *Harvard Business Review, 70*(10), 94–101.

Krugman, M., MacLauchlan, M., Riippi, L., & Grubbs, J. (2002). A multidisciplinary financial education research project. *Nursing Economic$, 20*(6), 273–278.

Lagoe, J., Arnold, K., & Noetscher, C. (1999). Benchmarking hospital lengths of stay using histograms. *Nursing Economic$, 17*(2), 75–85.

Lathrop, J. (1993). *Restructuring health care: The patient-focused paradigm.* San Francisco: Jossey-Bass.

Lefever, G. (1999). Invisible costs, visible savings. *Nursing Management, 30*(8), 29–32.

Meyer, M. (2002). Avoid PCU bottlenecks with proper admission and discharge criteria. *Nursing Management, 33*(6), 31–35.

Posner, B. (1987). Margin management. *INC.*, 117–118.

Rigby, D. (2002, April). Look before you lay off. Downsizing in a downturn can do more harm than good. *Harvard Business Review*, 20–21.

Rosenfeld, B. (2000). A remote possibility. *Cost & Quality*, 38–39.

Schonfeld, E. (1998). Can computers cure health care? *Fortune, 137*(6), 111–116.

Shortell, S., & Selberg, J. (2002). Working differently: The IOM's call to action. *Healthcare Executive, 17*(1), 6–10.

Simonsen-Anderson, S. (2002). Safe and sound. Telephone triage and home care recommendations save lives and money. *Nursing Management, 33*(6), 41–44.

CHAPTER **18**

An Overview of Case Management

Patricia A. Hayes, PhD, RN

Key Terms

☞ Case Management   ☞ Case Management Certification

Introduction

Case management, a health care delivery strategy, has experienced a renaissance with the rise of managed care during the last decade. Building on a rich history in public health nursing and social work, case management has evolved since the turn of the century from community service coordination to approaches that coordinate and deliver health care services across the care continuum. These settings include acute and subacute care, home care, and long-term care. This evolution has led to the development of new models and standards for case management practice. The models are diverse, growing in number and changing as health care systems continue to transform.

Within this context of evolving models, the definitions of case management often lack consensus. However, two major definitions have emerged, one specific to the discipline of nursing and the other interdisciplinary.

According to the American Nurses Credentialing Center (ANCC, 1998):

> Case management is a dynamic and systematic collaborative approach to providing and coordinating healthcare services to a defined population. It is a participative process to identify and facilitate options and services for meeting individuals' health needs, while decreasing fragmentation and duplication of care and enhancing quality, cost-effective clinical outcomes (p. 3).

This definition is grounded in the nursing process and focuses on collaboration and client populations as important elements for nursing case management.

The interdisciplinary definition, developed by the Case Management Society of America (CMSA, 2002), describes case management as a "collaborative process which assesses, plans, implements, coordinates, monitors and evaluates options and services to meet an individual's health needs through communication and available resources to promote quality, cost-effective outcomes" (p. 8). The major difference between the two definitions is ANCC's focus on the health needs of populations and CMSA's focus on the health needs of individuals.

From these two definitions have come common goals for case management models:

- quality of care demonstrated by therapeutic and beneficial patient outcomes
- length of stay focused on cost control through rapid movement of inpatients through the system

- resource utilization achieved through protocols or critical pathways derived from research and evaluation of patient outcomes
- continuity of care achieved through the integration of services across the illness episode by a familiar case manager (Flarey, 1996; Taylor, 1999).

How organizations operationalize these goals depends on the case management model they select to guide their particular case management delivery system.

Models of Case Management in Nursing: Past and Present

In the last decade many models of case management have appeared in the literature. A number of them have come and gone, primarily because they lacked sound theoretical underpinnings or failed to generate research findings that supported the core concepts within the models. Readers who are interested in the progression of nursing case management knowledge can find excellent descriptions and synthesis of key case management models in such textbooks as those by Cohen and Cesta (2005) and Flarey and Blancett (1996).

These textbooks, and other nursing literature, commonly categorize case management models into within-the-walls (hospital-based) and beyond-the-walls (community-based) classifications. Fitting into these classifications are two models introduced in the 1980s that have withstood the test of time and have been studied extensively, adopted, and/or adapted by health care organizations across the country: The New England Medical Center Hospitals within-the-walls model and the Carondelet St. Mary's Hospital beyond-the-walls model, often referred to as the Arizona model. Both models have a strong theoretical basis, and research data have shown the models to be effective in controlling institutional costs by achieving decreased hospital lengths of stay and decreased readmissions while maintaining quality patient care (Ethridge, 1997; Ethridge & Lamb, 1989; Zander, 1988a).

The New England Medical Center Hospitals model was developed by Zander in 1985 (Zander, 1988b, 1988c) and was the first initiation of within-the-walls case management. According to Zander, the model structures care of clients experiencing acute illness episodes. The focus of this conceptual model is on outcomes; it is a synthesis of primary nursing care and nursing process and introduces critical pathways and case management plans as essential concepts in structuring the episode of care. Unit-based primary care was selected as a core concept because it was known to facilitate nursing accountability, continuity, and satisfaction for patients. The nursing process, an applied scientific method, was included in the model because this process solves problems and leads to outcome definition (Zander, 1996). Case management adopts a critical pathway linked with a case management plan that creates methods for structuring, coordinating, and assessing the patients' progress. Critical pathways have proven to be one of the most innovative concepts of the model, and 15 years later they have been widely adapted (Renholm, Leino-Kilpi, & Suominen, 2002) and have become a symbol of case management. Zander defines a critical pathway[1] as follows:

> A tool that helps practitioners manage an episode of care for a patient population or condition by providing a timeline of the expected course of care with expected patient outcomes. The critical pathway is designed to improve quality of patient care and promote efficient utilization of resources (1988b, p. 28).

In this model, the case management plan is conceptualized as a comprehensive document. The document is designed to function as a tool that integrates the nursing process and the critical pathway and

---

[1] An example of a critical pathway is given in Dunham-Taylor and Pinczuk (2006).

to deal with variance analysis (deviations from the pathway). In addition, the document is used to record the caregiver relationship of caregiver interventions with patient outcomes along a timeline. This plan enables primary nurse case managers to coordinate a patient's entire episode of care across hospital units.

When a patient enters a hospital unit at the New England Medical Center, a primary nurse formulates a case management plan and becomes the patient's primary caregiver. If the patient transfers to another hospital unit, a new primary nurse is assigned to deliver direct care and the initial primary nurse continues to administer the patient's case management plan. Care coordination is facilitated through team meetings, case consultation, and interdisciplinary communication, focused by critical pathways. Because the model is grounded in primary nursing and nursing process, it has been applied easily to a variety of within-the-wall settings.

Zander (1996) described the episode of illness as finite and the continuum of care as infinite. According to Zander, the infinite continuum, which links within-the-wall and beyond-the-wall models, will, in the future, focus on wellness/prevention services that promote higher levels of care. She believes the concepts contained within her hospital-based case management model will flourish in this expanded continuum of health care. This model will culminate in a need for more primary nurse case managers skilled in developing and using critical pathways, now called careMaps, across the continuum of health care and in applying them to direct care for populations of clients (Zander, 2002). This present view of case management more closely reflects the professional nurse case management model developed at Carondelet St. Mary's Hospital in Tucson, Arizona.

In 1985 Carondelet St. Mary's Hospital developed the first beyond-the-walls case management model (Ethridge, 1987). Changing reimbursement patterns, due to Medicare cost-containment measures and the growing number of clients enrolled in managed care, resulted in patients being discharged while still in the early stages of recovery. Thus a need to provide care after discharge emerged. Rising to the challenge, nurse administrators at St. Mary's sought to meet this need by creating the professional nurse case management model. It was designed to offer case-managed nursing services to chronically ill and high-risk clients across hospital and community settings, moving care beyond the episode of illness into the continuum of care. One of the dominant values of the Carondelet St. Mary's Hospital model is the belief that a continuum of care encompasses all of life and death experiences (Doerge & Hagenow, 1995). The goals of the model are to offer case-managed services that improve and promote a person's health or peaceful death and assist individuals to learn new ways of managing their illness situations.

Three qualitative studies exploring Carondelet's professional nurse case management model theory-practice link have been reported in the literature (Forbes, 1999; Lamb & Stemple, 1994; Newman, Lamb, & Michaels, 1991). Findings identify the nurse case manager–client relationship as the concept in the model most integral to achieving quality and cost outcomes. Outcomes include "improved self-care skills, fewer hospitalizations and enhanced quality of life" (Lamb & Stemple, 1994, p. 12). Evidence from the studies suggests that the emphasis placed on building caring therapeutic nurse–client relationships motivates clients to engage in self-care strategies and thereby improves functional performance.

St. Mary's used these outcome data to negotiate managed care contracts and, as a result, launched the first nursing health maintenance organization (HMO). Contracts were negotiated using a capitated reimbursement system that extended community case management services to approximately 22,000 HMO members who were experiencing chronic illnesses, disease complications, and recurring institutionalizations. Preliminary findings showed that nursing case management reduced hospitalizations and home health visits to below the national average, increased knowledge of health-promoting behaviors over time, and motivated more than 50% of the HMO enrollees to attend annual health screening programs, which contributed to decreased health risks (Ethridge, 1997). In this integrated delivery model, one professional nurse case manager may work for several months (or years) with a chronically ill individual, caring for him or her in the hospital, in the long-term care facility, in the home, or in wellness centers located within retirement complexes. Professional nurse case managers procure needed resources, provide screening, counsel, make referrals to physicians, and engage in wellness education. This broader approach to nursing practice acknowledges the interconnectedness of life and illness situations and recognizes the individual without losing sight of the evolving whole.

Both The New England Medical Center Hospitals and Carondelet St. Mary's Hospital models are prototypes for within- and beyond-the-walls case management models, represent pioneering efforts credited with refocusing the spotlight on case management, and demonstrate its effectiveness on lowering use and cost of services. These innovative professional practice models are restructuring case management and the case manager role, are proven successful in affecting continuity of care and health maintenance, have ensured accountable resource use, have achieved cost containment goals, and have more effectively bridged transitions among hospital-based units and integrated health care networks.

Practicing Case Management: Role and Functions of a Case Manager

A common response when one speaks of case management and the case manager role as new strategies for health care delivery is that nurses have been case managing clients for years. However, this response fails to recognize the unique body of knowledge and skills emerging over the last decade that underpins the functional role of case management. Case managers see the big picture of client care. That is, they fully integrate the total spectrum of acute to chronic phases of care within clients' lived experience rather than simply possessing knowledge and skills limited to direct care delivery in one setting.

Practicing from this perspective requires nurses to have expert knowledge and skills in the following domains:

1. Providing direct care
2. Procuring community resources
3. Coordinating care across hospital units and health care delivery networks
4. Evaluating health care services for cost-effectiveness
5. Building therapeutic nurse–client long-term relationships

Four of these five domains of case management knowledge have been identified from a national study by the National Case Management Task Force (as cited in Bower, 2000) that surveyed certified case managers about key areas of knowledge they used to perform their case management functions. The fifth domain, building therapeutic nurse–client long-term relationships, emerged from studies that examined the processes of nursing case management (Lamb & Stemple, 1994; Newman et al., 1991).

In the first domain, providing direct care, the case manager's knowledge and skills include assessment and planning. Because knowledge development in clinical nursing is grounded in holistic assessment and care planning, nurses are well prepared to assess the interrelationships among medical, psychological, social, and behavioral components of clients' illness situations. These assessment findings are used to plan, intervene, and reassess how the components impact the client.

Although assessment and planning are already core functions of nursing, from a case management perspective assessment is an ongoing, continual process that seeks to understand patients' illness situation within the context of their total health care experiences. This expanded view of assessment provides consistency between planning and delivering care, because care of case-managed clients often occurs at multiple points of service.

Thus nurses practicing as case managers must shift their thinking and knowing from a focus on delivering and managing episodes of illness events within one service setting to providing and managing care within a broader service context, one that includes the community. Thinking and knowing from a community perspective requires a nurse case manager to develop new levels of community consciousness and a new level of community connection to provide direct care more effectively.

Community awareness and connection also enable a case manager to procure and manage resources, the second domain. Knowing what resources are available in the community for case management clients, as well as building relationships with referral agencies that provide these resources, are essential functions of a case manager (Berg-Weger & Tebb, 1998; Mick & Ackerman, 2002). One reason it is important to have knowledge of community agencies and resources is to fill gaps in care left by family support systems and insurance. Resource identification and service planning may involve skills in linking clients to needed services. This can include such things as transportation to medical appointments, assistive devices, home health care, meal delivery, skilled nursing services, personal emergency response systems, and restorative therapies (Schraeder, 2001). Wise allocation of resources, a goal of case management, requires a case manager to make sound clinical judgments about client needs and use of resources. To be successful in these functions, the case manager must possess a variety of skills, including the ability to assess the client's present and future needs, plan creatively, solve problems, collaborate with multiple professionals, understand benefit structures, and coordinate services (Taylor, 1999).

Coordinating care and services across health care units and health care delivery networks, the third domain, is a key role of the case manager. Here the case manager must design tools that define case management responsibilities and interventions. A case manager often uses tools like critical pathways, case management plans, and protocols to support clinical reasoning, goal, and outcome development and to coordinate care across provider settings. Coordinating care by using case management tools entails tracking a client's progress, monitoring for early signs of problems, gathering and analyzing data, and communicating the results to health care organizations, providers, and consumers (Lagoe, 1998). Professional case managers who demonstrate skills in continual assessment, administration of case management tools, interpretation of data, and communication are stewards of health care resources and dollars and add to client satisfaction by reducing the frustration that comes from negotiating care at multiple service sites (Berg-Weger & Tebb, 1998; Kegel, 1996; Lagoe, 1998; Lamb & Stemple, 1994; Salazar, 2000).

Successful performance depends on excellent communication with other disciplines, especially physicians. Efforts to improve communication and collaboration between physicians and case managers were the focus of a summit convened in 2003 by the CMSA. Physicians and case managers from across the country attended. Barriers and solutions to effective communication were identified and used to establish a framework for successful collaboration between the two groups. This framework and other summit outcomes were reported in a consensus paper entitled, "Exploring Best Practices in Physician & Case Management Collaboration to Improve Patient Care," which is available online at www.cmsa.org/Professional/Collaboration.

Coordinating a multidisciplinary plan that moves clients across the continuum of care, whether between hospital units or into other service settings, is the most important function of the nurse case manager (Novak, 1998). Lack of coordination within and among health care settings contributes to increased hospital readmission rates and costs of care (Burns, Lamb, & Wholey, 1996). To overcome ineffective coordination requires strong skills to negotiate with payers and providers to ensure smooth transitions and to sustain continuity of care for clients. By making communication and collaboration between physicians and case managers a priority, the CMSA summit has potentially made the coordination role of the case manager an easier function.

The fourth knowledge domain is managing financial matters. There are two aspects to this role: the first is to understand the payer systems and the second is to develop and apply methods for evaluating quality service and cost-effective care. Understanding common payer systems, such as HMOs, preferred provider organizations, point of service plans, and Medicare and Medicaid, is essential. By being aware of the advantages and disadvantages of the numerous reimbursement methods within payer delivery systems, the case manager is able to bridge the gap between provider and payer, allowing them to effectively coordinate care and secure services for clients. Case managers working with specific populations learn the criteria for eligibility, benefits, and the specific process for accessing services from payer sources commonly used in these populations. Maneuvering through the provider and payer system requires the case manager to assess the client's existing health care coverage and determine if it is adequate or if other sources of funding for services are available. Knowing how the process works helps when communicating with individuals in charge of referral authorization and prevents unnecessary or excessive charges.

The second aspect of this knowledge domain is concerned with the case manager's responsibility to build his or her knowledge about the financial performance of the case management program(s) and to build support for case management services. To accomplish these functions, a case manager needs to design outcomes and use cost analysis methods to evaluate the cost-effectiveness of case management services. A case manager must understand financial and budgeting methods and be able to apply outcome measures that result in a valid, reliable, and thorough assessment (Kleinpell-Nowell, 1999; Terra, 2007). In her article Kleinpell-Nowell (1999) compiles a helpful list of commonly used outcome measures and sources of research-based outcome instruments appropriate for evaluating case management effectiveness.

In a cost-analysis evaluation, consider factors such as external performance referents, including benchmarking or comparing the assessment results with those of another organization(s), to add validity to evaluation findings (Ketchen, Palmer, & Gamm, 2001). In the view of Ketchen et al. (2001), it is only when compared with a point of reference that cost-benefit analysis findings have meaning. This method may also reveal additional insights about the strategy used, or additional strategies to use, to facilitate cost containment. Using performance referents external to the organization can affect the future viability of a particular health care delivery strategy such as case management. For example, integrated hospital delivery systems that case manage high-risk populations of patients with chronic conditions could compare their cost-benefit analysis performance with licensed external disease management organizations specializing in case managing similar populations of patients.

It is challenging to have the knowledge and skills necessary to practice in a cost-effective manner and to have expertise in choosing appropriate outcome performance measures and tools that assess the financial performance of case management. When successfully managed, the role of case manager can be sustained and case management remains a vehicle for the delivery of quality cost-effective care in a managed care financing system.

The focus of the final knowledge domain of case management is building meaningful nurse–client relationships. Although nurse theorists' works have long touted the importance of building meaningful client–nurse relationships, a current research refocus examines client relationships in the nursing case management process. The result has been that nurse case managers have become more concerned, or need to be more concerned, with the importance and benefits of forming relationships with clients.

For example, McWilliam, Stewart, Brown, Desai, and Coderre (1996) explored the experiences of individuals living with chronic illness. The researchers discovered that clients wished to be involved in mutual knowing (mutual relationships) between client and nurse and believed that being known enhanced their personal knowledge and in turn their ability to follow through with self-care. The authors concluded that more attention needed to be placed on continuity of the caregiver rather than on the continuity of the care plan.

Lamb and Stemple (1994) discovered that clients who believed they were in partnerships felt empowered to assume an active role in their health care, thus resulting in renewed efforts to become involved in health maintenance and promotion strategies. These authors grounded their research in Newman's theory of expanding consciousness, which describes a nurse as one who "enters into a partnership with the client with the mutual goal of participating in an authentic relationship, trusting that in the process of its evolving, both will grow and become healthier in the sense of higher levels of consciousness" (Newman, 1986, p. 68).

Practicing case management from this perspective enables clients to become partners with case managers and meets one of the goals of case management—to optimize the client's self-care ability (Taylor, 1999). Creating an atmosphere that builds respectful relationships requires a case manager to develop and use the skills of active listening and being present; these skills enable clients to become their own "insider-experts in self-care" (Lamb & Stemple, 1994, p. 12).

On the whole, the five knowledge domains of the case manager role outlined above describe the new knowledge and skills needed to perform the role of case manager, contrasted with the basic practice of nurses. As nursing case management has evolved, there have been increased opportunities for nurses to move from basic nursing practice into this expanded role, which provides more autonomy and possibly more job enrichment (Goode, 1995; Reimanis, Cohen, & Redman, 2001).

Case Management Certification

The case management certification process ensures a common baseline of knowledge and gives the professional and public assurance of a certain degree of competence and higher quality of case management services. There are numerous licensure, certification, and certificate programs available for case managers working in various fields of health care. Listing each is beyond the scope of this chapter; rather, three key certifications are described.

The Commission for Case Manager Certification (CCMC) is an independent credentialing agency that sponsors and oversees one of the major case management certifications. The CCMC, nationally accredited by the National Commission for Certifying Agencies, is the only national accreditation body for private certification organizations in all disciplines. Since the CCMC began certifying case managers in 1993, more than 20,000 case managers have earned the Certified Case Manager (CCM) credential. This credential is designed as an adjunct to other professional credentials in health and human resources.

To earn the designation of CCM, applicants must

- Possess a good moral character
- Meet acceptable standards of practice
- Accomplish specific educational requirements, including a post-secondary degree program in a field that promotes the psychosocial or vocational well-being of consumers
- Provide a job description for each case management position held
- Meet the Continuum of Care requirement
- Hold a license that is based on the applicant having taken an examination in the area of educational specialization

- Ensure that the license grants the ability to practice without the supervision of another licensed professional
- Perform the six essential activities of case management:
  - Assessment
  - Coordination
  - Planning
  - Monitoring
  - Implementation
  - Evaluation in multiple environments over a minimum of five of the six core components:
    - process and relationships
    - health care management
    - community resources and support
    - service delivery
    - psychosocial intervention
    - rehabilitation case management
- Satisfy the necessary employment experience
- Demonstrate that they possess acceptable minimum knowledge by achieving a passing score on the CCM examination (www.ccmcertification.org/pages/121body.html)

The CCM examination is research based and covers competencies and job functions in six major domains of knowledge as listed above. It is administered semiannually in June and December; testing sites are usually located within each state.

The ANCC, the credentialing arm of the American Nurses Association, offers a second method of certification (www.nursingworld.org/ancc). In 1997 the Center began certifying nursing case managers and providing them with the (RN, cm) credential. Candidates for the exam must have a registered nurse license and a baccalaureate or higher degree. A core specialty is also desired; however, individuals without a core specialty are eligible but need 4,000 hours of registered nurse experience as opposed to the 2,000 hours of case management experience needed by those individuals who already hold a core nursing specialty certification. The framework for Nursing Case Management used by ANCC consists of the following five components: assessment, planning, implementation, evaluation, and interaction.

Both the CCM and ANCC require ongoing continuing education for recertification, which is required every 5 years. Each of the credentialing agencies provides written resource materials for case managers. The CCMC study guide is available through the CMSA (see www.ccmcertification.org). The ANCC published a book for individuals who are entering into case management practice or for experienced case managers who may have practiced in only one setting (Llewellyn, 2005). Each chapter in the book includes review questions and answers, as well as rationales, to assist with preparation for the national examination.

Certification for case management administrators is sponsored by the Center for Case Management and can be obtained from the Credentialing Advisory Board. Eligibility for the certification exam occurs by meeting one of three broad categories: a baccalaureate or higher degree with experience as a case manager, a certification in a core specialty, and/or a faculty in an academic setting teaching graduate-level courses or content in case management. The exam covers content about high-risk populations, assessment, strategy development, leadership, strategic planning, human resource management, and outcome management. For more information about this certification, contact the Center for Case Management at www.cfcm.com/certification.html.

Trends and Issues in Case Management

The dynamic nature of health care has set the stage for the many new trends and issues now emerging in case management. After a decade of movement into fully integrated delivery systems, health care organizations have created interdependent interactive structures designed to coordinate care across the continuum, with the goal of containing cost and maintaining or increasing quality. By default, if not by design, case management has emerged as the primary strategy to coordinate services, to provide care, and to communicate across these multiorganizational systems. This trend provides an unprecedented opportunity for nurses to showcase their leadership and their accomplishments in using nursing case management as a model to both promote quality and achieve cost reductions in health care.

The recent implementation of an evaluative study of coordinated care programs, sponsored by the Centers for Medicare and Medicaid Services, was implemented by the Mathematica Policy Research organization. This study has the potential to generate measurable data that confirm nursing case management's successful impact on cost and quality. Fifteen integrated health care delivery systems from across the country were selected in January 2004 to participate. Two-thirds of these systems use case managers to coordinate care. They design and initiate interventions with physicians, and a mix of other health care professionals, for chronically ill Medicare-recipient clients.

The participating institutions have designed some very innovative programs that require new, advanced skills for practice. For instance, many programs use telemedicine, in-home monitoring devices, and the Internet for counseling and interactive communication with clients. The electronic links allow important client data to be sent to the case manager for evaluation and action or shared with the primary physician for redesign of medical care. Further, tracking client data may help to transition clients more efficiently across organizations' multiple service settings. The organizations and case managers participating in this study hope that coordinating services across the continuum and using new technologies will produce outcomes that reflect a decrease in fragmented care, an increase in client knowledge and self-care, improved client satisfaction, and, of course, reduce Medicare expenditures for chronically ill individuals. The Centers for Medicare and Medicaid Services demonstration projects are funded for 4 years and evaluated every 2 years.

A recent trend within government programs has included using the case management strategy in the management of Medicaid beneficiaries. It is a central feature of Florida's, North Carolina's, and Oklahoma's approach to health care delivery for this population (Silberman et al., 2003). These programs are raising professional and public awareness of case management and are creating increased employment opportunities for nurses who desire to function in this specialty role.

The programs, however, also cause concern for many members of the profession (Daiski, 2000) because they often adopt disease management models as guides for nursing case management practice. These models focus on medical diagnosis, illness, and treatment, whereas nursing models focus on health wellness, prevention, and illness within the context of the patients' experience and cultural background.

After reviewing the literature on nursing case management models, my impression is that a substantial number of case management models guided by nursing theories exist that are useful for practice in all health care settings. As more government programs adopt case management as their strategy for health care, and there is every indication they will, it is imperative that nurse case managers advocate the use of case management models that move beyond functions of medical necessity to models with nursing functions that reflect the values of health embedded within the discipline of nursing's theories. Only in this way can we hope to shape health care policy. Thus we advocate that case management models emphasize the values of nursing and are guided by nursing theories.

The inclusion of monitoring devices, electronic links, and the Internet as sources of information reflects a trend throughout health care systems, both public and private. From a case management perspective, Internet connectivity has the power to link case managers to client's insurance plans, pharmacies, and physician offices as well as to track previous medical and nursing information about clients from the multiple service sites within the integrated system (Robinson, 2001).

The advent of Internet technology has also propelled consumers toward a greater use of technology (Adams, 2000). The consulting firm of Cyber Dialogue reported survey results estimating that 40 million U.S. adults use the Internet to access health information and that by 2005 this number will increase to 88 million (Oermann, Lesley, & Kuefler, 2002). These figures suggest the consumer is seeking information beyond that provided by his or her health caregivers.

Nursing case managers could develop and share a diary of reliable Internet sites with their client populations to answer questions about their health care situations or to connect them with others who are experiencing similar illness situations. Adams (2000) believes that case managers could deliver care as an integrated package of personal services, combined with education and knowledge tailored to the patient, via the Internet. Discussions of the many revolutionary new ways e-health, and other technologies, can be used to improve health care delivery in general, and case management in particular, can be found in a number of publications.[2]

The phenomenal growth of case management information systems and Internet technology has fostered a new culture of health care, one that empowers health care providers and consumers to track clinical decisions and access and compare information (Mastrian, 2007; Meadows, 2001). It will eventually move all health care professionals to embrace these tools to gain greater access to information, obtain better clinical outcomes (Carver, 2001; McGonigle, Mastrian, & Pavelekovsky, 2007), and meet the expectations of their clients.

These trends—fully integrated health systems delivering coordinated care using multiple information technologies as mechanisms to both facilitate and measure the effectiveness of this care—produce serious issues. First, with the widespread use of Internet technology in health care organizations, protecting data confidentiality has become a major issue. This public consumer concern prompted legislators to enact the Health Insurance Portability and Accountability Act (HIPAA) of 1996, an effort designed to achieve better electronic security of personal health information (Waldo, 2000).

The HIPAA legislation includes standards and regulations for information transmitted or exchanged electronically and impacts any organization, provider, or payer that handles individually identifiable health information. Under these HIPAA rules the case manager may need to obtain written authorization from the individual before requesting or transmitting information from providers or payers and most definitely needs to identify which transactions do or do not meet the HIPAA guidelines. Whether this will create barriers to the continuum model of case management, such as delaying the coordination of care and resource access and delaying or preventing electronic information exchange, is still unclear.

Second, the trend toward providing coordinated care across the continuum and over the life span of clients is congruent with the client's expectations and satisfaction with health care (Dunn, Sohl-Kreiger, & Marx, 2001; Lamb & Stemple, 1994). How the case manager, and the organization, transitions the client from one site to another has become an issue for both providers and clients. The Institute of Medicine (2001) report identified gaps in safety and care in patients as they transfer to different levels of care. Stanton (2008) consulted 10 experts in the field of case management

---

[2] Some excellent resources include: Adams, J. (2000). Applying e-health to case management. *Lippincott's Case Management, 5*(4), 168–171; and Meadows, G. (2001). The internet promise: A new look at e-health opportunities. *Nursing Economic$, 19*(6), 294–295.

to determine future trends that identified transitions of care as an area of major concern and as an area in which case management can have the greatest impact.

The literature suggests that clients prefer one provider across all settings and that this approach is the best method for clinical integration and coordination of all aspects of care (Lamb & Stemple, 1994; McWilliam et al., 1996). At this time, however, case managers and organizations rarely follow this approach; rather, it is more common to link acute care case managers with community-based case managers. Within this type of system, case managers need to be adept at sharing information about the clients' past and current illness situations to ensure both continuity and satisfaction with care as clients transition from the illness episode to the continuum of care. The shared information needs to include clients' preferences and successful strategies for promoting a relationship that fosters client goal attainment and produces client satisfaction outcomes.

Third, the preparation of nurses to practice case management using both continuum delivery models and effective technology has become an issue. It is generally agreed among nurse researchers and educators that there is a need for formal educational preparation of the nurse case manager, including preventive health care perspectives (Hallberg, 2004) and appropriate computer skills for the role. Presently, there are inadequacies in the academic approach (Cicatiello, 2000; Hallberg, 2004; Halstead, 2000; Sowell & Young, 1997). Agreement ends and disagreement begins, however, when these nurse scholars discuss curricula content and debate which educational level, undergraduate or graduate, is required to prepare case managers for entry into practice.

The reality is that all nurses need content and clinical practice experiences in case management and need to acquire skills in accessing information and managing databases via the Internet (Halstead, 2000; Stanton, 2008). Often, both staff nurses and advanced practice nurses are expected to become members of interdisciplinary case management teams and to make client care decisions based on case management concepts and electronic client data.

Sowell and Young (1997) believe that to meet the changing job expectations the baccalaureate graduate should have the expertise to be an effective case management team member, with knowledge of both databased clinical paths and of the quality/financial issues that influence care coordination. The advanced practice nurse graduate, on the other hand, must obtain the expertise needed to perform the case manager role for a caseload of clients within a specialized target population. This view of case management education reflects the current trend in Schools of Nursing (Haw, 1996).

According to Haw's (1996) national survey of case management education in universities, 95% of nursing schools are beginning to prepare the undergraduate in basic case management concepts and processes including community resource referral, health team collaboration, client progress monitoring, and technology health services (Halstead, 2000). Haw's survey (1996) also indicates that the emphasis in graduate case management education is on role performance behaviors, and therefore the graduate curriculum incorporates many more clinical practicum experiences than offered in undergraduate education. Findings and conclusions by Haw suggest that nurse educators view the case manager role as an advanced practice role even though employers usually list the undergraduate degree as a requirement for hire. In the end, whether case management education is included at the undergraduate level or graduate level, there is an overall trend toward more formal case management preparation in nursing academia (Haw, 1996; Stanton, Swanson, Sherrod, & Packa, 2005).

Finally, the emerging era of coordinating care across continuums creates issues for both integrated health system providers and case managers alike. It has been established that case managers need skills in accessing and managing patient care data across many different settings. Accurate tracking of patient visits, patient outcomes, and costs are necessary to plan for the delivery of services and the allocation of resources across the continuum. As case managers acquire these skills, there is mounting pressure for integrated health care delivery systems to provide these data. However, case management information systems that accurately track these data are costly (Mastrian, 2007; Noone & McKillip, 1996), and purchasing these new technologies requires sufficient profit margins. Unfortunately, integrated health care systems that are coordinating much of their services in community rather than acute care settings are discovering that capitated reimbursement practices by commercial and federal payers have reduced their profit margins (Lamb & Zazworsky, 2000). Unless financial incentives are aligned with service coordination initiatives, the trend toward coordinating care across the continuum by case managers cannot be sustained.

However, the ongoing research initiatives by the federal government are encouraging. The studies suggest that coordinating care across the continuum for Medicare patients does successfully reduce health care costs; thus future capitated reimbursement structures may increasingly cover these services and be sufficient to support the cost of developing and maintaining data systems.

Anticipating the Future of Case Management

The rapid and ongoing transformation of health care systems has made anticipating the future of case management as unpredictable as the ever-changing patterns of a kaleidoscope where the crystals rearrange to form new and exciting patterns. However, this change also creates an environment where nursing case management can flourish. As health care systems pursue their goals of promoting client satisfaction, fostering client loyalty, and becoming indispensable to the community, case management is becoming the dominant strategy selected by these systems to meet their goals. In the future it is easy to imagine that integrated health care delivery systems will link case managers to one another across their multiple service sites and make arrangements for the same person to manage the client's care, creating client trust and confidence in both the health care system and in the case management approach.

Further twisting of the kaleidoscope creates a future in which all clients will be health managed, and the role of the health manager will expand to include an emphasis on prevention and reducing recidivism. The overall trend of managed care toward expanded benefits that include complementary alternative medicine, prevention, and long-term care in the home support this vision.

Consumers today are beginning to demand that health care manage their health as well as their disease and satisfy their individual preferences over the life cycle. These expanded benefits for consumers support and subsidize the future development of wellness models of case management.

Health managers will be expected to provide care in a variety of settings and at various levels of care; the goal will be to manage health risks in the community rather than in acute care settings. In the near future case managers will be challenged to provide ways to offset the depersonalization and threat to client–nurse relationships caused by the greater use of technology for assessment and lack of communication with clients.

In the end, the shape that case management takes will depend on the diligence of both integrated delivery systems and case managers to search for new possibilities, reflect, question, and create images of care that capture the client's perspective. This reflection and partnership between the system and case manager will create new kaleidoscope of colors and patterns, creating health management models that illuminate a bright future for both the care providers and the client.

Discussion Questions

1. What would you consider the major differences between The New England Medical Center Hospitals and the Carondelet St. Mary's Hospital models?

2. Why do you believe that certification in case management is beneficial for you and how will it benefit your patients?
3. What is case management participation in a fully integrated health care delivery system? How do you participate in this process?
4. The Internet will play a major part in the delivery of health care. What precautions should be taken by using this tool and how comfortable should a manager be using it?
5. What role will HIPAA legislation play in case management in the future?

Glossary of Terms

Case Management—The interdisciplinary definition, developed by the Case Management Society of America (CMSA, 1995), describes case management as a "collaborative process which assesses, plans, implements, coordinates, monitors and evaluates options and services to meet an individual's health needs through communication and available resources to promote quality, cost-effective outcomes" (p. 8).

Case Management Certification—The Commission for Case Manager Certification (CCMC) is an independent credentialing agency that sponsors and oversees one of the major case management certifications. The American Nurses Credentialing Center (ANCC) offers a second method of certification (www.nursingworld.org/ancc). The ANCC is the credentialing arm of the American Nurses Association. Certification for case management administrators (CMAC) is sponsored by the Center for Case Management and can be obtained from the Credentialing Advisory Board (CAB).

References

Adams, J. (2000). Applying e-health to case management. *Lippincott's Case Management, 5*(4), 168–171.

American Nurses Credentialing Center. (1998). *Nursing case management catalogue.* Washington, DC: ANCC.

Berg-Weger, M., & Tebb, S. (1998). Caregiver well-being: A strengths-based case management approach. *Journal of Case Management, 7*(2), 67–73.

Bower, S. (2000). *Case management: A practical guide to success in managed care* (2nd ed.). New York: Lippincott.

Burns, L., Lamb, G., & Wholey, D. (1996). Impact of integrated community nursing services on hospital utilization and costs in a Medicare risk plan. *Inquiry, 33*, 30–41.

Carver, T. (2001). Continuum-based care coordination via the web. *Care Management, 17*(2), 14–20.

Case Management Society of America. (2002). *Standards of practice for case management.* Little Rock, AR: CMSA.

Cicatiello, J. (2000). A perspective of health care in the past—Insights and challenges for a health care system in the new millennium. *Nursing Administration Quarterly, 25*(1), 18–29.

Cohen, E., & Cesta, T. (2005). *Nursing case management* (4th ed.). St. Louis, MO: Elsevier Mosby.

Daiski, I. (2000). The road to professionalism in nursing: Case management or practice based in nursing theory? *Nursing Science Quarterly, 13*(1), 74–79.

Doerge, J., & Hagenow, N. (1995). Management restructuring. *Nursing Management, 26*(12), 32–37.

Dunham-Taylor, J., & Pinczuk, J. (2006). *Health care financial management for nurse managers: Applications from hospitals, long-term care, home care, and ambulatory care.* Sudbury, MA: Jones and Bartlett.

Dunn, S., Sohl-Kreiger, R., & Marx, S. (2001). Geriatric case management in an integrated care system. *Journal of Nursing Administration, 31*(2), 60–62.

Ethridge, P. (1987). Nurse accountability program improves satisfaction, turnover. *Health Progress, 68*, 44–49.

Ethridge, P. (1997). The Carondelet experience. *Nursing Management, 28*(3), 26–28.

Ethridge, P., & Lamb, G. (1989). Professional nursing case management improves quality, access and costs. *Nursing Management, 20*(3), 30–35.

Flarey, D. (1996). Case management: Delivering care in the age of managed care. In D. Flarey & S. Blancett (Eds.), *Handbook of nursing case management*. Gaithersburg, MD: Aspen.

Flarey, D., & Blancett, S. (Eds.). (1996). *Handbook of nursing case management*. Gaithersburg, MD: Aspen.

Forbes, M. (1999). The practice of professional nurse case management. *Nursing Case Management, 4*(1), 28–33.

Goode, C. (1995). Impact of a careMap and case management on patient satisfaction and staff satisfaction, collaboration, and autonomy. *Nursing Economic$, 13*(6), 337–348.

Hallberg, I. (2004). Preventive home care of frail older people: A review of recent case management studies. *Journal of Clinical Nursing, 13*(6b), 112–120.

Halstead, J. (2000). Implementing web-based instruction in a school of nursing: Implications for faculty and students. *Journal of Professional Nursing, 16*(5), 273–281.

Haw, M. (1996). Case management education in universities: A national survey. *Journal of Care Management, 2*(6), 10–23.

Institute of Medicine, Committeee on Quality of Health Care in America. (2001). *Crossing the quality chasm: A new health system for the 21st century*. Washington, DC: National Academics Press.

Kegel, L. (1996). Case management, critical pathways, and myocardial infarction. *Critical Care Nurse, 16*(2), 97–114.

Ketchen, D., Palmer, T., & Gamm, L. (2001). The role of performance referents in health services organizations. *Health Care Management Review, 26*(4), 19–26.

Kleinpell-Nowell, R. (1999). Measuring advanced practice nursing outcomes. *AACN Clinical Issues, 10*(3), 356–368.

Lagoe, R. (1998). Basic statistics for clinical pathway evaluation. *Nursing Economic$, 16*(3), 125–131.

Lamb, G., & Stemple, J. (1994). Nurse case management from the client's view: Growing as insider-expert. *Nursing Outlook, 42*(1), 7–14.

Lamb, G., & Zazworsky, D. (2000). The Carondelet case management program. In E. Cohen & T. Cesta (Eds.), *Nursing case management* (3rd ed.). St. Louis, MO: Mosby.

Llewellyn, A. (2005). *The case management review and resource manual: The essence of case management* (2nd ed.). Washington, DC: ANA.

Mastrian, K. (2007). Tips, tools & techniques. *Professional Case Management, 12*(3), 181–183.

McGonigle, D., Mastrian, K., & Pavelekovsky, K. (2007). Information systems and case management practice series, Part II: case management information systems goals, benefits, and system selection or development. *Professional Case Management, 12*(4), 239–241.

McWilliam, C., Stewart, M., Brown, J., Desai, K., & Coderre, P. (1996). Creating health with chronic illness. *Advances in Nursing Science, 18*(3), 1–15.

Meadows, G. (2001). The internet promise: A new look at e-health opportunities. *Nursing Economic$, 19*(6), 294–295.

Mick, D., & Ackerman, M. (2002). New perspectives on advanced practice nursing case management for aging patients. *Critical Care Nursing Clinics of North America, 14*, 281–291.

Newman, M. (1986). *Health as expanding consciousness*. St. Louis, MO: Mosby.

Newman, M., Lamb, G., & Michaels, C. (1991). Nurse case management: The coming together of theory and practice. *Nursing & Health Care, 12*(8), 404–408.

Noone, C., & McKillip, C. (1996). Data management through information systems. In D. Flarey & S. Blancett (Eds.), *Handbook of nursing case management*. Gaithersburg, MD: Aspen.

Novak, D. (1998). Nurse case managers' opinions of their role. *Nursing Case Management, 3*(6), 231–237.

Oermann, M., Lesley, M., & Kuefler, S. (2002). Using the Internet to teach consumers about quality care. *Journal of Quality Improvement, 28*(2), 83–89.

Reimanis, C., Cohen, E., & Redman, R. (2001). Nurse case manager role attributes: Fifteen years of evidence-based literature. *Lippincott's Case Management, 6*(6), 230–242.

Renholm, M., Leino-Kilpi, H., & Suominen, T. (2002). Critical pathways. *Journal of Nursing Administration, 32*(4), 196–201.

Robinson, J. (2001). The end of managed care. *Journal of the American Medical Association, 285*(20), 2622–2632.

Salazar, M. (2000). Maximizing the effectiveness of case management service delivery. *The Case Manager, 11*(3), 58–63.

Schraeder, C. (2001). Discharge planning. *Hospital Case Management, 9*(10), 155–156.

Sowell, R., & Young, S. (1997). Case management in the nursing curriculum. *Nursing Case Management, 2*(4), 173–176.

Stanton, M. (2008). The "wins" of change: Evaluating the impact of predicted changes on case management practice. *Professional Case Management, 13*(3), 161–168.

Stanton, M., Swanson, M., Sherrod, R., & Packa, D. (2005). Case management evolution: From basic to advanced practice role. *Lippincott's Case Management, 10*(6), 274–284.

Taylor, P. (1999). Comprehensive nursing case management: An advanced practice model. *Nursing Case Management, 4*(1), 2–10.

Terra, S. (2007). An evidence-based approach to case management model selection for an acute care facility. *Professional Case Management, 12*(3), 147–157.

Waldo, B. (2000). HIPPA: The next frontier. *Information Systems and Technology, 18*(1), 49–50.

Zander, K. (1988a). Nursing group practice: The Cadillac in continuity. *Definition, 3*(2), 1–2.

Zander, K. (1988b). Managed care within acute care settings: Design and implementation via nursing case management. *Health Care Supervisor, 6*(2), 24–43.

Zander, K. (1988c). Nursing care management: Strategic management of cost and quality outcomes. *Journal of Nursing Administration, 18*(5), 23–30.

Zander, K. (1996). The early years: The evolution of nursing case management. In D. Flarey & S. Blancett (Eds.), *Handbook of nursing case management.* Gaithersburg, MD: Aspen.

Zander, K. (2002). Nursing case management in the 21st century: Intervening where margin meets mission. *Nursing Administration Quarterly, 24*(5), 58–68.

PART VII

Finance/Accounting Issues

Although a nurse manager may never need to learn accounting and finance basics, we have included some beginning information about them in this book. We hope this helps the nurse manager to have a greater appreciation for the finance side of the organization. We thought it would be helpful for a nurse manager to be able to read a financial statement for a health care organization, explained in Chapter 19 on Accounting for Health Care Entities, as well as to learn more about certain financial ratios commonly used in health care organizations, found in Chapter 20 on Financial Analysis. If you would like more detailed background in these topics, we suggest that you take additional accounting or finance courses.

CHAPTER 19

Accounting for Healthcare Entities

Paul Bayes, DBA Accounting, MS Economics,
BS Accounting

Key Terms

- Accounts (Patients) Receivable Represents Future Cash Collection
- Accounts Payables
- Accumulated Depreciation
- Activity-Based Costing (ABC)
- Assets
- Average Costs
- Balance Sheet
- Buildings
- Cash Flow Statement
- Construction in Progress
- Costs and Expenses
- Current Assets
- Deferred Taxes
- Depreciation
- Equipment
- Financial Activities
- Fund Balance
- Goodwill
- Income Statement
- Intangible Assets
- Inventory
- Investment Activities
- Investments
- Liabilities
- Long-term Debt
- Marginal Costs
- Net Assets or Fund Balances
- Net Worth
- Operating Activities
- Preferred or Common Stock
- Provision for Doubtful Accounts
- Relevant Range
- Retained Earnings
- Schedule of Changes in Equity
- Tangible Assets
- Temporary Investments

Introduction

Accounting has been called the language of business because accounting information provides direction for action. Health care organizations can be classified as either for-profit or not-for-profit, but much of the information is the same and requires similar decision making. Each organization has assets and liabilities. The difference occurs in the area defined as either stockholder's equity (for-profit) or unrestricted, temporarily restricted, and permanently restricted funds (not-for-profit).

The financial synopsis of management's actions is contained in the financial statements (see Appendix for examples of a profit-oriented and not-for-profit entity). Excerpts from these statements are used as examples throughout this chapter. Years ago, it was uncommon for health care entities to have financial problems. However, changing economic conditions and revenue-limiting measures by third-party providers (insurance companies/government) require a more proactive look at the financial condition of a business. The failure to do so may result in what has happened to many "dot-com," as well as established, companies in recent years.

Financial statements are required every year, and publicly traded health care entities must also issue quarterly financial statements. These financial statements consist of the statement of financial position (balance sheet), the income statement (also called statement of activities—income and expenses or statement of earnings), and statement of cash flows. In recent years more attention has focused on the statement of cash flows because cash is the lifeblood of a business. To be an informed decision maker, you must understand how to use financial statements, but you do not necessarily have to know how to prepare these financial statements. Thus the focus of this chapter is on the understanding and use of financial information.

Accounting Framework

One of the basic frameworks of for-profit accounting is the accounting equation: assets = liabilities + equity. *Assets* are those items that provide future cash flow or have future economic benefit. If you were to prepare a personal financial statement for a bank loan, you would list those items that have value (assets) and can be sold in case of default on the loan. For business organizations, assets are used to generate revenue for the firm. *Liabilities* are claims on the assets of an organization. The claims are those of creditors who have provided resources such as buildings and equipment but have not been fully paid. Using the example of a personal loan, liabilities include credit card, car, or home mortgage balances. The difference between the assets and liabilities of an organization is the equity, or in the personal loan application example, *net worth*. Examples of these items follow. All amounts are in millions except for earnings per share.

In not-for-profit organizations, the result of subtracting liabilities from assets is called *net assets* or *fund balances*. Not-for-profit entities return the excess amount to the sponsoring organization if they cease to continue stated purposes. The accounting framework for a not-for-profit organization would be assets = liabilities + net assets or fund balances. Examples of these differences are illustrated as follows.

Statement of Financial Position (Balance Sheet)

Assets

The *balance sheet*—consisting of the assets, liabilities, and equity—is a "snapshot" of the health care entity and is dated for a 1-day period of time. The assets, liabilities, and equity or fund balances reflect only the amounts as of a certain date. Traditional examples use December 31 as the ending day, but firms have other ending time periods. The asset portion of Hospital Anywhere USA, which is dated as of December 31, appears in **Exhibit 19–1**. Complete financial statements are found in the Appendix.

Assets may be classified as current versus long term or, more specifically, *current assets, property and equipment (tangible), investments,* and *intangible assets* such as patents. Current assets are those items that will be used to generate revenue in either 1 year or the operating period, whichever is longer (most often this is 1 year).

Generally, the first item listed on the statement of financial position is cash, although many times it is combined with temporary investments, which are considered *cash equivalents*. Temporary investments are cash equivalents because they can be sold quickly with little or no loss in value.

Exhibit 19–1 Asset Section of Balance Sheet

(Dollars in millions)

Assets	2004	2003
Current assets		
Cash and cash equivalents	$314	$190
Accounts receivable, less allowance for doubtful accounts of $1,583 and $1,567	2,211	1,873
Inventories	396	383
Income taxes receivable	197	178
Other	1,335	973
Total current assets	**4,453**	**3,597**
Property and equipment at cost		
Land	793	813
Buildings	6,021	6,108
Equipment	7,045	6,721
Construction in progress	431	442
Total property and equipment	**14,290**	**14,084**
Accumulated depreciation	(5,810)	(5,594)
	8,480	8,490
Investments of insurance subsidiary	1,371	1,457
Investments in and advances to affiliates	779	654
Intangible assets, net of accumulated amortization of $785 and $644	2,155	2,319
Other	330	368
Total assets	**$17,568**	**$16,885**

This is the reserve needed to meet the operational needs of the organization such as salaries and to meet other obligations as they arise.

An important source of future cash is generically identified as *accounts (patients) receivable*. These may be represented by amounts owed by either patients to which the organization has provided services or by claims filed with third-party providers such as insurance companies. These provide future cash flows, and therefore it is imperative these insurance claims are filed quickly and accurately. Reducing the collection period provides cash more quickly for operations. This amount is often reported as a "net" number, reflecting amounts that will not be collected or reductions from third-party providers.

Other current assets of the organization consist of *inventory* items such as drugs in the pharmacy, surgical supplies, items maintained at nursing stations, and drinks and/or food in the cafeteria. The alternative inventory cost measures are not discussed in this text. The income taxes receivable account is the equivalent of receiving a tax refund but waiting for the check.

PROPERTY AND EQUIPMENT

The largest item on a for-profit health care entity's balance sheet is probably buildings and equipment. This may also be defined as *tangible assets. Land* on which a health care facility is located is one item included in this section. Land is not written off, unless there is something that impairs value such as pollution of the land site. Other tangible assets, such as buildings and equipment, have skyrocketing costs because of the complexity of equipment and more rigorous *building codes and regulations. Buildings* are the physical facilities in which patient services are provided. *Equipment* may be items such as x-ray and computed tomography (CT) machines or less complex items such as patient beds. The increased costs require either the availability of large amounts of funds for purchases (cash) or credit-granting sources. *Construction in progress* is an account indicating buildings that have not been completed but are being built. The account indicates progress toward completion. *Depreciation* is an accounting charge wherein the balance of the equipment and buildings is systematically written off over a period of time. *Accumulated depreciation*, which is the sum of the annual depreciation charges, is then subtracted from the plant and equipment balance, providing a net figure. This number does not relate to current market value but rather is book value only, which is the original cost minus accumulated depreciation.

INVESTMENTS

Investments are classified as long term in nature in that they are held for income purposes. These may be a result of using excess cash to either invest in items such as other organizations, joint ventures, purchase stocks, or bonds of other organizations or donations received from external parties. As in the case of Hospital Anywhere USA, they are investments in other organizations (affiliates of Hospital Anywhere USA) or loans made to affiliate organizations.

INTANGIBLE ASSETS

Intangible assets generally are those items that have no physical presence but do have value in the form of legal rights to use or sell an asset. One example is patents that have been developed by employees of the organization. Use of a patent may provide a strategic advantage over competing facilities or may reduce your firm's costs below that of competitors. One item that is harder to define as an intangible asset is *goodwill*. Goodwill occurs when an entity purchases another organization and there is an excess amount paid for the net assets of the purchased entity that exceeds market value. This excess amount is goodwill.

   Most intangible assets are also systematically written off over a period of time like that of depreciation but the process is called *amortization*. Goodwill must be evaluated each year, and a determination must be made for impairment of value. If value declines, goodwill must be reduced ("written down") by this amount.

Liabilities

To begin our discussion of liabilities, please refer to **Exhibit 19–2**.

CURRENT LIABILITIES

Accounts payables are claims on assets. These are short term in nature and are generally expected to be paid in 30 to 120 days based on the type of claim but can be unpaid up to 1 year. The purchase of operating supplies such as surgical staples and food items are examples.

   Accrued liabilities (i.e., salaries) are those that have been incurred in the course of business but have not yet been paid. For example, if employees are paid on the fifth of the month for effort in the previous month, then it is an accrued expense. Employers owe employees for services provided but have not yet made payment. Accounting recognizes expenses when incurred, not necessarily

Exhibit 19–2 Liabilities Section of Balance Sheet

(Dollars in millions, except for per share amount)

Liabilities	2004	2003
Current liabilities		
Accounts payable	693	657
Accrued salaries	352	403
Other accrued expenses	1,135	897
Government settlement accrual	840	
Long-term debt due within 1 year	1,121	1,160
Total current liabilities	**4,141**	**3,117**
Long-term debt	5,631	5,284
Professional liability risks, deferred taxes and other liabilities	2,050	2,104
Minority interests in equity of consolidated entities	572	763
Forward purchase contracts and put options	769	
Total liabilities	**13,163**	**11,268**

when paid. Other accrued expenses could include interest incurred on debt but not paid or taxes owed to government entities.

Most organizations finance equipment or a building that requires a large outlay of resources over a long period of time, with some financing arrangements lasting up to 40 years. Each year as that portion of the debt becomes due in the current year, it is considered a current liability.

LONG-TERM LIABILITIES (DEBT)

Long-term debt examples include such items as mortgages and bonds issued to borrow money. This debt is not paid in the current year or operating period. Other items identified as long-term debt could include professional liability risks such as unsettled lawsuits resulting from malpractice claims and employee work-related injuries. *Deferred taxes* are the differences between income reported in financial statements and that paid to the U.S. Treasury.

Stockholder's Equity

For-profit corporate firms raise funds by issuing either *preferred* or *common stock*. **Exhibit 19–3** provides an example. These stocks represent ownership shares in an organization. Both stocks generally have a par value and sell for more than this base amount (*capital in excess of par value*). The *par value* is arbitrarily established as a low amount and is used for accounting records.

Preferred stock is not used as extensively as common stock but is one possible source of funds. The stock gets its name from the preference over common stock in either payments of dividends or distribution of liquidation proceeds in case of the firm ceasing business. Three additional financial items are found in the stockholder's equity section of Hospital Anywhere USA.

The final item found on the statement of financial position is *retained earnings*. The name is misleading because there is no actual money in this account. Retained earnings is an account used by the accounting function to balance the books at the end of the year. The amount carried to retained earnings is the difference between all revenue sources, expenses and costs, and dividends paid. The equivalent section of the stockholder's equity of a not-for-profit is called a fund balance.

Exhibit 19–3 Stockholder's Equity Section of Balance Sheet

(Dollars in millions)

Stockholder's equity:		
Common stock $.01 par; authorized 1,600,000,000 voting shares 50,000,000 nonvoting shares; outstanding 521,991,700 voting shares and 21,000,000 shares and 21,000,000 nonvoting shares—2004 and 543,272,900 voting shares and 21,000,000 nonvoting shares—2003	5	6
Capital in excess of par value		951
Other	9	8
Accumulated other comprehensive income	52	53
Retained earnings	4,339	4,599
Total stockholder's equity	4,405	5,617
Total liabilities and stockholder's equity	**$17,568**	**$16,885**

Income Statement

The *income statement* is a financial statement that captures information about revenue sources, expenses, and costs of doing business during a period of time. For example, a yearly income statement would be labeled for the year ended. Hospital Anywhere USA shows years ended December 31, 2004, 2003, and 2002 (**Exhibit 19–4**).

Exhibit 19–4 Income Statement

(Dollars in millions)

	2004	2003	2002
Revenues	**$16,670**	**$16,657**	**$18,681**
Salaries and benefits	6,639	6,694	7,766
Supplies	2,640	2,645	2,901
Other operating expenses	3,085	3,251	3,816
Provision for doubtful accounts	1,255	1,269	1,442
Depreciation and amortization	1,033	1,094	1,247
Interest expense	559	471	561
Equity in earnings of affiliates	(126)	(90)	(112)
Settlement with federal government	840	0	0
Gains on sales of facilities	(34)	(297)	(744)
Impairment of long-lived assets	117	220	542
Restructuring of operations and investigation related costs	62	116	111
Total expenses	**16,070**	**15,373**	**17,530**

Most revenue sources come from providing patient services. The problem with these sources is that the amount billed is not the amount received. For example, using the prospective payment system established in the early 1990s, many of the major insurance companies pay only between 50% and 60% of the amount billed. For Medicare and state health plans, such as Medicaid, this amount is even lower—it could be as low as 25%. This has led to major changes in the accounting of health care providers, such as more accuracy in billing. If a claim is filed with a third-party provider, payment must be received as soon as possible. Many health care providers found that claims collection was taking as many as 90 days. This means services were provided, resulting in expenditures, but the health care provider has only a piece of paper representing a claim. Many providers have improved their claims collection through improved accuracy of coding and by using electronic filing. The sooner the payment is received, the sooner the health care entity can use the funds to pay its own claims for services provided by creditors and purchase new equipment or replacement equipment for improved diagnosis.

Additional revenue may take the form of providing services for other health care facilities or through the investment of funds. One example of additional services is that of a health care facility, such as Healthy Hospital, doing laundry service for other hospitals. One section of Hospital Anywhere USA asset section illustrated the category called investments. Revenues from invested funds in the form of interest or dividends can also supplement basic operations.

Reductions in payments by third-party providers, including government entities, have forced many health care facilities to establish an active foundation so additional funds are directed to the foundation. These additional sources of funds can be used to either cover shortfalls in revenues or can be invested to provide interest or other forms of additional revenue.

Costs and Expenses

Deductions from the revenue sources take the form of either *costs* or *expenses*. Costs and expenses, in the income statement, are those items used up or incurred in the generation of revenues. For Hospital Anywhere USA, the largest of these expenses is generally salaries and benefits paid to employees.

The second largest category of expenses is supplies and services, as shown in Exhibit 19–4. Each patient for whom services are rendered requires some use of supplies (i.e., forms for patient information, swabs for testing, testing supplies, or food and beverages provided through food services).

The third largest item is the provision for doubtful accounts (*bad debt expense/provision for bad debts*), which is the adjustment for patient services that are expected not to be collected. Bad debt expense is the charge for not being able to collect patient accounts. Charges filed with third-party payers are reduced according to payment schedules established by these firms. This reduces the amount of revenue from the gross (full) amount billed to the net amount. The amount over that paid by the third-party payers is expected to be collected from the patient to whom services were provided. This refers to *deductibles* and *copayments*, which are amounts the patient pays over the reasonable and customary charges, discussed in Chapter 10, which provides a health care economic overview. However, with Medicare and Medicaid patients, it is illegal to go back and bill the patients for whatever Medicare and Medicaid doesn't pay. In some cases, the patient will not be able to make payments. These must be taken as further charges in the form of bad debts.

Depreciation is a deduction allowed by the Internal Revenue Service. This is a paper and pencil amount (accounting) and is not an actual use of cash sources. Once a building or piece of equipment is acquired, it may be "written off" over a designated period of time. The cost of the equipment is allocated to a specific time period and is used to reduce the net revenue and thus reduce taxes. For example, if a piece of diagnostic equipment having a 10-year life span is purchased for

5 million dollars, using one of the many methods allowed for the calculation of depreciation (straight-line), the depreciation amount per year would be $500,000 ($5,000,000 ÷ 10 years = $500,000 depreciation per year). As stated previously, this reduces income and will lead to fewer taxes being paid.

Depending on the size of the health care facility, additional costs may be incurred.

Cash Flow

As stated previously, cash is the lifeblood of a business. The *cash flow statement* shows one part of the financial stability of a firm. If all transactions were cash based, then this statement would be easy to prepare and interpret. For-profit entities are required by generally accepted accounting principles (GAAP) to report on an *accrual basis*. This means that revenue must be reported when earned, not necessarily when payment is received, and expenses are recognized when incurred, not paid. This requires several estimates during the reporting period. For example, if a service has been provided and a health care entity has a reasonable expectation of collection and can identify the amount to be collected, then it must be reported as revenue. Cash for the service may not be received until the next period.

If employees are paid every Friday and the reporting period ends on Thursday, then salaries must be accrued. For simplicity let us assume those salaries are $100,000 per week and no one works on the weekends. Each week the health care entity makes cash payments of $100,000 until the final week of the year. Since the reporting period ends on Thursday, the firm owes the employees $80,000 (4 days of pay) for services rendered. This amount must be recorded as an expense in the current period but does not require cash expenditure until the next reporting period.

The *bad debt expense* must likewise be estimated at the end of the year. The total amount of bad debts will not be known until all efforts to collect an account have been exhausted. This requires recognition of the bad debt expense for the reporting period (quarterly or yearly). The estimate is based on past experience in collection of accounts receivable, necessitated by adjustments for economic conditions. If 2% of the accounts receivable have been identified as bad in previous years and there was a major plant closing in the current reporting period, it could be expected that the amount collected would decrease and the bad debt expense would increase.

Preparation of the cash flow statement requires a thorough knowledge of the financial statements. Taking the cash balance at the beginning of the period and subtracting the ending cash balance provides the change in cash. The cash flow statement provides information explaining why cash changed. Financial statement items causing changes in cash are identified as operating, financing, and investing activities.

OPERATING ACTIVITIES

Operating activities focus on the current portion of financial statements. They are the most important part of the cash flow analysis. Operating activities focus on the cash inflows and outflows from events that occur in the current operating period (**Exhibit 19–5**). Financing and investing activities can provide funds but are limited to the extent of the time to which they can provide cash flow. There are upper limits on the amount of debt that can be issued (borrowed) on stock that can be sold. Likewise, there is a limited amount of investments that can be sold to provide cash inflow. There is also a limit on the number of long-term assets that can be sold, and much like personal debt, there is a limit to the amount of money that can be borrowed.

Cash flow can be calculated in two ways, but the one preferred by most entities starts with the net income or loss from the income statement. All current assets and liabilities from the balance sheet must be analyzed to determine the impact on cash flow. If accounts receivable increases, how

Exhibit 19–5 Cash Flow Operating Activities Section

(Dollars in millions)			
Cash flows from continuing activities	**2004**	**2003**	**2002**
Net income	$219	$657	$379
Adjustments to reconcile net income to net cash provided by continuing operating activities			
Provision for doubtful accounts	1,255	1,269	1,442
Depreciation and amortization	1,033	1,094	1,247
Income taxes	(219)	(66)	351
Settlement with federal government	840	0	0
Gains on sales of facilities	(34)	(297)	(744)
Impairment of long-lived assets	117	220	542
Loss from discontinued operating assets	0	0	153
Increase (decrease) in cash from operating assets and liabilities			
Accounts receivable	(1,678)	(1,463)	(1,229)
Inventories and other assets	90	(119)	(39)
Accounts payable and accrued expenses	(147)	(110)	(177)
Other	71	38	(9)
Net case provided by continuing operating activities	**$1,547**	**$1,223**	**$1,916**

is cash impacted? Cash would decrease. If the amount of current assets represented by accounts receivable increases, you now have more paper and less cash coming in. From the perspective of the income statement, when services were provided you recorded the item as income. Net income is therefore higher than the cash generated from revenue, leading to the adjustment in net income on the cash flow statement. The same is true for all other current assets. There is an inverse relationship between the change in current assets and the impact on cash flow. If current assets increase, they will be deducted from net income. Or, vice versa, if current assets decrease, they will be added back to net income.

Current liabilities have the opposite effect. If any current liability increases, this adds to the cash balance. What is the impact on cash if current liabilities increase? The firm has acquired either goods or services without having a cash outflow. The cash balance is improved by acquisition of assets without having a cash outflow. All current liabilities have a direct relationship with the impact on cash flow. Increases are added to net income, and decreases are subtracted from net income. The result of adding or deducting changes in current assets and liabilities to net income provides cash flow from operating activities.

FINANCING ACTIVITIES

The second portion of the cash flow statement is the *financing activities*, which focuses on long-term liabilities (those having a due date of longer than 1 year) or equity in the form of common or preferred stock (**Exhibit 19–6**). If long-term liabilities increase during the year, it provides

Exhibit 19–6 Cash Flow Financing Activities Section

(Dollars in millons)			
Cash flows from financing activities	2004	2003	2002
Issuance of long-term debt	$2,980	$1,037	$3
Net change in bank borrowing	(500)	200	(2,514)
Repayment of long-term debt	(2,058)	(1,572)	(147)
Issuance (repurchase) of common stock, net	(677)	(1,884)	8
Payment of cash dividends	(44)	(44)	(52)
Other	(37)	8	3
Net cash used in financing activities	($336)	($2,255)	($2,699)

cash inflow. The firm is borrowing money to use in the business. If long-term liabilities decrease, then this implies that the liabilities are being paid off, leading to a decrease in cash. Stock operates in the same manner. If either the common or preferred stock accounts increase, then the implication is that stock is used to finance firm activities. If they decrease, then stock is being repurchased and cash is leaving the firm. Likewise the payment of dividends on stock decreases cash outflow.

INVESTING ACTIVITIES

The last part of the cash flow statement concerns the *investing activities* of an organization, as shown in **Exhibit 19–7**. This focuses mainly on the long-term assets of a business. If these assets are sold, cash inflows occur. On the other hand, if long-term assets are acquired, then cash is presumed to decrease. An increase in investments is shown as having a decrease in cash. A summary of these activities is presented in Exhibit 19–7 to indicate the change in cash and cash equivalents.

Adding each category, continuing operating, financing, and investing provides the change in cash and cash equivalents. Added to or subtracted from (if cash flow is negative as in 2003) cash and cash equivalents at the beginning of the period provides the amounts found on the balance sheet. The

Exhibit 19–7 Cash Flow Investing Activities Section

(Dollars in millions)			
Cash flows from investing activities	2004	2003	2002
Purchase of property and equipment	($1,155)	($1,287)	($1,255)
Acquisitions of hospitals and health care entities	(350)	0	(215)
Spin-off of facilities to stockholders	0	886	0
Disposal of hospitals and health care entities	327	805	2,060
Change in investments	106	565	(294)
Investment in discontinued operations, net	0	0	677
Other	(15)	(44)	(3)
Net cash provided by (used in) investing activities	($1,087)	$925	$970

Exhibit 19–8 Summary of Cash Flows and Changes in Cash and Cash Equivalents

| | (Dollars in millions) | | |
	2004	2003	2002
Net case provided by continuing operating activities	**$1,547**	**$1,223**	**$1,916**
Net cash provided by (used in) investing activities	**($1,087)**	**$925**	**$970**
Net cash used in financing activities	**($336)**	**($2,255)**	**($2,699)**
Change in cash and cash equivalents	124	(107)	187
Cash and cash equivalents at beginning of period	190	297	110
Cash and cash equivalents at end of period	$314	$190	$297

cash and cash equivalents account increased in both 2004 and 2002 and decreased in 2003, as shown in **Exhibit 19–8**, which provides a summary of all activities.

Schedule of Changes in Equity

The *Schedule of Changes in Equity* is required for all publicly reporting companies (governed by stock markets such as those sold on the New York Stock Exchange) and presents information for the reader to evaluate all changes in the owner's portion of the balance sheet.

Internal Accounting Information

Cost/Managerial Accounting

Although public-reporting, for-profit health care entities must issue financial statements to external users, not-for-profit entities are not required to report to the general public. Accounting information used for internal or management decisions is not available to the general public but is used by management and others working within an organization. This information may be as specific as the pay rate for individual employees or the costs to operate a function of the firm such as laboratories. For many health care workers, this is the area where management asks for employee input. This information is also used to evaluate the current operations of the organization and to solicit employee input to improve future operations. As previously mentioned, the amount of payments from third-party payers has declined in recent years. Health care facilities used to receive reimbursements based on costs of operation. However, with the advent of prospective payment systems, these amounts have generally been reduced. Thus input from employees is needed to reduce costs and to improve customer services. As one nurse stated to the author, "I know the technical part of my job but I am being asked to serve on committees that are looking at changing and improving business operations." Thus the nurse needs to understand accounting information and how it can be used to support these changes.

Costs

Costs to be considered in making management decisions include differentiating between fixed and variable, direct and indirect, and marginal costs. Included in the discussion of costs is the term "relevant range." To most, *relevant range* refers to the likely operating activity level expected to be incurred by a health care entity. For example, current staff can handle between 100 and 150 patients per day, which is the average use of our facilities. If the number of patients is either above or below these numbers, costs must be reconsidered (i.e., reduce or add employees to provide services).

From a revenue perspective, previous discussion centered on correct coding and use of diagnosis-related groups and resource utilization groups. Discussion also centered on the collection of these revenue items and the impact on financial statements. When health care facilities were forced to more carefully evaluate their operations, they found many services offered were losing money. Since revenues were capped, cost containment became the issue.

Fixed Versus Variable Costs

Evaluating operations begins with the evaluation of the costs involved. First is the distinction between fixed and variable costs. *Fixed costs* do not change with levels of services. If you are dealing with a facility that has 100 beds, building costs such as depreciation will be the same regardless if there is 1 patient or 100 patients occupying the bed(s). *Variable costs* do change with the increase of facility use. As more patients occupy the facility, costs such as food, medicines, and staff increases. These costs are variable because they change as the volume (number of patients or procedures) changes. Fixed and variable costs were previously discussed in Chapter 12.

Direct Versus Indirect Costs

The second cost distinction is indirect versus direct costs. For an example, let's use the costs of laboratory services. The cost of the lab assistant who draws blood for analysis is a *direct cost*. Likewise, needles and other supplies are direct costs. The staff person who manages the facility, handles the paperwork for the patient upon arrival, or files the claim is an *indirect cost*.

Marginal costs are those costs related to providing additional services. Again, using the laboratory example, assume that the lab can handle 20 patients a day. If the lab is currently offering services to 15 patients, how much will it cost to provide additional services to one more patient? There will be no additional costs for the person drawing the blood sample; thus there is no marginal cost associated with this service. There will be additional costs associated with the use of needles, bandages, and testing supplies. These are marginal costs. As long as revenue for these services increases more than the costs, services should be expanded.

Average costs are those costs divided by the total number of services provided. Let us assume that it costs $500 per day to maintain the lab. If the lab performs only one test on this day, then the average cost will be $500. However, if the lab performs five tests today, the average cost will be $100 per test. You can operate up to a certain point without expanding facilities, personnel, or equipment. As the number of tests increases, the average cost decreases (this is the relevant range). Let us assume that the facility expands these services to reach 40 tests per day but can process only 20 per day with the current number of employees. The relevant range would be up to 20 tests. Over 20 tests would require the addition of personnel or equipment. Direct, indirect, and marginal costs were previously discussed in Chapter 12.

Activity-Based Costing

Once the types of costs are identified, they need to be allocated to the specific services performed. With the limitations on cost recovery (revenue) imposed by third-party payers, health care entities must be aware of the costs to provide these services. Why should a facility pay $1.5M for a magnetic resonance imaging machine and incur the other costs to maintain and staff the center when the revenues will not cover the costs? Recently, one area of thought in accounting has been introduced to help users of accounting information focus on the specific costs of providing services. This is called *activity-based costing (ABC)*.

Activity-based costing (ABC) requires that you identify the cost drivers behind an activity. It requires that you break all services into specific functions and identify the costs associated with each activity. Assume you work in a physician's office and you need to determine the costs of a patient visit for a general exam. What activities are associated with the cost of providing these services? Let us assume the following, which is not a comprehensive example, for purposes of illustration:

- A general practitioner is paid $80,000 per year and spends on the average 15 minutes with each patient, seeing 24 patients per day. The physician works 45 weeks per year.
- A nurse is paid $35,000 per year and also spends 15 minutes with the patient.
- The receptionist is paid $24,000 and spends 5 minutes per patient in taking appointment calls and answering patient questions in the reception area.
- The cashier is paid $24,000 and spends 5 minutes per patient recording doctor information and verifying information for billing.
- All claims are entered electronically, and it takes a data recorder 10 minutes to fill out the electronic filing version. This person is paid $20,000.
- A bookkeeper is paid $25,000 per year to capture accounting information for the facility. The bookkeeper spends 10 minutes per patient on the average collecting and reporting data for management of the facility.
- A stethoscope costs $100 and lasts 2 years.
- Each tongue depressor costs $.01.
- Each pair of latex gloves costs $.01.
- Each of the above-mentioned individuals in the physician's office has a computer that costs $2,000 and is used for 2 years.
- Utility service per patient is $1.00.
- The cost per patient for building (facility) in the form of depreciation is $1.50.

Based on the previous information, the following provides an analysis of the cost of providing patient services for a general physical examination. In the example shown in **Exhibit 19–9**, the patient is the cost driver.

The diagnosis-related group code for medium intervention activity is billed at $50.00. A third-party payer remits, on the average, 56% of billed amount, yielding a payment of $35.60. Additional amounts may be collected from the patient, but that is not assumed in this case. (As mentioned earlier, this is true for coinsurance, deductibles, and what is above the reasonable and customary costs with regular insurance. However, with Medicaid and with Medicare, other than billing the deductible and coinsurance, it is illegal to bill the patient for the amount of reimbursement not paid by the government.) Given the cost of the service at $41.21, there is a loss of $5.61 for each patient seen by the physician. This is where decision making using accounting data can improve the profitability of services, whether this is done by a single physician, nursing home, or hospital. What would you suggest to reduce the costs of the above or improve the revenue? The physician and nurse spend 15 minutes per patient, but the others spend less time. Could the time the physician spends with each patient be reduced to increase the number of patients examined per year? Could there be additional physicians or nurse practitioners employed to increase the workload of others such as the receptionist and bookkeeper, thus reducing the costs of others such as the receptionist and cashier? If the number of patients seen increases, the building and computer cost per patient would be

Exhibit 19–9 Activity-Based Costing Example

(Dollars in millions)

Cost Driver	Cost	Cost Per Patient	Comments
Physician	$80,000	$14.81	15 minutes per patient/24 patients per day/45 weeks
Nurse	$35,000	$6.48	15 minutes per patient/24 patients per day/45 weeks
Receptionist	$24,000	$4.44	5 minutes per patient/24 patients per day/ 45 weeks
Cashier	$24,000	$4.44	5 minutes per patient/24 patients per day/ 45 weeks
Data Recorder	$20,000	$3.70	10 minutes per patient/24 patients per day/45 weeks
Bookkeeper	$25,000	$4.62	10 minutes per patient/24 patients per day/45 weeks
Utility Services		$1.00	
Computers	$12,000	$.19	6 computers/$2,000 per computer cost/ life of 2 years
Gloves		.01	
Tongue Depressor		.01	
Building Depreciation		$1.50	
Stethoscope	$100	.01	$100/lasts 2 years
Total		**$41.21**	

decreased. Another alternative is to either expand the nurse's responsibilities or to hire additional nurses to reduce the physician's time with patients.

One solution would be to evaluate the use of each part of the cost structure. In the previous example, the physician was limited to seeing 5,400 patients per year. This is also the limitation for each of the other members of the physician's organization and is the cost driver. If the time spent with patients can be reduced to 10 minutes per patient, then the number of patients the physician can examine will be increased to 36 patients per day, or 8,100 per year. This causes a decrease in the physician cost per patient to $9.88, and receptionist cost per patient to $2.96. The overall effect causes cost to be reduced to a level below the third-party payment that now exceeds cost.

Previously, different types of costs were defined. Using the previous example, we now illustrate the costs. Fixed costs are those that do not change in total as volume (number of patients) increases. All costs except utilities, gloves, and tongue depressors are fixed. These costs are variable in that they change as the number of patients increases. As seen in the revenue and cost comparison, the physician's salary is fixed and as the number of patients increased, the physician's cost per patient decreased (average cost decreases). As with any fixed costs, you want to maximize the use and lower the costs to the lowest level.

Direct costs are those related to the generation of revenues. In this case, the physician and nurse are considered direct costs of providing services, as are the gloves and tongue depressors. The other costs are considered indirect because they are not directly related to production of revenue. Why is this distinction needed? If you are trying to determine whether or not to expand services, you might want to look at the direct costs. Can you cover the direct costs of providing services? If so, then each patient or procedure will add to the profitability of the health care entity. For example, in the original illustration, if you can cover the direct costs (physician, nurse, gloves, and tongue depressor—$21.31), then additional amounts received can be applied to the indirect costs. The fixed costs will remain if a facility operates or closes for the weekend or vacations. If you can cover the direct cost, then any excess amount would be used to help cover fixed costs.

Marginal costs are those that increase as additional services are provided. Which costs in the illustration change as additional patients are added? Only the costs of the gloves and tongue depressor are marginal costs. What will it cost to provide service for one additional patient? When evaluating whether or not to accept additional patients, you need to consider the impact on the organization. If no new costs are added for providing additional services, as long as the additional revenue exceeds the additional cost, then the service should be provided. To clarify this point, assume that a third-party insurer approaches your organization offering a new client base consisting of local county employees. However, the insurer will pay a lower amount than that provided by other insurers. If you can determine the marginal costs of the services to be provided, the marginal costs may be less than the revenue received, increasing the contribution to firm profitability. This would benefit the organization.

Conclusion

Employees of health care facilities are being asked to improve patient services by generating additional revenue and becoming a valuable member of the management team. Correctly identifying services before filing claims with third parties can improve revenue collection. Additionally, making recommendations for more efficient use of services to minimize costs of these services is important for continuing organizational success. Can the health care entity substitute services for those currently being offered? Can someone in an organization provide the same quality services as others? For example, can I use a licensed practical nurse in place of a registered nurse? (This decision would be best only if the work performed by the person was appropriate at the licensed practical nurse level.) This is one of the major issues affecting health care today.

Discussion Questions

1. Why should you be familiar with the balance sheet? Why is it important to the organization? And what area of the balance sheet would you consider the most critical?
2. Comparing costs in this chapter, which costs do you have little control over and why? Which costs would be most important if you are expanding your services?
3. How would you know if the organization is a for-profit or a not-for-profit based on the information available from the balance sheet and the income statement?
4. Goodwill and patents are considered what types of assets?
5. Which asset is considered the lifeblood of the organization, and why?

Glossary of Terms

Accounts (Patients) Receivable Represents Future Cash Collection—These may be represented by amounts owed by either patients to whom the organization has provided services or by claims filed with third party providers such as insurance companies.

Accounts Payables—are claims on assets. These are short term in nature and are generally expected to be paid in 30–120 days based on the type of claim, but can be unpaid up to one year.

Accumulated Depreciation—is the sum of the annual depreciation charges, subtracted from the plant and equipment balance providing a net figure.

Activity-Based Costing (ABC)—requires that you break all services into specific functions and identify the cost drivers associated with each activity

Assets—are those items that provide future cash flow or have future economic benefit.

Average Costs—are those costs divided by the total number of services provided

Balance Sheet—consists of the assets, liabilities, and equity.

Buildings—are the physical facilities in which patient services are provided.

Cash Flow Statement—provides information explaining why cash changed. Financial statement items causing changes in cash are identified as operating, financing, and investing activities.

Construction in Progress—is an account indicating buildings that have not been completed but are being built. The account indicates progress toward completion.

Costs and Expenses—in the income statement, are those items used up or incurred in the generation of revenues

Current Assets—are those items that will be used to generate revenue in either one year of the operating period, whichever is longer (most often this is one year).

Deferred Taxes—are the differences between income reported in financial statements and that paid to the U.S. Treasury

Depreciation—is an accounting charge wherein the balance of the equipment and buildings is systematically written off over a period of time.

Equipment—may be items such as X-ray, CT machines, or less complex items such as patient beds.

Financial Activities—focuses on long-tem liabilities (obligations have a due date of longer than one year) or equity in the form of common or preferred stock

Fund Balance—section of the stockholder's equity of a not-for-profit organization.

Goodwill—occurs when an entity purchases another organization and there is an excess amount paid for the net assets of the purchased entity that exceeds market value. This excess amount is goodwill.

Income Statement—is a financial statement that captures information about revenue sources, expenses, and costs of doing business during a period of time.

Intangible Assets—generally are those items that have no physical presence but do have value in the form of legal rights to use or sell an asset.

Inventory—items such as drugs in the pharmacy, surgical supplies, items maintained in nursing stations and drinks and/or food in the cafeteria.

Investment Activities—focus mainly on the long-term assets of an organization.

Investments—are classified as long-term in nature in that they are held for income purposes. These may be a result of using excess cash to either invest in items such as other organizations, joint ventures, purchase stocks, or bonds of other organizations, or donations received from external parties.

Liabilities—are claims on the assets of an organization. The claims are those of creditors who have provided resources such as buildings and equipment but have not been fully paid.

Long-term Debt—include such items as mortgages and bonds issued to borrow money. This debt will not be paid in the current year or operating period

Marginal Costs—are those costs that are related to providing additional services

Net Assets or Fund Balances—in not-for-profit organizations the result of subtracting liabilities from assets.

Net Worth—difference between the assets and liabilities of an organization is the equity, or in the personal loan application example.

Operating Activities—focus on the cash inflows and outflows from events that occur in the current operating period

Preferred or Common Stock—For-profit corporate firms raise funds by issuing these stocks. These stocks represent ownership shares in an organization.

Provision for Doubtful Accounts—is the adjustment for patient services that are expected not to be collected

Relevant Range—refers to the likely operating activity level expected to be incurred by a health care entity

Retained Earnings—is an account used by the accounting function to balance the books at the end of the year.

Schedule of Changes in Equity—is required for all publicly reporting companies and present information for the reader to evaluate all changes in the owner's portion of the balance sheet

Tangible Assets—The largest item on a for-profit health care entity's balance sheet is probably buildings and equipment.

Temporary Investments—are cash equivalents because they can be sold quickly with little or no loss in value.

APPENDIX

(All amounts are dollars in millions, except per share amounts.)

Hospital Anywhere USA Consolidated Balance Sheets, December 31, 2004 and 2003

Assets	2004	2003
Current Assets:		
Cash and cash equivalents	$314	$190
Accounts receivable, less allowance for doubtful accounts of $1,583 and $1,567	2,211	1,873
Inventories	396	383
Income taxes receivable	197	178
Other	1,335	973
Total Current Assets	**4,453**	**3,597**
Property and equipment at cost:		
Land	793	813
Buildings	6,021	6,108
Equipment	7,045	6,721
Construction in progress	431	442
Total Property and Equipment	**14,290**	**14,084**
Accumulated depreciation	(5,810)	(5,594)
	8,480	8,490
Investments of insurance subsidiary	1,371	1,457
Investments in and advances to affiliates	779	654
Intangible assets, net of accumulated amortization of $785 and $644	2,155	2,319
Other	330	368
Total Assets	**$17,568**	**$16,885**
Liabilities	2004	2003
Current Liabilities:		
Accounts payable	693	657
Accrued salaries	352	403
Other accrued expenses	1,135	897
Government settlement accrual	840	
Long-term debt due within one year	1,121	1,160
Total Current Liabilities	**4,141**	**3,117**
Long-term debt	5,631	5,284
Professional liability risks, deferred taxes, and other liabilities	2,050	2,104
Minority interests in equity of consolidated entities	572	763
Forward purchase contracts and put options	769	
Total Liabilities	**13,163**	**11,268**
Stockholders equity:		
Common stock $.01 par; authorized 1,600,000,000 voting shares,		
50,000,000 nonvoting shares; outstanding 521,991,700 voting shares		
and 21,000,000 nonvoting shares—2004 and 543,272,900 voting shares		
and 21,000,000 nonvoting shares—2003	5	6
Capital in excess of par value		951
Other	9	8
Accumulated other comprehensive income	52	53
Retained earnings	4,339	4,599
Total Stockholder's Equity	**4,405**	**5,617**
Total Liabilities and Stockholder's Equity	**$17,568**	**$16,885**

Hospital Anywhere USA Consolidated Statement of Cash Flow for the Years Ended December 31, 2004, 2003, and 2002

Cash Flows from Continuing Activities:	2004	2003	2002
Net Income	$219	$657	$379
Adjustments to reconcile net income to net cash provided by continuing operating activities:			
Provision for doubtful accounts	1,255	1,269	1,442
Depreciation and amortization	1,033	1,094	1,247
Income taxes	(219)	(66)	351
Settlement with Federal government	840	0	0
Gains on sales of facilities	(34)	(297)	(744)
Impairment of long-lived assets	117	220	542
Loss from discontinued operating assets	0	0	153
Increase (decrease) in cash from operating assets and liabilities:			
Accounts receivable	(1,678)	(1,463)	(1,229)
Inventories and other assets	90	(119)	(39)
Accounts payable and accrued expenses	(147)	(110)	(177)
Other	71	38	(9)
Net case provided by continuing operating activities	**$1,547**	**$1,223**	**$1,916**
Cash flows from financing activities:	**2004**	**2003**	**2002**
Issuance of long-term debt	$2,980	$1,037	$3
Net change in bank borrowing	(500)	200	(2,514)
Repayment of long-term debt	(2,058)	(1,572)	(147)
Issuance (repurchase) of common stock, net	(677)	(1,884)	8
Payment of cash dividends	(44)	(44)	(52)
Other	(37)	8	3
Net cash used in financing activities	**($336)**	**($2,255)**	**($2,699)**
Cash flows from investing activities:	**2004**	**2003**	**2002**
Purchase of property and equipment	($1,155)	($1,287)	($1,255)
Acquisitions of hospitals and health care entities	(350)	0	(215)
Spin-off of facilities to stockholders	0	886	0
Disposal of hospitals and health care entities	327	805	2,060
Change in investments	106	565	(294)
Investment in discontinued operations, net	0	0	677
Other	(15)	(44)	(3)
Net cash provided by (used in) investing activities	**($1,087)**	**$925**	**$970**

	2004	2003	2002
Net cash provided by continuing operating activities	1,547	1,223	1,916
Net cash provided by (used in) investing activities	(1,087)	925	970
Net cash used in financing activities	(336)	(2,255)	(2,699)
Change in cash and cash equivalents	124	(107)	187
Cash and cash equivalents at beginning of period	190	297	110
Cash and cash equivalents at end of period	**$314**	**$190**	**$297**
Interest payments	$489	$475	$566
Income tax payments, net of refunds	$516	$634	($139)

Hospital Anywhere USA Consolidated Income Statements for the Years Ended December 31, 2004, 2003, and 2002

	2004	2003	2002
Revenues	$ 16,670	$ 16,657	$ 18,681
Salaries and benefits	6,639	6,694	7,766
Supplies	2,640	2,645	2,901
Other operating expenses	3,085	3,251	3,816
Provision for doubtful accounts	1,255	1,269	1,442
Depreciation and amortization	1,033	1,094	1,247
Interest expense	559	471	561
Equity in earnings of affiliates	(126)	(90)	(112)
Settlement with Federal government	840	0	0
Gains on sales of facilities	(34)	(297)	(744)
Impairment of long-lived assets	117	220	542
Restructuring of operations and investigation related costs	62	116	111
Total expenses	**16,070**	**15,373**	**17,530**
Income from continuing operations before minority interests and income taxes	66	1,284	1,151
Minority interests in earnings of consolidated entities	84	57	70
Income from continuing operations before income taxes	516	1,227	1,081
Provision for income taxes	297	570	549
Income from continuing operations	219	657	532
Discontinued operations:			
Loss from operations of discontinued businesses, net of income tax benefit of $26			(80)
Loss of disposals of discontinued businesses			(73)
Net income	$219	$657	$379
Basic earnings per share:			
Income from continuing operations	$0.39	$1.12	$0.82
Discontinued operations:			
Loss from operations of discontinued businesses			(.12)
Loss on disposals of discontinued businesses			(.11)
Net income	**$0.39**	**$1.12**	**$0.59**
Diluted earnings per share:			
Income from continuing operations	$0.39	$1.12	$0.82
Discontinued operations:			
Loss from operations of discontinued businesses			(.12)
Loss on disposals of discontinued businesses			(.11)
Net income	**$0.39**	**$1.12**	**$0.59**

CHAPTER 20

Financial Analysis: Improving Your Decision Making

Paul Bayes, DBA Accounting, MS Economics,
BS Accounting

Key Terms

- ☞ Accounts Receivable Collection Period
- ☞ Activity Ratios
- ☞ Benchmarking
- ☞ Cash on Hand
- ☞ Common Size Financial Statements
- ☞ Current Ratio
- ☞ Debt Ratio
- ☞ Fixed Asset Turnover
- ☞ Forward Purchase Contract
- ☞ Inventory Turnover

- ☞ Leverage Ratios, also called Capital Structure Ratios
- ☞ Liquidity Ratios
- ☞ Operating Profit Margin
- ☞ Profitability Ratios
- ☞ Program Service Ratio
- ☞ Put Option
- ☞ Quick or Acid-test Ratio
- ☞ Total Asset Turnover
- ☞ Trade or Cash Conversion Cycle Ratio

Numbers by themselves are data, not information. To be an informed and effective decision maker you must be able to convert raw data (numbers) into information. Putting financial data in a format that allows comparisons whether within your organization or between firms makes the information meaningful.

Benchmarking is a process that provides comparisons with the best practices of other organizations. These firms do not have to be within the same industry, but traditionally comparisons are based within specific industries. This is a limiting factor in identifying best practices but simplifies the comparisons.

The purpose of this chapter is to introduce you to financial analysis and to improve your understanding of the accounting information presented earlier. An improved understanding of financial information leads to better future policies and strategic plans. Analysis may be either qualitative (nonfinancial) or quantitative (financial). Most of this chapter focuses on quantitative analysis because this information is more readily available. Qualitative analysis examples are provided within the text of quantitative examples. All examples use the financial statements of Hospital Anywhere USA, a for-profit entity, which were provided in Chapter 19. Selected information from

Children's Hospital, a not-for-profit entity, is provided as a contrast to that of Hospital Anywhere USA. The financial statements of Retirement Homes, Inc. facility, a not-for-profit firm, are also provided as an example of a different type of not-for-profit facility. Differences in operating not-for-profit entities versus for-profit are noted.

Qualitative analysis requires a search of not only information in financial statements but also information from external sources. Stockholders' annual reports, not included in this book, along with financial statements, provide information. For example, the section on Management Discussion and Analysis provides information not found elsewhere in the financial statements, including strategic impetus and changes in the market structure. Other parts of the annual reports yield information as to accounting practices (footnotes), segment information, and risk. If an organization has subsidiaries (parts of the firm either partially or wholly owned by the parent company), information on segment information reveals reliance on operations of certain products, services, or geographic areas. The Securities and Exchange Commission (SEC) for publicly traded stock companies requires supplementary information. Additional information at the SEC Edgar Database can be found at http://www.sec.gov/edgarhp.htm. Information in Form 10-K and Form 10-Q reports is more comprehensive than the annual reports. In 10-Q (quarterly) reports, you can find information reported for each quarter of a firm. Rather than waiting until annual reports are issued, analysts can better track a firm's progress using these quarterly reports. Although the financial statements are the main focus of annual reports, they only make up a small portion. To illustrate, the annual report of Hospital Anywhere USA totals 51 pages of which the basic financial statements, including summaries, equal 7 pages.

Common Size Balance Sheets

Most of the focus in this chapter is quantitative and based on financial statements and the standard ratios found in both accounting and finance literature. One example of financial analysis is the use of common size financial statements. In the balance sheet and income statement, analysts select one number and then divide into all other numbers in the statement. Total assets (balance sheets) are used as the baseline figure in balance sheets. Either gross revenue (sales) or net revenue (sales) (income statement) is used as the basis for income statements. Gross revenue is the total sales made by a firm. The difference with the net figure is deductions such as discounts and returns have been removed. Dividing all items in this set of financial statements and comparing several years provides a quick method to evaluate trends (changes). The caveat is that a 2-year time frame may not be long enough to fully evaluate changes in operations (**Exhibit 20–1**).

Exhibit 20–1 illustrates some minor changes in the assets, liabilities, and stockholders' equity from 2003 to 2004. The cash and cash equivalents increased from 1.13% in 2003 to 1.79% in 2004. This trend indicates that Hospital Anywhere USA had more cash and cash equivalents as a percent of total assets in 2004 than they had in 2003. This increase may be due to management anticipation of a need for more cash or a better job of collecting patient accounts. Management may have also reduced expenses, thus improving cash flow. However, the accounts receivable percentages increased from 11.09% to 12.59%, indicating an increase in the amount of "paper" held and collection slowed. This point illustrates that the person doing the financial analysis may have to perform further evaluations rather than look at one piece of information. Total current assets also increased as a percent of total assets indicating that Hospital Anywhere USA was holding more liquid assets (ones that can be converted into cash quickly) in 2004 than in 2003.

Exhibit 20–1 Hospital Anywhere USA Consolidated Balance Sheets, December 31, 2004 and 2003

Dollars in Millions

Assets	2004		2003	
Current Assets				
Cash and cash equivalents	$314	1.79%	$190	1.13%
Accounts receivable, less allowance for doubtful accounts of $1,583 and $1,567	2,211	12.59%	1,873	11.09%
Inventories	396	2.25%	383	2.27%
Income taxes receivable	197	1.12%	178	1.05%
Other	1,335	7.6%	973	5.76%
Total Current Assets	**4,453**	**25.35%**	**3,597**	**21.30%**
Property and equipment at cost:				
Land	793	4.51%	813	4.81%
Buildings	6,021	34.27%	6,108	36.17%
Equipment	7,045	40.10%	6,721	39.80%
Construction in progress	431	2.45%	442	2.62%
Total Property and Equipment	**14,290**	**81.34%**	**14,084**	**83.41%**
Accumulated depreciation	-5,810	-33.07%	-5,594	-33.13%
	8,480	48.27%	8,490	50.28%
Investments of insurance subsidiary	1,371	7.8%	1,457	8.63%
Investments in and advances to affiliates	779	4.43%	654	3.87%
Intangible assets, net of accumulated amortization of $785 and $644	2,155	12.27%	2,319	13.73%
Other	330	1.88%	368	2.18%
Total Assets	**$17,568**	**100%**	**$16,885**	**100%**
Liabilities				
Current Liabilities				
Accounts payable	693	3.94%	657	3.89%
Accrued salaries	352	2.00%	403	2.39%
Other accrued expenses	1,135	6.46%	897	5.31%
Government settlement accrual	840	4.78%		
Long-term debt due within one year	1,121	6.38%	1,160	6.87%
Total Current Liabilities	**4,141**	**23.57%**	**3,117**	**18.46%**
Long-term debt	5,631	32.05%	5,284	31.29%
Professional liability risks, deferred taxes, and other liabilities	2,050	11.67%	2,104	12.46%
Minority interests in equity of consolidated entities	572	3.26%	763	4.92%
Forward purchase contracts and put options	769	4.38%		0%
Total Liabilities	**13,163**	**74.93%**	**11,268**	**66.73%**
Stockholders equity				
Common stock $.01 par; authorized 1,600,000,000 voting shares; 50,000,000 nonvoting shares; outstanding 521,991,700 voting shares and 21,000,000 nonvoting shares—2004 and 543,272,900 voting shares and 21,000,000 nonvoting shares—2003	5	.03%	6	.04%
Capital in excess of par value			951	5.63%
Other	9	0%	8	0%
Accumulated other comprehensive income	52	.30%	53	.31%
Retained earnings	4,339	24.07%	4,599	27.24%
Total Stockholders' Equity	4,405	25.07%	5,617	33.27%
Total Liabilities and Stockholders Equity	**$17,568**	**100%**	**$16,885**	**100%**

Three changes occurred in the items defined as long-term assets. First, the buildings account decreased from 36.17% to 34.27% of total assets, which indicates that Hospital Anywhere USA may have sold off some of its buildings. As this account illustrates, the dollar value of buildings in fact declined from $6,108 to $6,021. Footnotes accompanying the financial statements state that three properties were sold. The second change indicates construction in progress decreased slightly, which might provide evidence of some building projects either being completed or abandoned. The third change in these assets occurred in intangible assets, which showed a decrease of 1.46% from the previous year. This could be due to

- Selling off of parts of the organization, thereby reducing goodwill
- Selling off of some patents
- Expired patent rights
- A more aggressive manner used to write off existing patents or other intangible assets

One item that appears in conjunction with this account is that the amortization, systematic writing off of intangible assets, increased from $644 to $785. This explains, at least in part, the decrease in intangible assets but does not provide evidence as to the reason for the increase in write-offs. This would come with additional research in the schedules and notes accompanying the statements.

Current liabilities show one item changing drastically. The government settlement accrual went from zero in 2003 to $840 in 2004, indicating the settlement with the government over billing charges that cost the firm $840. The percentage change was from zero to 4.78%. Long-term debt, forward purchase contracts, and put options also went from zero to $769, making a percentage change from zero to 4.38%. A forward purchase contract is where one party agrees to buy a commodity at a specific price on a specific future date and the other party agrees to make the sale. In this case the agreement was for the repurchase of a limited number of common shares of Hospital Anywhere USA. A put option provides the right to sell stock at a specified price in the future. This again was related to the repurchase of the stock from a third party. In both instances a third party purchased shares of Hospital Anywhere USA stock in the market, and the hospital entered into a contract to purchase a set number of shares at a specified price from this third-party entity. Total liabilities also increased from 66.73% to 74.93%, indicating that a larger proportion of the business was financed using debt.

Analysis of stockholders equity indicates that the capital in excess of par values declined from $951 to zero going from 5.63% to zero. Although no information is directly available, a schedule that accompanies the financial statements provides information concerning this issue. Hospital Anywhere USA repurchased 21,281,200 shares of stock. Part of that repurchase plan would eliminate this account. A second item that negatively impacted the capital in excess of par value account was the reclassification of forward purchase contracts and put options to temporary equity. This was a result of action taken by the Financial Accounting Standards Board, which regulates reporting practices. Retained earnings declined from 27.24% to 24.70% as a result, partially, of the aforementioned reclassification.

Common Size Income Statements

Information in income statements is calculated in the same manner. The baseline number for analysis is either the gross revenue or net revenue. All items in the income statement are divided by this base figure, which converts the information into a common basis to detect trends (changes) in operations (**Exhibit 20–2**).

Exhibit 20–2 Hospital Anywhere USA Consolidated Income Statements for the Years Ended December 31, 2004, and 2003

Dollars in Millions

	2004		2003	
Revenues	$16,670	100.00%	$16,657	100.00%
Salaries and Benefits	6,639	39.83%	6,694	40.19%
Supplies	2,640	15.84%	2,645	15.88%
Other operating expenses	3,085	18.51%	3,251	19.52%
Provision for doubtful accounts	1,255	7.53%	1,269	7.62%
Depreciation and amortization	1,033	6.20%	1,094	6.57%
Interest expense	559	3.35%	471	2.83%
Equity in earnings of affiliates	-126	-0.76%	-90	-0.54%
Settlement with Federal government	840	5.04%	0	0.00%
Gains on sales of facilities	-34	-0.20%	-297	-1.78%
Impairment of long-lived assets	117	0.70%	220	1.32%
Restructuring of operations and investigation related costs	62	0.37%	116	0.70%
Total Expenses	**16,070**	**96.40%**	**15,373**	**92.29%**
Income from continuing operations before minority interests and income taxes	66	0.40%	1,284	7.71%
Minority interests in earnings of consolidated entities	84	0.50%	57	0.34%
Income from continuing operations before income taxes	516	3.10%	1,227	7.37%
Provision for income taxes	297	1.78%	570	3.42%
Income from continuing operations	219	1.31%	657	3.94%
Discontinued operations:				
Loss from operations of discontinued businesses, net of income tax benefit of $26				
Loss of disposals of discontinued businesses		0.00%		
Net Income	$219	1.31%	$657	3.94%
Basic earnings per share:				
Income from continuing operations	$0.39	0.00%	$1.12	0.01%
Discontinued operations:				
Loss from operations of discontinued businesses				
Loss on disposals of discontinued businesses				
Net income	**$0.39**	**0.00%**	**$1.12**	**0.01%**
Diluted earnings per share:				
Income from continuing operations	$0.39	0.00%	$1.12	0.01%
Discontinued operations:				
Loss from operations of discontinued businesses				
Loss on disposals of discontinued businesses				
Net income	**$0.39**	**0.00%**	**$1.12**	**0.01%**

Salaries and benefits decreased slightly, which indicates that Hospital Anywhere USA may have undertaken some cost control or containment measures during the 2004 reporting period. Other operating expenses also decreased from 19.52% to 18.51%. These would include items such as utilities, property taxes, professional fees (legal and accounting), maintenance, rent, and lease expenses. Interest expense and settlement with the federal government increased during this time period. With the aforementioned increase in debt financing, from the balance sheet analysis, there may be an increase in interest expenses. Unless a firm can negotiate a lower rate than that used in previous financing arrangements, the increased use of debt raises the risk to creditors, which causes the interest rate to increase. A simple explanation is that as more debt is issued, even at the same rate, there will be an increase in interest cost. The settlement with the federal government went from zero to 5.04%. This had a major impact on the profitability of the firm. The only remaining item that had a major change, other than summative categories, such as income from continuing operations before taxes and income from continuing operations, was provision for income taxes. This amount decreased from 3.42% to 1.78%. This may be a result of lower income or having either tax credits or deferred taxes that can be used to reduce the current year's taxable income. Tax credits are provided in the tax laws and allow firms to carry losses incurred in any year back for 2 years and forward for 20 years. Deferred taxes are a result of differences between financial reporting tax requirements and those used for reporting taxes to local, state, and federal government units. In some cases alternative inventory and depreciation may be used for reporting, thus creating a difference in the amounts owed and the payments may be deferred (postponed).

Financial Ratio Analysis

Key financial ratios can be classified into five categories:

1. Liquidity ratios
2. Activity ratios
3. Leverage ratios
4. Profitability ratios
5. Net trade cycle

Each category provides an analysis of different aspects of the organization and indicates how well the firm is managed. The following ratios are limited in number, and use varies by type of organization. The ones presented here are considered the more standard ratios for most businesses. Industry specific ratios would be used to provide additional information. The names used are the standard ones, and those used by different firms and professional organizations may be different. To provide a more complete analysis, the calculated ratios should be compared with industry averages. There are several services that provide this information on a for-fee basis. When making the comparisons, you must evaluate each firm by both size and type. For hospitals, the data are provided by size and geographic regions. The information can be obtained from sources for other types of not-for-profit organizations.

Liquidity Ratios

Liquidity ratios are concerned with short-term (current) items. The two most frequently used liquidity ratios are the current ratio and quick or acid-test ratio. The *current ratio* divides the current assets by current liabilities. This provides one measure of a firm's ability to pay short-term obligations, which arise in the course of operations or within one operating cycle (usually 1 year). For example, if the calculated ratio is two, this is interpreted to mean that you have 2 dollars in current assets for every 1 dollar in current liabilities. The limitation is that this ratio does not measure the true ability to pay obligations. A skewed example might be useful for improved understanding of this limitation. If current assets are $2M and current liabilities are $1M, then there are twice as many dollars in assets as there are in liabilities. However, let us assume that the current assets consist of $1 in cash and inventories make up the remainder. All current liabilities are due tomorrow. The original answer shows that obligations can be met, but, as the skewed example shows, the current debt cannot be met.

Now let's figure the actual liquidity ratio:

Ratio	How Calculated	2004	2003
Current Ratio	Current Assets/ Current Liabilities	$4,453/$4,141 = 1.08	$3,597/$3,117 = 1.15
Quick Ratio	Current Assests- Inventories/ Current Liabilities	$4,057/$4,141 = .98	$3,214/$3,117 = 1.03

The current ratio declined from 1.15 to 1.08 in the above results, indicating the ability to pay short-term obligations has weakened since 2003. Either current liabilities grew faster than current assets or current assets declined more rapidly than current liabilities. The common size balance sheet shows that current liabilities increased faster than current assets.

The *quick* or *acid-test ratio* provides additional information to evaluate the ability to meet short-term obligations. To compute this ratio, inventory must be subtracted from current assets. Sometimes items defined as "prepaid" may also be subtracted. The reason for the elimination of inventory from the numerator is that these items cannot be converted into cash quickly without a loss in value.

In the previous example the current and quick ratio both decreased. However, most current assets of Hospital Anywhere USA can be defined as quick assets (91.1% and 89.3%, respectively, for 2004 and 2003) so the current assets are highly liquid. If items other than cash and cash equivalents plus accounts receivable are eliminated, the quick ratio becomes 0.61 and 0.67, respectively, for 2004 and 2003. Two years is not enough time to make a completely informed judgment about the trends, but the trend is showing a decline. This is one indication of a decline in the ability of the hospital to meet its current obligations.

Activity Ratios

Activity ratios measure the liquidity and efficiency of asset management. The accounts receivable collection period measures the average time it takes a firm to collect its accounts (patient/insurance) receivable. The quicker a firm can convert the receivables to cash, the quicker it can pay its obligations or have cash for opportunities that may arise. This ratio is calculated by dividing the accounts receivable by the average daily revenue. Average daily revenue is calculated by dividing the revenue from the income statement by 365. This measures on the average how many times the organization has converted the receivables into cash.

Inventory turnover is found by dividing the cost of goods sold by inventory (accounting) or revenue by inventory (finance). This measures how quickly inventory is sold and is important for firms with products that deteriorate or have a short shelf life (drugs, surgical supplies).

Ratio	How Calculated	2004	2003
Accounts Receivable Collection Period	Accounts Receivable/ [(Revenue)/365]	$2,211/[($16,670)/365] = 45.67 Days	$1,873/[($16,657)/365] = 45.63 Days
Inventory Turnover	Cost of Goods Sold/ Inventory or Revenue/ Inventory	$16,670/$396 = 42.09	$16,657/$383 = 43.49

The above ratios for Hospital Anywhere USA indicate that the collection of accounts receivable takes an average of approximately 45 days. Once a patient leaves a facility after receiving medical services, the hospital is waiting for money from either the patient or a third-party payer 45 days before the claim is settled. Inventory turnover, from an accounting perspective, cannot be calculated for this hospital because cost of goods sold is not separately reported and cannot be calculated. This ratio is usually provided as supplemental information to the financial statements. If they had a subsidiary that sold medical items or the information was provided in the income statements, then the accounting ratio could be calculated. This is a standard ratio in all accounting literature. Finance literature supports a different calculation. As indicated previously, revenue is divided by the inventory. The turnover has increased slightly. For similar firms to Hospital Anywhere USA, this number would be quite high compared with standard manufacturing organizations.

Management's effectiveness in using assets to generate revenues can be measured by using two ratios. First, fixed asset turnover measures how well management is using the long-term assets of the organization to generate revenue. As the balance sheet shows in Chapter 19, this asset consists primarily of buildings and equipment used for providing patient services. For a health care organization this is important in that supplying beds and using equipment creates billable revenue. Fixed asset turnover is found by dividing net revenues by net property, plant, and equipment (cost of property, plant, and equipment minus accumulated depreciation). Total asset turnover measures how management is using all assets of the organization to generate revenue. The measure is found by dividing net revenues by all assets.

Ratio	How Calculated	2004	2003
Fixed Asset Turnover	Net Revenue/Net Property, Plant and Equipment	$16,670/$8,480 = 1.966	$16,657/$8,490 = 1.96
Total Asset Turnover	Net Revenue/Total Assests	$16,670/$17,568 = .949	$16,657/$16,885 = .986

Evaluation of the above indicates a minor change in the use of assets to generate revenue. Fixed asset turnover was relatively stable, whereas total asset turnover has declined slightly. However, this may be due to the increase in current assets as previously discussed.

Leverage Ratios

Leverage ratios, also called *capital structure ratios*, are one measure of how an organization is financed. For-profit firms can either borrow funds using a debt instrument (notes payable or bonds) or sell shares of stock (equity financing). Creditors look at this important ratio to determine if they will provide more funds to an organization or if the cost of funds (interest) will be changed. Remember from Chapter 19 that A = L + K. If an organization fails to continue in business due to financial setbacks (bankruptcy), the assets of the organization will be sold and distributed first to the creditors. If there is a remainder, the owners (those holding shares of stock) receive this amount. Thus the more debt that you have, the more risk you take on. This risk limits the amount of debt that creditors are willing to extend and raises the cost to finance projects.

However, on the positive side, debt can be used to improve the investment of stockholders (owners) of an organization. For instance, if you can borrow funds at 6% and invest at 10%, then the stockholders receive the differential. Profits are increased, and these are reinvested in the firm. For Hospital Anywhere USA the following three ratios provide an analysis of how much debt is used to finance the organization and the amount of debt compared with equity used to fund the operations and long-term projects of the firm:

Ratio	How Calculated	2004	2003
Debt Ratio	Total liabilities/total assets	$13,163/$17,568 = .749	$11,268/$16,885 = .667
Long-Term Debt to Total Capitalization	Long-term debt/ (Long-term debt + Stockholders' equity)	$9,022/($9,022 + $4,405) = .672	$8,151/($8,151 + $5,617) = .592
Debt to Equity	Total liabilities/ Stockholders' equity	$13,163/4,405 = 2.988	$11,268/$5,617 = 2.006

The *debt ratio* measures how much of the total assets have been financed using debt (obligations to pay a future amount of funds). The trend from 2003 to 2004, up from 66.7% to 74.9%, shows an increase, which indicates that more of the operations were financed using debt and a future outflow of funds either in interest costs or repayment of debt will be required. This debt may also increase the interest rate charged on these funds based on the increased risk. Remember that analysis of the common size income statement revealed that interest costs were higher in 2004 than in 2003. The other ratios confirm this trend in that debt has increased in relation to total funding (L + K) and compared with the use of equity financing (stocks).

Long-term debt to total capitalization (long-term debt divided by long-term debt plus stockholders equity) shows that more long-term debt is being used for financing (67.2% up from 59.2%). This number ($9,022 for 2004) is found by subtracting total current liabilities from total liabilities and dividing by long-term debt ($9,022) plus $4,405.

Debt to equity also indicates a larger use of debt financing in the business. This ratio indicates that debt was used approximately twice as often as equity in 2003 and almost three times as much in 2004. Firms with stable revenues can borrow more (increase their debt) than others with revenues that fluctuate. However, there is generally a limitation on the amount of funds that will be provided for operations.

Profitability Ratios

Profitability ratios measure how well a firm is doing in its basic operations. These ratios measure the percent that revenues minus certain costs exceed the revenues. They also determine how well the assets of the organization and owner's investment are being used. These ratios are the gross profit margin, operating profit margin, net profit margin, return on total assets, and return on equity.

Because Hospital Anywhere USA does not engage in selling physical assets, such as beds and drugs, and these items are not reported separately, the gross profit margin is not applicable. The gross profit amount is determined by subtracting from revenues the cost of goods sold. However, there is no cost of goods sold for this hospital—thus this amount cannot be calculated.

The operating profit margin is found by looking at the net revenues from the normal course of business, providing health care services, and subtracting all expenses of operations necessary to generate these revenues. This measure, sometimes called *EBIT (earnings before interest and taxes)*, indicates if the firm is covering its costs of operations. This amount is then divided by net revenues. Both 2004 and 2003 indicate a reasonable operating profit margin. For 2004 this means that Hospital Anywhere USA is covering operating costs and has approximately 12 cents on the dollar left to cover all other costs, including interest paid on debt and income taxes. The government settlement negatively impacted the earnings, but because of cost-reduction measures in 2004 other costs such as salaries were reduced, helping to alleviate impact on earnings.

The remaining three measures indicate that expenses were covered but there was little, percentage-wise, left to reinvest in the firm. Without knowing how others in the industry are doing, it becomes difficult to make a conclusion about the effectiveness of operations. The results presented indicate a decline in profitability of operations.

Ratio	How Calculated	2004	2003
Gross Profit Margin	Gross profit/Net revenue	N/A	N/A
Operating Profit Margin	Operating profit/Net revenue	$2,018/$16,670 = 12.1%	$1,704/$16,657 = 10.2%
Net Profit Margin	Net earnings/Net revenue	$219/$16,670 = 1.31%	$657/$16,657 = 4.18
Return on Total Assets or Return on Investment	Net earnings/Total assets	$219/$17,568 = 1.24%	$657/$16,885 = 3.89%
Return on Equity	Net earnings/ Stockholders' equity	$219/$4,405 = 4.97%	$657/$5,617 = 11.69%

Trade or Cash Conversion Cycle Ratio

The final group of standard ratios used to analyze a firm's operations evaluates the *trade or cash conversion cycle*. These measure, on the average, how long it takes to collect from either the patient or third-party providers or how long we are taking to pay our short-term obligations. The number of days in revenue is calculated as accounts receivable turnover previously discussed:

Ratio	How Calculated	2004	2003
Number of Days Revenue	Accounts receivable/(Revenue/365)	$2,211/($16,670/365) = 48.41	$1,873/($16,670/365) = 41.01
Number of Days Payable	Accounts payable/(Revenue/365)	$693/($16,670/365) = 15.17	$657/($16,657/365) = 14.38

If creditors provide 30 days in which to pay an obligation and your organization takes 40 days, a cash flow problem may exist. For Hospital Anywhere USA the number of days in payables, accounts payable divided by average daily revenues, increased from 14.38 to 15.17, which indicates that the hospital took longer to pay current obligations. This is a minor change, and anyone doing an evaluation would have to know the terms for payment that the hospital has with its creditors. This does, however, increase cash flow in that you retain cash longer by postponing the payment (cash outflow). A variation of this ratio is current liabilities divided by operating expenses minus depreciation divided by 365.

Not-for-Profit Comparisons

Not-for-profit entities have some differences that make comparisons more difficult from that of for-profit entities. Because profitability is not a mission of not-for-profit organizations, profitability ratios may not be calculated in the same manner. Health care organizations must provide an alternative performance indicator. This is normally in a footnote but must be clearly distinguished from other notes. It may take the form of either revenue over expenses, revenues and gains over expenses and losses, earned income, or performance income.

As the financial statements in **Exhibit 20–3** illustrate, there are differences between hospitals—especially between for-profit and not-for-profit firms. First, the dates of the statements are for June rather than December. The selection of a date is arbitrary. Second, other sources of revenue consist of government research grants and support provided to cover operating expenses. The latter is probably a result of donations by outside persons or organizations. The remaining accounts on the income statements are standard and would be expected to be found on both for-profit and not-for-profit organizations.

The balance sheet has one major difference with that of a for-profit entity. Instead of having stockholders (owners) of the firm, the accounts become unrestricted and temporarily restricted fund balances. *Unrestricted fund balances* are provided by others to support the mission of the hospital. *Temporarily restricted fund balances* are used for projects having a specific purpose and then returned to use for unrestricted purposes (**Exhibit 20–4**).

Exhibit 20–3 Children's Hospital Operating Revenues and Expenses June 30, 2004 and 2003

	2004	2003
Net Patient Services and Revenue	$238,736,833	$228,094,450
Other Sources of Revenue		
Government Research Grants	45,160,159	36,757,430
Support Provided to Cover Operating Expenses	100,137,765	82,342,438
Total Operating Revenues	**$384,034,757**	**$347,194,318**
Operating Expenses		
Salaries and Benefits	$195,621,776	$172,757,651
Services, Supplies, Other	146,371,984	131,094,528
Depreciation	28,116,508	24,262,840
Interest	5,899,845	5,492,360
Bad Debt Expense	3,048,592	6,182,778
Total Operating Expenses	**$383,268,634**	**$339,790,157**
Income (Loss) from Operations	**$769,123**	**$7,404,161**

Exhibit 20–4 Condensed Balance Sheets as of June 30, 2004 and 2003

	2004	2003
Assets		
Cash and Temporary Investments	$6,084,671	$3,767,117
Patient Accounts Receivable, Net of Allowances for Uncollectible Accounts	55,084,671	49,121,350
Other Current Assets	36,059,481	27,737,663
Current Assets	$97,388,219	$80,626,130
Plant and Equipment, Net of Accumulated Depreciation	$261,633,535	$223,695,756
Funds Held in Trust	82,118,866	42,568,303
Long-Term in Trust	110,292,993	101,245,215
Total Assets	**$551,433,613**	**$448,135,404**
Liabilities and Fund Balance		
Accounts Payable and Accrued Expenses	$44,489,716	$43,222,493
Current Portion of Long-Term Debt	4,884,203	4,540,418
Current Liabilities	**$49,373,919**	**$47,762,911**
Long-Term Debt	$212,548,645	$119,007,882
Other Long-Term Liabilities	21,664,716	24,468,880
Unrestricted Fund Balance	213,986,611	207,562,498
Temporarily restricted Fund Balance	53,859,722	49,333,233
Total Liabilities and Fund Balances	**$551,433,613**	**$448,135,404**

The four ratios presented in the following table are variations of those used in the analysis of Hospital Anywhere USA but are applied to that of Children's Hospital:

Ratio	How Calculated	2004	2005
Long-Term Debt to Total Capitalization	Long-term debt/(Long-term debt + Fund balances)	$234,213,357/ $502,059,690 = .4665	$143,476,762/ $400,372,493 = .3584
Debt to Fund Balances	Total liabilities/ Fund balances	$283,587,276/ $267,846,333 = 1.058	$191,239,673/ $256/895/731 = .744
Reported Income Index	Net Income/ Changes in Fund Balance	$786,123/ $10,950,602 = .072	N/A
Long-Term Debt to Fund Balances	Long-term debt/Fund balance	$234,213,357/ $267,846,333 = .874	$143,476,763/ $256,895,731 = .558

All three previously used ratios are smaller than those of Hospital Anywhere USA and declined in this time period, indicating this hospital does not use as much debt to finance operations as Hospital Anywhere USA. The reported income index was not directly applicable to Hospital Anywhere USA but is somewhat equivalent to profitability ratios that used net earnings computed for Hospital Anywhere USA. Again, a direct comparison should not be made with Hospital Anywhere USA but could be compared with other not-for-profit hospitals.

A further problem in comparing not-for-profit entities is the lack of standardized terminology or presentation formats. Some of these same problems exist with for-profit entities but the differences are not as glaring as that of not-for-profits. The last consideration in analyzing different not-for-profit firms is that information is not as readily available as that for publicly reporting firms.

The consolidated balance sheets and statement of activities (equivalent to for-profit income statements) of Retirement Homes, Inc. are introduced in **Exhibits 20–5** and **20–6**. Selected financial ratios follow the financial statements.

Retirement Homes, Inc. shows several differences between the previously reported organizations. In addition to being a smaller entity, they have permanently restricted funds; Children's Hospital does not. They also have gift fees and long-term obligations from advance payments from persons entering their facility. Patients may pay in advance, but until the retirement facility provides the services the income is not earned. The income statement format for Retirement Homes, Inc. also includes fund balance changes that were not included in previously presented income statements.

Current Ratios

Retirement Homes, Inc. shows an improvement in its ability to meet current obligations. In 2003 both ratios were below 1, whereas both improved to above 1 in 2004. How does this compare with the ratios presented for Hospital Anywhere USA? The ratios for Hospital Anywhere USA deteriorated, whereas those of Retirement Homes, Inc. improved. The trends can be compared, but a direct comparison cannot be made because the firms are in two different industries and operate as two different types of organizations (for-profit vs. not-for-profit).

Ratio	How Calculated	2004	2003
Current Ratio	Current Assets/ Current Liabilities	$2,045,481/ $1,601,510 = 1.28	$1,328,976/ $1,638,203 = .81
Quick Ratio	Current Assets- Inventories/Current Liabilities	$1,926,643/ $1,601,510 = 1.20	$1,183,812/ $1,683,203 = .70

ACTIVITY RATIOS

Notice in the following table that the number of days in the accounts receivable collection period increased, as did the inventory turnover. This indicates that the firm has slowed the time to make collections whereas inventory was being used faster. Again, a direct comparison cannot be made with Hospital Anywhere USA data. However, you can purchase industry comparison data (benchmarking) from either national services or associations and determine how well you are doing compared with others.

Exhibit 20–5 Retirement Homes, Inc. Consolidated Balance Sheet

	2000	1999
Assets		
Current Assets		
Cash and equivalents	$1,343,467	$557,494
Investments held by bond trustee	50,653	254,572
Accounts receivable, net of allowance for doubtful accounts of $166,200 and $45,200 in 2000 and 1999	444,396	371,746
Contributions and grants receivable	88,127	
Inventories	56,705	54,597
Prepaid expenses and other	62,133	90,567
Total current assets	**2,045,481**	**1,328,976**
Investments		
Held by bond trustee, net of amount requires to meet current obligations	4,845,585	4,562,685
Board designated funds	869,603	823,758
Foundation	1,832,579	1,637,170
	7,547,767	7,023,613
Property and equipment		
Land and improvements	2,630,999	2,537,686
Buildings and improvements	34,046,631	33,359,106
Equipment	1,679,668	1,513,251
Furniture and equipment	1,440,448	1,385,729
	39,797,746	38,795,772
Less accumulated depreciation	12,289,748	11,173,504
	27,507,998	27,622,268
Construction in progress	593,335	521,608
	28,101,333	28,143,876
Beneficial interest in charitable remainder trusts	72,250	
Net deferred charges:		
Marketing and consulting costs	1,568,833	1,758,238
Financing costs	2,437,811	2,774,112
Prepayment in lieu of taxes	210,000	280,000
	4,216,644	4,812,350
Other assets	21,500	21,500
Total assets	**$42,004,975**	**$41,330,315**
Current liabilities		
Accounts payable	$308,493	$399,480
Salaries, wages, and related liabilities	164,551	130,589
Accrued compensated absences	130,843	120,501
Accrued interest	81,580	83,561
Current portion of long-term debt	904,031	854,212
Other current liabilities	12,012	49,860
Total current liabilities	1,601,510	1,638,203
Other liabilities:		
Long-term obligations	33,247,449	34,163,586
Entrance fees received in advance and deposits	308,124	202,288
Gift annuities payable	377,079	254,184
Deferred entry fee revenue	23,022,153	22,865,940
	56,954,805	57,485,998
Net assets (deficit):		
Unrestricted	(18,014,253)	(19,176,458)
Temporarily restricted	1,415,676	1,382,572
Permanently restricted	47,237	
Total net assets (deficit)	(16,551,340)	(17,793,886)
Total liabilities and net deficit	**$42,004,975**	**$41,330,315**

Exhibit 20–6 Retirement Homes, Inc. Consolidated Statements of Activities Year Ended December 31

	2000	1999
Revenue and other support		
Resident services:		
Monthly service fees	$8,340,317	$8,111,191
Amortization of deferred revenues	3,345,893	3,075,632
Patient revenue from nonresidents	2,217,990	1,629,027
Interest income	258,845	322,954
Medicare and other	804,211	615,273
Net assets released from restriction	132,171	
Total revenue and other support	**15,099,427**	**13,754,077**
Expenses		
Salaries and wages	5,059,124	4,728,354
Employee benefits	733,960	691,892
Total employment expenses	5,793,084	5,420,246
Purchased services	1,534,747	1,082,729
Supplies	1,247,315	1,286,860
Provision for bad debts	123,404	5,000
Utilities	637,598	624,457
Rent	4,815	4,515
Insurance	204,503	42,417
Interest	2,410,079	2,426,461
Program expenses-foundation	116,924	
Foundation operating expenses	66,282	
Miscellaneous	369,046	
Depreciation and amortization	1,672,950	1,765,252
Total expenses	**14,180,747**	**13,073,233**
Excess of revenue over expenses	918,680	680,844
Net asset reclassification	172,018	
Net assets released from restriction for capital	78,896	
Net unrealized holding losses on investments	(7,389)	1,817
Increase in unrestricted assets	1,162,205	682,661
Temporarily restricted net assets:		
Net asset reclassification	(187,018)	
Contributions	308,263	127,066
Net unrealized holding losses on investments	(168,582)	(54,993)
Investment income	291,508	244,550
Net assets released from restrictions	(211,067)	(50,443)
Increase in temporarily restricted net assets	33,104	266,180
Permanently restricted net assets:		
Net Asset Reclassification	15,000	
Contributions	32,237	
Increase in permanently restricted net assets	47,237	
Increase in net assets	1,242,546	948,841
Net deficit, beginning of year	**(17,793,886)**	**(18,742,727)**
Net deficit, end of year	**$(16,551,340)**	**$(17,793,886)**

Ratio	How Calculated	2004	2003
Accounts Receivable Collection Period	Accounts Receivable/ [(Revenue)/365]	$444,396/ [($15,099,427)/365] = 10.7 Days	$371,746/ [($13,754,077)/365] = 9.86 Days
Inventory Turnover	Cost of Goods Sold/ Inventory or Revenue. Inventory	$15,099,427/ $56,705 = 266.3	$13,754,077/ $54,597 = 251.9

Notice again that both ratios improved but assets are not used as well to generate revenue for Retirement Homes, Inc. as they were for Hospital Anywhere USA. You are cautioned again not to make direct comparisons.

Ratio	How Calculated	2004	2003
Fixed Asset Turnover	Net Revenue/ Net Property, Plant and Equipment	$15,099,427/ $28,101,333 = .587	$13,754,077/ $28,143,876 = .488
Total Asset Turnover	Net Revenue/Total Assets	$15,099,427/ $42,004,975 = .359	$13,754,077/ $41,330,315 = .382

LEVERAGE RATIOS

In each case the amount of debt, long term and total, is greater than total assets and long-term debt plus net assets. Net assets, equivalent to for-profits stockholders equity, are negative. This negative figure is probably a result of losses in previous years of operation. As a result of this negative figure, the calculation is not applicable.

Ratio	How Calculated	2004	2003
Debt Ratio	Total liabilities/ Total assets	$56,954,805/ $42,004,975 = 1.356	$57,485,998/ $41,330,315 = 1.39
Long-Term Debt to Total Capitalization	Long-term debt/(Long-term debt + Net assets)	$55,353,295/ $38,801,955 = 1.43	$55,847,795,/ $38,053,909 = 1.47
Debt to Equity	Total liabilities/ Net assets	$56,954,805/ ($16,551,340) = N/A	$57,485,999/ ($17,793,886) = N/A

PROFITABILITY RATIOS

Two of the following ratios cannot be calculated either because of a lack of available data or because one part of the equation has a negative (deficit) balance. Two of the ratios (indicated with an *) are variations of those presented previously for Hospital Anywhere USA. These ratios use the increase in net assets because a not-for-profit does not report profits but rather looks at increases or decreases in assets. All three ratios that were calculated improved in year 2004 over that of 2003.

Ratio	How Calculated	2004	2003
Gross Profit Margin	Gross profit/Net revenue	N/A	N/A
Operating Profit Margin[*]	Excess of revenue over expenses/ Net revenue	$918,680/ $15,099,427 = 6%	$680,844/ $13,654,077 = 4.95%
Net Profit Margin[*]	Increase in net assets/ Net Revenue	$1,242,546/ $15,099,427 = 8.2%	$948,841/ $13,754,077 = 6.89%
Return on Total Assets or Return on Investment	Increase in Net assets/Total assets	$1,242,546/ $15,099,427 = 8.22%	$948, 841/ $13,754,077 = 6.89%
Return on Equity	Increase in net assets/Total net assets	$1,242,546/ ($16,551,340) = N/A	$948,841/ ($17,793,881) = N/A

ADDITIONAL FINANCIAL RATIOS

One ratio that can be applied to both not-for-profit and for-profit entities is the number of day's *cash on hand*. This is the amount of cash necessary to meet actual daily cash operating expenses. This measure excludes both bad debt and depreciation expenses from operating expenses. Remember, these are estimates and are a "paper and pencil" item only. They do not cause cash outflows. The calculation for this ratio follows:

$$Days \ of \ cash \ on \ hand = \frac{cash \ + \ marketable \ securities}{(operating \ expenses \ - \ bad \ debts \ - \ depreciation)/365}$$

One health care organization maintains 200 day's cash on hand. However, this amount is probably high for most firms. The more cash on hand, the less a firm has to invest in assets that have higher returns. A variation of the above ratio is the *cash flow coverage*. This measures how well you are able to cover required payments such as interest, rent, and debt payments. Information for calculation of this ratio would be found in the cash flow statements. Calculation of this ratio follows:

$$Cash \ flow \ coverage = \frac{cash \ from \ operations \ + \ interest \ + \ rent}{interest \ + \ rent \ + \ debt \ payments}$$

If the previous ratio is less than 1, it indicates that you are only able to make that percent of required payments. For example, if the above ratio was 0.8, you are only able to make 80% of required payments.

A ratio unique to not-for-profit organizations and one that only recently has been calculated is the *program service ratio*. This ratio is designed to determine what proportion of a firm's expenditures go directly into its program services (core business). This ratio is calculated by dividing program service expenses by total expenses. A firm should be spending a large proportion of its cash inflows on its mission.

$$Program\ service\ ratio = \frac{program\ services\ expenses}{total\ expenses}$$

Other financial ratios that might be computed for either for-profit or not-for-profit entities are

- Revenue per employee—net revenue/number of employees
- Net income per employee—net income/number of employees
- Price earnings ratio—market price of stock/earning per common share
- Growth rate of revenue—percentage change in revenue from previous time period

Ratios that are more applicable to not-for-profit and health care entities are

- Percent of deductibles—deductibles/gross patient service revenue
- Reported income index—net income/changes in fund balance
- Long-term debt to fund balance—long-term debt/fund balance

In any of the previously calculated ratios where stockholders equity numbers were used, the not-for-profit sector would use the fund balance as a replacement number for calculations. Deductibles are unique to the health care industry. As covered in Chapter 10, the industry is impacted negatively by third-party payment systems. Once a claim is filed, deductions based on contracted rates are removed from the expected payment. The actual amount received varies from amounts as low as 25 cents on the dollar to a high of around 60 cents on the dollar.

Conclusion

As with any comparisons that use ratios or common size financial statements, caution must be used. Comparisons must be made for a longer period than 2 years. Past results may not be indicative of future performance. Differences in management, risk aversive or risk takers, for one can affect how a firm is managed. Competition, geographic differences, and other factors can impact operations. Nonetheless, ratios and common size comparisons can provide indications of action that needs to be undertaken. Benchmarking allows a firm to judge how well it is doing in relation to other organizations in both the same industry and in other industries. Recall that benchmarking is looking at best practices, not just in firms in your industry but in all firms.

Discussion Questions

1. Which ratios would you consider most important in the daily and monthly operation of the organization? Why?
2. If you were analyzing an organization's ability to borrow money, which ratios would be most helpful?
3. Why is the accounts receivable turnover ratio important to the organization?
4. What process do organizations use to compare themselves with other organizations and how effective is this process?
5. When using common size financial statements, what number do analysts use for the balance sheet and what number is used for the income statements?

Glossary of Terms

Accounts Receivable Collection Period—measures the average time it takes an organization to collect its accounts (patient/insurance) receivable.

Activity Ratios—measure the liquidity and efficiency of asset management.

Benchmarking—is a process that provides comparisons with the best practices of other organizations. These firms do not have to be within the same industry but traditionally comparisons are based within specific industries. This is a limiting factor in identifying best practices but simplifies the comparisons.

Cash on Hand—applies to both not-for-profit and for-profit entities and computes the number of day's cash on hand. This is the amount of cash necessary to meet actual daily cash operating expenses. This measure excludes both bad debt and depreciation expenses from operating expenses.

Common Size Financial Statements—in the balance sheet and income statement, one number is selected and then divided into all other numbers in the statements.

Current Ratio—divides the current assets by current liabilities. This provides one measure of a firm's ability to pay short-term obligations.

Debt Ratio—measures how much of the total assets have been financed using debt (obligations to pay a future amount of funds).

Fixed Asset Turnover—measures how well management is using the long-term assets of the organization to generate revenue.

Forward Purchase Contract—where one party agrees to buy a commodity at a specific price on a specific future date and the other party agrees to make the sale.

Inventory Turnover—measures how quickly inventory is sold and is important for firms with products that deteriorate or have a short shelf life (drugs, surgical supplies).

Leverage Ratios, also called Capital Structure Ratios—are one measure of how an organization is financed.

Liquidity Ratios—are concerned with short-term (current items). The two most frequently used liquidity ratios are the current ratio and quick or acid-test ratio.

Operating Profit Margin—is found by looking at the net revenues from the normal course of business, providing health care services, and subtracting all expenses of operations necessary to generate these revenues. This measure, sometimes called EBIT (earnings before interest and taxes), indicates if the firm is covering their costs of operations.

Profitability Ratios—measure how well a firm is doing in its basic operations.

Program Service Ratio—A ratio unique to not-for-profit organizations and one that only recently has been calculated. This ratio is designed to determine what proportion of a firm's expenditures go directly into its program services (core business).

Put Option—provides the right to sell stock at a specified price in the future.

Quick or Acid-test Ratio—provides additional information to evaluate the ability to meet short-term obligations.

Total Asset Turnover—measures how management is using all assets of the organization to generate revenue. The measure is found by dividing net revenues by all.

Trade or Cash Conversion Cycle Ratio—measure, on the average, how long it takes to collect from either the patient or third party providers or how long the organization is taking to pay short-term obligations.

Index

A